Recent Progress in Tuberculosis Research

Recent Progress in Tuberculosis Research

Editor: Rupert Condron

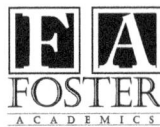

FOSTER
ACADEMICS

www.fosteracademics.com

www.fosteracademics.com

FA
FOSTER
ACADEMICS

Cataloging-in-Publication Data

Recent progress in tuberculosis research / edited by Rupert Condron.
    p. cm.
Includes bibliographical references and index.
ISBN 978-1-63242-695-6
1. Tuberculosis. 2. Tuberculosis--Research. 3. Chest--Diseases.
4. Lungs--Diseases. 5. Mycobacterial diseases. I. Condron, Rupert.
RC3114 .R43 2019
616.995--dc23

Foster Academics,
118-35 Queens Blvd., Suite 400,
Forest Hills, NY 11375, USA

ISBN 978-1-63242-695-6 (Hardback)

Contents

Permissions

List of Contributors

Index

Preface

In my initial years as a student, I used to run to the library at every possible instance to grab a book and learn something new. Books were my primary source of knowledge and I would not have come such a long way without all that I learnt from them. Thus, when I was approached to edit this book; I became understandably nostalgic. It was an absolute honor to be considered worthy of guiding the current generation as well as those to come. I put all my knowledge and hard work into making this book most beneficial for its readers.

Tuberculosis or TB, is an infectious disease which generally affects the lungs. It is caused by mycobacterium tuberculosis bacteria. It can affect the other body parts as well. Fever, night sweats, weight loss, lack of appetite and fatigue are some of its common symptoms. It spreads through air when people having active tuberculosis in their lungs cough, sneeze, spit or speak. Individuals with latent TB do not spread the disease. Chest X-rays and microscopic examination are usually used to diagnose active TB, whereas, tuberculin skin test or blood tests are useful in diagnosing latent TB. Bacillus Calmette–Guérin (BCG) vaccine is the most common vaccine used against tuberculosis. This book is a compilation of chapters that discuss the most vital concepts and emerging trends in the field of tuberculosis research. Different approaches, evaluations, methodologies and advanced studies on tuberculosis have been included in it. This book will prove immensely beneficial to students and researchers in this field.

I wish to thank my publisher for supporting me at every step. I would also like to thank all the authors who have contributed their researches in this book. I hope this book will be a valuable contribution to the progress of the field.

Editor

Early Therapeutic Drug Monitoring for Isoniazid and Rifampin among Diabetics with Newly Diagnosed Tuberculosis in Virginia, USA

Scott K. Heysell,[1] **Jane L. Moore,**[2] **Debbie Staley,**[2] **Denise Dodge,**[2] **and Eric R. Houpt**[1]

[1] *Division of Infectious Diseases and International Health, University of Virginia, P.O. Box 801340, Charlottesville, VA 22908-1340, USA*
[2] *Tuberculosis Control and Prevention, Virginia Department of Health, Richmond, VA, USA*

Correspondence should be addressed to Scott K. Heysell; skh8r@virginia.edu

Academic Editor: T. Ottenhoff

Slow responders to tuberculosis (TB) treatment in Virginia have prolonged treatment duration and consume more programmatic resources. Diabetes is an independent risk factor for slow response and low serum anti-TB drug concentrations. Thus, a statewide initiative of early therapeutic drug monitoring (TDM) for isoniazid and rifampin at 2 weeks after TB treatment was piloted for all diabetics with newly diagnosed TB. During the period of early TDM, 12/01/2011–12/31/2012, 21 diabetics had $C_{2\,hr}$ concentrations performed and 16 (76%) had a value below the expected range for isoniazid, rifampin, or both. Fifteen had follow-up concentrations after dose adjustment and 12 (80%) increased to within the expected range (including all for rifampin). Of 16 diabetic patients with pulmonary TB that had early TDM, 14 (88%) converted their sputum culture to negative in <2 months. Early TDM for diabetics was operationally feasible, may speed response to TB therapy, and can be considered for TB programs with high diabetes prevalence.

1. Introduction

Tuberculosis (TB) and diabetes mellitus have been described as the "convergence of two epidemics" and given the increasing rates of obesity and diabetes worldwide and the continued high rates of TB in low-income countries, it is estimated that the number of individuals with both TB and DM will increase dramatically [1]. Compared to those without diabetes, diabetics are at greater risk for incident TB [2, 3], where for instance, among Hispanic people aged 25–54 years, TB risk attributable to diabetes is estimated at 25% [1]. The largest meta-analysis to date demonstrated that diabetic patients were 3.1 times more likely to develop TB than nondiabetics, a risk which was amplified in regions outside North America [3].

Furthermore, when active TB disease develops, diabetes contributes to increased severity and poor treatment outcome [4]. Diabetics with TB appear more likely to die than non-diabetics with TB when adjusting for comorbid conditions

and have higher rates of relapse after treatment completion [5, 6]. In Virginia, diabetics were 7 times more likely to have slow response to TB therapy [7]. In addition to other complications of treatment, slow response prolongs infectiousness and often extends the treatment duration. While other comorbid immunosuppressing conditions or *Mycobacterium tuberculosis* drug resistance certainly contribute to slow response in Virginia, uniquely the majority of diabetics had serum anti-TB drug concentrations of isoniazid and rifampin below the expected range, and diabetes was an independent risk factor for low rifampin concentrations [7]. We further demonstrated that patients with similarly low serum concentrations of isoniazid or rifampin have impaired killing of their own *M. tuberculosis* isolate in a functional bioassay [8]. Yet in an individual diabetic, low serum concentrations cannot be reliably predicted and may be a consequence of inaccurate dosing, drug solubility, malabsorption, altered metabolism or protein binding, or drug-drug interactions [9]. In most instances, however, low serum concentrations of isoniazid and rifampin can be readily corrected with dose adjustment. We previously observed that low rifampin concentrations that were then corrected by dose adjustment in Virginia were not only well tolerated, but also those patients had a shorter duration of TB therapy compared to other slow responders [7]. Aside from early diagnosis and treatment of unrecognized diabetes in TB patients, few other interventions to improve treatment outcome have focused on this vulnerable population.

The measurement of anti-TB drug concentrations, termed therapeutic drug monitoring (TDM), has been in use in Virginia since 2007 [10]. Statewide guidelines for TDM have been developed for patients slow to respond to TB treatment at 4–6 weeks of therapy, specifically if the patient has persistent or worsening TB symptoms or for pulmonary TB patients, a lack of decrement in the mycobacterial burden in the sputum [11]. Once slow response is identified, serum is collected for TDM to isoniazid and rifampin at the time of estimated peak concentration (Table 2), and a single dose adjustment is made if a concentration is below the minimum of the expected range (e.g., rifampin 600 mg daily increased to 900 mg daily). Since the routine use of TDM, diabetics accounted for 10–15% of the annual TB cases, but 40% of those with slow response [10, 12]. As a consequence, a recent statewide initiative was begun to perform TDM at 2 weeks following TB treatment initiation (early TDM) in all diabetics with newly diagnosed TB in an effort to correct low drug concentrations and prevent slow response. The following report describes the programmatic results of the initiative.

2. Methods

2.1. Study Design. A retrospective analysis was performed of all patients in whom TDM was completed during the period of the early TDM initiative, 12/01/2011 to 12/31/2012. Specifically, diabetics with early TDM at 2 weeks were compared to non-diabetics that had standard TDM for slow response. Surveillance data were retrieved from the state TB registry and included demographics (age, sex, and country of origin), comorbidities including HIV and diabetes, prior TB history, and anatomic focus of current TB episode (pulmonary, extrapulmonary, or both). Laboratory report forms were reviewed for drug concentration results for isoniazid and rifampin. Non-diabetic patients that had TDM for reasons other than slow response and those with TDM for second-line medications used in the treatment of drug-resistant TB were excluded. For diabetics with pulmonary TB, the time in days to sputum culture conversion was also assessed as a marker for prevention of slow response, given that the intensive phase of treatment and/or the total treatment duration were commonly extended for patients that fail to convert their sputum culture to negative in <2 months. Standard procedure was for sputum collection weekly until smear conversion and monthly until culture conversion. The study was given exempt approval by the Institutional Review Board at the University of Virginia and the Virginia Department of Health.

2.2. Early TDM Initiative. In Virginia, all cases of active TB are reported to the State Department of Health, and each case is assigned to a nurse manager. Directly observed therapy is administered by the nurse case manager or a trained outreach worker. Diabetes is determined by self-report of the patient or caregiver to nurse case managers. During the early TDM initiative, nurse case managers also queried for use of insulin among diabetics. The use or type of oral hypoglycemic was not routinely recorded. Laboratory markers of disease severity such as glycosylated hemoglobin (HbA1c) were not available for analysis. Patients with diabetes had early TDM for isoniazid and rifampin at or as close to 2 weeks from treatment initiation for drug-susceptible TB, the earliest time point at which steady state concentrations are observed (Figure 1). The standard procedure for TDM was to directly administer medication and then collect venous blood 2 hours later at the time of estimated peak concentration ($C_{2\,hr}$) [11]. Serum was then separated by centrifugation at the Local Health Department before being transported on dry ice to the Regional Referral Laboratory. High performance liquid chromatography (HPLC) results were available within 48 hours of receipt of specimen and reported in reference to the expected μg/mL range [9]. For concentrations of either isoniazid or rifampin below the $C_{2\,hr}$ expected range, a single dose increase was performed with plan to recheck the drug concentration following dose adjustment. For daily dosed rifampin of 600 mg, the dose was increased to 900 mg; for daily dosed isoniazid of 300 mg, the dose was increased to 450 mg. Intermittent dosing of rifampin was unchanged from daily dose adjustment, while isoniazid of 900 mg (typical intermittent dosing) was increased to 1200 mg. Providers were encouraged to initiate therapy with daily dosing for diabetic patients, but initial decisions were determined by the individual provider.

Following TDM, patients were further monitored for slow response as defined by state guidelines [11] and if later identified, then referral was made to a state TB consultant (Figure 1). Patients without diabetes had TDM performed for isoniazid and rifampin only after the development of slow response. If drug concentrations remained below the expected range following dose adjustment in non-diabetic slow responders, then similar referral was made to a state TB consultant. Complications with dose adjustment or major toxicity were reported to the state TB control program.

2.3. Statistical Analysis. Demographic and clinical characteristics were compared between diabetics with early TDM and non-diabetics with standard TDM for slow response with the χ^2 statistic or for continuous variables, the Student t-test, or the Mann-Whitney U test when appropriate. $C_{2\,hr}$ values were dichotomized into "normal" if were within or above the expected range or "low" if were below the expected range. The biweekly or thrice weekly dosing used in some patients for isoniazid and rifampin was categorized as intermittent. Bivariate logistic regression analysis was used to determine additional risk factors for either a low isoniazid or a low rifampin concentration among diabetics. All tests of significance were two-sided.

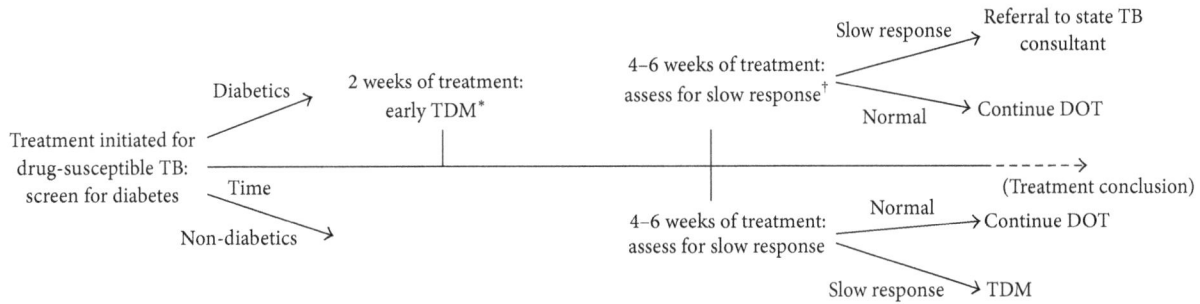

FIGURE 1: Statewide guidelines for the use of therapeutic drug monitoring (TDM). Diabetes identified by patient self-report or review or chart review by tuberculosis (TB) nurse case managers. *TDM: an estimated peak concentration ($C_{2\,hr}$) for isoniazid and rifampin is collected following directly observed therapy (DOT) and if below the expected range, then a single dose adjustment is made as per guidelines (e.g., rifampin 600 mg daily increased to 900 mg daily or isoniazid 300 mg daily increased to 450 mg daily) [11]. †Slow response defined as persistent or worsening symptoms of TB or lack of decrement in mycobacterial burden in sputum for pulmonary TB patients [11].

TABLE 1: Baseline characteristics of adults with drug-susceptible tuberculosis referred for therapeutic drug monitoring (TDM) based on slow response or early TDM if diabetic.

Characteristic	Diabetes (early TDM) $N = 21$	Slow response (standard TDM) $N = 14$	P value
Age, mean years ± SD	57 ± 17	46 ± 12	$P = 0.04$
Gender, male (%N)	15 (71)	11 (79)	$P = 0.69$
Prior episode of TB, n (%N)	0	2 (14)	$P = 0.17$
Pulmonary TB only, n (%N)	17 (81)	8 (57)	$P = 0.65$
Foreign born (%N with confirmed status*)	15 (79)	12 (92)	$P = 0.63$
HIV infected (%N with confirmed status*)	0	1 (11)	$P = 0.43$
Insulin dependence, n (%N)	10 (48)	N/A	N/A
Days to TDM from treatment initiation, median days (IQR)	23 ± 16	88 ± 54	$P = 0.003$

Slow response patients did not include diabetics (see Figure 1). *Missing values include foreign born status in 2 diabetics and 1 patient with slow response and HIV status in 4 patients with slow response. N/A: not applicable.

3. Results

During the study period, 266 cases of active TB were on treatment. Seven (3%) patients were excluded from the analysis as TDM was performed for reasons other than diabetes or slow response, such as the use of second-line drugs in the treatment of drug-resistant TB or first-line drug intolerance. Twenty-one diabetics (81% of total eligible diabetics) had early TDM with complete lab report forms available for review, and 14 non-diabetics had standard TDM for slow response (Table 1). Diabetics were older with mean age of 57 ± 17 years compared to slow responders, 46 ± 12 years ($P = 0.04$). The majority of patients in whom TDM was performed were male, foreign born, and with pulmonary TB, but without significant difference in these proportions between diabetics and slow responders. Ten (48%) of diabetics were insulin dependent. No diabetic had HIV or a prior history of TB. The median time to TDM after treatment initiation in diabetics was 23.4 ± 16 days and expectedly differed from slow responders, 88 ± 54 days ($P = 0.003$).

Initial TDM for isoniazid was successfully performed in all patients, including 4 (19%) of diabetics and 6 (43%) of slow responders on intermittent dosing schedules; and for rifampin it was performed in 20 (95%) of diabetics and all slow responders. Mean $C_{2\,hr}$ values of daily dosed isoniazid were 2.13 ± 1.5 μg/mL for diabetics compared to 3.1 ± 1.1 μg/mL in slow responders (expected range 3–6 μg/mL) ($P = 0.11$). While mean values for intermittent doses were 6.0 ± 3.0 μg/mL for diabetics compared to 11.3 ± 2.5 μg/mL in slow responders (expected range 9–18 μg/mL) ($P = 0.03$). Fourteen (67%) of diabetics had a low isoniazid $C_{2\,hr}$ compared to 6 (50%) slow responders ($P = 0.29$). A low rifampin $C_{2\,hr}$ was observed in 12 (60%) diabetics, including 7 (70%) of insulin-dependent diabetics, compared to 5 (41%) of slow responders ($P = 0.31$).

Overall, 16 (76%) of diabetics had a low isoniazid or rifampin $C_{2\,hr}$. Insulin use was not additionally predictive of a low concentration of either medication among diabetics in bivariate analysis; odds ratio were 2.3 (0.37–14.6) ($P = 0.37$) for rifampin and 1.3 (0.21–8.3) ($P = 0.76$) for isoniazid. Age, gender or extrapulmonary TB also did not predict a low concentration in bivariate analysis. Patient weight was not available in all patients for stratification by mg/kg dosing. Fifteen patients had follow-up concentrations after dose adjustment and 12 (80%) increased to the expected

TABLE 2: Distribution of estimated peak concentrations (C_{2hr}) for isoniazid and rifampin.

Drug	Diabetics (early TDM)	Nondiabetic slow responders (standard TDM)	P value
Rifampin (expected range 8–24 μg/mL)	$N = 20$	$N = 14$	
Mean C_{2hr} μg/mL ± SD	6.6 ± 4.3	8.2 ± 6.2	$P = 0.40$
Below expected range (%N)	12 (60)	4 (41)	$P = 0.31$
Isoniazid (daily) (expected range 3–6 μg/mL)	$N = 17$	$N = 8$	
Mean C_{2hr} μg/mL ± SD	2.1 ± 1.5	3.1 ± 1.1	$P = 0.11$
Below expected range (%N)	11 (65)	5 (63)	$P = 0.92$
Isoniazid (intermittent) (expected range 9–18 μg/mL)	$N = 4$	$N = 6$	
Mean C_{2hr} μg/mL ± SD	6.0 ± 3.0	11.3 ± 2.5	$P = 0.03$
Below expected range (%N)	3 (75)	1 (17)	$P = 0.19$

TDM: therapeutic drug monitoring (see Figure 1).

range (including all for rifampin). No complications or major toxicity from dose adjustment were reported.

Of 16 diabetic patients with pulmonary TB, 14 (88%) converted their sputum culture to negative in <2 months, including 9 of 11 (82%) patients for whom either rifampin or isoniazid was dose increased. There were no deaths reported over a median follow-up time of 10.5 months (IQR 8–12.25 months). The two diabetics that failed to culture convert in two months were both foreign born males of advanced age (88 and 71 years); one of whom had low C_{2hr} isoniazid and rifampin where each medication was corrected to the expected range, and the other with low C_{2hr} rifampin in whom a repeat concentration was not repeated after dose increase. Including the diabetics with pulmonary TB that failed to culture convert in <2 months or those with extra-pulmonary TB that were later deemed to have slow response, the mean number of slow responders was 1.2 per month (12.5% diabetic) during the early TDM period, decreased from preintervention rates of 1.6 per month (40% diabetic) [7].

4. Discussion

A statewide initiative of early TDM in diabetics starting anti-TB therapy found that the majority have a low serum C_{2hr} value of isoniazid or rifampin that corrected to the expected range with a single dose increase. The process was operationally feasible and accepted by health departments with capture of more than 80% of all diabetics treated for active TB. The target of performing early TDM at 2 weeks after treatment initiation was closely approximated in most diabetics.

To our knowledge, this is the first programmatic initiative to correct low isoniazid and rifampin concentrations routinely in all diabetics. The few observational studies that have examined anti-TB pharmacokinetics specifically in diabetics did not include dose correction and focused on rifampin. For example, rifampin exposure, as measured by sampling of serum throughout the daily dosing interval, was 2-fold lower in diabetic patients compared to age and gender matched controls from Indonesia when performed during the continuation phase of treatment [13]. However, these findings were not reproduced when studied in a similar cohort of subjects

during the first two weeks of therapy, but the comparator group also had a high proportion with low rifampin exposure and the authors suggest that patient's weight and hepatic induction may be more contributory to the lower rifampin concentrations they had previously observed during the later stage of the treatment course [14]. Similarly, a recent study of C_{2hr} and C_{6hr} concentrations of rifampin from Peru found that the majority of diabetics have low rifampin concentrations though not significantly different than non-diabetics, but nearly 85% of the total population studied had peak concentrations below the expected range, including a notable proportion with undetectable C_{2hr} values, which may have made differences in the diabetic and non-diabetic populations difficult to detect [15]. Furthermore, rifampin solubility is affected by gastric pH and transit time, conditions which are influenced by chronic hyperglycemia and can fluctuate significantly within an individual patient [16, 17]. Thus, while the programmatic initiative of checking only a C_{2hr} concentration may miss a proportion of those with a delayed peak concentration, the operational decision to test for both isoniazid and rifampin at single time point was found most feasible in our setting. Additionally, the lack of significant side effects with a single dose correction of either medication suggests that a delayed time to peak, if present, was not clinically significant.

Therefore, given the high frequency of low anti-TB drug concentrations in diabetics, a randomized trial of TDM with dose correction may be the best means of quantifying the contribution of pharmacokinetic optimization to both early and late markers of treatment outcome. For instance, a low rifampin concentration may not be sufficient to affect late markers such as cure or relapse in a subject with a highly rifampin susceptible *M. tuberculosis* isolate or adequate concentrations of the other anti-TB drugs in the regimen. However, dose correction to the higher range of expected peak concentrations may hasten the early treatment response [18]. This may be particularly important for subjects with *M. tuberculosis* isolates with higher minimum inhibitory concentrations still considered susceptible by conventional testing [8]. The early TDM initiative found fewer diabetics with low rifampin concentrations compared to our prior study in Virginia when TDM was restricted to only those patients with slow response, and low isoniazid and rifampin

$C_{2\,hr}$ concentrations were found in 63% and 76% of diabetics, respectively [7]. We speculate this may be an indication of the relative importance of rifampin in the rapidity of treatment response for diabetics in our setting. Indeed, recent attention to the optimization of rifampin concentrations demonstrates significantly improved bactericidal activity with dose increase as measured by sputum colony counts, and promising clinical trials are underway to study higher dose rifampin for shortening treatment duration [18–20]. Therefore, following the outcomes of these trials, diabetics may be an ideal subpopulation in which consider a higher initial dose of rifampin.

A high proportion of diabetics with early TDM had a favorable time to sputum culture conversion of <2 months. The time to culture conversion has been modestly delayed in other studies of diabetics when compared to non-diabetic controls likely related to a higher bacillary burden at presentation [5, 21, 22]. While our current study did not permit comparison of time to culture conversion in TB cases for whom TDM was not performed, the decreased total number of slow responders during the period of the early TDM initiative and the decreased proportion of diabetics that developed slow response compared to historical norms provide support that early correction of low drug concentrations may avert slow response in some diabetics. This finding is of considerable programmatic value as the total treatment duration depends upon the microbiological and symptomatic response in the first two months of therapy. Given current financial constraints placed on state TB control programs, avoiding an extended duration of directly observed therapy can be resource sparing and cost saving.

Diabetes is currently identified by patient self-report or chart review by the state TB control program. Yet in studies of active screening by fasting blood glucose or HbA1c in new TB patients without a known history of diabetes, the rate of identification of new cases of diabetes ranged from 2 to 35% depending on the population of study [23]. In the Indian state of Kerala for instance, only 4 new TB cases were needed to be screened by HbA1c in order to identify 1 new case of diabetes [24]. Thus, the burden of diabetes among slow responders to anti-TB treatment may be underestimated in our setting. Active screening for diabetes in all new TB patients may identify a subset of patients otherwise eligible for early TDM. Consequently, plans to start active screening for diabetes with HbA1c are now underway in Virginia.

There are several limitations to this study given the necessity for retrospective study of an initiative in place for all diabetics and the inability to randomize diabetics to early TDM or the prior standard of care. While a drop in the total number of slow responders compared to preinitiative rates was observed, nurse case managers or TB clinicians may have possessed an unintended bias and preferentially failed to identify a diabetic patient as slow to respond once early TDM had been performed. If occurring, however, the bias would largely be limited to patients without the objective finding of sputum culture conversion. In addition, a minority of eligible diabetics did not have early TDM performed, and while they were not later identified as having slow response,

the reasons for lack of the implementation of the initiative in these patients were not known.

Furthermore, sputum culture conversion and identification of slow response were used as proxy for predicting total treatment duration and the intensity of programmatic resources required in management. Thus, further cost-effectiveness analysis would require long-term followup and comprehensive comparison of data from matched non-diabetic controls that were not currently available. Lastly, while insulin use did not further risk stratify for low drug concentrations among diabetics, little else was known about diabetic disease severity. Furthermore, details of comorbid medical conditions, patient weight, or medication use may have additionally refined the interpretation of low drug concentrations or markers of treatment response such as sputum culture conversion.

5. Conclusions

In summary, early TDM in diabetics starting anti-TB therapy revealed that the majority had a low isoniazid or rifampin serum concentration corrected to the expected range with a single dose increase and no major reported toxicity. Diabetics with early TDM and pulmonary TB had a favorable time to sputum culture conversion and the total statewide burden of slow response appeared to be minimized during the period of the initiative. Thus, early TDM for diabetics can be considered in settings of high diabetes/TB coprevalence where slow response and prolonged treatment duration are programmatic concerns.

Acknowledgments

Scott K. Heysell was supported by the National Institutes of Health Grant K23AI099019 and the Burroughs Wellcome Fund/American Society of Tropical Medicine and Hygiene. Eric R. Houpt was also supported in part by the National Institutes of Health Grant R01AI093358 and the Virginia Department of Health.

References

[1] K. E. Dooley and R. E. Chaisson, "Tuberculosis and diabetes mellitus: convergence of two epidemics," *The Lancet Infectious Diseases*, vol. 9, no. 12, pp. 737–746, 2009.

[2] C. R. Stevenson, N. G. Forouhi, G. Roglic et al., "Diabetes and tuberculosis: the impact of the diabetes epidemic on tuberculosis incidence," *BMC Public Health*, vol. 7, article 234, 2007.

[3] C. Y. Jeon and M. B. Murray, "Diabetes mellitus increases the risk of active tuberculosis: a systematic review of 13 observational studies," *PloS Medicine*, vol. 5, no. 7, article e152, 2008.

[4] B. Alisjahbana, E. Sahiratmadja, E. J. Nelwan et al., "The effect of type 2 diabetes mellitus on the presentation and treatment

response of pulmonary tuberculosis," *Clinical Infectious Diseases*, vol. 45, no. 4, pp. 428–435, 2007.

[5] K. E. Dooley, T. Tang, J. E. Golub, S. E. Dorman, and W. Cronin, "Impact of diabetes mellitus on treatment outcomes of patients with active tuberculosis," *The American Journal of Tropical Medicine and Hygiene*, vol. 80, no. 4, pp. 634–639, 2009.

[6] M. A. Baker, A. D. Harries, C. Y. Jeon et al., "The impact of diabetes on tuberculosis treatment outcomes: a systematic review," *BMC Medicine*, vol. 9, article 81, 2011.

[7] S. K. Heysell, J. L. Moore, S. J. Keller, and E. R. Houpt, "Therapeutic drug monitoring for slow response to tuberculosis treatment in a state control program, Virginia, USA," *Emerging Infectious Diseases*, vol. 16, no. 10, pp. 1546–1553, 2010.

[8] S. K. Heysell, C. Mtabho, S. Mpagama et al., "Plasma drug activity assay for treatment optimization in tuberculosis patients," *Antimicrobial Agents and Chemotherapy*, vol. 55, no. 12, pp. 5819–5825, 2011.

[9] C. A. Peloquin, "Therapeutic drug monitoring in the treatment of tuberculosis," *Drugs*, vol. 62, no. 15, pp. 2169–2183, 2002.

[10] S. K. Heysell, J. L. Moore, D. Dodge, D. Staley, and E. Houpt, "Guidelines for the use of therapeutic drug level monitoring in Virginia: the first year," in *Proceedings of the Annual Meeting of the National Tuberculosis Controller's Association*, Atlanta, Ga, USA, 2012.

[11] Virginia Department of Health, "Recommendations and procedures for the use of therapeutic drug monitoring in clients with drug-susceptible tuberculosis receiving directly-observed therapy," http://www.vdh.virginia.gov/epidemiology/DiseasePrevention/Programs/Tuberculosis/documents/TDM-RecommendationsandProceduresRrevised082013Final.pdf.

[12] Virginia Department of Health, Office of Epidemiology, and Division of Disease Prevention, *2011 Annual Tuberculosis Surveillance Report*, 2012.

[13] H. M. J. Nijland, R. Ruslami, J. E. Stalenhoef et al., "Exposure to rifampicin is strongly reduced in patients with tuberculosis and type 2 diabetes," *Clinical Infectious Diseases*, vol. 43, no. 7, pp. 848–854, 2006.

[14] R. Ruslami, H. M. J. Nijland, I. G. N. Adhiarta et al., "Pharmacokinetics of antituberculosis drugs in pulmonary tuberculosis patients with type 2 diabetes," *Antimicrobial Agents and Chemotherapy*, vol. 54, no. 3, pp. 1068–1074, 2010.

[15] A. Requena-Méndez, G. Davies, A. Ardrey et al., "Pharmacokinetics of rifampin in Peruvian tuberculosis patients with and without comorbid diabetes or HIV," *Antimicrobial Agents and Chemotherapy*, vol. 56, no. 5, pp. 2357–2363, 2012.

[16] P. R. Gwilt, R. R. Nahhas, and W. G. Tracewell, "The effects of diabetes mellitus on pharmacokinetics and pharmacodynamics in humans," *Clinical Pharmacokinetics*, vol. 20, no. 6, pp. 477–490, 1991.

[17] Y. Ashokraj, K. J. Kaur, I. Singh et al., "In vivo dissolution: predominant factor affecting the bioavailability of rifampicin in its solid oral dosage forms," *Clinical Research and Regulatory Affairs*, vol. 25, no. 1, pp. 1–12, 2008.

[18] M. J. Boeree, A. H. Diacon, R. Dawson, A. Venter et al., "What is the "right" dose of rifampin?, abstract #148LB," in *Proceedings of the Conference on Retroviruses and Opportunistic Infections*, Atlanta, Ga, USA, 2013.

[19] A. H. Diacon, R. F. Patientia, A. Venter et al., "Early bactericidal activity of high-dose rifampin in patients with pulmonary tuberculosis evidenced by positive sputum smears," *Antimicrobial Agents and Chemotherapy*, vol. 51, no. 8, pp. 2994–2996, 2007.

[20] J. van Ingen, R. E. Aarnoutse, P. R. Donald et al., "Why do we use 600 mg of rifampicin in tuberculosis treatment?" *Clinical Infectious Diseases*, vol. 52, no. 9, pp. e194–e199, 2011.

[21] S. Maâlej, N. Belhaoui, M. Bourguiba et al., "Pulmonary tuberculosis and diabetes: retrospective study of 60 patients in Tunisia," *La Presse Médicale*, vol. 38, no. 1, pp. 20–24, 2009.

[22] B. I. Restrepo, S. P. Fisher-Hoch, B. Smith, S. Jeon, M. H. Rahbar, and J. B. McCormick, "Mycobacterial clearance from sputum is delayed during the first phase of treatment in patients with diabetes," *The American Journal of Tropical Medicine and Hygiene*, vol. 79, no. 4, pp. 541–544, 2008.

[23] C. Y. Jeon, A. D. Harries, M. A. Baker et al., "Bi-directional screening for tuberculosis and diabetes: a systematic review," *Tropical Medicine and International Health*, vol. 15, no. 11, pp. 1300–1314, 2010.

[24] S. Balakrishnan, S. Vijayan, S. Nair, J. Subramoniapillai et al., "High diabetes prevalence among tuberculosis cases in Kerala, India," *PLoS ONE*, vol. 7, no. 10, Article ID e46502, 2012.

Barriers and Delays in Tuberculosis Diagnosis and Treatment Services: Does Gender Matter?

Wei-Teng Yang,[1] Celine R. Gounder,[2] Tokunbo Akande,[1] Jan-Walter De Neve,[3]
Katherine N. McIntire,[2] Aditya Chandrasekhar,[1] Alan de Lima Pereira,[1] Naveen Gummadi,[4]
Santanu Samanta,[5] and Amita Gupta[1,2,6]

[1] Johns Hopkins Bloomberg School of Public Health, Baltimore, MD 21205, USA
[2] Department of Medicine, Johns Hopkins University School of Medicine, Baltimore, MD 21287, USA
[3] Harvard School of Public Health, Boston, MA 02115, USA
[4] Narayana Hrudayalaya Hospital, Hyderabad 500055, India
[5] All India Institute of Medical Sciences, New Delhi 110029, India
[6] Center for Clinical Global Health Education, 600 North Wolfe Street, Phipps 540B, Baltimore, MD 21287, USA

Correspondence should be addressed to Amita Gupta; agupta25@jhmi.edu

Academic Editor: Edward A. Graviss

Background. Tuberculosis (TB) remains a global public health problem with known gender-related disparities. We reviewed the quantitative evidence for gender-related differences in accessing TB services from symptom onset to treatment initiation. *Methods.* Following a systematic review process, we: searched 12 electronic databases; included quantitative studies assessing gender differences in accessing TB diagnostic and treatment services; abstracted data; and assessed study validity. We defined barriers and delays at the individual and provider/system levels using a conceptual framework of the TB care continuum and examined gender-related differences. *Results.* Among 13,448 articles, 137 were included: many assessed individual-level barriers (52%) and delays (42%), 76% surveyed persons presenting for care with diagnosed or suspected TB, 24% surveyed community members, and two-thirds were from African and Asian regions. Many studies reported no gender differences. Among studies reporting disparities, women faced greater barriers (financial: 64% versus 36%; physical: 100% versus 0%; stigma: 85% versus 15%; health literacy: 67% versus 33%; and provider-/system-level: 100% versus 0%) and longer delays (presentation to diagnosis: 45% versus 0%) than men. *Conclusions.* Many studies found no quantitative gender-related differences in barriers and delays limiting access to TB services. When differences were identified, women experienced greater barriers and longer delays than men.

1. Introduction

Tuberculosis (TB) remains a significant global public health issue. Significantly, the TB disease burden is unequally distributed among men and women. Of the estimated 8.7 million incident TB cases and 1.4 million deaths caused by TB globally in 2011, roughly one-third occurred among women (2.9 million incident TB cases and 0.5 million deaths) [1]. Currently, it is unclear whether these disparities are due to sex-related differences (i.e., biology), gender-based differences (i.e., sociocultural practices and different social roles of men and women), or both [2–4]. Until recently, gender-related differences in the epidemiology, diagnosis,

treatment, outcomes, and socioeconomic costs of TB have received relatively little attention. To address this knowledge gap, the World Health Organization (WHO) has proposed a framework and priorities for research on gender and TB [5].

To date, gender-based research supports that men and women respond differently to illness and face different barriers when accessing TB diagnostic and treatment services [2]. Barriers that limit access to TB services occur at the individual and provider/system levels. Individual-level barriers involve physical (distance to TB services and access to transport), financial (the direct and indirect costs of seeking TB services), stigma (stigma surrounding TB and its association with HIV), health literacy (TB-related knowledge and education), and sociocultural (gender roles and status in the family) factors, whereas provider/system-level barriers include provider degree of suspicion for TB, the number and types of providers seen before TB diagnosis, provider adherence to national TB program guidelines, and patient satisfaction with TB services. A comprehensive understanding of gender-related differences in barriers and delays at each level is needed so that researchers and policymakers can formulate and prioritize gender-specific interventions to improve the global impact of TB services.

Although several reviews have examined gender-related barriers and delays in seeking TB care [2, 3, 6–11], none have simultaneously assessed the contribution of both barriers and delays in a systematic manner. Furthermore, previous reviews have assessed a narrow study population. Currently, no review has captured the full continuum of TB care by including studies that have surveyed the general population, high-risk populations (e.g., homeless or HIV-infected persons), TB suspects who may not have sought care (e.g., untreated individuals with chest symptoms in the community), and TB patients and suspects presenting for care.

Our review aims to address these limitations. Using a partially-adopted, published framework [5], we systematically reviewed the literature to examine the quantitative evidence for gender-related differences in the barriers and delays that limit access to TB services along the continuum of care from symptom onset to treatment initiation. In this report, we present the findings from our quantitative review, which have important implications for TB service programs, research, and policymakers alike.

2. Methods

2.1. Systematic Review Process

2.1.1. Search Strategy. We searched 12 electronic databases for human and English articles published between January 1953 and October 2010. We developed our search strategy for MEDLINE using PubMed with a combination of controlled vocabulary and keyword terms and phrases (see Supplementary Material available online at http://dx.doi.org/10.1155/2014/461935). The strategy was then translated for the Excerpta Medica Database (EMBASE), the Cumulative Index to Nursing and Allied Health Literature (CINAHL), Global Health, Popline, Africa Wide, LILACS, Web of Science, and the inclusive databases of the Cochrane Library using their respective thesaurus terms, synonyms, and keywords. Citations from each database were imported into a reference management system, and duplicates were removed.

2.1.2. Study Selection Criteria. We included quantitative studies that reported on gender-related differences in barriers to and/or delays in accessing TB diagnostic and treatment services and studied human participants aged 15 years or older. Studies that did not provide a gender comparison as well as case reports, editorials, review articles, commentaries, practice guidelines, and studies of treatment compliance and/or outcomes were excluded. Participants were

defined as persons with diagnosed or suspected TB, persons from either the general population or high-risk populations (e.g., HIV-infected, homeless, and prisoner), or health care providers. Diagnosed TB included both pulmonary and extrapulmonary forms, and TB diagnosis could be made by sputum smear microscopy, culture, or chest X-ray using histopathological or clinical criteria.

2.1.3. Study Selection Process. Following deduplication, studies were reviewed sequentially by title, abstract, and in full-text form (Figure 1). At each stage, two reviewers independently evaluated each study against study selection criteria. Articles were included or excluded only when both reviewers were in agreement, and conflicts were resolved by a third, independent reviewer (AC, AG, or CRG). To ensure sufficient concordance between reviewers, a pilot review and reviewer discussion were conducted at each stage before proceeding with the remaining studies. Six reviewers conducted the title screen (ADP, JWDN, NG, SS, TA, and WTY), and four reviewers conducted the abstract screen and the full-text screen (ADP, JWDN, TA, and WTY). Following the full-text screen, included articles underwent the full-text assessment, which included data abstraction and a study validity assessment.

2.1.4. Data Abstraction. Four reviewers (ADP, JWDN, TA, and WTY) independently abstracted quantitative data from each included full-text article in duplicate, and any conflicts were resolved through discussion with a third, independent reviewer (AG or CRG). Abstracted summary measures included differences in means or proportions, risk ratios, odds ratios, and hazards ratios.

2.1.5. Validity Assessment. We used validity assessment tools to examine the quality of studies that inform our review; the assessment was not used to exclude studies. We assessed observational studies using items adopted from the methods and results sections of the Strengthening the Reporting of Observational Studies in Epidemiology (STROBE) checklist [148]. We used items adopted from the Consolidated Standards of Reporting Trials (CONSORT) checklist extension for clustered randomized trials to assess an included clustered randomized trial [149] and a pragmatic randomized controlled trial [150]. Two reviewers independently assessed the validity of each study using the adopted items (TA and WTY), and conflicts were resolved through discussion and arbitration with a third reviewer (CRG).

2.2. Outcomes and Definitions. Outcomes were quantitative associations between gender and both barriers and delays that limit access to TB services along the full continuum of TB care from symptom onset through diagnosis and treatment initiation. Figure 2 presents the conceptual framework that we used to define barriers and delays at the individual and provider/system levels at various time points along the continuum of TB care. Individual-level barriers were defined to be financial (the direct or indirect costs of TB care, including costs of travel, diagnosis, and/or treatment as well as the opportunity costs of lost employment, compensation, or

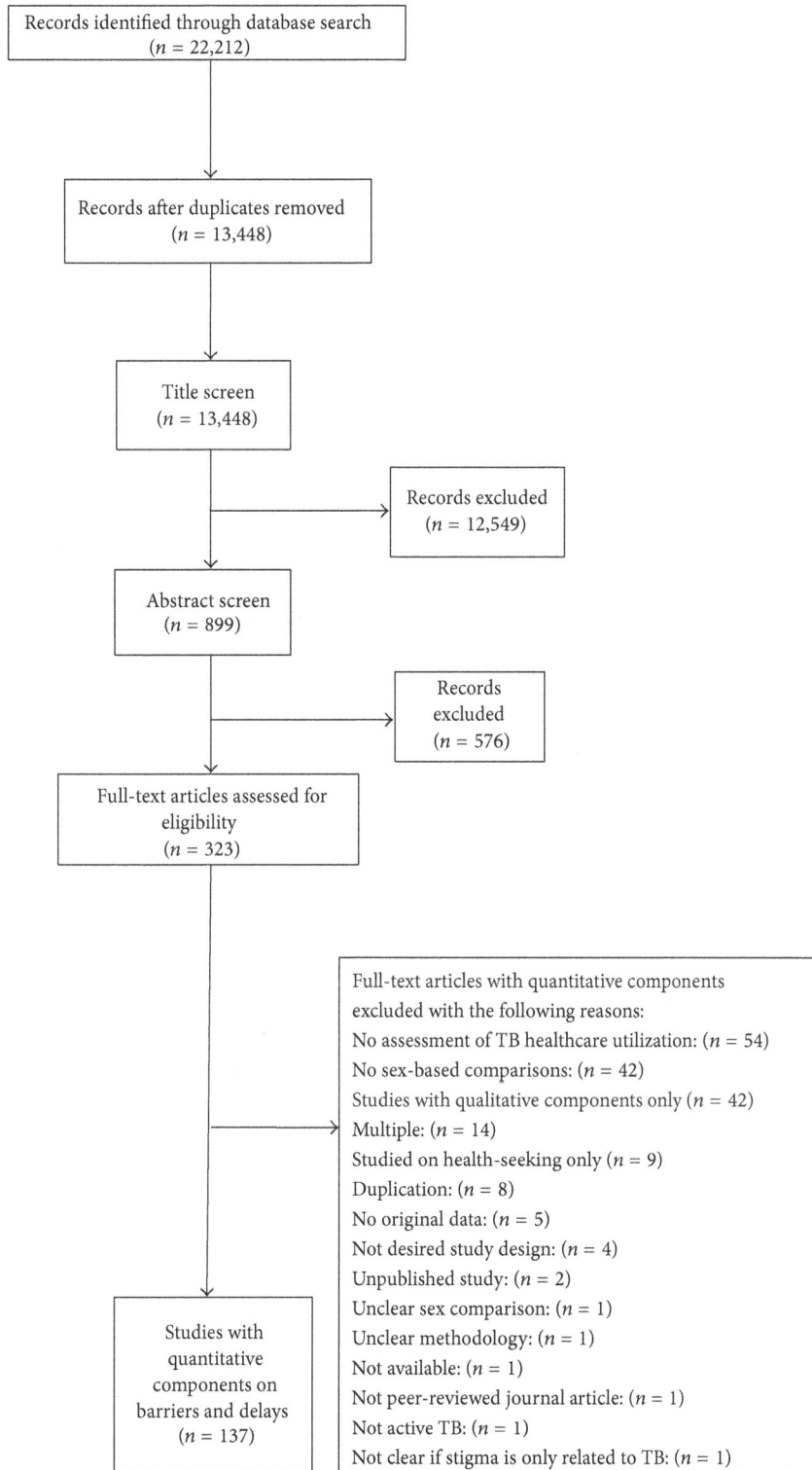

FIGURE 1: Study selection process.

household work); physical (distance, travel logistics, and/or access to TB care facilities); stigma (TB-specific sociocultural barriers arising from community or individual prejudice related to TB diagnosis or treatment, including social isolation, marriage prospects, fertility concerns, and association with HIV); health literacy (TB-related knowledge and education); and sociodemographic (age, race, rural versus urban residence, social caste, norms of practice, and social hierarchies). Provider-/system-level barriers were defined as any of the following: provider degree of suspicion for TB, number

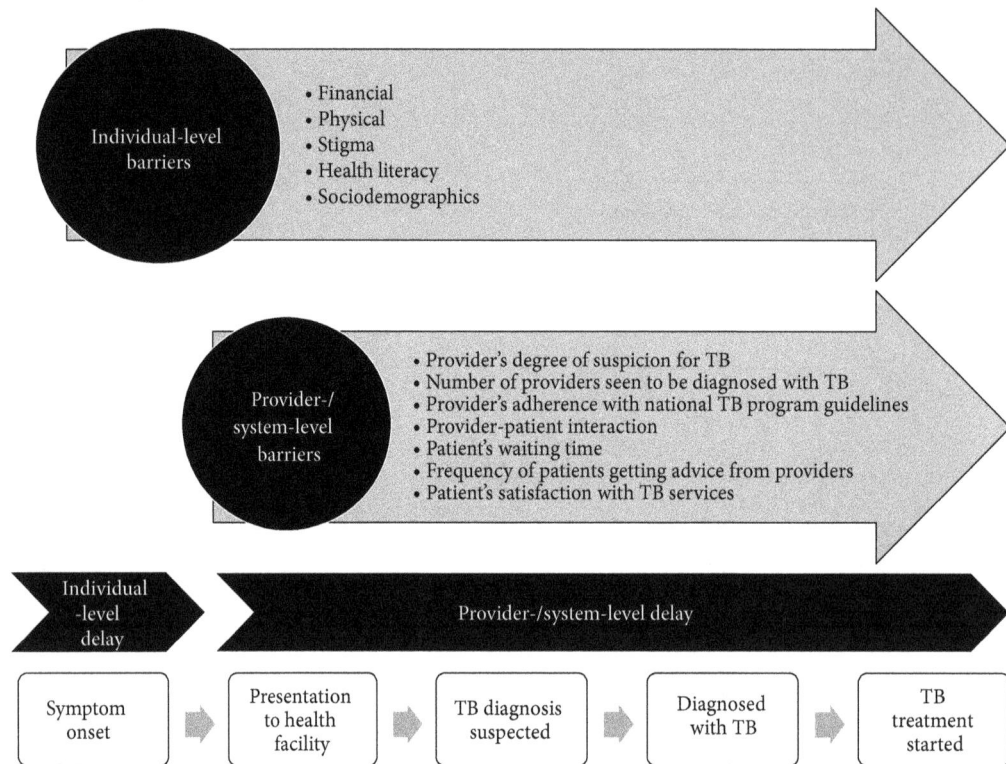

FIGURE 2: Conceptual framework illustrating barriers and delays that limit access to TB diagnostic and treatment services. The figure illustrates the conceptual framework of the tuberculosis (TB) care continuum from symptom onset to treatment initiation that we used to define barriers and delays that limit access to TB diagnostic and treatment services at the individual and provider/system levels. Individual-level barriers impact access to TB services along the full continuum of TB care, and provider-/system-level barriers impact access to TB services from patient presentation to any health care provider through TB treatment initiation. Barriers may contribute to delays between each step along the TB care continuum. Accordingly, we define individual-level delay as the delay between symptom onset and presentation to any health care provider; provider/system delay as the delay between presentation to any health care provider and diagnosis, the delay between presentation to any health care provider and treatment initiation or the delay between diagnosis and treatment initiation; and combined individual/provider/system delay as the delay between symptom onset and diagnosis or the delay between symptom onset and treatment initiation.

of providers seen before TB diagnosis, provider adherence to national TB program guidelines, provider-patient interaction, patient waiting time, frequency of getting advice, and patient satisfaction with TB services. Delay was defined as any time period between points along the TB care pathway under our conceptual framework from symptom onset to TB treatment initiation (Figure 2). Although barriers and delays are highly interrelated, few studies assess the contribution of barriers to delays quantitatively. Therefore, we present results for barriers and delays separately. We presented the impact of certain barriers on delays whenever possible.

3. Results

3.1. Study Characteristics. Our search strategy yielded 13,448 citations. Of these, 323 articles were reviewed in full-text form, and 137 studies met our selection criteria and were included in our review (Figure 1). Among the included studies, there was one (<1%) cluster-randomized clinical trial [91], one (<1%) pragmatic randomized controlled trial [55], eight (6%) cohort studies [33, 37, 67, 68, 87, 92, 136, 137], one

(<1%) case-control study [69], and 126 (92%) cross-sectional studies [12–32, 34–36, 38–54, 56–66, 70–86, 88–90, 93–135, 138–147, 151]. Most studies (76%) assessed persons presenting for care with diagnosed or suspected TB, and the median sample size was 335 (IQR 190–1000) with women comprising less than half of the study population (median, interquartile range [IQR]: 42%, 34–49%). Most studies were published between 2000 and 2010, and two-thirds were conducted in Africa and Asia (Table 1).

3.2. Outcomes. Overall, the included studies reported on gender-related barriers and delays at the individual, provider/system, and combined individual/provider/system levels. Specifically, 71 (52%) studies assessed individual-level barriers, 19 (14%) studies assessed provider-/system-level barriers, and 7 (5%) studies assessed combined individual-/provider-/system-level barriers. Individual-level delays were assessed by 58 (42%) studies, 37 (27%) studies assessed provider/system-level delays, and 25 (18%) studies assessed combined individual-/provider-/system-level delays. Key findings are summarized below by outcome type (barrier or

TABLE 1: Characteristics of included studies.

Study characteristic	Description
Study design: n (%)	Clustered randomized trial: 1 (<1%); pragmatic randomized clinical trial: 1 (<1%); cohort study: 8 (6%); case-control study: 1 (<1%); cross-sectional study: 126 (92%)
Study population: n (%)	Individuals with diagnosed/suspected TB who presented to care: 76%; individuals in the community or population: 24%
Year of publication: n (%)	2000–2010: 123 (90%); 1990–1999: 11 (8%); 1980–1989: 2 (1%); 1970–1979: 1 (1%)
WHO regional distribution: n (%)	AFRO: 37 (27%); SEARO: 31 (23%); WPRO: 25 (18%); AMRO: 17 (13%); EMRO: 12 (9%); EURO: 11 (8%); multiple regions: 4 (3%)
Sample size	Range: 39–209,560,379; median (IQR): 335 (190–1,000)
Proportion of women	Range: 23–73%; median (IQR): 42% (34–49%)

AFRO: African region; AMRO: region of the Americas; EMRO: Eastern Mediterranean region; EURO: European region; IQR: interquartile range; SEARO: South East Asia region; TB: tuberculosis; WHO: World Health Organization; WPRO: Western Pacific region.

delay) and level of impact (individual, provider/system, combined individual/provider/system) (Table 2 and Supplementary Table S1).

3.3. Individual-Level Barriers

3.3.1. Financial. Of 137 studies, 21 (15%) examined gender-related financial barriers to accessing TB services. Overall, a large number of studies found that women faced more financial barriers to seeking TB service than men. Fewer studies found either no difference in financial barriers between men and women or men faced greater financial barriers to accessing care (e.g., the opportunity cost of lost wages or income). While both men and women reported financial barriers to seeking TB services, the nature of these barriers differed. Women were more likely to be financially dependent on others [19, 26], unemployed, or without income [16, 17, 20]. Women also experienced greater healthcare seeking costs due to transport or the need for an escort [12, 17, 31], which may impact a woman's autonomy in seeking care. One study found that women may have also experienced greater financial barriers than men because they were more likely to see private providers than public providers [18]. The total direct costs of seeking TB diagnostic services as a proportion of income were higher for women than men in urban Zambia, largely because women had lower monthly incomes than men [13]. In Malawi, the indirect household costs of seeking care were higher for women [15].

3.3.2. Physical. Of 137 studies, only nine (7%) explored gender-related physical barriers to accessing TB services. All nine studies found that distance and travel time to a health facility were similar for men and women. However, one study

noted that distance to a clinic was more likely to result in delayed diagnosis among women than men [14].

3.3.3. Stigma. Of 137 studies, 18% investigated gender-related differences in TB-related stigma as a barrier to accessing TB diagnostic and treatment services. Of these, 12 found no gender-related differences in stigma, 11 found that women reported greater TB-related stigma than men, and two studies found that men experienced greater TB-related stigma than women. Only two studies specifically examined the impact of TB-related stigma on gender-based differences in individual-level delays in seeking TB services; one study found that the impact of stigma on delay was greater among women than men [47], and the other study found no gender-based difference [48]. Four studies examined the impact of TB-related stigma on marriage and marital prospects, and all reported that women were more likely than men to believe that TB would have an adverse impact on marriage prospects and marriage [35, 39, 43, 44].

3.3.4. Health Literacy. Of 137 studies, 36% described gender-related differences in TB-related knowledge and education as barriers to accessing TB services, and the majority of these (80%) examined differences in knowledge of the etiology, transmission, symptoms, diagnosis, and/or treatment of TB.

Of the 39 studies that assessed TB-related health literacy, 18 found that men and women had similar levels of TB-related knowledge, and, among those, six were conducted strictly in urban settings, and five were conducted in both urban and rural settings. Fourteen studies found that men had higher levels of TB-related knowledge than women; nine of these were conducted in strictly rural settings, and four were conducted in both rural and urban settings. Seven studies found that women had higher levels of TB-related knowledge than men; only one of these was conducted in a strictly rural setting. In addition, among ten studies that examined general educational attainment and literacy as barriers to accessing TB services, seven found that men were more educated and/or had higher literacy rates than women, and the remaining three studies found no gender-related differences.

Only two studies looked at the impact of TB-related knowledge and education on individual-level delays in presenting to TB services; one found that women suffered longer delays than men due to poor TB-related knowledge and education [14], and one found no gender-related differences [59]. One intervention trial found that, compared to women who did not receive brief instruction before submitting sputum samples, women who received instruction yielded significantly increased rates of both sputum positivity and return for submission of a second sputum sample. However, no significant changes were found among men who received such instruction [55]. This suggests that the intervention removed poor knowledge as a barrier for women to provide good sputum samples and to return for second sputum submission. Among two studies that examined the impact of TB-related knowledge on the likelihood of seeking tertiary-level care, one found that TB-related knowledge was more predictive of seeking hospital care among men than among women [41], and one found no gender-related difference [61].

TABLE 2: Summary of quantitative gender-related findings by outcome type.

| Outcome type | Number of studies | Gender difference | | | | No gender difference | |
| | | Women > Men | | Men > Women | | | |
		n (%)	List of studies	n (%)	List of studies	n (%)	List of studies
Individual-level barriers							
Financial	21[a]	11 (52%)	[12–14], [15][a], [16–22]	5 (24%)	[23, 24], [15][a], [25, 26]	6 (29%)	[27–32]
Physical	9	1 (11%)	[14]			8 (89%)	[26, 30–36]
Stigma[b]	25	11 (44%)	[17, 18, 22, 37–44]	2 (8%)	[45, 46]	12 (48%)	[24–26, 35, 47–54]
Health literacy	49	17 (35%)	[26, 34–36, 38, 41, 44, 50, 55–63]	8 (16%)	[24, 28, 40, 42, 43, 64–66]	24 (50%)	[14, 20, 22, 25, 30, 37, 45–47, 51–53, 67–78]
Sociodemographic	6	4 (67%)	[17, 79–81]			2 (33%)	[36, 71]
Provider-/system- level barriers	19	8 (42%)	[17, 29, 37, 82–86]			11 (58%)	[15, 28, 34, 35, 52, 73, 75, 87–90]
Combined individual-, provider-, and system-level barriers	7	5 (72%)	[29, 91–94]	1 (14%)	[95]	1 (14%)	[18]
Individual-level delay	58	13 (22%)	[14, 17, 21, 51, 73, 79, 96–102]	7 (12%)	[37, 61, 103–107]	38 (66%)	[16, 18–20, 28, 30–32, 36, 56, 71, 81, 108–133]
Provider-/system-level delay	37	11 (30%)	[14, 19, 20, 36, 81, 85, 120, 128, 131, 134, 135]	2 (5%)	[35, 101]	24 (65%)	[16, 18, 32, 33, 79, 96, 99, 100, 104, 106, 107, 113, 115, 117, 118, 121, 122, 124, 132, 133, 136–139]
Combined individual-, provider-, and system-level delay	25[c]	9 (36%)	[140], [141][c], [27, 32, 36, 79, 100, 142, 143]	1 (4%)	[141][c]	17 (68%)	[33, 69, 110], [141][c], [35, 86, 114, 117, 124, 129, 131–133, 144–147]

[a]This study is included in both gender difference categories as it reported that the direct costs of seeking care were higher for men and that the household costs of seeking care were higher for women.

[b]One study was not included because the direction of association between gender and stigma could not be assessed [30].

[c]This study is included in all three gender-related finding columns as it is a multicountry study and reported gender-related findings that differed from country to country.

3.3.5. Sociodemographic. Only six (4%) studies explored gender-related differences in sociodemographic barriers (factors of older age, family size, marital status, or caste) to accessing TB services. Older women were more likely than older men to either delay or not seek care [79–81]. Compared to men, lower caste was more likely to predict individual-level delays among women [80], but family size had no gender-related differential impact on delays in seeking care [36]. Two studies explored the impact of being unmarried, separated, divorced, or widowed on seeking TB care [17, 71]. Among TB patients in Kenya, there was no gender-related difference in the impact of marital status on seeking care for TB [71]. However, in Bangladesh, women were more likely to be adversely affected than men [17].

3.4. Provider-/System-Level Barriers. Of 137 studies, 19 (14%) assessed gender-related barriers to accessing TB services at the provider and system levels. Overall, these studies were highly heterogeneous both in the barriers that were assessed and the findings.

Barriers to accessing diagnostic and/or treatment services at the provider and system levels were examined by nine (47%) studies. Of these, eight studies examined gender-related barriers to TB diagnosis and screening. In Thailand, it was found that providers were more likely to adhere to TB diagnostic guidelines among males with suspected TB compared to females with suspected TB [83]. In Malawi, males and females with suspected TB made a similar number of visits to a health facility before being diagnosed with TB [15, 90], and, in India, males and females with suspected TB were offered sputum smear microscopy with similar frequency [89]. In contrast, women in Gambia sought care from a larger number of healthcare providers to obtain a TB diagnosis than men [86], and, in Vietnam, women took more health-seeking actions for their symptoms than men but were offered sputum smear examinations significantly less often [21]. Among patients hospitalized and diagnosed with TB in the United States, women faced greater provider-/system-level delays in undergoing sputum smear microscopy than men [85]. However, among HIV-infected patients in the

United States, men and women were screened for TB with similar frequency [87]. Only one study assessed gender-related barriers to TB treatment following a diagnosis of TB and found no differences between male and female patients with respect to provider-related factors [28].

Gender-related differences in patient satisfaction with TB services were examined by seven (37%) studies [17, 34, 35, 37, 52, 73, 84]. In Nepal and Egypt, males and females with suspected TB had similar levels of satisfaction with TB services [34, 35]. However, women in Egypt were less satisfied with drug availability than men, and women in Bangladesh and Syria were less satisfied with TB clinic hours, providers, and services than men, all of which were also predictors of health-seeking [17, 35, 37]. Compared to men, a greater proportion of women in Tanzania reported that a good provider-patient relationship was an important factor in their satisfaction with TB services [73]. Vietnamese TB patients reported no gender-related differences in the health education they received about their disease [52]. In another Tanzanian study where patients were randomized to community-based versus clinic-based TB treatment, male patients were more satisfied with community-based treatment than female patients [84]. Divided opinion regarding venue of treatment was noted in the study. Some patients preferred community-based treatment due to convenience, reduced transport costs, saved time, and reduced lost wages, whereas others preferred clinic-based treatment because it led to greater access to other clinical services and health education [84].

The remaining three studies reported on gender-related differences in health literacy among providers and TB-related hospitalization. Two studies assessed gender-based differences in TB-related knowledge among health workers and found no gender-based differences among providers in Oman and Iraq where patients may be more likely to seek care from providers of the same sex [75, 88]. One study in Tajikistan found that male TB patients were more likely to be hospitalized for treatment than female TB patients; other predictors of hospitalization in this study included positive sputum smear and availability of hospital beds [82].

3.5. Combined Individual-/Provider-/System-Level Barriers. Seven (5%) studies assessed gender-related differences in TB case detection rates, which were impacted by combined individual-/provider-/system-level barriers. Community-based active case finding was one strategy used to overcome combined level barriers to accessing TB diagnostic services [152, 153]. Seven studies compared community-based active case finding versus passive case finding (i.e., self-referral). Of these, five found that community-based active case finding increased TB case detection rates more significantly among women than men [29, 91–94]; one found greater increases in case detection rates among men than women [95]; and one found no difference in the change of case detection rates between men and women [18].

3.6. Individual-Level Delays. Almost half of the included studies (42%) appraised gender-related differences in individual-level delays. Of these, 38 found that symptomatic women were as likely as symptomatic men to delay or

not seek TB services. However, among the 20 studies that found gender-related differences, 13 found that symptomatic women were more likely to delay or not seek TB services than symptomatic men, whereas seven studies found that symptomatic women were less likely to delay or not seek TB services than symptomatic men. The majority of studies were performed among study populations of persons who had already presented for care with diagnosed or suspected TB. Only five studies assessed persons with suspected TB in the general population. Of these, one study found that women were quicker to seek care for a prolonged cough [61], two studies found that women were slower to seek care [21, 97], and two studies found no difference in delay by gender [56, 111].

3.7. Provider-/System-Level Delays. Of 137 studies, 37 (27%) assessed gender-related differences in provider-/system-level delays in accessing TB services. The time between the presentation of a person with suspected TB to a health facility and TB diagnosis was most commonly assessed. Of 22 studies, 55% found no gender-related difference in the delay from presentation to TB diagnosis. All of the remaining 10 studies found that women experienced longer delays than men. Among 13 studies that examined the delay from presentation to TB treatment initiation, nine found no gender-related difference, three found that women had longer delays than men [14, 81, 135], and only one study found that men experienced longer delays than women [101]. Similarly, among seven studies that measured the delay between TB diagnosis and TB treatment initiation, four found no gender-related difference [33, 79, 104, 137], two found that women had longer delays than men [14, 19], and only one found that men had longer delays than women [35].

3.8. Combined Individual-/Provider-/System-Level Delays. Of 137 studies, 25 (18%) reported on gender-related differences in combined individual /provider /system level delays. The delay between symptom onset and TB treatment initiation was most commonly assessed, and 13 out of these 18 (68%) studies found no gender-related difference. When a gender-related difference was observed, women faced longer delays than men [27, 79, 100, 140, 143]. One multicountry study found that, compared to men, women experienced longer delays in Yemen and shorter delays in Egypt but similar delays in other countries [141]. Among nine studies that assessed gender-related differences in the delay between symptom onset and TB diagnosis, 5 found no gender-related difference [33, 35, 114, 133, 146], whereas four studies found that women experienced longer delays than men [32, 36, 79, 142].

3.9. Quality of Included Studies. We assessed 126 cross-sectional studies, one case-control study, and eight cohort studies using the STROBE criteria [148], and we assessed two randomized trials using the CONSORT criteria [149, 150]. The majority of studies suffered from poor quality reporting of research design, methods, analyses, and results (see Supplementary Tables S2 and S3). Key weaknesses specific to and pervasive among the cross-sectional studies (92% of included studies) were inadequate reporting regarding the numbers of males and females at each study stage from eligibility assessment through enrollment, participation, follow-up, and analysis; explanation of nonparticipation for males and females at each stage; information on prevalence of exposures and confounders among the male and female participants; presentation of unadjusted and confounder-adjusted estimates for males and females; and explanation for selection of confounders for adjustment.

4. Discussion

Guided by a systematic review process, our review aimed to assess the quantitative evidence for gender-related differences in the barriers and delays that impact access to TB diagnostic and treatment services at the individual and provider/system levels. While, collectively, the included studies reported on barriers and delays at each level, more studies examined individual-level barriers and delays, and most studies surveyed persons presenting for care with diagnosed or suspected TB and were conducted in Africa and Asia. Overall, our review identified that many studies found no quantitative gender-related differences. However, when differences were reported, more studies found that women experienced greater barriers and longer delays at each level than men. In particular, many studies reported gender-related differences in financial, stigma, and health literacy barriers, which are interrelated and represent potential targets for gender-specific interventions that may be integrated into current and future TB service strategies.

While both genders experienced financial barriers to accessing TB services, the majority of studies that found gender-related differences reported that women experienced greater financial barriers than men, and the identified barriers were gender-specific. Specifically, the male role of primary income earner in many households prevented men from leaving work to access TB services, whereas, for women, their financial dependence on spouses and families limited access to TB services. Similar gender-related differences have been observed in financial barriers that limit access to diagnostic and treatment services for HIV and malaria [154–157]. Instituting more flexible hours and locations for TB services may help overcome the opportunity cost of lost wages and may improve case detection and treatment initiation among men. For women, barriers due to financial dependence may be compounded by the deprioritization of women's health care within the household below the needs of men and children. Because maternal health is prioritized by some households [158], efforts to integrate TB services with maternal healthcare may overcome some financial barriers and facilitate access to TB services among some women.

Regarding TB-related stigma, our review found that women were fearful of having a diagnosis of TB disclosed to their spouse, family, or community. Women experienced greater stigma than men, when gender-related differences were found. The impact of disease-related stigma has been well studied in the context of HIV, where anticipated or experienced stigma may lead patients to conceal symptoms, avoid or delay seeking care, hide their diagnoses, and be nonadherent with treatment [159–163]. Specifically, TB has

been associated with dirtiness, immorality, substance abuse, and sexual promiscuity or deviancy [164–166], and, in communities with high rates of TB/HIV coinfection, TB may be further stigmatized by its association with HIV [167]. In addition to the psychosocial consequences of a TB diagnosis, our review also found that women were concerned about marital prospects and rejection by their spouse or families. Thus, TB-related stigma may also manifest as a financial barrier among those women who depend on spouses and family for financial support.

While stigma barriers may be addressed by interventions to improve TB-related health literacy, our review suggests that such programs may be particularly beneficial for women in rural areas. Among the included studies that reported gender difference in TB-related knowledge, men had greater TB-related knowledge and higher general literacy rates than women, and the majority of these (64%) were conducted in rural settings. It may be important to examine the interaction between female literacy and the impact of poverty on care seeking as this interaction has impacted care seeking among women in the context of other health services [168, 169].

Although only a few studies assessed the impact of barriers on delays, individual-level barriers appear to impact individual-level delays in TB care seeking in gender-specific ways. Symptomatic women were more likely to delay or not seek care than symptomatic men when gender-related differences in individual-level delays were reported. Individual-level TB-related stigma can represent both an obstacle and a motivation to seeking care [48], and marital status, which is intimately interlinked with issues of financial and social dependency as well as spousal and family support or rejection, also had a variable impact on gender-related differences in access to services [17, 71]. Regarding sociodemographic barriers, older age was a more significant barrier to accessing TB services among women than men [79, 81]. Given the complexity of these relationships, it is important to go beyond comparing the frequency and severity of individual-level barriers among women and men. Researchers and policymakers must also understand the impact of individual-level barriers on individual-level delays and how these barriers cause delays in accessing TB services among women and men. Qualitative studies may play an invaluable role here and inform researchers on the mechanisms of barriers and delays, which can be the points of intervention in the future.

Similarly, it is important to understand gender-related differences in provider-/system-level barriers and delays. In our review, fewer studies assessed barriers and delays at the provider/system level. However, when disparities were found, women were more likely to face barriers to accessing TB services than men. In addition, gender-specific individual barriers, such as financial and stigma barriers, may also impact the provider/system level but were not assessed by the studies included in our review. Surprisingly, in the context of other diseases, there are few reports on gender-related disparities in barriers and delays that limit access to care, particularly at the provider/system levels among patients in resource-limited settings. Provider-/system-level barriers and delays that lead to gender-related disparities in health often result from the lack of attention to the different needs of men and women while planning and providing health services, particularly with respect to service availability (e.g., geographical location, transportation available, service hours, and waiting time), affordability, acceptability (e.g., social and cultural competency, respect, privacy, confidentiality, and autonomy), and accountability [170, 171]. Furthermore, health providers and health systems may compound individual-level and community-level disparities by failing to recognize that gender-based differences exist or by failing to acknowledge the need for corrective interventions [1].

In addition to the paucity of data on barriers and delays at the provider/system levels, our review revealed several other research gaps. To comprehensively identify gender-related barriers and delays, study populations need to include persons with suspected TB who have not presented for care. There is also an urgent need for more granular analyses of gender disparities in accessing TB services for each step along the diagnostic and treatment continuum (i.e., symptom onset to symptom recognition; symptom recognition to seeking care; seeking care to TB diagnosis; TB diagnosis to notification; and notification to treatment initiation) at all levels. More generally, prospectively designed gender analyses are needed, and standardized ethnographic and cultural epidemiologic tools [5] also need to be used prospectively to systematically collect and compare gender-related socio-cultural variables across studies, which may help to identify common as well as unique gender-related barriers.

The studies included in our review span different continents and differ among degree of urbanization and type of study population. Therefore, it is important to recognize heterogeneity while summarizing our findings. While most of the included studies were conducted in the Africa, South East Asia, and West Pacific regions, the frequency of some reported barriers by gender was not always proportional to numbers of studies from these regions. For example, financial barriers and delays at the individual and provider/system levels were reported proportionally by region, regardless of gender. However, women in South East Asia were noted to face more stigma, and women in West Pacific and both men and women in South East Asia had lower health literacy than persons from Africa (see Supplementary Table S4). These findings implicate region-specific priorities in interventions to improve access to TB care. Regarding study population type, included studies that assessed the general population (one quarter of the included studies) almost exclusively reported on stigma and health literacy barriers. Compared to studies among persons with diagnosed or suspected TB that found gender disparities, studies that assessed the general population were less likely to report that women face greater stigma and more likely to report that women have lower health literacy than men (see Supplementary Table S5). There is very little data to assess barriers and delays in different degrees of urbanization, as high percentage of studies were conducted in mixed urban and rural setting. However, studies from rural areas more frequently reported on worse health literacy among women (see Supplementary Table S6). The implication was already discussed above.

Many have called for more research on gender-related disparities in TB [4, 5, 8, 172, 173]. Accordingly, our systematic review aimed to assess the quantitative gender-related differences in barriers and delays that limit access to TB diagnostic and treatment services, which have been recognized as important for optimal TB control. However, a number of biases may have impacted our results and the individual studies that were included in our review. Although we strove to capture all high-quality studies addressing the topic of this review, some studies may have been missed, particularly those that were not published because they failed to document gender-related differences in accessing TB services, which may have resulted in an over representation of studies that demonstrated a difference (i.e., publication bias). In addition, our review was subject to biases introduced by the exclusion of non-English articles as studies from countries where English is not a primary language, particularly Latin American countries or East Asia, may be underrepresented. A noted limitation of the included studies was that the majority was cross-sectional studies and assessed patients with a confirmed TB diagnosis and/or those presenting for TB care. Those experiencing the greatest barriers to TB services are also least likely to be diagnosed with TB. Because persons presenting for care have already surmounted many individual-level barriers, comparisons of gender-related differences in these study populations will suffer from selection bias. In addition, sample size among the included studies was highly variable, and the quality of study reporting was generally poor. Finally, the summary measures and definitions of barriers and delays were inconsistently used, making it difficult to weigh the relative importance of findings from the included studies or to conduct a meta-analysis or stratified analysis.

5. Conclusions

Overall, the scientific community is recognizing that gender-related differences in health may be greater than is known and is increasingly prioritizing the need for routine gender-related analyses [174–177]. Notably, the WHO has developed a strategy to mainstream the analysis of the role of gender in health and to monitor and address systemic gender-related health inequities [178]. In the context of TB, gender analyses are critical to inform interventions to optimize the global impact of TB services. Our systematic review indicated that, when gender-related differences were found, women experienced greater barriers and longer delays than men and identified several gender-specific components within individual-level financial, stigma, and health literacy barriers that are amenable to intervention. However, our review also revealed research gaps and clearly highlighted that well-designed gender analyses are critical. Finally, qualitative accounts of the gender differences presented here would inform mechanisms of barriers and provide insight for interventions.

Authors' Contribution

Wei-Teng Yang, Celine R. Gounder, and Katherine N. McIntire wrote the manuscript and analyzed data. Wei-Teng Yang, Tokunbo Akande, and Jan-Walter De Neve abstracted data and made supplementary tables. Amita Gupta and Celine R. Gounder wrote the grant for funding from the World Health Organization. Aditya Chandrasekhar, Alan de Lima Pereira, Naveen Gummadi, and Santanu Samanta were involved in the title and abstract screening. All authors commented on and approved the paper.

Acknowledgment

This study was funded in part by a grant from the World Health Organization. The funders had no role in study design, data collection and analysis, preparation of the paper, or decision to publish. Wei-Teng Yang and Celine R. Gounder have joint first authorship.

References

[1] WHO, *Global Tuberculosis Control 2012*, WHO, 2012.

[2] P. Hudelson, "Gender differentials in tuberculosis: the role of socio-economic and cultural factors," *Tubercle and Lung Disease*, vol. 77, no. 5, pp. 391–400, 1996.

[3] A. Thorson and V. K. Diwan, "Gender inequalities in tuberculosis: aspects of infection, notification rates, and compliance," *Current Opinion in Pulmonary Medicine*, vol. 7, no. 3, pp. 165–169, 2001.

[4] C. B. Holmes, H. Hausler, and P. Nunn, "A review of sex differences in the epidemiology of tuberculosis," *International Journal of Tuberculosis and Lung Disease*, vol. 2, no. 2, pp. 96–104, 1998.

[5] WHO, *Gender and Tuberculosis*, Gender and Health Research Series, WHO, 2004.

[6] M. Connolly and P. Nunn, "Women and tuberculosis," *World Health Statistics Quarterly*, vol. 49, no. 2, pp. 115–119, 1996.

[7] D. G. Storla, S. Yimer, and G. A. Bjune, "A systematic review of delay in the diagnosis and treatment of tuberculosis," *BMC Public Health*, vol. 8, article 15, 2008.

[8] M. W. Uplekar, S. Rangan, M. G. Weiss, J. Ogden, M. W. Borgdorff, and P. Hudelson, "Attention to gender issues in tuberculosis control," *International Journal of Tuberculosis and Lung Disease*, vol. 5, no. 3, pp. 220–224, 2001.

[9] J. Ogden, S. Rangan, M. Uplekar et al., "Shifting the paradigm in tuberculosis control: illustrations from India," *International Journal of Tuberculosis and Lung Disease*, vol. 3, no. 10, pp. 855–861, 1999.

[10] I. Bates, C. Fenton, J. Gruber et al., "Vulnerability to malaria, tuberculosis, and HIV/AIDS infection and disease—part 1: determinants operating at individual and household level," *The Lancet Infectious Diseases*, vol. 4, no. 5, pp. 267–277, 2004.

[11] B. Vissandjee and M. Pai, "The socio-cultural challenge in public health interventions: the case of tuberculosis in India," *International Journal of Public Health*, vol. 52, no. 4, pp. 199–201, 2007.

[12] M. M. Mesfin, J. N. Newell, R. J. Madeley et al., "Cost implications of delays to tuberculosis diagnosis among pulmonary tuberculosis patients in Ethiopia," *BMC Public Health*, vol. 10, article 173, 2010.

[13] A. Aspler, D. Menzies, O. Oxlade et al., "Cost of tuberculosis diagnosis and treatment from the patient perspective in Lusaka, Zambia," *International Journal of Tuberculosis and Lung Disease*, vol. 12, no. 8, pp. 928–935, 2008.

[14] S. G. Mfinanga, B. K. Mutayoba, A. Kahwa et al., "The magnitude and factors associated with delays in management of smear positive tuberculosis in Dar es Salaam, Tanzania," *BMC Health Services Research*, vol. 8, article 158, 2008.

[15] J. R. Kemp, G. Mann, B. N. Simwaka, F. M. L. Salaniponi, and S. B. Squire, "Can Malawi's poor afford free tuberculosis services? Patient and household costs associated with a tuberculosis diagnosis in Lilongwe," *Bulletin of the World Health Organization*, vol. 85, no. 8, pp. 580–585, 2007.

[16] M. S. Kiwuwa, K. Charles, and M. K. Harriet, "Patient and health service delay in pulmonary tuberculosis patients attending a referral hospital: a cross-sectional study," *BMC Public Health*, vol. 5, article 122, 2005.

[17] G. Ahsan, J. Ahmed, P. Singhasivanon et al., "Gender difference in treatment seeking behaviors of tuberculosis cases in rural communities of Bangladesh," *Southeast Asian Journal of Tropical Medicine and Public Health*, vol. 35, no. 1, pp. 126–135, 2004.

[18] R. Balasubramanian, R. Garg, T. Santha et al., "Gender disparities in tuberculosis: report from a rural DOTS programme in south India," *International Journal of Tuberculosis and Lung Disease*, vol. 8, no. 3, pp. 323–332, 2004.

[19] M. R. Masjedi, A. Cheragvandi, M. Hadian, and A. A. Velayati, "Reasons for delay in the management of patients with pulmonary tuberculosis," *Eastern Mediterranean Health Journal*, vol. 8, no. 2-3, pp. 324–329, 2002.

[20] J. Ngamvithayapong, H. Yanai, A. Winkvist, and V. Diwan, "Health seeking behaviour and diagnosis for pulmonary tuberculosis in an HIV-epidemic mountainous area of Thailand," *International Journal of Tuberculosis and Lung Disease*, vol. 5, no. 11, pp. 1013–1020, 2001.

[21] A. Thorson, N. P. Hoa, and N. H. Long, "Health-seeking behaviour of individuals with a cough of more than 3 weeks," *The Lancet*, vol. 356, no. 9244, pp. 1823–1824, 2000.

[22] R. Rajeswari, R. Balasubramanian, M. Muniyandi, S. Geetharamani, X. Thresa, and P. Venkatesan, "Socio-economic impact of tuberculosis on patients and family in India," *International Journal of Tuberculosis and Lung Disease*, vol. 3, no. 10, pp. 869–877, 1999.

[23] A. Vassall, A. Seme, P. Compernolle, and F. Meheus, "Patient costs of accessing collaborative tuberculosis and human immunodeficiency virus interventions in Ethiopia," *International Journal of Tuberculosis and Lung Disease*, vol. 14, no. 5, pp. 604–610, 2010.

[24] M. G. Weiss, D. Somma, F. Karim et al., "Cultural epidemiology of TB with reference to gender in Bangladesh, India and Malawi," *International Journal of Tuberculosis and Lung Disease*, vol. 12, no. 7, pp. 837–847, 2008.

[25] S. R. Atre, A. M. Kudale, S. N. Morankar, S. G. Rangan, and M. G. Weiss, "Cultural concepts of tuberculosis and gender among the general population without tuberculosis in rural Maharashtra, India," *Tropical Medicine and International Health*, vol. 9, no. 11, pp. 1228–1238, 2004.

[26] M. A. H. Salim, E. Declercq, A. van Deun, and K. A. R. Saki, "Gender differences in tuberculosis: a prevalence survey done in Bangladesh," *International Journal of Tuberculosis and Lung Disease*, vol. 8, no. 8, pp. 952–957, 2004.

[27] M. Lambert, R. Delgado, G. Michaux, A. Volz, N. Speybroeck, and P. van der Stuyft, "Delays to treatment and out-of-pocket

medical expenditure for tuberculosis patients, in an urban area of South America," *Annals of Tropical Medicine and Parasitology*, vol. 99, no. 8, pp. 781–787, 2005.

[28] R. Dandona, L. Dandona, A. Mishra, S. Dhingra, K. Venkatagopalakrishna, and L. S. Chauhan, "Utilization of and barriers to public sector tuberculosis services in India," *National Medical Journal of India*, vol. 17, no. 6, pp. 292–299, 2004.

[29] A. Thorson, N. P. Hoa, N. H. Long, P. Allebeck, and V. K. Diwan, "Do women with tuberculosis have a lower likelihood of getting diagnosed? Prevalence and case detection of sputum smear positive pulmonary TB, a population-based study from Vietnam," *Journal of Clinical Epidemiology*, vol. 57, no. 4, pp. 398–402, 2004.

[30] P. Godfrey-Faussett, H. Kaunda, J. Kamanga et al., "Why do patients with a cough delay seeking care at Lusaka urban health centres? A health systems research approach," *International Journal of Tuberculosis and Lung Disease*, vol. 6, no. 9, pp. 796–805, 2002.

[31] H. Sadiq and A. D. Muynck, "Health care seeking behavior of pulmonary tuberculosis patients visiting TB Center Rawalpindi," *Journal of the Pakistan Medical Association*, vol. 51, no. 1, pp. 10–16, 2001.

[32] M. Yamasaki-Nakagawa, K. Ozasa, N. Yamada et al., "Gender difference in delays to diagnosis and health care seeking behavior in a rural area of Nepal," *International Journal of Tuberculosis and Lung Disease*, vol. 5, no. 1, pp. 24–31, 2001.

[33] M. Jiménez-Corona, L. García-García, K. DeRiemer et al., "Gender differentials of pulmonary tuberculosis transmission and reactivation in an endemic area," *Thorax*, vol. 61, no. 4, pp. 348–353, 2006.

[34] S. K. Tiwari and E. J. Love, "Gender and tuberculosis control in armed conflict areas in Nepal," *International Medical Journal*, vol. 14, no. 4, pp. 265–271, 2007.

[35] M. I. Kamel, S. Rashed, N. Foda, A. Mohie, and M. Loutfy, "Gender differences in health care utilization and outcome of respiratory tuberculosis in Alexandria," *Eastern Mediterranean Health Journal*, vol. 9, no. 4, pp. 741–756, 2003.

[36] N. H. Long, E. Johansson, K. Lönnroth, B. Eriksson, A. Winkvist, and V. K. Diwan, "Longer delays in tuberculosis diagnosis among women in Vietnam," *International Journal of Tuberculosis and Lung Disease*, vol. 3, no. 5, pp. 388–393, 1999.

[37] H. Bashour and F. Mamaree, "Gender differences and tuberculosis in the Syrian Arab Republic: patients' attitudes, compliance and outcomes," *Eastern Mediterranean Health Journal*, vol. 9, no. 4, pp. 757–768, 2003.

[38] A. Deribew, G. Abebe, L. Apers et al., "Prejudice and misconceptions about tuberculosis and HIV in rural and urban communities in Ethiopia: a challenge for the TB/HIV control program," *BMC Public Health*, vol. 10, article 400, 2010.

[39] V. K. Dhingra and S. Khan, "A sociological study on stigma among TB patients in Delhi," *Indian Journal of Tuberculosis*, vol. 57, no. 1, pp. 12–18, 2010.

[40] M. Berisha, V. Zheki, D. Zadzhmi, S. Gashi, R. Hokha, and I. Begoli, "Level of knowledge regarding tuberculosis and stigma among patients suffering from tuberculosis," *Georgian Medical News*, no. 166, pp. 89–93, 2009.

[41] N. P. Hoa, N. T. K. Chuc, and A. Thorson, "Knowledge, attitudes, and practices about tuberculosis and choice of communication channels in a rural community in Vietnam," *Health Policy*, vol. 90, no. 1, pp. 8–12, 2009.

[42] S. M. Marks, N. Deluca, and W. Walton, "Knowledge, attitudes and risk perceptions about tuberculosis: US national health

interview survey," *International Journal of Tuberculosis and Lung Disease*, vol. 12, no. 11, pp. 1261–1267, 2008.

[43] F. Karim, A. M. R. Chowdhury, A. Islam, and M. G. Weiss, "Stigma, gender, and their impact on patients with tuberculosis in rural Bangladesh," *Anthropology and Medicine*, vol. 14, no. 2, pp. 139–151, 2007.

[44] H. Getahun and D. Aragaw, "Tuberculosis in rural northwest Ethiopia: community perspective," *Ethiopian Medical Journal*, vol. 39, no. 4, pp. 283–291, 2001.

[45] R. X. Armijos, M. M. Weigel, M. Qincha, and B. Ulloa, "The meaning and consequences of tuberculosis for an at-risk urban group in Ecuador," *Pan American Journal of Public Health*, vol. 23, no. 3, pp. 188–197, 2008.

[46] M. S. Westaway, "Knowledge, beliefs and feelings about tuberculosis," *Health Education Research*, vol. 4, no. 2, pp. 205–211, 1989.

[47] J. M. Cramm, H. J. Finkenflügel, V. Møller, and A. P. Nieboer, "TB treatment initiation and adherence in a South African community influenced more by perceptions than by knowledge of tuberculosis," *BMC Public Health*, vol. 10, article 72, 2010.

[48] P. Pungrassami, A. M. Kipp, P. W. Stewart, V. Chongsuvivatwong, R. P. Strauss, and A. van Rie, "Tuberculosis and AIDS stigma among patients who delay seeking care for tuberculosis symptoms," *International Journal of Tuberculosis and Lung Disease*, vol. 14, no. 2, pp. 181–187, 2010.

[49] S. Atre, A. Kudale, S. Morankar, D. Gosoniu, and M. G. Weiss, "Gender and community views of stigma and tuberculosis in rural Maharashtra, India," *Global Public Health*, vol. 6, no. 1, pp. 56–71, 2011.

[50] S. H. Lu, B. C. Tian, X. P. Kang et al., "Public awareness of tuberculosis in China: a national survey of 69253 subjects," *International Journal of Tuberculosis and Lung Disease*, vol. 13, no. 12, pp. 1493–1499, 2009.

[51] S. A. Qureshi, O. Morkve, and T. Mustafa, "Patient and health system delays: health-care seeking behaviour among pulmonary tuberculosis patients in Pakistan," *Journal of the Pakistan Medical Association*, vol. 58, no. 6, pp. 318–321, 2008.

[52] N. P. Hoa, V. K. Diwan, N. V. Co, and A. E. K. Thorson, "Knowledge about tuberculosis and its treatment among new pulmonary TB patients in the north and central regions of Vietnam," *International Journal of Tuberculosis and Lung Disease*, vol. 8, no. 5, pp. 603–608, 2004.

[53] T. K. Koay, "Knowledge and attitudes towards tuberculosis among the people living in Kudat district, Sabah," *Medical Journal of Malaysia*, vol. 59, no. 4, pp. 502–511, 2004.

[54] N. Shetty, M. Shemko, and A. Abbas, "Knowledge, attitudes and practices regarding tuberculosis among immigrants of Somalian ethnic origin in London: a cross-sectional study," *Communicable Disease and Public Health*, vol. 7, no. 1, pp. 77–82, 2004.

[55] M. S. Khan, O. Dar, C. Sismanidis, K. Shah, and P. Godfrey-Faussett, "Improvement of tuberculosis case detection and reduction of discrepancies between men and women by simple sputum-submission instructions: a pragmatic randomised controlled trial," *The Lancet*, vol. 369, no. 9577, pp. 1955–1960, 2007.

[56] J. M. Wang, Y. Fei, H. B. Shen, and B. Xu, "Gender difference in knowledge of tuberculosis and associated health-care seeking behaviors: a cross-sectional study in a rural area of China," *BMC Public Health*, vol. 8, article 354, 2008.

[57] N. Sharma, R. Malhotra, D. K. Taneja, R. Saha, and G. K. Ingle, "Awareness and perception about tuberculosis in the general

population of Delhi," *Asia-Pacific Journal of Public Health*, vol. 19, no. 2, pp. 10–15, 2007.

[58] T. H. Zhang, X. Y. Liu, H. Bromley, and S. L. Tang, "Perceptions of tuberculosis and health seeking behaviour in rural Inner Mongolia, China," *Health Policy*, vol. 81, no. 2-3, pp. 155–165, 2007.

[59] J. Date and K. Okita, "Gender and literacy: factors related to diagnostic delay and unsuccessful treatment of tuberculosis in the mountainous area of Yemen," *International Journal of Tuberculosis and Lung Disease*, vol. 9, no. 6, pp. 680–685, 2005.

[60] M. Agboatwalla, G. N. Kazi, S. K. Shah, and M. Tariq, "Gender perspectives on knowledge and practices regarding tuberculosis in urban and rural areas in Pakistan," *Eastern Mediterranean Health Journal*, vol. 9, no. 4, pp. 732–740, 2003.

[61] N. P. Hoa, A. E. K. Thorson, N. H. Long, and V. K. Diwan, "Knowledge of tuberculosis and associated health-seeking behaviour among rural Vietnamese adults with a cough for at least three weeks," *Scandinavian Journal of Public Health*, vol. 62, pp. 59–65, 2003.

[62] R. Malhotra, D. K. Taneja, V. K. Dhingra, S. Rajpal, and M. Mehra, "Awareness regarding tuberculosis in a rural population of Delhi," *Indian Journal of Community Medicine*, vol. 27, no. 2, pp. 62–68, 2002.

[63] J. S. Marinac, S. K. Willsie, D. McBride, and S. C. Hamburger, "Knowledge of tuberculosis in high-risk populations: survey of inner city minorities," *International Journal of Tuberculosis and Lung Disease*, vol. 2, no. 10, pp. 804–810, 1998.

[64] B. Chimbanrai, W. Fungladda, J. Kaewkungwal, and U. Silachamroon, "Treatment-seeking behaviors and improvement in adherence to treatment regimen of tuberculosis patients using intensive triad-model program, Thailand," *Southeast Asian Journal of Tropical Medicine and Public Health*, vol. 39, no. 3, pp. 526–541, 2008.

[65] S. Promtussananon and K. Peltzer, "Perceptions of tuberculosis: attributions of cause, suggested means of risk reduction, and preferred treatment in the Limpopo province, South Africa," *Journal of Health, Population and Nutrition*, vol. 23, no. 1, pp. 74–81, 2005.

[66] R. L. Ailinger, H. Lasus, and M. Dear, "Americans' knowledge and perceived risk of tuberculosis," *Public Health Nursing*, vol. 20, no. 3, pp. 211–215, 2003.

[67] C. K. Liam, K. H. Lim, C. M. M. Wong, and B. G. Tang, "Attitudes and knowledge of newly diagnosed tuberculosis patients regarding the disease, and factors affecting treatment compliance," *International Journal of Tuberculosis and Lung Disease*, vol. 3, no. 4, pp. 300–309, 1999.

[68] R. Rajeswari, M. Muniyandi, R. Balasubramanian, and P. R. Narayanan, "Perceptions of tuberculosis patients about their physical, mental and social well-being: a field report from south India," *Social Science and Medicine*, vol. 60, no. 8, pp. 1845–1853, 2005.

[69] A. C. Crampin, J. R. Glynn, S. Floyd et al., "Tuberculosis and gender: exploring the patterns in a case control study in Malawi," *International Journal of Tuberculosis and Lung Disease*, vol. 8, no. 2, pp. 194–203, 2004.

[70] M. U. Mushtaq, M. A. Majrooh, W. Ahmad et al., "Knowledge, attitudes and practices regarding tuberculosis in two districts of Punjab, Pakistan," *International Journal of Tuberculosis and Lung Disease*, vol. 14, no. 3, pp. 303–310, 2010.

[71] P. O. Ayuo, L. O. Diero, W. D. Owino-Ong'or, and A. W. Mwangi, "Causes of delay in diagnosis of pulmonary tuberculosis in patients attending a referral hospital in Western Kenya," *East African Medical Journal*, vol. 85, no. 6, pp. 263–268, 2008.

[72] P. Brassard, K. K. Anderson, D. Menzies, K. Schwartzman, and M. E. Macdonald, "Knowledge and perceptions of tuberculosis among a sample of urban aboriginal people," *Journal of Community Health*, vol. 33, no. 4, pp. 192–198, 2008.

[73] A. M. Kilale, A. K. Mushi, L. A. Lema et al., "Perceptions of tuberculosis and treatment seeking behaviour in Ilala and Kinondoni Municipalities in Tanzania," *Tanzania Journal of Health Research*, vol. 10, no. 2, pp. 89–94, 2008.

[74] A. Katamba, D. B. Neuhauser, K. A. Smyth, F. Adatu, E. Katabira, and C. C. Whalen, "Patients perceived stigma associated with community-based directly observed therapy of tuberculosis in Uganda," *East African Medical Journal*, vol. 82, no. 7, pp. 337–342, 2005.

[75] D. S. Hashim, W. Al Kubaisy, and A. Al Dulayme, "Knowledge, attitudes and practices survey among health care workers and tuberculosis patients in Iraq," *Eastern Mediterranean Health Journal*, vol. 9, no. 4, pp. 718–731, 2003.

[76] E. R. Wandwalo and O. Morkve, "Knowledge of disease and treatment among tuberculosis patients in Mwanza, Tanzania," *International Journal of Tuberculosis and Lung Disease*, vol. 4, no. 11, pp. 1041–1046, 2000.

[77] J. P. Tulsky, M. C. White, J. A. Young, R. Meakin, and A. R. Moss, "Street talk: knowledge and attitudes about tuberculosis and tuberculosis control among homeless adults," *International Journal of Tuberculosis and Lung Disease*, vol. 3, no. 6, pp. 528–533, 1999.

[78] D. Jenkins, "Tuberculosis: the Native Indian viewpoint on its prevention, diagnosis, and treatment," *Preventive Medicine*, vol. 6, no. 4, pp. 545–555, 1977.

[79] F. Karim, M. A. Islam, A. M. R. Chowdhury, E. Johansson, and V. K. Diwan, "Gender differences in delays in diagnosis and treatment of tuberculosis," *Health Policy and Planning*, vol. 22, no. 5, pp. 329–334, 2007.

[80] A. Kaulagekar and A. Radkar, "Social status makes a difference: tuberculosis scenario during national family health survey-2," *The Indian Journal of Tuberculosis*, vol. 54, no. 1, pp. 17–23, 2007.

[81] J. Ward, V. Siskind, and A. Konstantinos, "Patient and health care system delays in Queensland tuberculosis patients, 1985–1998," *International Journal of Tuberculosis and Lung Disease*, vol. 5, no. 11, pp. 1021–1027, 2001.

[82] C. Thierfelder, K. Makowiecka, T. Vinichenko, R. Ayé, P. Edwards, and K. Wyss, "Management of pulmonary tuberculosis in Tajikistan: which factors determine hospitalization?" *Tropical Medicine and International Health*, vol. 13, no. 11, pp. 1364–1371, 2008.

[83] W. Thongraung, V. Chongsuvivatwong, and P. Pungrassamee, "Multilevel factors affecting tuberculosis diagnosis and initial treatment," *Journal of Evaluation in Clinical Practice*, vol. 14, no. 3, pp. 378–384, 2008.

[84] E. Wandwalo, E. Makundi, T. Hasler, and O. Morkve, "Acceptability of community and health facility-based directly observed treatment of tuberculosis in Tanzanian urban setting," *Health Policy*, vol. 78, no. 2-3, pp. 284–294, 2006.

[85] J. Rozovsky-Weinberger, J. P. Parada, L. Phan et al., "Delays in suspicion and isolation among hospitalized persons with pulmonary tuberculosis at public and private US hospitals during 1996 to 1999," *Chest*, vol. 127, no. 1, pp. 205–212, 2005.

[86] C. Lienhardt, J. Rowley, K. Manneh et al., "Factors affecting time delay to treatment in a tuberculosis control programme in a

sub-Saharan African country: the experience of the Gambia," *International Journal of Tuberculosis and Lung Disease*, vol. 5, no. 3, pp. 233–239, 2001.

[87] T. L. Box, M. Olsen, E. Z. Oddone, and S. A. Keitz, "Healthcare access and utilization by patients infected with human immunodeficiency virus: does gender matter?" *Journal of Women's Health*, vol. 12, no. 4, pp. 391–397, 2003.

[88] A. A. Al-Maniri, O. A. Al-Rawas, F. Al-Ajmi, A. de Costa, B. Eriksson, and V. K. Diwan, "Tuberculosis suspicion and knowledge among private and public general practitioners: questionnaire Based Study in Oman," *BMC Public Health*, vol. 8, article 177, 2008.

[89] G. Fochsen, K. Deshpande, V. Diwan, A. Mishra, V. K. Diwan, and A. Thorson, "Health care seeking among individuals with cough and tuberculosis: a population-based study from rural India," *International Journal of Tuberculosis and Lung Disease*, vol. 10, no. 9, pp. 995–1000, 2006.

[90] A. D. Harries, T. E. Nyirenda, P. Godfrey-Faussett, and F. M. Salaniponi, "Defining and assessing the maximum number of visits patients should make to a health facility to obtain a diagnosis of pulmonary tuberculosis," *International Journal of Tuberculosis and Lung Disease*, vol. 7, no. 10, pp. 953–958, 2003.

[91] D. G. Datiko and B. Lindtjørn, "Health extension workers improve tuberculosis case detection and treatment success in southern Ethiopia: a community randomized trial," *PLoS ONE*, vol. 4, no. 5, Article ID e5443, 2009.

[92] A. Cassels, E. Heineman, S. LeClerq, P. K. Gurung, and C. B. Rahut, "Tuberculosis case-finding in Eastern Nepal," *Tubercle*, vol. 63, no. 3, pp. 175–185, 1982.

[93] S. Yimer, C. Holm-Hansen, T. Yimaldu, and G. Bjune, "Evaluating an active case-fi nding strategy to identify smear-positive tuberculosis in rural Ethiopia," *International Journal of Tuberculosis and Lung Disease*, vol. 13, no. 11, pp. 1399–1404, 2009.

[94] M. C. Becerra, I. F. Pachao-Torreblanca, J. Bayona et al., "Expanding tuberculosis case detection by screening household contacts," *Public Health Reports*, vol. 120, no. 3, pp. 271–277, 2005.

[95] T. Santha, G. Renu, T. R. Frieden et al., "Are community surveys to detect tuberculosis in high prevalence areas useful? Results of a comparative study from Tiruvallur District, South India," *International Journal of Tuberculosis and Lung Disease*, vol. 7, no. 3, pp. 258–265, 2003.

[96] R. Basnet, S. G. Hinderaker, D. Enarson, P. Malla, and O. Mørkve, "Delay in the diagnosis of tuberculosis in Nepal," *BMC Public Health*, vol. 9, article 236, 2009.

[97] K. A. Rumman, N. A. Sabra, F. Bakri, A. Seita, and A. Bassili, "Prevalence of tuberculosis suspects and their healthcare-seeking behavior in urban and rural Jordan," *The American Journal of Tropical Medicine and Hygiene*, vol. 79, no. 4, pp. 545–551, 2008.

[98] Y. Wang, Q. Long, Q. Liu, R. Tolhurst, and S. L. Tang, "Treatment seeking for symptoms suggestive of TB: comparison between migrants and permanent urban residents in Chongqing, China," *Tropical Medicine and International Health*, vol. 13, no. 7, pp. 927–933, 2008.

[99] C. T. Chang and A. Esterman, "Diagnostic delay among pulmonary tuberculosis patients in Sarawak, Malaysia: a cross-sectional study," *Rural and Remote Health*, vol. 7, no. 2, p. 667, 2007.

[100] N. T. Huong, M. Vree, B. D. Duong et al., "Delays in the diagnosis and treatment of tuberculosis patients in Vietnam: a cross-sectional study," *BMC Public Health*, vol. 7, article 110, 2007.

[101] T. Wondimu, K. W. Michael, K. Wondwossen, and G. Sofonias, "Delay in initiating tuberculosis treatment and factors associated among pulmonary tuberculosis patients in East Wollega, Western Ethiopia," *Ethiopian Journal of Health Development*, vol. 21, no. 2, pp. 148–156, 2007.

[102] M. Díez, M. J. Bleda, J. Alcaide et al., "Determinants of patient delay among tuberculosis cases in Spain," *European Journal of Public Health*, vol. 14, no. 2, pp. 151–155, 2004.

[103] C. M. Ford, A. M. Bayer, R. H. Gilman et al., "Factors associated with delayed tuberculosis test-seeking behavior in the Peruvian Amazon," *The American Journal of Tropical Medicine and Hygiene*, vol. 81, no. 6, pp. 1097–1102, 2009.

[104] G. Meintjes, H. Schoeman, C. Morroni, D. Wilson, and G. Maartens, "Patient and provider delay in tuberculosis suspects from communities with a high HIV prevalence in South Africa: a cross-sectional study," *BMC Infectious Diseases*, vol. 8, article 72, 2008.

[105] L. Pehme, K. Rahu, M. Rahu, and A. Altraja, "Factors related to patient delay in pulmonary tuberculosis in Estonia," *Scandinavian Journal of Infectious Diseases*, vol. 38, no. 11-12, pp. 1017–1022, 2006.

[106] R. Rajeswari, V. Chandrasekaran, M. Suhadev, S. Sivasubramaniam, G. Sudha, and G. Renu, "Factors associated with patient and health system delays in the diagnosis of tuberculosis in South India," *International Journal of Tuberculosis and Lung Disease*, vol. 6, no. 9, pp. 789–795, 2002.

[107] L. N. Hooi, "Case-finding for pulmonary tuberculosis in Penang," *Medical Journal of Malaysia*, vol. 49, no. 3, pp. 223–230, 1994.

[108] A. A. Gele, G. Bjune, and F. Abebe, "Pastoralism and delay in diagnosis of TB in Ethiopia," *BMC Public Health*, vol. 9, article 5, 2009.

[109] M. M. Mesfin, J. N. Newell, J. D. Walley, A. Gessessew, and R. J. Madeley, "Delayed consultation among pulmonary tuberculosis patients: a cross sectional study of 10 DOTS districts of Ethiopia," *BMC Public Health*, vol. 9, article 53, 2009.

[110] E. S. Ngadaya, G. S. Mfinanga, E. R. Wandwalo, and O. Morkve, "Delay in Tuberculosis case detection in Pwani region, Tanzania. A cross sectional study," *BMC Health Services Research*, vol. 9, article 196, 2009.

[111] S. Yimer, C. Holm-Hansen, T. Yimaldu, and G. Bjune, "Health care seeking among pulmonary tuberculosis suspects and patients in rural Ethiopia: a community-based study," *BMC Public Health*, vol. 9, article 454, 2009.

[112] X. Lin, V. Chongsuvivatwong, A. Geater, and R. Lijuan, "The effect of geographical distance on TB patient delays in a mountainous province of China," *International Journal of Tuberculosis and Lung Disease*, vol. 12, no. 3, pp. 288–293, 2008.

[113] N. Lorent, P. Mugwaneza, J. Mugabekazi et al., "Risk factors for delay in the diagnosis and treatment of tuberculosis at a referral hospital in Rwanda," *International Journal of Tuberculosis and Lung Disease*, vol. 12, no. 4, pp. 392–396, 2008.

[114] F. Maamari, "Case-finding tuberculosis patients: diagnostic and treatment delays and their determinants," *Eastern Mediterranean Health Journal*, vol. 14, no. 3, pp. 531–545, 2008.

[115] J. M. Selvam, F. Wares, M. Perumal et al., "Health-seeking behaviour of new smear-positive TB patients under a DOTS programme in Tamil Nadu, India, 2003," *International Journal of Tuberculosis and Lung Disease*, vol. 11, no. 2, pp. 161–167, 2007.

[116] B. Xu, V. K. Diwan, and L. Bogg, "Access to tuberculosis care: what did chronic cough patients experience in the way of

healthcare-seeking?" *Scandinavian Journal of Public Health*, vol. 35, no. 4, pp. 396–402, 2007.

[117] M. G. Farah, J. H. Rygh, T. W. Steen, R. Selmer, E. Heldal, and G. Bjune, "Patient and health care system delays in the start of tuberculosis treatment in Norway," *BMC Infectious Diseases*, vol. 6, article 33, 2006.

[118] M. Rojpibulstit, J. Kanjanakiritamrong, and V. Chongsuvivatwong, "Patient and health system delays in the diagnosis of tuberculosis in Southern Thailand after health care reform," *International Journal of Tuberculosis and Lung Disease*, vol. 10, no. 4, pp. 422–428, 2006.

[119] M. J. van der Werf, Y. Chechulin, O. B. Yegorova et al., "Health care seeking behaviour for tuberculosis symptoms in Kiev City, Ukraine," *International Journal of Tuberculosis and Lung Disease*, vol. 10, no. 4, pp. 390–395, 2006.

[120] G. Cheng, R. Tolhurst, R. Z. Li, Q. Y. Meng, and S. Tang, "Factors affecting delays in tuberculosis diagnosis in rural China: a case study in four counties in Shandong Province," *Transactions of the Royal Society of Tropical Medicine and Hygiene*, vol. 99, no. 5, pp. 355–362, 2005.

[121] B. Xu, Q. W. Jiang, Y. Xiu, and V. K. Diwan, "Diagnostic delays in access to tuberculosis care in counties with or without the national tuberculosis control programme in rural China," *International Journal of Tuberculosis and Lung Disease*, vol. 9, no. 7, pp. 784–790, 2005.

[122] S. Yimer, G. Bjune, and G. Alene, "Diagnostic and treatment delay among pulmonary tuberculosis patients in Ethiopia: a cross sectional study," *BMC Infectious Diseases*, vol. 5, article 112, 2005.

[123] O. O. Odusanya and J. O. Babafemi, "Patterns of delays amongst pulmonary tuberculosis patients in Lagos, Nigeria," *BMC Public Health*, vol. 4, article 18, 2004.

[124] S. Paynter, A. Hayward, P. Wilkinson, S. Lozewicz, and R. Coker, "Patient and health service delays in initiating treatment for patients with pulmonary tuberculosis: retrospective cohort study," *International Journal of Tuberculosis and Lung Disease*, vol. 8, no. 2, pp. 180–185, 2004.

[125] G. Sudha, C. Nirupa, M. Rajasakthivel et al., "Factors influencing the care-seeking behaviour of chest symptomatics: a community-based study involving rural and urban population in Tamil Nadu, South India," *Tropical Medicine and International Health*, vol. 8, no. 4, pp. 336–341, 2003.

[126] M. Demissie, B. Lindtjorn, and Y. Berhane, "Patient and health service delay in the diagnosis of pulmonary tuberculosis in Ethiopia," *BMC Public Health*, vol. 2, no. 1, p. 23, 2002.

[127] V. K. Dhingra, S. Rajpal, D. K. Taneja, D. Kalra, and R. Malhotra, "Health care seeking pattern of tuberculosis patients attending an urban TB clinic in Delhi," *Journal of Communicable Diseases*, vol. 34, no. 3, pp. 185–192, 2002.

[128] P. M. Pronyk, M. B. Makhubele, J. R. Hargreaves, S. M. Tollman, and H. P. Hausler, "Assessing health seeking behaviour among tuberculosis patients in rural South Africa," *International Journal of Tuberculosis and Lung Disease*, vol. 5, no. 7, pp. 619–627, 2001.

[129] E. R. Wandwalo and O. Mørkve, "Delay in tuberculosis case-finding and treatment in Mwanza, Tanzania," *International Journal of Tuberculosis and Lung Disease*, vol. 4, no. 2, pp. 133–138, 2000.

[130] S. Asch, B. Leake, R. Anderson, and L. Gelberg, "Why do symptomatic patients delay obtaining care for tuberculosis?" *The American Journal of Respiratory and Critical Care Medicine*, vol. 157, no. 4, pp. 1244–1248, 1998.

[131] S. D. Lawn, B. Afful, and J. W. Acheampong, "Pulmonary tuberculosis: diagnostic delay in Ghanaian adults," *International Journal of Tuberculosis and Lung Disease*, vol. 2, no. 8, pp. 635–640, 1998.

[132] S. Enkhbat, M. Toyota, N. Yasuda, and H. Ohara, "Differing influence on delays in the case-finding process for tuberculosis between general physicians and specialists in mongolia," *Journal of Epidemiology*, vol. 7, no. 2, pp. 93–98, 1997.

[133] T. Mori, T. Shimao, B. W. Jin, and S. J. Kim, "Analysis of case-finding process of tuberculosis in Korea," *Tubercle and Lung Disease*, vol. 73, no. 4, pp. 225–231, 1992.

[134] F. Yan, R. Thomson, S. L. Tang et al., "Multiple perspectives on diagnosis delay for tuberculosis from key stakeholders in poor rural China: case study in four provinces," *Health Policy*, vol. 82, no. 2, pp. 186–199, 2007.

[135] M. Díez, M. J. Bleda, J. Alcaide et al., "Determinants of health system delay among confirmed tuberculosis cases in Spain," *European Journal of Public Health*, vol. 15, no. 4, pp. 343–349, 2005.

[136] N. H. Long, V. K. Diwan, and A. Winkvist, "Difference in symptoms suggesting pulmonary tuberculosis among men and women," *Journal of Clinical Epidemiology*, vol. 55, no. 2, pp. 115–120, 2002.

[137] T. L. Creek, S. Lockman, T. A. Kenyon et al., "Completeness and timeliness of treatment initiation after laboratory diagnosis of tuberculosis in Gaborone, Botswana," *International Journal of Tuberculosis and Lung Disease*, vol. 4, no. 10, pp. 956–961, 2000.

[138] L. Pehme, K. Rahu, M. Rahu, and A. Altraja, "Factors related to health system delays in the diagnosis of pulmonary tuberculosis in Estonia," *International Journal of Tuberculosis and Lung Disease*, vol. 11, no. 3, pp. 275–281, 2007.

[139] L. F. Sherman, P. I. Fujiwara, S. V. Cook, L. B. Bazerman, and T. R. Frieden, "Patient and health care system delays in the diagnosis and treatment of tuberculosis," *International Journal of Tuberculosis and Lung Disease*, vol. 3, no. 12, pp. 1088–1095, 1999.

[140] C. E. French, M. E. Kruijshaar, J. A. Jones, and I. Abubakar, "The influence of socio-economic deprivation on tuberculosis treatment delays in England, 2000–2005," *Epidemiology and Infection*, vol. 137, no. 4, pp. 591–596, 2009.

[141] A. Bassili, A. Seita, S. Baghdadi et al., "Diagnostic and treatment delay in tuberculosis in 7 countries of the Eastern Mediterranean Region," *Infectious Diseases in Clinical Practice*, vol. 16, no. 1, pp. 23–35, 2008.

[142] G. D. Gosoniu, S. Ganapathy, J. Kemp et al., "Gender and socio-cultural determinants of delay to diagnosis of TB in Bangladesh, India and Malawi," *International Journal of Tuberculosis and Lung Disease*, vol. 12, no. 7, pp. 848–855, 2008.

[143] D. M. Needham, S. D. Foster, G. Tomlinson, and P. Godfrey-Faussett, "Socio-economic, gender and health services factors affecting diagnostic delay for tuberculosis patients in urban Zambia," *Tropical Medicine and International Health*, vol. 6, no. 4, pp. 256–259, 2001.

[144] Y. Mahendradhata, B. M. Syahrizal, and A. Utarini, "Delayed treatment of tuberculosis patients in rural areas of Yogyakarta province, Indonesia," *BMC Public Health*, vol. 8, article 393, 2008.

[145] S. Saly, I. Onozaki, and N. Ishikawa, "Decentralized dots shortens delay to TB treatment significantly in Cambodia," *Kekkaku*, vol. 81, no. 7, pp. 467–474, 2006.

[146] K. Sarmiento, Y. Hirsch-Moverman, P. W. Colson, and W. El-Sadr, "Help-seeking behavior of marginalized groups: a study

of TB patients in Harlem, New York," *International Journal of Tuberculosis and Lung Disease*, vol. 10, no. 10, pp. 1140–1145, 2006.

[147] M. A. P. S. dos Santos, M. F. P. M. Albuquerque, R. A. A. Ximenes et al., "Risk factors for treatment delay in pulmonary tuberculosis in Recife, Brazil," *BMC Public Health*, vol. 5, article 25, 2005.

[148] J. P. Vandenbroucke, E. von Elm, D. G. Altman et al., "Strengthening the reporting of observational studies in epidemiology (STROBE): explanation and elaboration," *PLoS Medicine*, vol. 4, no. 10, pp. 1628–1654, 2007.

[149] M. K. Campbell, D. R. Elbourne, and D. G. Altman, "CONSORT statement: extension to cluster randomised trials," *The British Medical Journal*, vol. 328, no. 7441, pp. 702–708, 2004.

[150] M. Zwarenstein, S. Treweek, J. J. Gagnier et al., "Improving the reporting of pragmatic trials: an extension of the CONSORT statement," *The British Medical Journal*, vol. 337, Article ID a2390, 2008.

[151] D. Somma, B. E. Thomas, F. Karim et al., "Gender and sociocultural determinants of TB-related stigma in Bangladesh, India, Malawi and Colombia," *International Journal of Tuberculosis and Lung Disease*, vol. 12, no. 7, pp. 856–866, 2008.

[152] E. L. Corbett, T. Bandason, T. Duong et al., "Comparison of two active case-finding strategies for community-based diagnosis of symptomatic smear-positive tuberculosis and control of infectious tuberculosis in Harare, Zimbabwe (DETECTB): a cluster-randomised trial," *The Lancet*, vol. 376, no. 9748, pp. 1244–1253, 2010.

[153] A. C. Miller, J. E. Golub, S. C. Cavalcante et al., "Controlled trial of active tuberculosis case finding in a Brazilian favela," *International Journal of Tuberculosis and Lung Disease*, vol. 14, no. 6, pp. 720–726, 2010.

[154] D. M. Tuller, D. R. Bangsberg, J. Senkungu, N. C. Ware, N. Emenyonu, and S. D. Weiser, "Transportation costs impede sustained adherence and access to HAART in a clinic population in Southwestern Uganda: a qualitative study," *AIDS and Behavior*, vol. 14, no. 4, pp. 778–784, 2010.

[155] A. P. Hardon, D. Akurut, C. Comoro et al., "Hunger, waiting time and transport costs. time to confront challenges to ART adherence in Africa," *AIDS Care—Psychological and Socio-Medical Aspects of AIDS/HIV*, vol. 19, no. 5, pp. 658–665, 2007.

[156] M. Lubega, X. Nsabagasani, N. M. Tumwesigye et al., "Policy and practice, lost in transition: reasons for high drop-out from pre-antiretroviral care in a resource-poor setting of Eastern Uganda," *Health Policy*, vol. 95, no. 2-3, pp. 153–158, 2010.

[157] R. Levine, A. Glassman, and M. Schneidman, *La Salud de la Mujer en América Latina y el Caribe*, Inter-American Development Bank, Washington, DC, USA, 2001.

[158] S. S. Gopalan and V. Durairaj, "Addressing women's non-maternal healthcare financing in developing countries: what can we learn from the experiences of rural indian women?" *PLoS ONE*, vol. 7, no. 1, Article ID e29936, 2012.

[159] I. M. Kigozi, L. M. Dobkin, J. N. Martin et al., "Late-disease stage at presentation to an HIV clinic in the era of free antiretroviral therapy in Sub-Saharan Africa," *Journal of Acquired Immune Deficiency Syndromes*, vol. 52, no. 2, pp. 280–289, 2009.

[160] M. Charurat, M. Oyegunle, R. Benjamin et al., "Patient retention and adherence to antiretrovirals in a large antiretroviral therapy program in Nigeria: a longitudinal analysis for risk factors," *PLoS ONE*, vol. 5, no. 5, Article ID e10584, 2010.

[161] M. Chileshe and V. A. Bond, "Barriers and outcomes: TB patients co-infected with HIV accessing antiretroviral therapy in rural Zambia," *AIDS Care—Psychological and Socio-Medical Aspects of AIDS/HIV*, vol. 22, supplement 1, pp. 51–59, 2010.

[162] C. Jasseron, L. Mandelbrot, C. Dollfus et al., "Non-disclosure of a pregnant woman's HIV status to her partner is associated with non-optimal prevention of mother-to-child transmission," *AIDS and Behavior*, vol. 17, no. 2, pp. 488–497, 2013.

[163] J. Ostermann, E. A. Reddy, M. M. Shorter et al., "Who tests, who doesn't, and why? Uptake of mobile HIV counseling and testing in the kilimanjaro region of Tanzania," *PLoS ONE*, vol. 6, no. 1, Article ID e16488, 2011.

[164] S. V. Eastwood and P. C. Hill, "A gender-focused qualitative study of barriers to accessing tuberculosis treatment in the Gambia, West Africa," *International Journal of Tuberculosis and Lung Disease*, vol. 8, no. 1, pp. 70–75, 2004.

[165] R. Liefooghe, N. Michiels, S. Habib, M. B. Moran, and A. de Muynck, "Perception and social consequences of tuberculosis: a focus group study of tuberculosis patients in Sialkot, Pakistan," *Social Science and Medicine*, vol. 41, no. 12, pp. 1685–1692, 1995.

[166] R. Liefooghe, J. B. Baliddawa, E. M. Kipruto, C. Vermeire, and A. O. de Munynck, "From their own perspective. A Kenyan community's perception of tuberculosis," *Tropical Medicine and International Health*, vol. 2, no. 8, pp. 809–821, 1997.

[167] A. Daftary, "HIV and tuberculosis: the construction and management of double stigma," *Social Science and Medicine*, vol. 74, no. 10, pp. 1512–1519, 2012.

[168] S. McTavish, S. Moore, S. Harper, and J. Lynch, "National female literacy, individual socio-economic status, and maternal health care use in sub-Saharan Africa," *Social Science and Medicine*, vol. 71, no. 11, pp. 1958–1963, 2010.

[169] P. K. Nirmalan, A. Padmavathi, and R. D. Thulasiraj, "Sex inequalities in cataract blindness burden and surgical services in south India," *The British Journal of Ophthalmology*, vol. 87, no. 7, pp. 847–849, 2003.

[170] L. Gilson, J. Doherty, R. Loewenson, and V. Francis, *Challenging Inequity Through Health Systems*, WHO Commission on the Social Determinants of Health, 2007.

[171] G. Sen, P. Östlin, and A. George, *Unequal, Unfair, Ineffective and Inefficient-Gender Inequlty in Health: Why It Exists and How We Can Change It*, WHO Commission on Social Determinants of Health, 2007.

[172] V. K. Diwan and A. Thorson, "Sex, gender, and tuberculosis," *The Lancet*, vol. 353, no. 9157, pp. 1000–1001, 1999.

[173] H. Getahun, D. Sculier, C. Sismanidis, M. Grzemska, and M. Raviglione, "Prevention, diagnosis, and treatment of tuberculosis in children and mothers: evidence for action for maternal, neonatal, and child health services," *Journal of Infectious Diseases*, vol. 205, supplement 2, pp. S216–S227, 2012.

[174] L. Nieuwenhoven and I. Klinge, "Scientific excellence in applying sex- and gender-sensitive methods in biomedical and health research," *Journal of Women's Health*, vol. 19, no. 2, pp. 313–321, 2010.

[175] "Taking sex into account in medicine," *The Lancet*, vol. 378, no. 9806, p. 1826, 2011.

[176] "Manifesto for integrated action on the gender dimension in research and innovation," http://www.gender-summit.eu/index .php?option=com_content&view=article&id=278&Itemid=42.

[177] Gendered Innovations in Science, Health & Medicine, and Engineering, 2011, http://genderedinnovations.eu.

[178] WHO, *Strategy for Integrating Gender Analysis and Actions into the Work of WHO*, WHO, 2009.

3

Tuberculosis Is Not a Risk Factor for Primary Biliary Cirrhosis: A Review of the Literature

Daniel S. Smyk,[1] Dimitrios P. Bogdanos,[1, 2, 3] Albert Pares,[4] Christos Liaskos,[2] Charalambos Billinis,[5] Andrew K. Burroughs,[6] and Eirini I. Rigopoulou[3]

[1] Institute of Liver Studies, King's College Hospital and Division of Transplantation Immunology and Mucosal Biology, School of Medicine, King's College London, London SE5 9RS, UK
[2] Cellular Immunotherapy and Molecular Immunodiagnostics, Center for Research and Technology Thessaly, 41222 Larissa, Greece
[3] Department of Medicine, University Hospital of Larissa, University of Thessaly School of Medicine, 41110 Larissa, Greece
[4] Liver Unit, Hospital Clínic de Barcelona, IDIBAPS, CIBERehd, University of Barcelona, 08036 Barcelona, Spain
[5] Faculty of Veterinary Science, University of Thessaly, 43100 Karditsa, Greece
[6] The Royal Free Sheila Sherlock Liver Centre, Royal Free Hospital and Department of Surgery, University Collegue London, London NW32QG, UK

Correspondence should be addressed to Dimitrios P. Bogdanos, dimitrios.bogdanos@kcl.ac.uk

Academic Editor: Juraj Ivanyi

Primary biliary cirrhosis (PBC) is a progressive cholestatic liver disease characterised serologically by cholestasis and the presence of high-titre antimitochondrial antibodies, and histologically by chronic nonsuppurative cholangitis and granulomata. As PBC is a granulomatous disease and *Mycobacterium tuberculosis* is the most frequent cause of granulomata, a causal relation between tuberculosis and PBC has been suggested. Attempts to find serological evidence of PBC-specific autoantibodies such as AMA have been made and, conversely, granulomatous livers from patients with PBC have been investigated for molecular evidence of *Mycobacterium tuberculosis*. This paper discusses in detail the reported data in support or against an association between *Mycobacterium tuberculosis* infection and PBC. We discuss the immunological and microbiological data exploring the association of PBC with exposure to *Mycobacterium tuberculosis*. We also discuss the findings of large epidemiologic studies investigating the association of PBC with preexistent or concomitant disorders and the relevance of these findings with tuberculosis. Genome-wide association studies in patients with tuberculosis as well as in patients with PBC provide conclusive hints regarding the assumed association between exposure to this mycobacterium and the induction of PBC. Analysis of these data suggest that *Mycobacterium tuberculosis* is an unlikely infectious trigger of PBC.

1. Introduction

Primary biliary cirrhosis (PBC) is a chronic cholestatic, autoimmune liver disease characterised by progressive inflammatory destruction of the small and medium intrahepatic bile ducts and subsequent fibrosis, cirrhosis [1–5], and eventually liver failure [6, 7]. The disease predominantly affects middle-aged women and is practically absent in children or youngsters [8–11]. PBC affects more than one member within the same family, and several reports indicate that first degree relatives of PBC patients have an increased risk of developing the disease [12, 13]. The prevalence of the disease varies among countries, with a recent systematic review indicating prevalence to be 1.91–40.2 per 100,000 inhabitants, and the incidence to be 0.33–5.8 per 100,000 inhabitants/year, in European and North American cohorts (although a breakdown of ethnicity was not provided) [14]. There is a consensus, however, that despite the heterogeneity in the estimated prevalence and incidence amongst ethnic groups, the incidence and prevalence of PBC is increasing [14–18]. The reasons for this increase are poorly understood. Whether there is a true increase or it is due to the awareness for the disease amongst clinicians and the meticulous diagnostic assessment, such a disease-specific autoantibody testing remains to be seen.

Several autoantibody profiles have been found to be specific for the disease [19] and aid in the diagnostic workup of PBC. These include antimitochondrial antibodies (AMA) [20–24] and/or disease-specific antinuclear antibody (ANA) [25–27], which are found in both symptomatic and asymptomatic patients [28]. Most common symptoms at presentation are nonspecific and include fatigue, pruritus, Sicca symptomatology, and arthralgias. Autoimmune rheumatic diseases such as Sjögren's syndrome and systemic sclerosis, as well as other extrahepatic autoimmune manifestations such as autoimmune thyroiditis frequently coexist with PBC [2, 29, 30]. In more severe cases, symptoms relate to portal hypertension and hepatic decompensation (jaundice, ascites, or variceal bleeding), which may indicate the need for liver transplantation [2, 5, 31]. The progression of PBC is generally slow in the majority of the cases [6, 31].

The widely accepted diagnostic criteria of PBC consists of three components: (1) biochemical evidence of cholestasis in the form of elevated levels of alkaline phosphatase (ALP) and γGT, (2) seropositivity for disease-specific antimitochondrial antibodies, and (3) histological features on liver biopsy compatible with or diagnostic of PBC [2]. The diagnosis of PBC is probable when at least two of these criteria are met [2, 4]. Most cases have elevated levels of immunoglobulin M (IgM) [2, 4, 32].

The diagnostic hallmark of PBC is the presence of high-titre AMA mainly targeting the E2 subunits of the oxo-acid dehydrogenase complexes (OADC), and in particular that of pyruvate dehydrogenase complex (PDC-E2) [21, 24, 28, 33]. Only 3–10% of patients with PBC lack these antibodies and are considered true AMA-negative PBC patients [28, 34–37]. These autoantibodies are practically nonexistent in patients with other liver diseases unrelated to PBC [38, 39]. Also, true AMA seropositivity in patients with autoimmune rheumatic diseases indicates the current or future development of PBC [23, 40]. Prospective studies have shown that the presence of AMA predicts the future development of PBC in asymptomatic, cholestatic, or acholestatic individuals [22, 41]. ANA specific for the disease can also be present in approximately 50% of patients [42–44]. Published data support the notion that PBC-specific ANA reactivities may have prognostic significance [27, 44–47]. Various other autoantibody specificities have been reported in patients with PBC [48–51].

The most prominent histological features of PBC include chronic nonsuppurative cholangitis with or without granulomata demonstrating destruction of biliary epithelial cells and loss of small bile ducts with portal inflammatory cell infiltration (see below) [2, 4, 5]. Genetic factors and environmental triggers have been considered important for the induction of autoimmune disease, such as PBC [8, 52–57]. Several infectious and noninfectious triggers have been implicated in the pathogenesis of PBC [8, 12, 52, 55, 58–64].

Because *Mycobacterium tuberculosis* (*M. tuberculosis*) [65] is the most frequent cause of granulomas [66], and

in view of reports indicating serological evidence of PBC-specific AMA in patients with tuberculosis, it has been suggested that tuberculosis/*M. tuberculosis* may be a cause of PBC (Table 1). Indeed, *M. tuberculosis* has been indicated as a potential cause of other autoimmune disease such as systemic lupus erythematosus (SLE) [67–74]. This paper will critically analyse the epidemiological, clinical, immunological, and experimental data in support or against the notion that tuberculosis and PBC may be pathogenetically linked.

2. Granulomas in PBC

Up to 15% of liver biopsy material contains evidence of granulomas [82–86]. An analysis of 12,161 liver biopsies revealed the presence of granulomas in 442 (3.6%) [87] cases, including 215 diagnosed with PBC, representing 48.7% of all biopsies with granulomas and 1.8% of all biopsies analysed [87]. Molecular evidence of infectious agents by PCR was found in just 15 samples (3.4%) and *M. tuberculosis* has been detected in three of the 15 (20%) but it is not clear whether the *M. tuberculosis*-positive cases were from livers of patients with PBC [87]. The fact that three or less of the 215 granulomatous livers from PBC cases had molecular evidence of *M. tuberculosis* argues against the notion that this mycobacterium is a trigger for the development of this enigmatic disease. Other studies have also noted and reported a diagnosis of PBC in 24–62% of livers with evidence of granulomas [82, 83, 88]. However, only a small proportion of the PBC granulomata had evidence of mycobacteria, again pointing towards the lack of an association of *M. tuberculosis* with PBC.

Irrespective of the relation of PBC granulomas with *M. tuberculosis* infections, attempts have been made by researchers to delineate the role of immunity in the development of PBC granulomas. A recent comprehensive immuno-histochemical analysis by You et al. [89] has shown that CD11c, the classical dendritic cell marker, is highly expressed in PBC granulomas. It also appears that CD11c-positive epitheliod granulomas are more prevalent in patients with PBC at early disease stages. Finally, the expression of CD11c in PBC granulomas is associated with higher IgM levels. These findings further support the notion that the influence of antigenic stimulation to professional antigen presenting cells largely influences the formation of granulomas in PBC. You et al. [89] suggested that PBC liver granulomas may result from the interaction between immature dendritic cells and IgM, but this needs to be addressed at the experimental level. On the other hand, in human tuberculosis the formation of granulomas is considered either as an attempt to contain *M. tuberculosis* infection or an early effort by the pathogenic mycobacteria to assist the spreading of bacteria to uninfected macrophages that are recruited at the site of inflammation [66, 90]. This perception raises the notion that granulomas in human tuberculosis may have a beneficial or catastrophic potential for the host depending on the timing of their formation [91, 92].

2.1. Evidence of Mycobacterial Infection in PBC. Tanaka et al. searched for evidence of infectious agents by PCR in livers

TABLE 1: Summary of the major findings of studies investigating the role of *Mycobacterium tuberculosis* as a trigger of PBC. The findings are presented in relation to Koch's postulates. To date, no conclusive evidence has been presented which links *Mycobacterium tuberculosis* with PBC.

Koch's postulates	Finding	Study
Infectious aetiology Microorganism must be present in every case of diseased individuals	Positive staining for mycobacterial hsp65 in PBC cases has been demonstrated, but hsp65 is conserved among all mycobacterial species and it is unclear whether this staining is *Mycobacterium tuberculosis*-specific and characteristic for PBC patients with granulomata	[75]
Isolation The microorganism must be isolated and grown in pure cultures	No such data exist	
Disease causality Pure cultures inoculated in healthy animals must reproduce the disease	No such data exist Only one case report of a female that developed PBC following tuberculosis infection has been published There is no epidemiological or evidence linking tuberculosis with PBC, including vaccination against tuberculosis	[76] [77–80]
Reproducibility The microorganism must be recovered from the diseased animal	No such data exist	
Other data indirectly relevant to Koch's postulates	PBC specific AMA was detected in 43% of tuberculosis patients, but in low titres, and did not show the typical indirect immunofluorescent patterns of antimitochondrial antibodies seen in PBC. These patients do not have clinical features of PBC.	[19, 21, 22, 81]

tissues from 29 patients with PBC. Mycobacterial DNA was not detected in any of these samples [93]. Other attempts to provide evidence of mycobacteria DNA in livers from PBC cases have provided inconclusive data. Broome et al. [75] demonstrated positive staining for mycobacterial hsp65 using a monoclonal antibodies in nine of the ten PBC cases [75]. O'Donohue and colleagues [94] studied liver biopsy specimen from eleven PBC cases. Five lymph nodes from patients with tuberculous lymphadenopathy were used as positive controls [94]. Three of the positive controls also had liver biopsies taken for concurrent tuberculous hepatitis. Four of the five positive controls had detectable mycobacterial DNA. Mycobacterial DNA was undetectable in the tissues obtained from patients with PBC [94].

2.2. PBC-Specific Autoantibodies in Patients with Tuberculosis.
An early study by Klein et al. [81] reported the presence of PBC-specific AMA in 12/28 (43%) of patients with tuberculosis. Immunoblotting demonstrated that these sera recognized PDC-E2 based on purified mitochondrial fraction derived from beef heart mitochondrial as an antigenic source. Only 2% of sera from individuals with other viral and bacterial infections showed reactivity with PDC-E2, and there was no reaction with sera from healthy controls [81]. As well, the titres of anti-PDC-E2 antibodies were low [81]. Additionally, none of the anti-PDC-E2 antibody positive sera (1/10 dilution) gave an immunofluorescent pattern typical of PBC by indirect immunofluorescence [19, 21, 22, 81]. This contrasts to what is normally seen in most patients with PBC, where titers of PDC-E2 targeting AMA give typical and strong immunofluorescent staining at dilutions as high as 1/100,000. Amongst the 12 AMA positive cases

with active tuberculosis, six had abnormal levels of γGT and four had elevated levels of alkaline phosphatase, with only two of the twelve cases having increased IgM levels. None of the patients had increased bilirubin levels or evidence of impaired synthetic function. Liver biopsies were not performed and it is not known what has happen to these individuals over the years, and whether they have developed clinically overt liver disease. There was no information as to whether other causes of abnormal liver biochemistry such as drug-induced hepatotoxicity were excluded.

Patients with *M. tuberculosis* and AMA positivity show reactivity to PDC-E2, which has not been observed in those infected with other forms of mycobacteria [81, 95]. Gilburd et al. [95] suggested sequence homology between *M. leprae* antigens and the 35, 41, and 54 kDa subunits of OADC, implying that molecular mimicry and immunological cross-reactivity between *M. leprae* and human mitochondrial autoantigens may be responsible for the induction of AMA in patients with leprosy.

2.3. Mycobacteria and PBC: The Role of Molecular Mimicry.
It is unclear as to whether a negative result for *M. tuberculosis* also rules out the effects of a previous and nonactive infection. It has been suggested that mycobacteria and other infectious agents may be involved in the initiation of autoimmunity by microbial/self-immunological cross-reactivity, where infection and clearance of the infection occur before the onset of clinical disease [96–100]. The role of molecular mimicry has been studied by several groups [96, 101–107] and immunological cross-reactivity has been documented [108–113] as a mechanism responsible for the induction of autoantigen-specific immune responses in

microbial-triggered autoimmunity [107, 114–117] in susceptible individuals [118, 119]. Impairment in the immunosuppressory functions of the host appears to be important for the induction and perpetuation of autoaggression induced via molecular mimicry or other mechanisms [120, 121]. Indeed, our group has studied molecular mimicry as a potential inducer of autoimmunity in several autoimmune liver and gastrointestinal diseases [97, 104, 110, 122, 123]. Most of the microbial/self-homologues are not targets of cross-reactive responses, and this underlines the importance of disease-specific pairs targeted by antibodies [99, 100, 111, 113, 124, 125]. Of relevance to mycobacteria, Vilagut et al. [126] has reported that hsp65 kDa *M. gordonae* and human OADC antigens, including human PDC-E2, are cross-reactive [127]. They also reported the presence of mycobacterial DNA in livers from patients with PBC. We have attempted to better define the extent of this cross-reactivity at the peptidyl level and through amino-acid comparison database searches, and we have identified an amino-acid homology between human PDC-E2, and mycobacterial hsp65 [124]. Thus, the hexameric motif [GDL(IL)AE)] is present in hsp65$_{94-99}$ and the major PBC-specific mitochondrial autoepitopes, namely, the inner lipoyl PDC-E2$_{216-221}$ and the outer lipoyl domain human PDC-E2$_{102-107}$ [124]. The hsp65 mimic was not restricted to *M. gordonae*, but was conserved amongst mycobacteria (including *M. tuberculosis*). The SxGDL[IL]AE motif is virtually unique to mycobacterial hsp, and human PDC-E2 is the only known human sequence containing it [124]. We also obtained data to suggest that peptides spanning the homologous mycobacterial hsp65 and human PDC-E2 sequences are targets of cross-reactive responses when serum samples from patients with PBC are tested. These data support the notion that mycobacterial infection could initiate antimycobacterial responses against hsp65, which in turn could cross-react with human PDC-E2. The relevance of the biological significance of these data in the immunopathogenesis of microbial-induced PBC remains unaddressed.

If there is a link between tuberculosis and PBC, it would be expected that areas where *M. tuberculosis* is endemic would have high rates of PBC, but this is not the case. For example, southern Africa is endemic for tuberculosis, but PBC is relatively rare in those regions [128, 129]. The same could be said for India and China, which have relatively high rates of tuberculosis but low rates of PBC [130–132]. Also, epidemiological studies assessing susceptibility to PBC would be expected to identify tuberculosis as a risk factor.

3. Risk Factors of PBC: Epidemiological Studies

Several epidemiological studies have been conducted to investigate risk factors for the development of PBC [77–80]. These studies have largely been based on questionnaires addressing geographical and lifestyle factors, as well as personal and familial medical and surgical histories. However, very few of these studies specifically mention infection with *M. tuberculosis*. A study by Parikh-Patel and colleagues

[79] administered a standardized US National Health and Nutrition Examination Study (NHANES) questionnaire to 241 PBC patients from the USA, in addition to 261 of their siblings and 141 friends as controls. Within the medical histories, it was found that 2 patients with PBC (1.2%) reported having tuberculosis as adults, compared to none of the siblings, and one friend (0.8%) [79]. A larger study conducted by Gershwin et al. [78] was also based on an NHANES questionnaire. The cohort in that study consisted of 1032 PBC patients from 23 tertiary care centres in the USA, 1041 controls selected from a random-digit-dialling protocol, which were sex, age, race, and geographically matched. All participants were administered the questionnaire by trained professionals, but it was not indicated as to whether specific questions were asked regarding tuberculosis [78]. However, it appears that questions were raised as to whether participants had been vaccinated for tuberculosis [78]. Despite this, it does not appear that any significant link was found in regards to tuberculosis and/or tuberculosis infection [78]. Prince et al. [80] conducted an epidemiological study involving 318 PBC patients from an epidemiological study and 2258 from a PBC support group, in addition to 2438 controls. There was no indication as to whether specific questions were raised in regards to tuberculosis [80]. Corpechot and colleagues [77] administered a standardized questionnaire to 222 PBC patients and 509 age, sex, and residentially matched controls [77]. Although no history of previous tuberculosis infection was indicated, it appears that questions regarding immunization for tuberculosis were asked, as 1% of PBC cases reported vaccination, although 1% of controls also reported vaccination [77]. Based on the epidemiological evidence, it does not appear that infection with *M. tuberculosis* is linked with PBC. However, it should also be noted that it is not clear as to whether history of tuberculosis infection and/or vaccination was investigated in some studies. In those which do, there was no significantly higher incidence of PBC infection among patients compared to controls, and there was no significantly higher incidence of vaccination against tuberculosis in PBC patients. An association between vaccination and the development of PBC has been reported for other microbial agents, and in particular Lactobacilli, and the mechanism of molecular mimicry has been proposed to account for the induction of PBC-specific autoreactivity [97, 98].

4. Case Studies of PBC and Tuberculosis

A PubMed search for case reports in of patients with tuberculosis who developed PBC (search terms: "primary biliary cirrhosis, tuberculosis" and "primary biliary cirrhosis, *mycobacterium tuberculosis*") revealed one case [76]. That case reports of a 70-year-old Tunisian patient who developed antimitochondrial antibodies and anti-ADN during urogenital tuberculosis. There were clinical and biological signs of primary biliary cirrhosis and systemic lupus erythematosus in that patient [76]. If there was a link between tuberculosis and PBC, it would be expected that several case reports of patients developing PBC, or AMA positivity following infection with *M. tuberculosis*.

5. Genome-Wide Association Studies in Tuberculosis and in PBC

Genome-wide association studies (GWAS) have recently shed light on the genetic background of PBC and pulmonary tuberculosis. Genes implicated in PBC lay within both HLA and non-HLA regions (Table 2) [133–140]. GWAS have led to the identification of several genes that infer susceptibility to developing active pulmonary tuberculosis l [141, 142] including JAG1, DYNLRB2, EBF1, TMEFF2, CCL17, HAUS6, PENK, and TXNDC4. If tuberculosis is a risk factor for the development of PBC, it would be reasonable to infer that both conditions would share several susceptibility genes [143]. However, no significant overlapping of genes conferring susceptibility to both PBC and tuberculosis has been identified (Table 2). Also depending on the geographical region, environmental exposures related to tuberculosis may differ, as well as strong associations between different evolutionary lineages of *Mycobacterium tuberculosis* with specific geographical regions have been noted [144]. Such differences have been extensively studied in tuberculosis patients, such as those originating from Indonesian patients living in Jakarta and Bandung compared to other regions/islands. The extent by which genetic co-evolution and phylogenetic difference involving *M. tuberculosis* participate in the dysregulation of host's immune response is worthy for further investigation.

6. Tuberculosis in Other Autoimmune Diseases

PBC is not the only autoimmune disease in which *M. tuberculosis* has been implicated. *M. Tuberculosis* has also been noted to be involved in a more common autoimmune disease, SLE, and specifically to disease flares. An early study by Shoenfeld and colleagues [73] examined whether murine monoclonal anti-TB antibodies reacted with ssDNA, dsDNA, and other polynucleotides and found that monoclonal anti-DNA autoantibodies from humans and mouse SLE models bound to three glycolipids shared among mycobacteria. Incubation of the antibodies with ssDNA and/or polynucleotides or glycolipid antigens was found to inhibit binding [73]. This suggests a possible explanation for the production of autoantibodies in mycobacterial infections. Sela and colleagues [145] examined the sera from 57 patients with untreated TB for the anti-DNA idiotype 16/6 and found that 60% had increased levels of the idiotype compared to 4% of controls. As well, there were also increased levels of autoantibodies such as those to ssDNA, dsDNA, polynucleotides, and cardiolipin [145]. A study by Amital-Teplizki et al. [67] examined the binding of human lupus anti-DNA antibodies and murine antimycobacterial antibodies to human cortical brain tissue. That group found that antimycobacterial and anti-DNA antibodies competed on the binding site of a common neuronal membrane

TABLE 2: Major susceptibility genes associated with tuberculosis [141, 142] and primary biliary cirrhosis [133–140], as reported through genome wide association studies. Note that no positive associations are significantly shared between primary biliary cirrhosis (PBC) and pulmonary tuberculosis (TB).

Gene	PBC	TB
HLA		
DR8	+	−
DQB1	+	−
DRB1	+	−
DQA1	+	−
DQA2	+	−
Non-HLA		
STAT4	+	−
SPIB	+	−
IRF5	+	−
IL12A	+	−
IL12RB	+	−
MMEL1	+	−
CXCR5	+	−
NFKB1	+	−
JAG1	−	+
DYNLRB2	−	+
EBF1	−	+
TMEFF2	−	+
CCL17	−	+
HAUS6	−	+
PENK	−	+
TXNDC4	−	+

epitope, indicating the presence of a shared antigen between mycobacteria and DNA [67].

In addition to the above molecular findings, a link between SLE flares and TB have also been noted. Ribeiro and colleagues [74] describe the development of TB infection in parallel with lupus flares in four females. The site of mycobacterial infection/detection in the women included a positive urine culture for mycobacterial spp., a nodular pulmonary lesion with subsequent positive tuberculin cutaneous test, a positive acid-fact bacilli test on bronchoalveolar lavage, and one case of disseminated TB [74]. In all four women, SLE flares did not improve on administration of antirheumatic treatment and immunosuppression but did improve after the administration of antituberculosis treatment [74]. Those authors suggest that *M. tuberculosis* stimulated the production of autoantibodies with shared affinity for mycobacterial and human antigens, which in turn may have led to the SLE flare [74]. These cases indicate a possible link between SLE and TB, but it should also be noted that the immunosuppressive treatment given to SLE patients may in fact reactivate a latent TB infection.

7. Conclusion

The study of the role of *Mycobacterium tuberculosis* in PBC has been limited due to the scarcity of studies and data.

Multiple epidemiological studies have failed to indicate tuberculosis as a risk factor for the development of PBC, and there is an absence of case reports of tuberculosis infection followed by PBC in the literature. It would be expected that if *M. tuberculosis* was linked with PBC, there would be a higher incidence of PBC in areas which are endemic for tuberculosis. However, this does not appear to be the case [146]. It would also be expected that if *M. tuberculosis* was linked to PBC, several genes which predispose to one disease, would overlap with the other. However, with the advent of GWAS, this link has also been ruled out, with no genes being shared between the two conditions. Although more studies are needed to investigate a potential link, the existent data are highly suggestive of a lack of a causative link between tuberculosis and PBC. However, the observation of granulomatous lesion in PBC liver biopsies warrants further investigation, as the significance of these lesions in the liver of PBC patients is unknown.

Author's Contribution

E. I. Rigopoulou and D. P. Bogdanos conceived the idea for writing a review on this topic; D. S. Smyk, D. P. Bogdanos, and E. I. Rigopoulou wrote the first and subsequent drafts of the paper. All authors contributed to the editing of the first and subsequent versions of the paper. All authors have read and approved the final paper.

References

[1] S. Hohenester, R. P. J. Oude-Elferink, and U. Beuers, "Primary biliary cirrhosis," *Seminars in Immunopathology*, vol. 31, no. 3, pp. 283–307, 2009.

[2] M. M. Kaplan and M. E. Gershwin, "Primary biliary cirrhosis," *The New England Journal of Medicine*, vol. 353, no. 12, pp. 1261–1273, 2005.

[3] T. Kumagi and E. J. Heathcote, "Primary biliary cirrhosis," *Orphanet Journal of Rare Diseases*, vol. 3, no. 1, article no. 1, 2008.

[4] K. D. Lindor, M. E. Gershwin, R. Poupon, M. Kaplan, N. V. Bergasa, and E. J. Heathcote, "Primary biliary cirrhosis," *Hepatology*, vol. 50, no. 1, pp. 291–308, 2009.

[5] J. Neuberger, "Primary biliary cirrhosis," *The Lancet*, vol. 350, no. 9081, pp. 875–879, 1997.

[6] E. Jenny Heathcote, "Management of primary biliary cirrhosis. The American Association for the Study of Liver Diseases practice guidelines," *Hepatology*, vol. 31, no. 4, pp. 1005–1013, 2000.

[7] R. Poupon, "Primary biliary cirrhosis: a 2010 update," *Journal of Hepatology*, vol. 52, no. 5, pp. 745–758, 2010.

[8] D. S. Smyk, E. I. Rigopoulou, A. Pares et al., "Sex differences associated with primary biliary cirrhosis," *Clinical and developmental immunology*, vol. 2012, Article ID 610504, 2012.

[9] P. Invernizzi, M. G. Alessio, D. S. Smyk et al., "Autoimmune hepatitis type 2 associated with an unexpected and transient presence of primary biliary cirrhosis-specific antimitochondrial antibodies: a case study and review of the literature," *BMC Gastroenterology*, vol. 12, p. 92, 2012.

[10] C. A. Aoki, C. M. Roifman, Z. X. Lian et al., "IL-2 receptor alpha deficiency and features of primary biliary cirrhosis," *Journal of Autoimmunity*, vol. 27, no. 1, pp. 50–53, 2006.

[11] Y. Dahlan, L. Smith, D. Simmonds et al., "Pediatric-onset primary biliary cirrhosis," *Gastroenterology*, vol. 125, no. 5, pp. 1476–1479, 2003.

[12] D. Smyk, E. Cholongitas, S. Kriese, E. I. Rigopoulou, and D. P. Bogdanos, "Primary biliary cirrhosis: family stories," *Autoimmune Diseases*, vol. 2011, Article ID 189585, 2011.

[13] D. Smyk, E. I. Rigopoulou, A. Pares, M. Mytilinaiou, P. Invernizzi, and D. Bogdanos, "Familial primary biliary cirrhosis: like mother, like daughter?" *Acta Gastro-Enterologica Belgica*, vol. 75, pp. 203–209, 2012.

[14] K. Boonstra, U. Beuers, and C. Y. Ponsioen, "Epidemiology of primary sclerosing cholangitis and primary biliary cirrhosis: a systematic review," *Journal of Hepatology*, vol. 56, pp. 1181–1188, 2012.

[15] O. E. W. James, R. Bhopal, D. Howel, J. Gray, A. D. Burt, and J. V. Metcalf, "Primary biliary cirrhosis once rare, now common in the United Kingdom?" *Hepatology*, vol. 30, no. 2, pp. 390–394, 1999.

[16] W. R. Kim, K. D. Lindor, G. R. Locke et al., "Epidemiology and natural history of primary biliary cirrhosis in a U.S. community," *Gastroenterology*, vol. 119, no. 6, pp. 1631–1636, 2000.

[17] S. Sood, P. J. Gow, J. M. Christie, and P. W. Angus, "Epidemiology of primary biliary cirrhosis in Victoria, Australia: high prevalence in migrant populations," *Gastroenterology*, vol. 127, no. 2, pp. 470–475, 2004.

[18] C. Selmi, P. Invernizzi, E. B. Keefe et al., "Epidemiology and pathogenesis of primary biliary cirrhosis," *Journal of Clinical Gastroenterology*, vol. 38, no. 3, pp. 264–271, 2004.

[19] D. P. Bogdanos, G. Mieli-Vergani, and D. Vergani, "Autoantibodies and their antigens in autoimmune hepatitis," *Seminars in Liver Disease*, vol. 29, no. 3, pp. 241–253, 2009.

[20] D. P. Bogdanos, H. Baum, and D. Vergani, "Antimitochondrial and other autoantibodies," *Clinics in Liver Disease*, vol. 7, no. 4, pp. 759–777, 2003.

[21] D. P. Bogdanos, P. Invernizzi, I. R. Mackay, and D. Vergani, "Autoimmune liver serology: current diagnostic and clinical challenges," *World Journal of Gastroenterology*, vol. 14, no. 21, pp. 3374–3387, 2008.

[22] D. P. Bogdanos and L. Komorowski, "Disease-specific autoantibodies in primary biliary cirrhosis," *Clinica Chimica Acta*, vol. 412, no. 7-8, pp. 502–512, 2011.

[23] D. P. Bogdanos, C. Liaskos, E. I. Rigopoulou, and G. N. Dalekos, "Anti-mitochondrial antibodies in patients with systemic lupus erythematosus: revealing the unforeseen," *Clinica Chimica Acta*, vol. 373, no. 1-2, pp. 183–184, 2006.

[24] P. S. C. Leung, R. L. Coppel, A. Ansari, S. Munoz, and M. E. Gershwin, "Antimitochondrial antibodies in primary biliary cirrhosis," *Seminars in Liver Disease*, vol. 17, no. 1, pp. 61–69, 1997.

[25] D. P. Bogdanos, A. Pares, J. Rodés et al., "Primary biliary cirrhosis specific antinuclear antibodies in patients from Spain," *American Journal of Gastroenterology*, vol. 99, no. 4, pp. 763–765, 2004.

[26] D. P. Bogdanos, D. Vergani, P. Muratori, L. Muratori, and F. B. Bianchi, "Specificity of anti-sp100 antibody for primary biliary cirrhosis," *Scandinavian Journal of Gastroenterology*, vol. 39, no. 4, pp. 405–407, 2004.

[27] P. Invernizzi, M. Podda, P. M. Battezzati et al., "Autoantibodies against nuclear pore complexes are associated with more active and severe liver disease in primary biliary cirrhosis," *Journal of Hepatology*, vol. 34, no. 3, pp. 366–372, 2001.

[28] L. Muratori, A. Granito, P. Muratori, G. Pappas, and F. B. Bianchi, "Antimitochondrial antibodies and other antibodies

in primary biliary cirrhosis: diagnostic and prognostic value," *Clinics in Liver Disease*, vol. 12, no. 2, pp. 261–276, 2008.

[29] C. Rigamonti, D. P. Bogdanos, M. G. Mytilinaiou, D. S. Smyk, E. I. Rigopoulou, and A. K. Burroughs, "Primary biliary cirrhosis associated with systemic sclerosis: diagnostic and clinical challenges," *International Journal of Rheumatology*, vol. 2011, Article ID 976427, 12 pages, 2011.

[30] D. P. Bogdanos, C. Rigamonti, D. Smyk, M. G. Mytilinaiou, E. I. Rigopoulou, and A. K. Burroughs, "Emerging issues in the immunopathogenesis, diagnosis and clinical management of primary biliary cirrhosis associated with systemic sclerosis," in *Systemic Sclerosis—An Update on the Aberrant Immune System and Clinical Features*, T. Radstake, Ed., pp. 151–166, Intech, Rijeka, Croatia, 2012.

[31] T. Kumagi and M. Onji, "Presentation and diagnosis of primary biliary sirrhosis in the 21st century," *Clinics in Liver Disease*, vol. 12, no. 2, pp. 243–259, 2008.

[32] C. Duarte-Rey, D. P. Bogdanos, P. S. Leung, J. M. Anaya, and M. E. Gershwin, "IgM predominance in autoimmune disease: genetics and gender," *Autoimmun Rev*, vol. 11, pp. A404–A412, 2012.

[33] E. I. Rigopoulou, E. T. Davies, D. P. Bogdanos et al., "Antimitochondrial antibodies of immunoglobulin G3 subclass are associated with a more severe disease course in primary biliary cirrhosis," *Liver International*, vol. 27, no. 9, pp. 1226–1231, 2007.

[34] E. I. Rigopoulou, D. P. Bogdanos, C. Liaskos et al., "Antimitochondrial antibody immunofluorescent titres correlate with the number and intensity of immunoblot-detected mitochondrial bands in patients with primary biliary cirrhosis," *Clinica Chimica Acta*, vol. 380, no. 1-2, pp. 118–121, 2007.

[35] C. Dähnrich, A. Pares, L. Caballeria et al., "New ELISA for detecting primary biliary cirrhosis-specific antimitochondrial antibodies," *Clinical Chemistry*, vol. 55, no. 5, pp. 978–985, 2009.

[36] P. Invernizzi, A. Crosignani, P. M. Battezzati et al., "Comparison of the clinical features and clinical course of antimitochondrial antibody-positive and -negative primary biliary cirrhosis," *Hepatology*, vol. 25, no. 5, pp. 1090–1095, 1997.

[37] N. Bizzaro, G. Covini, F. Rosina et al., "Overcoming a "probable" diagnosis in antimitochondrial antibody negative primary biliary cirrhosis: study of 100 sera and review of the literature," *Clinical Reviews in Allergy and Immunology*, vol. 42, no. 3, pp. 288–297, 2012.

[38] W. Bernal, F. Meda, Y. Ma, D. P. Bogdanos, and D. Vergani, "Disease-specific autoantibodies in patients with acute liver failure: the King's College London experience," *Hepatology*, vol. 47, no. 3, pp. 1096–1097, 2008.

[39] P. S. C. Leung, L. Rossaro, P. A. Davis et al., "Antimitochondrial antibodies in acute liver failure: implications for primary biliary cirrhosis," *Hepatology*, vol. 46, no. 5, pp. 1436–1442, 2007.

[40] C. Liaskos, D. P. Bogdanos, E. I. Rigopoulou, and G. N. Dalekos, "Development of antimitochondrial antibodies in patients with autoimmune hepatitis: art of facts or an artifact?" *Journal of Gastroenterology and Hepatology*, vol. 22, no. 3, pp. 454–455, 2007.

[41] J. V. Metcalf, H. C. Mitchison, J. M. Palmer, D. E. Jones, M. F. Bassendine, and O. F. W. James, "Natural history of early primary biliary cirrhosis," *The Lancet*, vol. 348, no. 9039, pp. 1399–1402, 1996.

[42] C. Duarte-Rey, D. Bogdanos, C. Y. Yang et al., "Primary biliary cirrhosis and the nuclear pore complex," *Autoimmunity Reviews*, vol. 11, no. 12, pp. 898–902, 2012.

[43] S. Itoh, T. Ichida, T. Yoshida et al., "Autoantibodies against a 210 kDa glycoprotein of the nuclear pore complex as a prognostic marker in patients with primary biliary cirrhosis," *Journal of Gastroenterology and Hepatology*, vol. 13, no. 3, pp. 257–265, 1998.

[44] J. Wesierska-Gadek, H. Hohenauer, E. Hitchman, and E. Penner, "Autoantibodies from patients with primary biliary cirrhosis preferentially react with the amino-terminal domain of nuclear pore complex glycoprotein gp210," *Journal of Experimental Medicine*, vol. 182, no. 4, pp. 1159–1162, 1995.

[45] E. I. Rigopoulou, E. T. Davies, A. Pares et al., "Prevalence and clinical significance of isotype specific antinuclear antibodies in primary biliary cirrhosis," *Gut*, vol. 54, no. 4, pp. 528–532, 2005.

[46] D. P. Bogdanos, C. Liaskos, A. Pares et al., "Anti-gp210 antibody mirrors disease severity in primary biliary cirrhosis," *Hepatology*, vol. 45, no. 6, p. 1583, 2007.

[47] M. G. Mytilinaiou, W. Meyer, T. Scheper et al., "Diagnostic and clinical utility of antibodies against the nuclear body promyelocytic leukaemia and Sp100 antigens in patients with primary biliary cirrhosis," *Clinica Chimica Acta*, vol. 413, pp. 1211–1216, 2012.

[48] C. Liaskos, G. L. Norman, A. Moulas et al., "Prevalence of gastric parietal cell antibodies and intrinsic factor antibodies in primary biliary cirrhosis," *Clinica Chimica Acta*, vol. 411, no. 5-6, pp. 411–415, 2010.

[49] S. Gabeta, G. L. Norman, N. Gatselis et al., "IgA anti-b2GPI antibodies in patients with autoimmune liver diseases," *Journal of Clinical Immunology*, vol. 28, no. 5, pp. 501–511, 2008.

[50] P. Muratori, L. Muratori, M. Guidi et al., "Anti-Saccharomyces cerevisiae antibodies (ASCA) and autoimmune liver diseases," *Clinical and Experimental Immunology*, vol. 132, no. 3, pp. 473–476, 2003.

[51] E. I. Rigopoulou, D. Roggenbuck, D. S. Smyk et al., "Asialoglycoprotein receptor (ASGPR) as target autoantigen in liver autoimmunity: lost and found," *Autoimmunity Reviews*. In press.

[52] D. P. Bogdanos, D. S. Smyk, E. I. Rigopoulou et al., "Twin studies in autoimmune disease: genetics, gender and environment," *Journal of Autoimmunity*, vol. 38, pp. J156–J169, 2012.

[53] C. Selmi, P. S. Leung, D. H. Sherr et al., "Mechanisms of environmental influence on human autoimmunity: a national institute of environmental health sciences expert panel workshop," *Journal of Autoimmunity*. In press.

[54] F. W. Miller, K. M. Pollard, C. G. Parks et al., "Criteria for environmentally associated Autoimmune Dis," *Journal of Autoimmunity*. In press.

[55] D. S. Smyk, E. I. Rigopoulou, L. Muratori, A. K. Burroughs, and D. P. Bogdanos, "Smoking as a risk factor for autoimmune liver disease: what we can learn from primary biliary cirrhosis," *Annals of Hepatology*, vol. 11, pp. 7–14, 2012.

[56] D. S. Smyk, M. G. Mytilinaiou, P. Milkiewicz, E. I. Rigopoulou, P. Invernizzi, and D. P. Bogdanos, "Towards systemic sclerosis and away from primary biliary cirrhosis: the case of PTPN22," *Autoimmunity Highlights*, vol. 3, pp. 1–9, 2012.

[57] D. S. Smyk, E. I. Rigopoulou, N. Bizzaro, and D. P. Bogdanos, "Hair dyes as a risk for autoimmunity: from systemic lupus

erythematosus to primary biliary cirrhosis," *Autoimmunity Highlights*. In press.

[58] D. Smyk, M. G. Mytilinaiou, E. I. Rigopoulou, and D. P. Bogdanos, "PBC triggers in water reservoirs, coal mining areas and waste disposal sites: from Newcastle to New York," *Disease Markers*, vol. 29, no. 6, pp. 337–344, 2010.

[59] D. S. Smyk, E. I. Rigopoulou, A. Lleo et al., "Immunopathogenesis of primary biliary cirrhosis: an old wives' tale," *Immunity & Ageing*, vol. 8, p. 12, 2011.

[60] E. I. Rigopoulou, D. S. Smyk, C. E. Matthews et al., "Epstein-barr virus as a trigger of autoimmune liver diseases," *Advances in Virology*, vol. 2012, Article ID 987471, 12 pages, 2012.

[61] D. S. Smyk, D. P. Bogdanos, S. Kriese, C. Billinis, A. K. Burroughs, and E. I. Rigopoulou, "Urinary tract infection as a risk factor for autoimmune liver disease: from bench to bedside," *Clinics and Research in Hepatology and Gastroenterology*, vol. 36, pp. 110–121, 2012.

[62] D. Smyk, E. I. Rigopoulou, H. Baum, A. K. Burroughs, D. Vergani, and D. P. Bogdanos, "Autoimmunity and environment: am i at risk?" *Clinical Reviews in Allergy and Immunology*, vol. 42, pp. 199–212, 2012.

[63] F. K. Varyani, J. West, and T. R. Card, "An increased risk of urinary tract infection precedes development of primary biliary cirrhosis," *BMC Gastroenterology*, vol. 11, p. 95, 2011.

[64] D. Smyk, E. I. Rigopoulou, Z. Yoh, A. Koutsoumpas, H. Baum, and D. P. Bogdanos, "Infectious triggers of primary biliary cirrhosis: do we know enough?" *Current Trends in Immunology*, vol. 11, pp. 35–49, 2010.

[65] G. Maartens and R. J. Wilkinson, "Tuberculosis," *The Lancet*, vol. 370, no. 9604, pp. 2030–2043, 2007.

[66] B. M. Saunders and W. J. Britton, "Life and death in the granuloma: immunopathology of tuberculosis," *Immunology and Cell Biology*, vol. 85, no. 2, pp. 103–111, 2007.

[67] H. Amital-Teplizki, I. Avinoach, A. R. M. Coates, O. Kooperman, M. Blank, and Y. Shoenfeld, "Binding of monoclonal anti-DNA and anti-TB glycolipids to brain tissue," *Autoimmunity*, vol. 4, no. 4, pp. 277–287, 1989.

[68] R. A. Asherson, K. Gunter, D. Daya, and Y. Shoenfeld, "Multiple autoimmune diseases in a young woman: tuberculosis and splenectomy as possible triggering factors? Another example of the "mosaic" of autoimmunity," *Journal of Rheumatology*, vol. 35, no. 6, pp. 1224–1227, 2008.

[69] M. Cutolo, C. Pizzorni, and A. Sulli, "Vitamin D endocrine system involvement in autoimmune rheumatic diseases," *Autoimmunity Reviews*, vol. 11, pp. 84–87, 2011.

[70] A. Dubaniewicz, "*Mycobacterium tuberculosis* heat shock proteins and autoimmunity in sarcoidosis," *Autoimmunity Reviews*, vol. 9, no. 6, pp. 419–424, 2010.

[71] Y. Shapira, N. Agmon-Levin, and Y. Shoenfeld, "*Mycobacterium tuberculosis*, autoimmunity, and vitamin D," *Clinical Reviews in Allergy and Immunology*, vol. 38, no. 2-3, pp. 169–177, 2010.

[72] M. A. B. Thomas, G. Frampton, D. A. Isenberg et al., "A common anti-DNA antibody idiotype and anti-phospholipid antibodies in sera from patients with schistosomiasis and filariasis with and without nephritis," *Journal of Autoimmunity*, vol. 2, no. 6, pp. 803–811, 1989.

[73] Y. Shoenfeld, Y. Vilner, and A. R. M. Coates, "Monoclonal anti-tuberculosis antibodies react with DNA, and monoclonal anti-DNA autoantibodies react with *Mycobacterium tuberculosis*," *Clinical and Experimental Immunology*, vol. 66, no. 2, pp. 255–261, 1986.

[74] F. M. Ribeiro, M. Szyper-Kravitz, E. M. Klumb et al., "Can lupus flares be associated with tuberculosis infection?" *Clinical Reviews in Allergy and Immunology*, vol. 38, no. 2-3, pp. 163–168, 2010.

[75] U. Broome, A. Scheynius, and R. Hultcrantz, "Induced expression of heat-shock protein on biliary epithelium in patients with primary sclerosing cholangitis and primary biliary cirrhosis," *Hepatology*, vol. 18, no. 2, pp. 298–303, 1993.

[76] M. Kallel Sellami, M. Zitouni, F. Zouiten, L. Laadhar, T. Ben Chaabane, and S. Makni, "Tuberculosis, primary biliary cirrhosis and autoimmunity," *Bulletin de la Societe de Pathologie Exotique*, vol. 94, no. 4, pp. 330–331, 2001.

[77] C. Corpechot, Y. Chrétien, O. Chazouillères, and R. Poupon, "Demographic, lifestyle, medical and familial factors associated with primary biliary cirrhosis," *Journal of Hepatology*, vol. 53, no. 1, pp. 162–169, 2010.

[78] M. E. Gershwin, C. Selmi, H. J. Worman et al., "Risk factors and comorbidities in primary biliary cirrhosis: a controlled interview-based study of 1032 patients," *Hepatology*, vol. 42, no. 5, pp. 1194–1202, 2005.

[79] A. Parikh-Patel, E. B. Gold, H. Worman, K. E. Krivy, and M. E. Gershwin, "Risk factors for primary biliary cirrhosis in a cohort of patients from the United States," *Hepatology*, vol. 33, no. 1, pp. 16–21, 2001.

[80] M. I. Prince, S. J. Ducker, and O. F. W. James, "Case-control studies of risk factors for primary biliary cirrhosis in two United Kingdom populations," *Gut*, vol. 59, no. 4, pp. 508–512, 2010.

[81] R. Klein, M. Wiebel, S. Engelhart, and P. A. Berg, "Sera from patients with tuberculosis recognize the M2a-epitope (E2-subunit of pyruvate dehydrogenase) specific for primary biliary cirrhosis," *Clinical and Experimental Immunology*, vol. 92, no. 2, pp. 308–316, 1993.

[82] D. R. Gaya, D. Thorburn, K. A. Oien, A. J. Morris, and A. J. Stanley, "Hepatic granulomas: a 10 year single centre experience," *Journal of Clinical Pathology*, vol. 56, no. 11, pp. 850–853, 2003.

[83] W. G. McCluggage and J. M. Sloan, "Hepatic granulomas in Northern Ireland: a thirteen year review," *Histopathology*, vol. 25, no. 3, pp. 219–228, 1994.

[84] I. K. Onal, O. Ersoy, M. Aydinli et al., "Hepatic granuloma in Turkish adults: a report of 13 cases," *European Journal of Internal Medicine*, vol. 19, no. 7, pp. 527–530, 2008.

[85] J. S. Sartin and R. C. Walker, "Granulomatous hepatitis: a retrospective review of 88 cases at the Mayo Clinic," *Mayo Clinic Proceedings*, vol. 66, no. 9, pp. 914–918, 1991.

[86] M. B. Satti, H. Al-Freihi, E. M. Ibrahim et al., "Hepatic granuloma in Saudi Arabia: a clinicopathological study of 59 cases," *American Journal of Gastroenterology*, vol. 85, no. 6, pp. 669–674, 1990.

[87] U. Drebber, H. U. Kasper, J. Ratering et al., "Hepatic granulomas: histological and molecular pathological approach to differential diagnosis-a study of 442 cases," *Liver International*, vol. 28, no. 6, pp. 828–834, 2008.

[88] S. P. Dourakis, R. Saramadou, A. Alexopoulou et al., "Hepatic granulomas: a 6-year experience in a single center in Greece," *European Journal of Gastroenterology and Hepatology*, vol. 19, no. 2, pp. 101–104, 2007.

[89] Z. You, Q. Wang, Z. Bian et al., "The immunopathology of liver granulomas in primary biliary cirrhosis," *Journal of Autoimmunity*, vol. 39, no. 3, pp. 216–221, 2012.

[90] J. L. Flynn, J. Chan, and P. L. Lin, "Macrophages and control of granulomatous inflammation in tuberculosis," *Mucosal Immunology*, vol. 4, no. 3, pp. 271–278, 2011.

[91] J. M. Davis and L. Ramakrishnan, "The role of the granuloma in expansion and dissemination of early tuberculous infection," *Cell*, vol. 136, no. 1, pp. 37–49, 2009.

[92] L. Ramakrishnan, "Revisiting the role of the granuloma in tuberculosis," *Nature Reviews Immunology*, vol. 12, pp. 352–366, 2012.

[93] A. Tanaka, T. P. Prindiville, R. Gish et al., "Are infectious agents involved in primary biliary cirrhosis? A PCR approach," *Journal of Hepatology*, vol. 31, no. 4, pp. 664–671, 1999.

[94] J. O'Donohue, H. Fidler, M. Garcia-Barcelo, K. Nouri-Aria, R. Williams, and J. McFadden, "Mycobacterial DNA not detected in liver sections from patients with primary billiary cirrhosis," *Journal of Hepatology*, vol. 28, no. 3, pp. 433–438, 1998.

[95] B. Gilburd, L. Ziporen, D. Zharhary et al., "Antimitochondrial (pyruvate dehydrogenase) antibodies in leprosy," *Journal of Clinical Immunology*, vol. 14, no. 1, pp. 14–19, 1994.

[96] J. Van de Water, H. Ishibashi, R. L. Coppel, and M. E. Gershwin, "Molecular mimicry and primary biliary cirrhosis: premises not promises," *Hepatology*, vol. 33, no. 4, pp. 771–775, 2001.

[97] D. Bogdanos, T. Pusl, C. Rust, D. Vergani, and U. Beuers, "Primary biliary cirrhosis following lactobacillus vaccination for recurrent vaginitis," *Journal of Hepatology*, vol. 49, no. 3, pp. 466–473, 2008.

[98] D. P. Bogdanos, H. Baum, M. Okamoto et al., "Primary biliary cirrhosis is characterized by IgG3 antibodies crossreactive with the major mitochondrial autoepitope and its lactobacillus mimic," *Hepatology*, vol. 42, no. 2, pp. 458–465, 2005.

[99] D. P. Bogdanos, H. Baum, U. C. Sharma et al., "Antibodies against homologous microbial caseinolytic proteases P characterise primary biliary cirrhosis," *Journal of Hepatology*, vol. 36, no. 1, pp. 14–21, 2002.

[100] D. P. Bogdanos and D. Vergani, "Bacteria and primary biliary cirrhosis," *Clinical Reviews in Allergy and Immunology*, vol. 36, no. 1, pp. 30–39, 2009.

[101] D. P. Bogdanos, H. Baum, P. Butler et al., "Association between the primary biliary cirrhosis specific anti-sp100 antibodies and recurrent urinary tract infection," *Digestive and Liver Disease*, vol. 35, no. 11, pp. 801–805, 2003.

[102] D. P. Bogdanos, H. Baum, D. Vergani, and A. K. Burroughs, "The role of *E. coli* infection in the pathogenesis of primary biliary cirrhosis," *Disease Markers*, vol. 29, no. 6, pp. 301–311, 2010.

[103] A. Koutsoumpas, D. Polymeros, Z. Tsiamoulos et al., "Peculiar antibody reactivity to human connexin 37 and its microbial mimics in patients with Crohn's disease," *Journal of Crohn's and Colitis*, vol. 5, no. 2, pp. 101–109, 2011.

[104] G. V. Gregorio, K. Choudhuri, Y. Ma et al., "Mimicry between the hepatitis C virus polyprotein and antigenic targets of nuclear and smooth muscle antibodies in chronic hepatitis C virus infection," *Clinical and Experimental Immunology*, vol. 133, no. 3, pp. 404–413, 2003.

[105] G. H. Haydon and J. Neuberger, "PBC: an infectious disease?" *Gut*, vol. 47, no. 4, pp. 586–588, 2000.

[106] H. Kita, S. Matsumura, X. S. He et al., "Analysis of TCR antagonism and molecular mimicry of an HLA-A*0201-restricted CTL epitope in primary biliary cirrhosis," *Hepatology*, vol. 36, no. 4 I, pp. 918–926, 2002.

[107] Y. Ma, D. P. Bogdanos, M. J. Hussain et al., "Polyclonal T-cell responses to cytochrome P450IID6 are associated with disease activity in autoimmune hepatitis type 2," *Gastroenterology*, vol. 130, no. 3, pp. 868–882, 2006.

[108] D. Polymeros, D. P. Bogdanos, R. Day, D. Arioli, D. Vergani, and A. Forbes, "Does cross-reactivity between mycobacterium avium paratuberculosis and human intestinal antigens characterize Crohn's disease?" *Gastroenterology*, vol. 131, no. 1, pp. 85–96, 2006.

[109] H. Baum, D. P. Bogdanos, and D. Vergani, "Antibodies to Clp protease in primary biliary cirrhosis: possible role of a mimicking T-cell epitope," *Journal of Hepatology*, vol. 34, no. 5, pp. 785–787, 2001.

[110] N. Kerkar, K. Choudhuri, Y. Ma et al., "Cytochrome P4502D6193-212: a new immunodominant epitope and target of virus/self cross-reactivity in liver kidney microsomal autoantibody type 1-positive liver disease," *Journal of Immunology*, vol. 170, no. 3, pp. 1481–1489, 2003.

[111] A. Koutsoumpas, M. Mytilinaiou, D. Polymeros, G. N. Dalekos, and D. P. Bogdanos, "Anti-Helicobacter pylori antibody responses specific for VacA do not trigger primary biliary cirrhosis-specific antimitochondrial antibodies," *European Journal of Gastroenterology and Hepatology*, vol. 21, no. 10, p. 1220, 2009.

[112] M. S. Longhi, M. J. Hussain, D. P. Bogdanos et al., "Cytochrome P450IID6-specific CD8 T cell immune responses mirror disease activity in autoimmune hepatitis type 2," *Hepatology*, vol. 46, no. 2, pp. 472–484, 2007.

[113] D. P. Bogdanos, H. Baum, F. Gunsar et al., "Extensive homology between the major immunodominant mitochondrial antigen in primary biliary cirrhosis and Helicobacter pylori does not lead to immunological cross-reactivity," *Scandinavian Journal of Gastroenterology*, vol. 39, no. 10, pp. 981–987, 2004.

[114] S. Hannam, D. P. Bogdanos, E. T. Davies et al., "Neonatal liver disease associated with placental transfer of antimitochondrial antibodies," *Autoimmunity*, vol. 35, no. 8, pp. 545–550, 2002.

[115] Y. Ma, M. Meregalli, S. Hodges et al., "Alcohol dehydrogenase: an autoantibody target in patients with alcoholic liver disease," *International Journal of Immunopathology and Pharmacology*, vol. 18, no. 1, pp. 173–182, 2005.

[116] Y. Ma, M. Okamoto, M. G. Thomas et al., "Antibodies to conformational epitopes of soluble liver antigen define a severe form of autoimmune liver disease," *Hepatology*, vol. 35, no. 3, pp. 658–664, 2002.

[117] Y. Ma, M. G. Thomas, M. Okamoto et al., "Key residues of a major cytochrome P4502D6 epitope are located on the surface of the molecule," *Journal of Immunology*, vol. 169, no. 1, pp. 277–285, 2002.

[118] L. Muratori, D. P. Bogdanos, P. Muratori et al., "Susceptibility to thyroid disorders in hepatitis C," *Clinical Gastroenterology and Hepatology*, vol. 3, no. 6, pp. 595–603, 2005.

[119] L. Wen, Y. Ma, D. P. Bogdanos et al., "Pédiatrie autoimmune liver diseases: the molecular basis of humoral and cellular immunity," *Current Molecular Medicine*, vol. 1, no. 3, pp. 379–389, 2001.

[120] M. S. Longhi, Y. Ma, D. P. Bogdanos, P. Cheeseman, G. Mieli-Vergani, and D. Vergani, "Impairment of CD4$^+$CD25$^+$ regulatory T-cells in autoimmune liver disease," *Journal of Hepatology*, vol. 41, no. 1, pp. 31–37, 2004.

[121] M. S. Longhi, Y. Ma, R. R. Mitry et al., "Effect of CD4+CD25+ regulatory T-cells on CD8 T-cell function in patients with autoimmune hepatitis," *Journal of Autoimmunity*, vol. 25, no. 1, pp. 63–71, 2005.

[122] D. P. Bogdanos, M. Lenzi, M. Okamoto et al., "Multiple viral/self immunological cross-reactivity in liver kidney microsomal antibody positive hepatitis C virus-infected patients is associated with the possession of HLA B51," *International Journal of Immunopathology and Pharmacology*, vol. 17, no. 1, pp. 83–92, 2004.

[123] D. Vergani, D. P. Bogdanos, and H. Baum, "Unusual suspects in primary biliary cirrhosis," *Hepatology*, vol. 39, no. 1, pp. 38–41, 2004.

[124] D. P. Bogdanos, A. Pares, H. Baum et al., "Disease-specific cross-reactivity between mimicking peptides of heat shock protein of mycobacterium gordonae and dominant epitope of E2 subunit of pyruvate dehydrogenase is common in Spanish but not British patients with primary biliary cirrhosis," *Journal of Autoimmunity*, vol. 22, no. 4, pp. 353–362, 2004.

[125] D. P. Bogdanos, K. Choudhuri, and D. Vergani, "Molecular mimicry and autoimmune liver disease: virtuous intentions, malign consequences," *Liver*, vol. 21, no. 4, pp. 225–232, 2001.

[126] L. Vilagut, J. Vila, O. Vinas et al., "Cross-reactivity of anti-Mycobacterium gordonae antibodies with the major mitochondrial autoantigens in primary biliary cirrhosis," *Journal of Hepatology*, vol. 21, no. 4, pp. 673–677, 1994.

[127] L. Vilagut, A. Parés, O. Viñas, J. Vila, M. T. Jiménez De Anta, and J. Rodés, "Antibodies to mycobacterial 65-kD heat shock protein cross-react with the main mitochondrial antigens in patients with primary biliary cirrhosis," *European Journal of Clinical Investigation*, vol. 27, no. 8, pp. 667–672, 1997.

[128] S. C. Robson, R. J. Hift, and R. E. Kirsch, "Primary biliary cirrhosis. A retrospective survey at Groote Schuur Hospital, Cape Town," *South African Medical Journal*, vol. 78, no. 1, pp. 19–22, 1990.

[129] L. Nesher, K. Riesenberg, L. Saidel-Odes, F. Schlaeffer, and R. Smolyakov, "Tuberculosis in African refugees from the Eastern Sub-Sahara region," *The Israel Medical Association Journal*, vol. 14, pp. 111–114, 2012.

[130] A. K. S. Samanta, A. G. Bhagwat, and M. Mukherjee, "Primary biliary cirrhosis in India," *Gut*, vol. 14, no. 6, pp. 448–450, 1973.

[131] S. K. Sarin, R. Monga, B. S. Sandhu, B. C. Sharma, P. Sakhuja, and V. Malhotra, "Primary biliary cirrhosis in India," *Hepatobiliary and Pancreatic Diseases International*, vol. 5, no. 1, pp. 105–109, 2006.

[132] H. Liu, Y. Liu, L. Wang et al., "Prevalence of primary biliary cirrhosis in adults referring hospital for annual health checkup in Southern China," *BMC Gastroenterology*, vol. 10, p. 100, 2010.

[133] G. M. Hirschfield and P. Invernizzi, "Progress in the genetics of primary biliary cirrhosis," *Seminars in Liver Disease*, vol. 31, no. 2, pp. 147–156, 2011.

[134] P. Invernizzi, "Human leukocyte antigen in primary biliary cirrhosis: an old story now reviving," *Hepatology*, vol. 54, no. 2, pp. 714–723, 2011.

[135] P. Invernizzi, M. Ransom, S. Raychaudhuri et al., "Classical HLA-DRB1 and DPB1 alleles account for HLA associations with primary biliary cirrhosis," *Genes and Immunity*, vol. 13, no. 6, pp. 461–468, 2012.

[136] P. Invernizzi, C. Selmi, F. Poli et al., "Human leukocyte antigen polymorphisms in Italian primary biliary cirrhosis: a multicenter study of 664 patients and 1992 healthy controls," *Hepatology*, vol. 48, no. 6, pp. 1906–1912, 2008.

[137] G. F. Mells, J. A. B. Floyd, K. I. Morley et al., "Genome-wide association study identifies 12 new susceptibility loci for primary biliary cirrhosis," *Nature Genetics*, vol. 43, no. 4, pp. 332–333, 2011.

[138] C. Selmi, N. J. Torok, A. Affronti, and M. E. Gershwin, "Genomic variants associated with primary biliary cirrhosis," *Genome Medicine*, vol. 2, no. 1, p. 5, 2010.

[139] A. Tanaka, P. Invernizzi, H. Ohira et al., "Replicated association of 17q12-21 with susceptibility of primary biliary cirrhosis in a Japanese cohort," *Tissue Antigens*, vol. 78, no. 1, pp. 65–68, 2011.

[140] A. Tanaka, H. Ohira, K. Kikuchi et al., "Genetic association of Fc receptor-like 3 polymorphisms with susceptibility to primary biliary cirrhosis: ethnic comparative study in Japanese and Italian patients," *Tissue Antigens*, vol. 77, no. 3, pp. 239–243, 2011.

[141] E. Png, B. Alisjahbana, E. Sahiratmadja et al., "A genome wide association study of pulmonary tuberculosis susceptibility in Indonesians," *BMC Medical Genetics*, vol. 13, p. 5, 2012.

[142] T. Thye, F. O. Vannberg, S. H. Wong et al., "Genome-wide association analyses identifies a susceptibility locus for tuberculosis on chromosome 18q11.2," *Nature Genetics*, vol. 42, no. 9, pp. 739–741, 2010.

[143] J. L. Casanova and L. Abel, "Genetic dissection of immunity to mycobacteria: the human model," *Annual Review of Immunology*, vol. 20, pp. 581–620, 2002.

[144] R. Van Crevel, I. Parwati, E. Sahiratmadja et al., "Infection with *Mycobacterium tuberculosis* Beijing genotype strains is associated with polymorphisms in SLC11A1/NRAMP1 in Indonesian patients with tuberculosis," *Journal of Infectious Diseases*, vol. 200, no. 11, pp. 1671–1674, 2009.

[145] O. Sela, A. El-Roeiy, and D. A. Isenberg, "A common anti-DNA idiotype in sera of patients with active pulmonary tuberculosis," *Arthritis and Rheumatism*, vol. 30, no. 1, pp. 50–56, 1987.

[146] J. A. Cayla and A. Orcau, "Control of tuberculosis in large cities in developed countries: an organizational problem," *BMC Medicine*, vol. 9, p. 127, 2011.

4

Acid-Fast Bacilli Other than Mycobacteria in Tuberculosis Patients Receiving Directly Observed Therapy Short Course in Cross River State, Nigeria

Benjamin Thumamo Pokam[1] and Anne E. Asuquo[2]

[1] *Department of Medical Laboratory Science, University of Buea, P.O. Box 63, Buea, Cameroon*
[2] *Department of Medical Laboratory Science, University of Calabar, Calabar, Nigeria*

Correspondence should be addressed to Benjamin Thumamo Pokam, thumamo@yahoo.fr

Academic Editor: Jeffrey R. Starke

The information on the contribution of non tuberculous mycobacteria (NTM) to mycobacterial infections in Africa is scarce due to limited laboratory culture for its isolation and identification. One hundred and thirty-seven sputum smear positive patients were recruited into a study on the molecular epidemiology of *Mycobacterium tuberculosis* in Cross River State. Following sputum culture, 97 pure isolates were obtained and identified using Capilia TB-Neo and further confirmed by the GenoType Mycobacterium CM kit. Of the 97 isolates, 81 (83.5%) isolates were Capilia TB-Neo positive while 16 (16.5%) were Capilia TB-Neo negative. Further confirmation with the GenoType Mycobacterium CM kit revealed that 4 (25%) of the 16 isolates belonged to NTM and included *M. fortuitum I, M. fortuitum II/M magaritense, M. abscessus,* and *M. avium* ssp. The remaining 12 (75%) Capilia TB-Neo negative isolates were not members of the genus *Mycobacterium* despite their AFB appearance. Six (33.3%) of the Capilia TB-Neo negative were from HIV positive tuberculosis patients. All subjects in this study were placed on DOTS shortly after the AFB results were obtained. The implication of isolation of 16.5% nontuberculous isolates further emphasizes the need for culture of sputum specimen especially in HIV positive patients prior to administration of antituberculosis therapy.

1. Introduction

Mycobacterium tuberculosis is the most important causative agent of tuberculosis (TB) while nontuberculous mycobacteria (NTM) may play a key role in etiology of TB-like syndromes [1].

Data on nontuberculous mycobacterial disease in sub-Saharan Africa are limited, due mainly to the lack of laboratory culture facilities for the identification of mycobacterial species. Consequently, many laboratories do not discriminate between *M. tuberculosis* and NTM for similar reasons [2–4]. Treatment of TB patients in most sub-Saharan African countries including Nigeria is based solely on the results of microscopic smear positivity. As such, all sputum smear positive diagnosed patients are indiscriminately placed on DOTS, the current international TB treatment strategy. The implication is that NTM is inappropriately managed with first-line antituberculous drug [4, 5], worsening the patient's condition and raising the risk of drug resistance. Although it is known that most sputum smear positive patients are truly TB patients [6], the continued increase in TB drug resistance raises the question on the impact of this indiscriminate use of TB drugs to treat all diagnosed sputum smear positive patients. In assessing the molecular epidemiology of *Mycobacterium tuberculosis* complex in the Cross River State of Nigeria, the data revealed the involvement of AFB other than mycobacteria in tuberculosis-like symptoms in the population.

2. Materials and Methods

2.1. Patients and Setting. The study was carried out in Cross River State, located in the South-South part of Nigeria. Patients included 137 smear positive patients from which 3 consecutive sputum specimens were collected. Patients were recruited over a period of 12 months (June 2008 to May 2009) from the major hospitals and TB care facilities in the north, central, and south senatorial districts of the state. Both genders and age groups of 10 to 70 years were included. Permission to carry out the work was obtained from the local ethical committee, and informed medical consent was equally obtained from all participating patients.

2.2. Sputum Cultures. Sputum specimen obtained from patients was preserved using sodium carbonate (75 mg) and/or refrigerated until cultured. Specimens were decontaminated using modified Petroff's method [7] and cultured using BACTEC 960 (Becton Dickinson, Franklin Lakes, NJ07417, USA). Smears were made from isolates obtained from the BACTEC MGIT tubes, stained by the Ziehl Neelsen staining method, and examined for the presence of acid-fast bacilli (AFB). The growth on AFB positive MGIT tubes was further inoculated into two Lowenstein-Jensen slants, one containing sodium pyruvate. The cultures were examined twice a week and their rate of growth and colonial morphologies recorded. Contaminated slants were further re-decontaminated and recultured. Negative cultures and discarded heavily contaminated slants reduced our working cultures to 97 pure isolates.

2.3. Identification of Isolates. Primary identification of organisms using Capilia TB-Neo (TAUNS Laboratories, Inc. Japan), an immunochromatographic method which can detect MPT64, a protein specifically secreted by *M. tuberculosis* complex and not produced by NTM, was performed according to the manufacturer's instructions (http://capilia .jp/english/capilia_tb_neo.html).

To determine the species of the Capilia TB-Neo negative isolates, the GenoType Mycobacterium CM kit, a test based on the DNA-STRIP technology that permits the identification of some mycobacterial species, was used according to the manufacturer's instructions (Hain Lifescience GmbH, Nehren, Germany). Briefly, DNA extraction was carried out by sonication on the cultured organisms, heat killed at 80°C for 30 minutes, followed by a multiplex amplification with biotinylated primers and a reverse hybridization. The hybridization included the chemical denaturation of the amplification products, hybridization of a single-stranded, biotin-labeled amplicons to membrane-bound probes, stringent washing, addition of a streptavidin/alkaline phosphatase conjugate, and an alkaline phosphatase mediated staining reaction. A template ensured the easy and fast interpretation of the banding pattern obtained. Three controls (conjugate, universal, and genus) are included in each strip.

3. Results

Following culture and identification of the 97 isolates in this study, 81 (83.5%) were identified as members of the *Mycobacterium tuberculosis* complex (data published [8]) using both immunochromatographic technique (Capilia TB-Neo positive) and GenoType Mycobacterium CM. Eighteen

TABLE 1: Association of mycobacteria genus and HIV status of subjects.

HIV status	Capilia TB-Neo		Total
	Positive (%)	Negative (%)	
Positive	12 (66.7)	6 (33.3)	18
Negative	50 (86.2)	8 (13.8)	58
Unknown	19 (90.5)	2 (9.5)	21
Total	81	16	97

TABLE 2: Genotype mycobacteria identification of Capilia TB-Neo negative isolates from sputum smear positive patients.

Isolates no.	Sex/Age	Strains	HIV status
0015IDH	F/25–34	NM	NEG
0033TH	F/25–34	NM	POS
0043TH	M/35–44	NM	NEG
0053TH	M/35–44	NM	POS
0073IDH	M/45–54	*M. fortuitum* I	POS
0082IDH	M/25–34	NM	UNK
0083IDH	F/25–34	NM	NEG
0086IDH	F/25–34	NM	POS
0089IDH	M/25–34	*M. fortuitum* II/ *M. magaritense*	NEG
0094IDH	F/25–34	NM	NEG
0105TH	F/15–24	NM	NEG
00111IDH	M/25–34	NM	POS
00113IDH	M/15–24	NM	NEG
00128TH	M/25–34	NM	NEG
00134TH	M/35–44	*M. abcessus*	POS
00407OG	F/35–44	*M. avium* ssp.	UNK

F: female; M: male; NM: not member of the genus mycobacteria; POS: positive; NEG: negative; UNK: unknown.

(18.6%) patients were HIV positive. However, 21 individuals did not know their HIV status at the time the study was carried out. Of the 18 HIV positive TB patients, 6 (33.3%) were Capilia negative ($P = 0.09$) (Table 1).

Of the 16 Capilia negative isolates, GenoType Mycobacterium CM molecular test identified 4 isolates as *M. fortuitum* I, *M. fortuitum* II/*M magaritense*, *M. abcessus*, and *M. avium* ssp. Two of the 4 isolates were obtained from HIV positive patients. Twelve AFB smear positive isolates were found not to be members of the genus mycobacteria, as shown in Table 2.

4. Discussion

In recent times, several newer immunochromatographic techniques have emerged (e.g., Capilia) making rapid differentiation between *M. tuberculosis* complex and NTM possible and less cumbersome, even though they cannot identify the NTM species. Although it has been shown that most cultures-positive mycobacteria are *M. tuberculosis* in regions where tuberculosis is highly prevalent [6, 9], NTM isolates have been increasing gradually. Up to 20–30% of AFB smear positive isolates have been identified as NTM in Korea [10]. These organisms can cause true infection and disease and can be important clinically [11]. In Africa, the contribution of NTM to such disease has been examined on a small scale only [1]. Two previous studies in Nigeria show that Fawcett and Watkins [12] did not isolate mycobacteria other than those causing tuberculosis in their study in the northern region of the country. However, 11% atypical Mycobacteria have been reported in Lagos in 1986 [6]. The latter authors classified six as *M. avium*, four as *M. kansasii*, and one as *M. fortuitum*. The four NTM species isolated in this study included *M. fortuitum* I, *M. fortuitum* II/*M. magaritense*, and *M. avium* species besides M. abscessus. Two studies carried in the country have equally isolated *M. fortuitum*, *M. intracellulare*, *M. chelonae*, *M. avium*, and *M. kansasi* among sputum smear positive samples/culture isolates [9, 13].

Most NTM disease cases involve species of *M. avium* complex, *M. abscessus*, *M. fortuitum*, and *M. kansasii*. *M. abscessus* is being seen with increasing frequency and is particularly difficult to treat medically [14], because the disease caused by *M. abscessus* often progresses slowly over years and because older adults are typically affected. In more developed countries, *M. avium* and *M. simiae* are responsible for disseminated disease in HIV-infected persons [15]. The HIV era has brought an increase of infection by these opportunistic human pathogens. Nontuberculous mycobacteria are involved in a range of diseases including pulmonary disease, hypersensitivity pneumonitis, cervical lymphadenitis, and disseminated infection. The disseminated infection is generally associated with HIV infection: AIDS and immunosuppression [16]. Though this study did not show any association between the NTM and HIV infection, this could be attributed to the number of patients that did not know their status at the time of specimen collection. In 2008, when patients in this study were being sampled, HIV counseling and testing in Nigeria were not compulsory for TB suspects or patients newly diagnosed with TB. Moreover, in 2007, only 3 percent of health facilities in Nigeria had HIV testing and counseling services [17].

Of the initial 16 NTM isolated in this study, molecular techniques showed that 12 were not members of the genus *Mycobacterium*, despite the fact that they were isolated from sputum smear positive patients. It may be that these organisms are *Nocardia* species or *Rhodococcus equi*, since their microscopic appearance was consistent with AFB. The incidence of nocardiosis especially the former *Nocardia asteroides* complex has been on the increase due to the increase in the number of immunosuppressed patients during recent decades [18]. More than 70% of patients with nocardial infection are immunocompromised, and disseminated nocardiosis is associated with several immunocompromising conditions. More recently, HIV infection has been described as a risk factor for disseminated nocardiosis [19]. Pulmonary nocardiosis is very often misdiagnosed as tuberculosis and treated with antitubercular drugs. Such cases may end fatally [20].

5. Conclusion

The challenge therefore in most African countries, and especially in Nigeria, still remains the introduction in a large scale of laboratory culture for the specific identification of the mycobacteria. The data obtained in this study provide some evidence of the role of nontuberculous AFB organisms and the public health implications of DOTS administration without sputum culture. Sputum culture should be performed in smear positive patients with known HIV positive status or HIV patients with clinical symptoms of tuberculosis, so as to identify the strains involved and thus avoid unnecessary administration of anti-TB drugs with risk of drug toxicity for the patients and increase drug resistance. Half (2/4) of the patients in this study with the identified NTM were HIV positive. Moreover, drug resistance should not be systematically considered as it is currently the case, especially in patients still AFB smear positive following intensive phase treatment in settings devoid of culture facilities, as such patients may be either infected by NTM or AFB not members of the genus mycobacteria.

Acknowledgment

The molecular work was carried out at the Dr. Nalin Rastogi's Mycobacteriology laboratory, Institut Pasteur of Guadeloupe, France.

References

[1] P. C. A. M. Buijtels, M. A. B. Van Der Sande, C. S. De Graaff et al., "Nontuberculous mycobacteria, Zambia," *Emerging Infectious Diseases*, vol. 15, no. 2, pp. 242–249, 2009.

[2] C. L. Chang, T. H. Park, M. N. Kim, N. Y. Lee, H. J. Lee, and J. T. Suh, "Survey on changes in mycobacterial testing practices in Korean laboratories," *Korean Journal of Clinical Microbiology*, vol. 4, pp. 108–114, 2001.

[3] M. N. Kim, S. H. Lee, S. E. Yang, and C. H. Pai, "Mycobacterial testing in hospital laboratories in Korea: results of a survey of 40 university or tertiary-care hospitals," *Korean Journal of Clinical Pathology*, vol. 19, pp. 86–91, 1999.

[4] W. J. Koh and J. Kwon, "Treatment of tuberculosis patients in the private sector in Korea," *Tuberculosis and Respiratory Diseases*, vol. 56, no. 5, pp. 443–449, 2004.

[5] J. J. Yim and S. K. Han, "Diagnosis and treatment of nontuberculous mycobacterial pulmonary diseases," *Journal of Korean Medical Association*, vol. 48, pp. 563–570, 2005.

[6] E. O. Idigbe, C. E. Anyiwo, and D. I. Onwujekwe, "Human pulmonary infections with bovine and typical mycobacteria in Lagos, Nigeria," *Journal of Tropical Medicine and Hygiene*, vol. 89, no. 3, pp. 143–148, 1986.

[7] WHO, *Laboratory Services in Tuberculosis Control. Part III. Culture*, WHO, Geneva, Switzerland, 1998.

[8] B. P. Thumamo, A. E. Asuquo, L. N. Abia-Bassey et al., "Molecular epidemiology and genetic diversity of *Mycobacterium tuberculosis* complex in the Cross River State, Nigeria," *Infection, Genetics and Evolution*, vol. 12, no. 4, pp. 671–677, 2012.

[9] O. Daniel, E. Osman, P. Adebiyi, G. Mourad, E. Declarcq, and R. Bakare, "Non tuberculosis mycobacteria isolates among new and previously treated pulmonary tuberculosis patients in Nigeria," *Asian Pacific Journal of Tropical Disease*, vol. 1, no. 2, pp. 113–115, 2011.

[10] W. J. Koh, O. J. Kwon, C. M. Yu et al., "Recovery rate of nontuberculous mycobacteria from acid-fast-bacilli smear-positive sputum specimens," *Tuberculosis and Respiratory Diseases*, vol. 54, no. 1, pp. 22–32, 2003.

[11] D. Wagner and L. S. Young, "Nontuberculous mycobacterial infections: a clinical review," *Infection*, vol. 32, no. 5, pp. 257–270, 2004.

[12] I. W. Fawcett and B. J. Watkins, "Initial resistance of *Mycobacterium tuberculosis* in Northern Nigeria," *Tubercle*, vol. 57, no. 1, pp. 71–73, 1976.

[13] J. D. Mawak, N. E. Gomwalk, C. S. S. Bello, and Y. T. Kandakai-Olukemi, "Human pulmonary infections with bovine and environment (Atypical) mycobacteria in Jos, Nigeria," *Ghana Medical Journal*, vol. 40, no. 4, pp. 132–136, 2006.

[14] D. E. Griffith, W. M. Girard, and R. J. Wallace, "Clinical features of pulmonary disease caused by rapidly growing mycobacteria: an analysis of 154 patients," *American Review of Respiratory Disease*, vol. 147, no. 5, pp. 1271–1278, 1993.

[15] J. A. Crump, J. Van Ingen, A. B. Morrissey et al., "Invasive disease caused by nontuberculous mycobacteria, Tanzania," *Emerging Infectious Diseases*, vol. 15, no. 1, pp. 53–55, 2009.

[16] D. E. Griffith, T. Aksamit, B. A. Brown-Elliott et al., "An official ATS/IDSA statement: diagnosis, treatment, and prevention of nontuberculous mycobacterial diseases," *American Journal of Respiratory and Critical Care Medicine*, vol. 175, no. 4, pp. 367–416, 2007.

[17] WHO, UNAIDS, UNICEF, "Towards universal access: scaling up priority HIV/AIDS Interventions in the health sector," 2008.

[18] F. Márquez-Diaz, L. E. Soto-Ramirez, and J. Sifuentes-Osornio, "Nocardiasis in patients with HIV infection," *AIDS Patient Care and STDs*, vol. 12, no. 11, pp. 825–832, 1998.

[19] S. V. S. Malladi, P. K. Ankathi, L. Vemu, and N. Rao, "Disseminated nocardiosis in an advanced AIDS patient," *Journal of Association of Physicians of India*, vol. 58, no. 5, pp. 317–318, 2010.

[20] V. Chopra, G. C. Ahir, and M. E. Grossman, "Cutaneous nocardiosis," *Journal of the American Academy of Dermatology*, vol. 48, p. 211, 1985.

5

Prevalence of Extensively Drug Resistant Tuberculosis among Archived Multidrug Resistant Tuberculosis Isolates in Zimbabwe

Tichaona Sagonda,[1,2] **Lucy Mupfumi,**[1] **Rumbidzai Manzou,**[1]
Beauty Makamure,[1] **Mqondisi Tshabalala,**[3] **Lovemore Gwanzura,**[1,2]
Peter Mason,[1,2] **and Reggie Mutetwa**[1]

[1] *Biomedical Research and Training Institute, Harare, Zimbabwe*
[2] *Department of Medical Laboratory Sciences, University of Zimbabwe, Harare, Zimbabwe*
[3] *Immunology Department, College of Health Sciences, University of Zimbabwe, P.O. Box A178,*
  Avondale, Harare, Zimbabwe

Correspondence should be addressed to Tichaona Sagonda; tichaonasagonda@gmail.com

Academic Editor: Paul R. Klatser

We conducted a cross-sectional study of second line drug resistance patterns and genetic diversity of MDR-TB isolates archived at the BRTI-TB Laboratory, Harare, between January 2007 and December 2011. DSTs were performed for second line antituberculosis drugs. XDR-TB strains were defined as MDR-TB strains with resistance to either kanamycin and ofloxacin or capreomycin and ofloxacin. Strain types were identified by spoligotyping. No resistance to any second line drugs was shown in 73% of the isolates, with 23% resistant to one or two drugs but not meeting the definition of XDR-TB. A total of 26 shared types were identified, and 18 (69%) matched preexisting shared types in the current published spoligotype databases. Of the 11 out of 18 clustered SITs, 4 predominant (>6 isolates per shared type) were identified. The most and least abundant types were SIT 1468 (LAM 11-ZWE) with 12 (18%) isolates and SIT 53 (T1) with 6 (9%) isolates, respectively. XDR-TB strains are rare in Zimbabwe, but the high proportion of "pre-XDR-TB" strains and treatment failure cases is of concern. The genetic diversity of the MDR-TB strains showed no significant association between SITs and drug resistance.

1. Introduction

Tuberculosis (TB) is second to human immunodeficiency virus (HIV) as the leading cause of death due to a single infectious agent in the world. Although the global prevalence of TB has been on the decline (from 13 million in 2010 to 12 million in 2011) [1], the burden of TB that remains is still very large. Geographically, America and Europe contribute only 7.3% of the total global burden, largely made possible by huge financial, infrastructural, and manpower resources channeled towards control efforts. However in resource limited settings the picture is drastically different. Asia and Africa contributed 59% and 29% of the global TB burden, respectively. In Asia, India and China have the highest TB burden with the two combined accounting for 38% [1] of the

global TB burden in 2011. In the African region, 9 countries (South Africa, Zimbabwe, DR Congo, Tanzania, Ethiopia, Kenya, Nigeria, Uganda, and Mozambique) are on the 22 high TB burden list with South Africa having the highest TB burden in the region in 2011. During the same period, HIV coinfection was estimated to be 13% of the global TB prevalence, with Sub-Saharan Africa accounting for 80% [1] of this burden. Deaths related to TB/HIV coinfection were estimated to be 0.4 million, about a third of the total TB related deaths reported in 2011 [1].

Extensively drug resistant TB is defined as multidrug resistant TB (MDR-TB) plus resistance to a fluoroquinolone and at least one of three injectable second line drugs (amikacin, kanamycin, or capreomycin). XDR-TB infections are very difficult to treat and characterized by high mortality.

As with any other public health problem, the emergence and spread of XDR-TB are thought to be due to many factors, though shortage of human resources, inappropriate health infrastructure, and insufficient medicines are probably the more significant causes. Globally the number of countries identifying XDR-TB increased from 58 in January 2010 [2] to 84 by the end of 2011 [1]. In 2008 a total of 23 760 XDR-TB cases were reported, with the number increasing to 27 900 in 2011.

Current TB global data estimates that 9.0% of all multidrug resistant TB (MDR-TB) cases are XDR-TB. Former States of the Soviet Union, India, and China have the greatest burden of XDR-TB globally [3–5], with Estonia reporting an XDR-TB burden of 18.7% among MDR-TB cases [1]. In Sub-Saharan Africa, 1st line drug sensitivity test (DST) coverage is very poor and 2nd line DST coverage is virtually nonexistent at national level. In 2011, it was estimated that only 0.2% of the 2.3 million new TB cases reported in Sub-Saharan Africa had a DST result [1]. To date only 16/53 African countries have reported at least one case of XDR-TB, the majority of which were from independent research activities rather than nationally acquired data. South Africa currently accounts for the highest XDR-TB in the region with outbreaks being reported in various provinces since 2006 [1, 6].

To date Zimbabwe has not reported any cases of XDR-TB, which is unusual given that four of her neighbors had reported at least one case of XDR-TB by late 2011 [1, 7]. Given the large population movements between Zimbabwe and her neighbors that resulted from the Economic Crisis of 2006–2008, it is expected that XDR-TB be reported in Zimbabwe. The lack of data on XDR-TB trends in the country could be a result of the poor DST coverage (currently 0.8 per 5 million) and the lack of second line DST in our TB culture laboratories [1]. Currently, there are two laboratories with TB culture facilities: The National TB Reference Laboratory (NTBRL) in Bulawayo and The National Microbiology Reference Laboratory (NMRL), TB section, in Harare.

2. Materials and Methods

2.1. Study Design.
This was a cross-sectional study where all available archived MDR-TB isolates were retrieved from the BRTI/NMRL TB Laboratory for further analysis.

2.2. Isolate Source.
A record review of laboratory DST records was done to find MDR-TB isolates identified at the BRTI/NMRL TB Laboratory between January 2007 and December 2011. The list of MDR-TB isolates generated from the record review was used to locate and retrieve the archived isolates form the laboratory repository. Only the first MDR isolate of a patient was included, excluding multiple isolates form the same patient. All of the available isolates were retrieved. Another record review of "request for examination" forms submitted to the laboratory along with the original patient specimen was done to collect patient demographics. Data on age, gender, TB treatment history, and province of origin were collected using a coded form.

2.3. MDR-TB Isolate Recovery from Storage Media.
Isolates were retrieved from the freezer and allowed to thaw to room temperature. Two loops full of the Trypticase Soy Broth (TSB), per isolate, were inoculated onto plain LJ slopes and incubated at 37°C. Slopes were incubated for a maximum of 8 weeks and checked weekly for growth. Pure colonies of positive isolates were harvested by scraping pure colonies of MTB from LJ slopes to use them as inoculum for 2nd line DST. The remaining pure colonies were harvested and stored in 0.5 mL of sterile distilled water at −80°C for later use in DNA extraction.

2.4. Second Line DST on 7H10 Middlebrook Agar.
Second line DST of revived isolates was performed using the proportion method on 7H10 Middlebrook agar [8]. The second line drugs used were capreomycin, kanamycin, ethionamide, and ofloxacin. One loopful of MTB colonies was added to 4.5 mL of 20% Tween 80 containing glass beads and placed on a vortex for 1-2 mins until a turbidity equal to number 1 McFarland's standard was obtained. A volume of 0.5 mL of the suspension was used to make serial dilutions of 10^{-1}, 10^{-2}, 10^{-3}, and 10^{-4} for each isolate. The 10^{-4} and 10^{-3} serial dilutions were inoculated onto two plain media quadrants (control) and the 10^{-2} dilution was used to inoculate the quadrants with the drug filled media. Each inoculated Petri dish was sealed in a polythene bag to maintain moisture, incubated at 37°C for a maximum of 4 weeks, and checked for growth weekly. Growth was indicated by the presence of smooth straw colored colonies. Resistance to drugs was interpreted as growth on drug filled media that was significantly more than growth of the 10^{-3} and 10^{-4} serial dilutions of the same isolate on drug-free media.

2.5. DNA Extraction.
To extract genomic DNA for use in spoligotyping, the frozen regrown MDR-TB isolates were defrosted on a thermomixer at 60°C. 70 μL of 10% SDS (Sigma, USA) and 50 μL of 10 mg/mL proteinase K (Sigma, USA) were added to the thawed sample and incubated for 1 hour at 60°C at 400 rpm on a thermomixer. 100 μL of 5 M NaCl and cetyltrimethylammonium bromide (CTAB) (preheated to 60°C in water bath) was added and mixed by inversion before further incubation for 1 hour at 60°C and 400 rpm. The mix was then incubated at −70°C for 15 minutes before being allowed to thaw and reincubated for 15 minutes at 60°C and 400 rpm. 700 μL of chloroform/isoamyl alcohol (Sigma, USA) (24 : 1) was added and the mixture was centrifuged for 10 mins at 13,000 rpm. The resulting upper aqueous phase was transferred into a clean tube containing 700 μL of cold isopropanol (Sigma, USA) and incubated at 4°C overnight. The next day the solution was centrifuged for 10 minutes at 13,000 rpm and the supernatant was discarded. The tube was washed with 100 μL of 80% ethanol (Sigma, USA) by centrifuging for 10 minutes at 13,000 rpm. The supernatant was discarded and the pellet DNA pellet was air-dried before being resuspended in 50 μL of DNase-free water and kept at −40°C.

2.6. Spoligotyping.
Spoligotyping of the MDR-TB isolates was performed using the spoligotyping kit from Ocimum

TABLE 1: MDR patient demographics.

Characteristics	Total n (%)	Routine specimens n (%)	Study specimens n (%)
	86	42 (48.8)	44 (51.2)
Gender			
Male	32 (37.2)	14 (33.3)	18 (40.9)
Age			
Median (Q1–Q3)	33 (25–40)	35 (31–45)	27.5 (24–35)
1st line resistance profile			
H + R only	24 (29.7)	4 (10.5)	20 (45.5)
H + R + E only	5 (6.1)	4 (10.5)	1 (2.3)
H + R + S only	8 (9.8)	5 (13.2)	3 (6.8)
H + R + E + S	45 (54.5)	25 (65.8)	20 (45.5)
TB treatment history			
New TB cases	3 (3.5)	—	3 (6.8)
Treatment failure case	33 (38.4)	17 (40.5)	16 (36.4)
TB relapse case	7 (8.1)	4 (9.5)	3 (6.8)
Treatment defaulter	1 (1.2)	—	1 (2.3)

H: isoniazid, R: rifampicin, E: ethambutol, and S: streptomycin.

BioSolutions (India) as previously described [9]. The spoligotype signatures that were generated were coded into binary format using the following codes: 1 = black dot and 0 = no black dot. The binary codes generated were entered into an Excel spreadsheet and compared with a published online spoligotype database MIRU-VNTRplus [10] where a search by similarity was performed to assign spoligotype based strain lineages and to search for similar types in the database.

3. Results

A total of 86 MDR-TB isolates were identified and retrieved from the BRTI/NMRL TB archive. Of these 42 (49%) were isolated from routine specimens (sent in from government referral hospitals) and 44 (51%) were isolated from study specimens (sent in from TB research study sites). Laboratory records of all 86 identified isolates were investigated for geodemographic data. Twenty (23%) isolates failed to grow after subculture onto fresh LJ media, and these were excluded from second line DST and spoligotyping experiments.

3.1. MDR-TB Patient Demographics. The study population consisted of 32 (37%) males and 36 (42%) females, with gender data not available for 18 (20.9%) of the patients. The median age and interquartile range (IQR) was 33 (25–40) years, with data on age missing for 23% of the patients. A total of 29 (34%) isolates were obtained from patients residing in Harare Metropolitan province; 11 (13%) were isolated from Manicaland province, 7 (8%) from Mashonaland West province, 8 (9%) from Mashonaland West province, 4 (5%) from Midlands province, 1 (1%) each from Matabeleland North and Bulawayo Metropolitan provinces, and 5 (6%) from patients in Matabeleland South province (see Table 1).

Fourteen (16%) of the isolates were resistant to isoniazid and rifampicin alone, 4 (5%) were resistant to isoniazid,

rifampicin, and ethambutol only, and 7 (8%) were resistant to isoniazid, rifampicin, and streptomycin only, with 46 (54%) being resistant to all four first line TB drugs. New TB cases accounted for 3 (4%) of the isolates, with 33 (38%) coming from treatment failure cases, 7 (8%) from TB relapse cases, and 1 (1%) from a treatment defaulter.

A total of 66 (77%) isolates were successfully subcultured onto LJ and subsequently tested for second line drug resistance. No resistance to any of the second line drugs was seen in 48 (73%) of the isolates. Resistance to kanamycin and ethionamide was seen in 3 (5%) of the isolates, whilst 1 (2%) isolate was resistant to ethionamide and ofloxacin. Fourteen isolates (21%) were resistant to ethionamide only.

3.2. Spoligotyping. A total of 24 SITs were identified and 18 (69%) matched preexisting shared types in the database. The remaining 6 shared types did not match any isolates in the MIRU-VNTRplus database [10]. The majority (11/18) of the identified shared types were clustered (2 or more isolates with same SIT), and of these 4 predominant (>6 isolates per shared type) clusters were identified. The largest were SIT 1468 (LAM 11-ZWE) with 12 (18%) isolates, SIT 1 (Beijing) with 8 (12%), SIT 60 (LAM 4) with 7 (11%), and SIT 53 (T1) with 6 (9%) isolates (Table 2). These 4 predominant shared types account for half of all the isolates that were genotyped. Three isolates with orphan shared types were identified as belonging to the East African Indian family, 3 from the LAM family, 1 from the Delhi/CAS family, and 1 from the Uganda 1 family.

3.3. Measures of Association. Table 3 shows spoligotype based MTB strain lineages stratified by 1st line DST pattern and TB treatment history. There was no significant association between MTB strain lineages and 1st line DST pattern (*P* value 0.57) and between MTB strain lineages and TB treatment history (*P* value 0.88).

TABLE 2: Spoligotyping signatures of MDR-TB isolates.

Shared international type (SIT)	Subclade	Octal codes	Total n (%)
1	Beijing	000000000003771	8 (11.9)
21	CAS1 KILI	703377400001771	2 (3.0)
25	CAS1 Delhi	703777740003171	1 (1.5)
34	S	776377777760771	3 (4.5)
37	T 3	777737777760771	2 (3.0)
42	LAM 9	777777607760771	3 (4.5)
53	T 1	777777777760771	6 (9.0)
54	MANU 2	777777777763771	1 (1.5)
59	LAM 11-ZWE	777777606060771	2 (3.0)
60	LAM 4	777777607760731	7 (10.5)
73	T 2	777737777760731	1 (1.5)
95	LAM 6	777777607560731	4 (6.0)
398	LAM 9	777777607760631	1 (1.5)
583	MANU 2	777737777763771	1 (1.5)
753	LAM 9	477777607760771	2 (3.0)
813	LAM 11-ZWE	777777606060631	1 (1.5)
1466	LAM 11-ZWE	757777606060771	1 (1.5)
1468	LAM 11-ZWE	077777606060671	12 (17.9)

TABLE 3: MTB strain lineages stratified by 1st line DST and TB treatment history.

	Total n (%)	Indo-Oceanic n (%)	East Asian n (%)	East African Indian n (%)	Euro-American n (%)	P value
1st line DST pattern[#]						
HR resistant	19 (28.4)	1 (5.3)	2 (10.5)	3 (15.8)	13 (68.4)	
HRE resistant	4 (6.0)	1 (25.0)	—	—	3 (75.0)	0.57
HRS resistant	5 (7.5)	—	—	1 (20.0)	4 (80.0)	
HRES resistant	38 (56.7)	1 (2.6)	6 (15.8)	—	30 (78.9)	
TB treatment history[*]						
New TB cases	3 (4.5)	—	—	—	3 (5.9)	
Treatment failure	27 (40.3)	1 (3.7)	2 (7.4)	3 (11.1)	20 (74.1)	0.88
TB relapse	3 (4.5)	—	—	—	3 (5.9)	

[#]$n = 1$ missing, [*]$n = 34$ missing, H: isoniazid, R: rifampicin, E: ethambutol, and S: streptomycin.

4. Discussion

The emergence of MDR-TB and XDR-TB is a major global health issue, as high rates of DR-TB have serious consequences for TB control activities, especially in high TB and HIV burden settings, where high mortality and morbidity have been strongly associated with XDR-TB/HIV coinfection. In 2011, global TB data reported an estimated 9.0% of all MDR-TB cases where XDR-TB however very little data is available on DR-TB in Africa due to limited capacity of laboratories in that region to perform DST. Considering that Africa contains 25% of the global TB burden, 80% of which is HIV coinfected, data on DR-TB prevalence in the region is thus essential to guide planning of TB control and management policies.

The TB patients whose MDR-TB isolates were analyzed in this study were predominately young, with a median age of 33 years (IQR: 25–40). Other studies in Africa show a similar age distribution [11, 12] among MDR-TB patients. Studies in Asia also report similar findings with MDR-TB patients having a mean age of 33. Drug resistance data stratified by age is very important in surveillance of drug resistant trends in a setting since a high proportion of drug resistant cases in young age groups could be indicative of recent transmission. In older age groups, high proportions of drug resistance could be an indicator of reactivation of old infections.

In this study, high proportion of "request for examination" forms omitted data on age (23.3%), gender (20.9%), geographic origin (24%), and TB treatment history (48.8%), highlighting poor data collection by nurses and clinicians requesting TB examination for their patients. This presents a challenge to effective monitoring and surveillance of drug resistance patterns and trends, as patient biographical and clinical data is essential in understanding the factors driving TB and possible risk factors for the disease. Effective reporting of such data reduces the need for resource limited countries, such as Zimbabwe, to conduct periodical surveys, which are costly and labour intensive. Routinely collected data is an easy and efficacious way of monitoring TB drug resistance patterns and trends over time, without the need for expensive surveys.

In our current study, the largest group (38%) of MDR-TB isolates was from TB treatment failure cases. By the end of 2012, it was estimated that 20% of global MDR-TB cases were from previously treated TB cases [1]. The proportion of MDR-TB among previously treated cases shown by this study is higher than the global average and this could be explained by a number of factors. The MDR-TB isolates analyzed in this study were archived between January 2007 and December 2011, a period during which Zimbabwe was going through an economic decline. This economic crisis affected health service delivery in the country. Shortage of drugs and trained personnel could have led to the high number of TB patients failing treatment. Zimbabwe is also a high HIV burden nation, with more than 70% of TB cases in the country being HIV coinfected. Studies have shown that, due to the immune compromised state of HIV patients, they are likely to have recurrent TB episodes. HIV patients receiving ART are also at high risk of poor TB treatment adherence due to the high pill burden they take. Some ART drugs have also been documented to have adverse outcomes when administered with anti-TB drugs. These factors combined increase the risk of failing treatment and developing MDR-TB.

A large proportion (53%) of the MDR-TB isolates showed resistance to all four first line drugs (isoniazid, rifampicin, streptomycin, and ethambutol). Poor patient adherence and interrupted drug supplies have been shown to contribute to the emergence of MDR-TB strains. Patients with such organisms pose a challenge for management and treatment to National TB programs. The internationally accepted practice when treating MDR-TB cases is to base the second line regimen on DST results [13]. Having a large proportion of MDR-TB patients resistant to all 1st line drugs places a huge financial burden on the nation as 2nd line drugs are often more expensive, require extended treatment periods, and are often toxic [13–15].

In this study, high proportion of "request for examination" forms omitted data on age (23.3%), gender (20.9%), and TB treatment history (48.8%), highlighting poor data collection by nurses and clinicians requesting TB examination for their patients. This presents a challenge to effective monitoring and surveillance of drug resistance patterns and trends, as patient biographical and clinical data is critical in understanding the factors driving TB and possible risk factors for the disease. Effective reporting of such data reduces the need for resource limited countries, such as Zimbabwe, to conduct periodical surveys, which are costly and labour intensive. Routinely collected data is an easy and efficacious

way of monitoring TB drug resistance patterns and trends over time, without the need for expensive surveys.

XDR-TB strains are defined as MTB strains that are resistant to isoniazid and rifampicin (i.e., MDR-TB), plus resistance to a fluoroquinolone and any second line anti-TB injectable aminoglycoside. In this study, the drugs evaluated were ofloxacin, aminoglycosides, kanamycin, and capreomycin. Therefore in the context of our study an XDR-TB strain would have been resistant either to kanamycin and ofloxacin or to capreomycin and ofloxacin. Our study did not identify such resistance patterns, and so there were no XDR-TB strains. A large proportion (73%) of the MDR-TB isolates showed susceptibility to all 2nd line drugs. The remaining 27% of the isolates were shown to be resistant to one or more of the 2nd line drugs but did not meet the definition of XDR-TB. TB strains that are resistant to isoniazid and rifampicin and either a fluoroquinolone or an aminoglycoside, but not both, are termed "pre-XDR-TB" strains.

By late 2011, all of Zimbabwe's neighbors (Botswana, Mozambique, South Africa, and Zambia) had identified at least one XDR-TB strain [1]. Due to the economic situation in Zimbabwe between 2007 and 2009, there was a lot of population movement to and from her neighbors, especially South Africa which is one of the high MDR-TB burden countries and has reported a number of XDR-TB outbreaks [12, 16–18]. Therefore this study hypothesizes that XDR-TB strains could have been imported into the country during this period and thus would be identified among MDR-TB isolates archived during that time. However this study's failure to identify any XDR-TB strains could be due to a number of factors.

There has been much debate on the diagnostic accuracy and reproducibility of some of the methods used to perform 2nd line DST [19–21]. This lack of consensus has led to the absence of an absolute gold standard for 2nd line DST. Second line DST is especially difficult since the critical concentrations of some of the 2nd line drugs are very close to the minimum inhibitory concentrations (MICs); hence the changes in MIC associated with resistance are very small [20, 22, 23]. A lot of research is needed towards standardizing the 2nd line MICs for the various DST methods available. The proportion method on 7H10 Middlebrook has been the gold standard for 2nd line DST in Europe and in America in the past 20 years, but recent WHO guidelines on 2nd line DST recommend the MGIT based DST method [13, 24–26].

This study showed a large proportion (27%) of pre-XDR-TB strains. Globally, the number of pre-XDR-TB strains being identified has increased. A recent study in Nigeria showed a pre-XDR prevalence of 17% [11]. Another study in India reported a pre-XDR-TB prevalence of 42% among MDR-TB cases [27]. The emergence of pre-XDR-TB is a major concern to the TB control program in Zimbabwe, as this highlights possible effects of the use of FQs and aminoglycosides in the treatment of nontubercular infections. However, the majority (14/18) of the pre-XDR-TB strains identified in the study were resistant to ethionamide. There are a number of issues concerning the use of ethionamide in 2nd line DST. The MIC of ethionamide has yet to be standardized [23, 28] and thus the reproducibility of its DST results is questionable. Also the thermoliable nature of ethionamide makes it prone to degradation during media preparation, thus increasing the likelihood of false positive results.

This study also related genetic diversity to the sample of MDR-TB isolates determined by genotyping. A total of 66 MDR-TB isolates were typed using spoligotyping and presented the LAM spoligotype family as the predominant strain type (50%), followed by the T family (13.6%) and finally by the Beijing family (11.9%). The LAM family showed the highest diversity with 9 SITs, LAM 11 ZWE (SIT 1468) being the predominant with 17.9%. The T family had 3 SITs (73, 53, 37), and the Beijing family strains all had SIT 1.

The predominance of the LAM 11 ZWE (SIT 1468) was expected as this SIT has been described as the predominant strain circulating in Zimbabwe by previous studies [29] while the LAM spoligotype family has also been described as the predominant strain circulating in countries neighboring Zimbabwe [7, 29–31]. The presence of the T family was also expected as it is one of the 3 strains reported by the literature to predominate TB infection in Africa [32], along with the Haarlem and LAM families. Studies describing diversity of MTB strain circulating in different parts of Africa also show similar predominance of the LAM spoligotype [33–35], though having different SITs.

Interestingly, the Beijing family had not been seen before in studies describing MTB strains circulating in Zimbabwe. This study however is expected to observe Beijing strains, as the global distribution of this strain is reported to be on the increase [36, 37]. This strain type has also been reported in countries neighboring Zimbabwe, with South Africa reporting a significant proportion of these strains having been isolated from MDR/XDR-TB cases [31, 38].

Much has been postulated in recent publications regarding the association between the Beijing strain and drug resistance [39–42], with observations showing increased bacterial fitness of drug resistant Beijing strains [39, 40]. However, mutations on the MTB genome causing drug resistance on Beijing strains result in reduced fitness cost [41, 43]. This reduced fitness cost explains why the Beijing strain has not taken over as the predominant strain in most drug resistant TB outbreaks and TB endemic populations. Interestingly this study showed that all strains classified as Beijing had the same SIT, which might show the same source of infection, or that the Beijing strain circulating in Zimbabwe is highly conserved resulting in low diversity of the family.

This study showed no significant associations when MTB strain types were stratified by TB treatment history ($P = 0.88$) and first line drug susceptibility profile ($P = 0.57$). These results were expected as no significant association between a particular strain type and drug resistance has been reported. The study was also limited in its power to detect a significant association between strain type and drug resistance due to the small sample size used in this study.

5. Conclusion

Despite the small sample size to generalize the study results, this study failed to identify any XDR-TB isolates, but the high proportion (27%) of pre-XDR-TB could be a possible indicator of the future emergence of XDR-TB in Zimbabwe. The SITs described in this study were not different from those reported previously in Zimbabwe. The study also failed to identify SITs reported to have caused XDR-TB and MDR-TB in neighboring countries.

Acknowledgments

Tichaona Sagonda was supported by the Fogarty International Center, National Institutes of Health (NIH-USA), through the International Clinical, Operational and Health Services and Training Award (ICOHRTA) Programme, BIMR (Award no. U2RTW007367). Tichaona Sagonda also received laboratory training from Professor R. J. Wilkinson, CIDRI Group, Institute of Infectious Diseases and Molecular Medicine, University of Cape Town, South Africa.

References

[1] WHO, *Global Tuberculosis Report*, 2012.

[2] WHO, *Multidrug and Extensively Drug-Resistant TB (M/XDR-TB)*, Global Report on Surveillance and Response, 2010.

[3] A. Ignatova, S. Dubiley, V. Stepanshina, and I. Shemyakin, "Predominance of multi-drug-resistant LAM and Beijing family strains among *Mycobacterium tuberculosis* isolates recovered from prison inmates in Tula Region, Russia," *Journal of Medical Microbiology*, vol. 55, no. 10, pp. 1413–1418, 2006.

[4] A. Bhargava, L. Pinto, and M. Pai, "Mismanagement of tuberculosis in India: causes , consequences , and the way forward," *Hypothesis*, vol. 9, pp. 1–13, 2012.

[5] C. H. Liu, H. M. Li, L. Li et al., "Anti-tuberculosis drug resistance patterns and trends in a tuberculosis referral hospital, 1997–2009," *Epidemiology and Infection*, vol. 139, no. 12, pp. 1909–1918, 2011.

[6] N. R. Gandhi, P. Nunn, K. Dheda et al., "Multidrug-resistant and extensively drug-resistant tuberculosis: a threat to global control of tuberculosis," *The Lancet*, vol. 6736, pp. 1–14, 2010.

[7] S. O. Viegas, A. MacHado, R. Groenheit et al., "Molecular diversity of *Mycobacterium tuberculosis* isolates from patients with pulmonary tuberculosis in Mozambique," *BMC Microbiology*, vol. 10, article 195, 2010.

[8] C. A. Sanders, R. R. Nieda, and E. P. Desmond, "Validation of the use of middlebrook 7H10 agar, BACTEC MGIT 960, and BACTEC 460 12B media for testing the susceptibility of *Mycobacterium tuberculosis* to levofloxacin," *Journal of Clinical Microbiology*, vol. 42, no. 11, pp. 5225–5228, 2004.

[9] M. Goyal, N. A. Saunders, and J. D. van Embden, "Differentiation of *Mycobacterium tuberculosis* isolates by spoligotyping and IS6110 restriction fragment length polymorphism," *Journal of Clinical Microbiology*, vol. 35, no. 3, pp. 647–651, 1997.

[10] C. Allix-Béguec, D. Harmsen, T. Weniger, P. Supply, and S. Niemann, "Evaluation and strategy for use of MIRU-VNTRplus, a multifunctional database for online analysis of genotyping data and phylogenetic identification of *Mycobacterium tuberculosis*

complex isolates," *Journal of Clinical Microbiology*, vol. 46, no. 8, pp. 2692–2699, 2008.

[11] O. Daniel, E. Osman, O. Oladimeji, and O. G. Dairo, "Pre-extensive drug resistant tuberculosis (Pre-XDR-TB) among MDR-TB patents in Nigeria," *Global Advanced Research Journal of Microbiology*, vol. 2, pp. 22–25, 2013.

[12] H. S. Cox, C. McDermid, V. Azevedo et al., "Epidemic levels of drug resistant tuberculosis (MDR and XDR-TB) in a high HIV prevalence setting in Khayelitsha, South Africa," *PLoS ONE*, vol. 5, no. 11, Article ID e13901, 2010.

[13] I. G. Sia and M. L. Wieland, *Current Concepts in the Management of Tuberculosis*, 2011.

[14] H. S. Schaaf, A. P. Moll, and K. Dheda, "Multidrug- and extensively drug-resistant tuberculosis in Africa and South America: epidemiology, diagnosis and management in adults and children," *Clinics in Chest Medicine*, vol. 30, no. 4, pp. 667–683, 2009.

[15] F. Drobniewski, Y. Balabanova, and R. Coker, "Clinical features, diagnosis, and management of multiple drug—resistant tuberculosis since 2002," *Current Opinion in Pulmonary Medicine*, vol. 10, no. 3, pp. 211–217, 2004.

[16] C. L. Kvasnovsky, J. P. Cegielski, R. Erasmus, N. O. Siwisa, K. Thomas, and M. L. V. Der Walt, "Extensively drug-resistant TB in Eastern Cape, South Africa: high mortality in HIV-negative and HIV-positive patients," *Journal of Acquired Immune Deficiency Syndromes*, vol. 57, no. 2, pp. 146–152, 2011.

[17] S. V. Shenoi, R. P. Brooks, R. Barbour et al., "Survival from XDR-TB is associated with modifiable clinical characteristics in rural South Africa," *PLoS ONE*, vol. 7, no. 3, Article ID e31786, 2012.

[18] N. R. Gandhi, N. S. Shah, J. R. Andrews et al., "HIV coinfection in multidrug- and extensively drug-resistant tuberculosis results in high early mortality," *The American Journal of Respiratory and Critical Care Medicine*, vol. 181, no. 1, pp. 80–86, 2010.

[19] J. Pasipanodya and S. Srivastava, "New susceptibility breakpoints and the regional variability of MIC distribution in *Mycobacterium tuberculosis* isolates," *Antimicrobial Agents and Chemotherapy*, vol. 56, no. 5428, 2012.

[20] G. Kahlmeter and S. E. Hoffner, "Challenging a dogma: antimicrobial susceptibility testing breakpoints for *Mycobacterium tuberculosis*," *Bulletin of the World Health Organization*, vol. 90, no. 9, pp. 693–698, 2012.

[21] G. Kahlmeter, D. F. J. Brown, F. W. Goldstein et al., "European Committee on Antimicrobial Susceptibility Testing (EUCAST) technical notes on antimicrobial susceptibility testing," *Clinical Microbiology and Infection*, vol. 12, no. 6, pp. 501–503, 2006.

[22] T. Gumbo, "New susceptibility breakpoints for first-line antituberculosis drugs based on antimicrobial pharmacokinetic/pharmacodynamic science and population pharmacokinetic variability," *Antimicrobial Agents and Chemotherapy*, vol. 54, no. 4, pp. 1484–1491, 2010.

[23] S. J. Kim, "Drug-susceptibility testing in tuberculosis: methods and reliability of results," *European Respiratory Journal*, vol. 25, no. 3, pp. 564–569, 2005.

[24] A. Martin, A. von Groll, K. Fissette, J. C. Palomino, F. Varaine, and F. Portaels, "Rapid detection of *Mycobacterium tuberculosis* resistance to second-line drugs by use of the manual mycobacterium growth indicator tube system," *Journal of Clinical Microbiology*, vol. 46, no. 12, pp. 3952–3956, 2008.

[25] A. Martin, P. M. Waweru, F. B. Okatch et al., "Implementation of the thin layer agar method for diagnosis of smear-negative pulmonary tuberculosis in a setting with a high prevalence of human immunodeficiency virus infection in Homa Bay, Kenya," *Journal of Clinical Microbiology*, vol. 47, no. 8, pp. 2632–2634, 2009.

[26] J. O'Grady, M. Maeurer, P. Mwaba et al., "New and improved diagnostics for detection of drug-resistant pulmonary tuberculosis," *Current Opinion in Pulmonary Medicine*, vol. 17, no. 3, pp. 134–141, 2011.

[27] A. Jain, P. Dixit, and R. Prasad, "Pre-XDR & XDR in MDR and Ofloxacin and Kanamycin resistance in non-MDR Mycobacterium tuberculosis isolates," *Journal of Tuberculosis*, vol. 92, pp. 404–406, 2012.

[28] E. C. Böttger, "The ins and outs of *Mycobacterium tuberculosis* drug susceptibility testing," *Clinical Microbiology and Infection*, vol. 17, no. 8, pp. 1128–1134, 2011.

[29] V. Chihota, L. Apers, S. Mungofa et al., "Predominance of a single genotype of *Mycobacterium tuberculosis* in regions of Southern Africa," *International Journal of Tuberculosis and Lung Disease*, vol. 11, no. 3, pp. 311–318, 2007.

[30] S. Lockman, J. D. Sheppard, C. R. Braden et al., "Molecular and conventional epidemiology of *Mycobacterium tuberculosis* in Botswana: a population-based prospective study of 301 pulmonary tuberculosis patients," *Journal of Clinical Microbiology*, vol. 39, no. 3, pp. 1042–1047, 2001.

[31] E. M. Streicher, R. M. Warren, C. Kewley et al., "Genotypic and phenotypic characterization of drug-resistant *Mycobacterium tuberculosis* isolates from rural districts of the Western Cape Province of South Africa," *Journal of Clinical Microbiology*, vol. 42, no. 2, pp. 891–894, 2004.

[32] E. M. Streicher, T. C. Victor, G. van der Spuy et al., "Spoligotype signatures in the *Mycobacterium tuberculosis* complex," *Journal of Clinical Microbiology*, vol. 45, no. 1, pp. 237–240, 2007.

[33] A. Ani, T. Bruvik, Y. Okoh et al., "Genetic diversity of *Mycobacterium tuberculosis* Complex in Jos, Nigeria," *BMC Infectious Diseases*, vol. 10, article 189, 2010.

[34] N. Saleri, G. Badoum, M. Ouedraogo et al., "Extensively drug-resistant tuberculosis, Burkina Faso," *Emerging Infectious Diseases*, vol. 16, no. 5, pp. 840–842, 2010.

[35] L. Tazi, J. El Baghdadi, S. Lesjean et al., "Genetic diversity and population structure of *Mycobacterium tuberculosis* in Casablanca, a Moroccan City with high incidence of tuberculosis," *Journal of Clinical Microbiology*, vol. 42, no. 1, pp. 461–466, 2004.

[36] J. R. Glynn, J. Whiteley, P. J. Bifani, K. Kremer, and D. Van Soolingen, "Worldwide occurrence of Beijing/W strains of *Mycobacterium tuberculosis*: a systematic review," *Emerging Infectious Diseases*, vol. 8, no. 8, pp. 843–849, 2002.

[37] B. Lu, P. Zhao, B. Liu et al., "Genetic diversity of *Mycobacterium tuberculosis* isolates from Beijing, China assessed by Spoligotyping, LSPs and VNTR profiles," *BMC Infectious Diseases*, vol. 12, article 372, 2012.

[38] C. K. Mlambo, R. M. Warren, X. Poswa, T. C. Victor, A. G. Duse, and E. Marais, "Genotypic diversity of extensively drug-resistant tuberculosis (XDR-TB) in South Africa," *International Journal of Tuberculosis and Lung Disease*, vol. 12, no. 1, pp. 99–104, 2008.

[39] M. Y. Lipin, V. N. Stepanshina, I. G. Shemyakin, and T. M. Shinnick, "Association of specific mutations in katG, rpoB, rps L and rrs genes with spoligotypes of multidrug-resistant *Mycobacterium tuberculosis* isolates in Russia," *Clinical Microbiology and Infection*, vol. 13, no. 6, pp. 620–626, 2007.

[40] D. A. Duong, N. T. H. Duyen, N. T. N. Lan et al., "Beijing genotype of *Mycobacterium tuberculosis* is significantly associated with high-level fluoroquinolone resistance in Vietnam," *Antimicrobial Agents and Chemotherapy*, vol. 53, no. 11, pp. 4835–4839, 2009.

[41] P. Bhatter, A. Chatterjee, and N. Mistry, "*Mycobacterium tuberculosis* "Beijing" epidemics: a race against mutations?" *Tuberculosis*, vol. 92, no. 1, pp. 92–94, 2012.

[42] J. Zhang, S. Heng, S. Le Moullec et al., "A first assessment of the genetic diversity of *Mycobacterium tuberculosis* complex in Cambodia," *BMC Infectious Diseases*, vol. 11, article 42, 2011.

[43] O. S. Toungoussova, D. A. Caugant, P. Sandven, A. O. Mariandyshev, and G. Bjune, "Impact of drug resistance on fitness of *Mycobacterium tuberculosis* strains of the W-Beijing genotype," *FEMS Immunology and Medical Microbiology*, vol. 42, no. 3, pp. 281–290, 2004.

6

Extensive Genetic Diversity among Clinical Isolates of *Mycobacterium tuberculosis* in Central Province of Iran

Saman Soleimanpour,[1,2] **Daryoush Hamedi Asl,**[1]
Keyvan Tadayon,[1,3] **Ali Asghar Farazi,**[4] **Rouhollah Keshavarz,**[1] **Kioomars Soleymani,**[1]
Fereshteh Sadat Seddighinia,[1] **and Nader Mosavari**[1]

[1] *PPD Tuberculin Department, Razi Vaccine & Serum Research Institute, Karaj 3197619751, Iran*
[2] *Antimicrobial Resistance Research Center, Mashhad University of Medical Sciences, Mashhad, Iran*
[3] *Aerobic Bacterial Research and Vaccine Production Department, Razi Vaccine & Serum Research Institute, Karaj, Iran*
[4] *Arak University of Medical Sciences, Arak, Iran*

Correspondence should be addressed to Nader Mosavari; n.mosavari@rvsri.ac.ir

Academic Editor: José R. Lapa e Silva

Human tuberculosis caused by *Mycobacterium tuberculosis* (*Mtb*) remains a significant disease in many countries. According to Iran's borders with Afghanistan and Pakistan, which are among the 22 high burden countries around the world, this study was conducted to analyze the current molecular epidemiology of tuberculosis and survey genetic diversity of *Mtb* strains in Markazi Province in center of Iran. In this experimental study, 75 sputum specimens and one gastric lavage from all smear-positive TB patients admitted to the public hospitals across the Markazi Province were cultured on specific mycobacterial culture media. Genomic DNA was digested by *Pvu*II and transferred to positively charged nylon membrane by southern blotting method and hybridization by PGRS and DR probes. Genotyping of the isolates by PGRS-RFLP and DR-RFLP displayed a wide range of genetic diversity as 25 and 26 genotypes were identified, respectively. Generally speaking, despite the relatively limited number of isolates in the study, high age of patients and also large heterogeneity found in the setting are both in opposition to active circulation of *Mtb* strains between patients under study either Iranian or Afghan nationals. Thus, it seems that reactivation of latent infection has had the main role in the spread of tuberculosis.

1. Introduction

Globally, tuberculosis (TB) remains one of the most prevalent and epidemiologically important diseases of all ages. For three decades since its initial introduction, molecular genotyping has provided the medical community with an enormous load of epidemiological information about TB. This has been materialized through help in identification of index (source) cases in TB outbreaks, detection of TB transmissions, differentiation between cases of relapse and reinfection, and finally effective assessment in antibiotic therapy. According to the World Health Organization report, the prevalence of tuberculosis in Iran in 2012 was estimated to be 33 cases per 100000 people [1]. Geographical spread, racial diversity with large differences in income, and socioeconomic status of people have changed this index in geographic regions and provinces in Iran. In Markazi Province, in 2006, prevalence of TB was estimated to be 10.3 cases per 100000 people which is lower than the national average [2]. Factors such as being neighbors with Tehran Province, located on the main road access to the western areas of the country and a large number of traditional manufacturing and service units that are good purpose of non-Iranian workforce including labor migrants and Afghan asylum seekers, lead to the fact that the province can accommodate a significant number of non-Iranian nationals. On the other hand, political adversity, weak central government, civil wars, terrorism, poverty, and weak health systems for a long time affect neighboring countries of Iran and the presence of nearly 4 million foreign nationals from these countries (about 6 percent of the current population of Iran) has put additional pressure on the structure of Iran health care. As a result, the transmission of infectious diseases like tuberculosis from these countries has changed epidemiological features of these diseases in Iran [3]. Despite numerous studies on molecular epidemiology of tuberculosis in different regions of Iran, there is little information in this regard in Markazi Province in center of Iran. Therefore, the present study was conducted in order to analyze the current epidemiology of TB in this province.

2. Materials and Methods

2.1. Sampling. 75 sputum specimens and one gastric lavage were collected during the period of February 2010 to September 2011 from all smear-positive TB patients (e.g., 72 Iranians and 4 Afghans) admitted to the public hospitals across the Markazi Province, center of Iran.

This study was approved by the Ethics Committee of Arak University of Medical Sciences, Arak, Iran. Study subjects were recruited after providing written informed consent.

2.2. Preferential Growth of Bacteria on LJ Medium Containing Glycerol as Compared with Pyruvate LJ Medium. The collected specimens were processed and cultured on glycerinated and also pyruvate traditional Lowenstein-Jensen (LJ) slopes according to the available standard protocols for preliminary identification of *M. bovis* isolates [4, 5].

2.3. Genomic Experiments

2.3.1. Genomic DNA Preparations. For IS6110-PCR, RD, and PCR-RFLP analyses, simply a loopful of bacterial growth was transferred to a microfuge tube containing $400 \mu L$ TB lyses buffer (Cinnagen, Tehran, Iran), heat-treated ($95°C$, 30 min), vortexed, and centrifuged ($4500 g$, 15 min) followed by transfer of the supernatant to a new tube and another round of heat treatment ($80°C$, 30 min). The tube content was then stored at $-20°C$ before use for PCRs. For PGRS-RFLP and DR-RFLP tests, the high quality genomic DNA was extracted as previously described [6].

2.3.2. PCR-16SrRNA. The method of Huard was employed to amplify a 543 bp long fragment of the 16SrRNA. The sequences of primers are shown in Table 1 [7].

2.3.3. PCR-IS6110. The method of McHugh was employed to amplify a 245 bp long fragment of the IS6110 marker using INS1 and INS2 primers (Table 1) [8].

2.3.4. RD-Typing. For the RD experiment, the Warren method was employed with brief modifications where 4 individual PCRs including RD1, RD4, RD9, and finally RD12 were performed by previously described primers to differentiate members of *M. tuberculosis* complex (Table 1) [9].

2.3.5. PGRS-RFLP and DR-RFLP. Internationally standardized protocol was employed to conduct these RFLP experiments [6]. In brief, 6 microgram of genomic DNA was

digested by *Pvu*II and incubated at $37°C$ overnight. DNA fragments were separated by gel electrophoresis and transferred onto a positively charged nylon membrane (southern blot). The digoxigenin tail-labelled PGRS ($5'$ CGG CCG TTG CCG CCG TTG CCG CCG TTG CCG CCG $3'$) or DR ($5'$ CCG AGA GGG GAC GGA AAC $3'$) probes were used for hybridization which was performed at $65°C$ using rolling bottle method (Table 2). The hybridized membrane was exposed to alkaline phosphatase-conjugated anti-DIG antibody solution and the hybridization signals were detected using substrate BCIP/NBT. Photography was with a scanner (Cannon Laser Base MF3110, Japan) and the acquired image was subsequently saved in JEPG format. The achieved RFLP patterns were carefully observed by two experienced members of the research team and analyzed using Gel-Pro (Media Cybernetics, Milan, Italy) [6, 10].

3. Results

3.1. Study Population. Out of the 76 specimens (e.g., 76 patients) incorporated in the study, bacterial culture was successfully resulted in collection of 62 mycobacterial isolates. Information of patients including age, gender, and nationality of them were extracted. The patients (culture-positive) include 32 men and 30 women that 4 persons of them were Afghan nationals (2 men and 2 women). Age of the patients varied from 27 to 93 and the average age was 62 years.

3.2. Microbial Culture on Glycerinated and Pyruvate LJ. 61 isolates had better growth on glycerinated LJ compared with pyruvate LJ that is a sign of *Mycobacterium tuberculosis*. Only one isolate was grown in a pyruvate LJ stronger than glycerinated LJ that showed that it is *Mycobacterium bovis*.

3.3. PCR-16SrRNA. All these isolates produced a 543 bp long typical fragment specific to members of Mycobacterium species.

3.4. PCR-IS6110 Test. In IS6110-PCR all these isolates produced a 245 bp long typical fragment specific to members of *M. tuberculosis* complex.

3.5. RD-Typing Test. When the RD typing results were observed, all but one of the isolates in the study setting showed patterns that were matching with *M. tuberculosis* while the non-*M. tuberculosis* isolates were understood to be *M. bovis*.

3.6. PGRS and DR RFLP. PGRS-RFLP using *Pvu*II was successfully conducted on 62 isolates and we classified them into 25 genotypic groups (P1 to P25) (Figure 1). This induced eight clustered and 17 orphan patterns. Sixty-two of the isolates were also subjected to RFLP typing using DR probe with *Pvu*II and produced 26 RFLP-DR types (D1 to D26) (Figure 2). This induced eight clustered and 18 orphan patterns. Unlike Iranian patients, none of the Afghan patient isolates had a genetic similarity. Eight isolates belonged to

TABLE 1: The primers sequences used.

Target genes	Primers	Annealing (°C)	Amplicon size (bp)	References
16S rRNA	ACGGTGGGTACTAGGTGTGGGTTTC TCTGCGATTACTAGCGACTCCGACTTCA	62	543	[7]
IS6110	CCTGCGAGCGTAGGCGTCGG CTCGTCCAGCGCCGC	68	123	[8]
RD1	AAGCGGTTGCCGCCGACCGACC CTGGCTATATTCCTGGGCCCGG GAGGCGATCTGGCGGTTTGGGG	62	146	[9]
RD4	ATGTGCGAGCTGAGCGATG TGTACTATGCTGACCCATGCG AAAGGAGCACCATCGTCCAC	62	172	[9]
RD9	CAAGTTGCCGTTTCGAGCC CAATGTTTGTTGCGCTGC GCTACCCTCGACCAAGTGTT	62	235	[9]
RD12	GGGAGCCCAGCATTTACCTC GTGTTGCGGGAATTACTCGG AGCAGGAGCGGTTGGATATTC	62	369	[9]

TABLE 2: Restriction enzyme and probes sequences used for RFLP.

Genes	Restriction enzyme	Probes	Annealing (°C)	References
PGRS	PvuII	CGGCCGTTGCCGCCGTTGCCGCCGTTGCCGCCG	65	[6]
DR		CCGAGAGGGGACGGAAAC	65	[6]

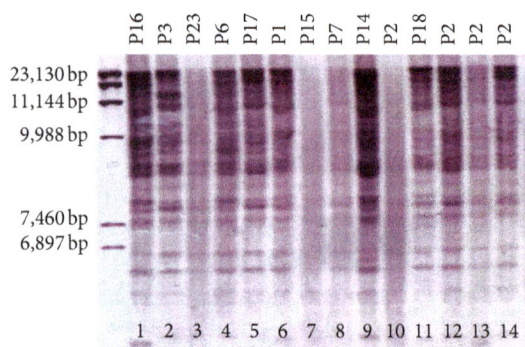

FIGURE 1: RFLP patterns of *M. tuberculosis* isolates from central province of Iran using *Pvu*II-digested DNA with the PGRS probe. Designations above the lanes represent RFLP-PGRS (P1, 2, 3, 6, 7, 14, 15, 16, 17, 18, and 23) patterns; left side bar is DNA size markers. Lane 1–14: *M. tuberculosis* isolates.

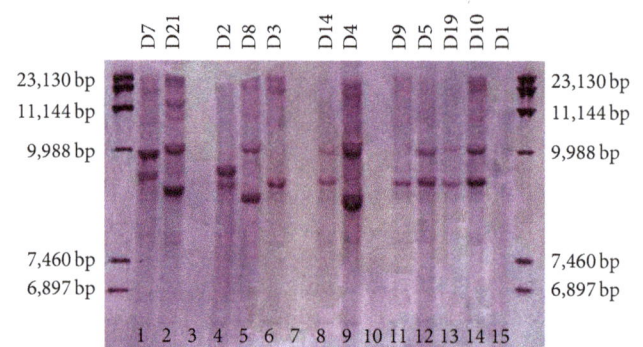

FIGURE 2: RFLP patterns of *M. tuberculosis* isolates from central province of Iran using *Pvu*II-digested DNA with the DR probe. Designations above the lanes represent DR-PGRS (D1, 2, 3, 4, 5, 7, 8, 9, 10, 14, 19, and 21) patterns; side bars are DNA size markers. Lane 1–14: *M. tuberculosis* isolates.

4 genotypes (2 isolates in per group) in both methods were placed in one group (P5-D1; P4-D6; P1-D11; P8-D20). Genetic patterns of *M. bovis* isolate (P20-D15) were entirely different with *M. tuberculosis* isolates and did not have any similarity with previously reported genotypes from Iran.

4. Discussion

Urbanization and industrialization of Central province of Iran caused the migration of many people in this province.

Client access to cheap foreign labor, the elimination of insurance costs, and the possibility of further mastery on Afghan workers because of their need to work more than the Iranian jobseekers have caused employers to use them. It leads to the fact that this province can accommodate a significant number of non-Iranian nationals. As a result, the transmission of tuberculosis from these immigrants has changed epidemiological features of this disease in Markazi Province in center of Iran.

In recent decades, molecular epidemiology of tuberculosis in different areas of Iran [11, 12] such as Tehran [13, 14], East Azarbaijan [15], and Khorasan [16] has been studied, but there is little information about Markazi Province. Thus, the present study was conducted in order to analyze the current epidemiology of TB in this province. A considerably large genetic diversity is seen in the population of *Mycobacterium tuberculosis* in Iran confirmed mutually by almost all the recently employed DNA typing systems [15, 17]. Although reactivation of disease due to infection in the past years appears to be explanatory of these epidemiological findings [17], conclusive evidence of this condition is still unknown. Interestingly different epidemiological features of *Mycobacterium bovis* population have been reported in Iran that show very little genetic diversity of this pathogen [18]. The findings of the present study are important from the four aspects. First, viewing 25 and 26 different genetic types by PGRS and DR-RFLP among a relatively small set of *Mycobacterium tuberculosis* isolates (62 isolates) showed considerable variation of this pathogen in Markazi Province. It is essential to note probably increase the number of isolates in further investigation show more polymorphism than the current value. Despite differences in the mechanisms of evolution and changes in PGRS and DR genetic markers, agreement between the results obtained by both typing methods confirms the accuracy of the present results which show a significant level of strain diversity in the Markazi Province. When findings of two genetic markers were merged, four combinational genotypes, namely, P5-D1, P1-D11, P4-D6, and P8-D20, were identified where each type was displayed by two isolates, an indication of their likely epidemiological link. On the other hand, these small cluster patterns indicate that there is reactivation cases TB rather than an epidemic transmission. Second, genetic dissimilarity between *Mycobacterium tuberculosis* strains isolated from Iranian (58 persons) and Afghan (4 persons) patients shows that contrary to popular perception, non-Persian minorities do not have an extensive role in infecting the citizens of Iran. It already has been considered by some authors [3, 17]. Nevertheless, a definite similarity between one Afghan isolate (from a 60-year-old woman) and an Iranian isolate (from a 75-year-old man) shows a single genotype (D11 and P1) therefore likely to be indicative of disease transmission and epidemic isolates. Since a thorough review of the social relationship between the two patients has been done, it was found that Afghan woman worked as a housekeeper in house of Iranian man. Third, considering the average age of patients in research was older than 62 years we believe this is more likely to be a reactivation case of tuberculosis rather than an epidemic transmission event as contact tracing strategy also confirms the explanation of other authors in Iran. Fourth, the only isolate of *Mycobacterium bovis* that was collected from an Iranian patient showed a completely different genetic pattern (P20-D15) compared to those of other *M. bovis* isolates previously genotyped in Iran by Mosavari and colleagues [10]. Considering the age (75-year-old female) and nationality (Iranian) of the patient hosting this specific isolate and the nature of zoonotic tuberculosis caused by *M. bovis* in humans, possibility of infection at an earlier time due to exposure to a strain that for some unknown reasons is no longer frequent or available in cattle farms appears to be explanatory as the most frequent bovine *M. bovis* strains have been exhaustively studied over the recent years in Iran. Therefore, this is more likely to be a reactivation case of zoonotic TB rather than an epidemic transmission event.

5. Conclusion

To conclude, in this region role of *M. bovis* in human tuberculosis is little and genetic diversity of *M. tuberculosis* is high, so it seems that more studies like MIRU-VNTR and IS*6110* are required to provide a reliable biogeographical map of TB in this province and Iran.

Ethical Approval

This study was reviewed and approved by the Institutional Ethics Review Committee of Razi Vaccine and Serum Research Institute, Karaj, Iran.

Authors' Contribution

Saman Soleimanpour, Daryoush Hamedi Asl, Keyvan Tadayon, Ali Asghar Farazi, Rouhollah Keshavarz, Kioomars Soleymani, Fereshteh Sadat Sedighinia, and Nader Mosavari participated in designing the study, data collection, laboratory work, statistical analysis, and reviewing of the paper. All the authors read and approved the final paper.

Acknowledgments

The Razi Vaccine and Serum Research Institute (RVSRI) and the Medical Sciences University of Arak are thanked for the funding and administrational supporting of the study. Doctors and laboratory staff at Karaj and Arak branches of RVSRI and also hospitals in Markazi Province who participated in this piece of work are acknowledged. Mehdi Ahmadi, Shojaat Dashti, and Samrand Reshadi are specifically thanked for their contribution in handling the clinical specimens. Saman Soleimanpour is a postgraduate student at RVSRI.

References

[1] World Health Organization (WHO), "Global Tuberculosis Report 2012. Country Profiles," Tech. Rep. WHO/HTM/TB/2012.6, WHO, Geneva, Switzerland, 2012.

[2] M. R. Masjedi, P. Farnia, S. Sorooch et al., "Extensively drug-resistant tuberculosis: 2 years of surveillance in Iran," *Clinical Infectious Diseases*, vol. 43, no. 7, pp. 841–847, 2006.

[3] A. A. Velayati, P. Farnia, M. Mirsaeidi, and M. Reza Masjedi, "The most prevalent *Mycobacterium tuberculosis* superfamilies among Iranian and Afghan TB cases," *Scandinavian Journal of Infectious Diseases*, vol. 38, no. 6-7, pp. 463–468, 2006.

[4] A. L. Gibson, G. Hewinson, T. Goodchild et al., "Molecular epidemiology of disease due to *Mycobacterium bovis* in humans in the United Kingdom," *Journal of Clinical Microbiology*, vol. 42, no. 1, pp. 431–434, 2004.

[5] J. Grange M, M. D. Yates, and I. de Kantor, *Guidelines for Speciation within the Mycobacterium Tuberculosis Complex*, Document WHO/EMC/ZOO/96.4, World Health Organization, Geneva, Switzerland, 2nd edition, 1996.

[6] D. van Soolingen, E. W. P. de Haas, and K. Kremer, *Restriction Fragment Length Polymorphism (RFLP) Typing of Mycobacteria*, National Institute of Public Health and the Environment, Bilthoven, The Netherlands, 2002.

[7] R. C. Huard, L. C. de Oliveira Lazzarini, W. R. Butler, D. Van Soolingen, and J. L. Ho, "PCR-based method to differentiate the subspecies of the *Mycobacterium tuberculosis* complex on the basis of genomic deletions," *Journal of Clinical Microbiology*, vol. 41, no. 4, pp. 1637–1650, 2003.

[8] T. D. McHugh, L. E. Newport, and S. H. Gillespie, "IS6110 homologs are present in multiple copies in mycobacteria other than tuberculosis-causing mycobacteria," *Journal of Clinical Microbiology*, vol. 35, no. 7, pp. 1769–1771, 1997.

[9] R. M. Warren, N. C. G. van Pittius, M. Barnard et al., "Differentiation of *Mycobacterium tuberculosis* complex by PCR amplification of genomic regions of difference," *International Journal of Tuberculosis and Lung Disease*, vol. 10, no. 7, pp. 818–822, 2006.

[10] N. Mosavari, M. M. Feizabadi, M. Jamshidian et al., "Molecular genotyping and epidemiology of *Mycobacterium bovis* strains obtained from cattle in Iran," *Veterinary Microbiology*, vol. 151, no. 1-2, pp. 148–152, 2011.

[11] D. Cousins, S. Williams, E. Liébana et al., "Evaluation of four DNA typing techniques in epidemiological investigations of bovine tuberculosis," *Journal of Clinical Microbiology*, vol. 36, no. 1, pp. 168–178, 1998.

[12] M. Doroudchi, K. Kremer, E. A. Basiri, M. R. Kadivar, D. Van Soolingen, and A. A. Ghaderi, "IS6110-RFLP and spoligotyping of *Mycobacterium tuberculosis* isolates in Iran," *Scandinavian Journal of Infectious Diseases*, vol. 32, no. 6, pp. 663–668, 2000.

[13] P. Farnia, F. Mohammadi, M. Mirsaedi et al., "Bacteriological follow-up of pulmonary tuberculosis treatment: a study with a simple colorimetric assay," *Microbes and Infection*, vol. 6, no. 11, pp. 972–976, 2004.

[14] M. M. Feizabadi, M. Shahriari, M. Safavi, S. Gharavi, and M. Hamid, "Multidrug-resistant strains of *Mycobacterium tuberculosis* isolated from patients in Tehran belong to a genetically distinct cluster," *Scandinavian Journal of Infectious Diseases*, vol. 35, no. 1, pp. 47–51, 2003.

[15] M. Asgharzadeh, M. Khakpour, T. Z. Salehi, and H. S. Kafil, "Use of mycobacterial interspersed repetitive unit-variable-number tandem repeat typing to study *Mycobacterium tuberculosis* isolates from East Azarbaijan Province of Iran," *Pakistan Journal of Biological Sciences*, vol. 10, no. 21, pp. 3769–3777, 2007.

[16] M. Rohani, P. Farnia, M. Nasab, R. Moniri, M. Torfeh, and M. M. Amiri, "Beijing genotype and other predominant *Mycobacterium tuberculosis* spoligotypes observed in Mashhad city, Iran," *Indian Journal of Medical Microbiology*, vol. 27, no. 4, pp. 306–310, 2009.

[17] P. Farnia, M. R. Masjedi, M. Varahram et al., "The recent-transmission of *Mycobacterium tuberculosis* strains among Iranian and Afghan relapse cases: a DNA-fingerprinting using RFLP and spoligotyping," *BMC Infectious Diseases*, vol. 8, article 109, 2008.

[18] K. Tadayon, N. Mosavari, F. Sadeghi, and K. J. Forbes, "Mycobacterium bovis infection in Holstein Friesian cattle, Iran," *Emerging Infectious Diseases*, vol. 14, no. 12, pp. 1919–1921, 2008.

7

Pastoralist Community's Perception of Tuberculosis: A Quantitative Study from Shinille Area of Ethiopia

Samuel Melaku,[1] **Hardeep Rai Sharma,**[2] **and Getahun Asres Alemie**[3]

[1] *Department of Public Health Nursing, Jijiga Health Science College, P.O. Box 504, Jijiga, Ethiopia*
[2] *Institute of Environmental Studies, Kurukshetra University, Kurukshetra, Haryana 136119, India*
[3] *Institute of Public Health, University of Gondar, P.O. Box 196, Gondar, Ethiopia*

Correspondence should be addressed to Hardeep Rai Sharma; hrsharma74@yahoo.co.in

Academic Editor: Jacques Grosset

Background. In Ethiopia the prevalence of all forms of TB is estimated at 261/100 000 population, leading to an annual mortality rate of 64/100 000 population. The incidence rate of smear-positive TB is 108/100 000 population. *Objectives.* To assess knowledge, attitudes, and practices regarding TB among pastoralists in Shinille district, Somali region, Ethiopia. *Method.* A community-based cross-sectional study was conducted among 821 pastoralists aged >18 years and above from February to May, 2011 using self-structured questionnaire. *Results.* Most (92.8%) of the study participants heard about TB, but only 10.1% knew about its causative agent. Weight loss as main symptom, transmittance through respiratory air droplets, and sputum examination for diagnosis were the answers of 34.3%, 29.9%, and 37.9% of pastoralists, respectively. The majority (98.3%) of respondents reported that TB could be cured, of which 93.3% believed with modern drugs. About 41.3% of participants mentioned covering the nose and mouth during sneezing and coughing as a preventive measure. The multivariate logistic regression analysis indicated that household income >300 Ethiopian Birr and Somali ethnicity were associated with high TB knowledge. Regarding health seeking behaviour practice only 48.0% of the respondents preferred to visit government hospital and discuss their problems with doctors/health care providers. *Conclusion.* This study observed familiarity with gaps and low overall knowledge on TB and revealed negative attitudes like discrimination intentions in the studied pastoral community.

1. Introduction

Tuberculosis continues to be one of the most important global public health threats. About one-third of the world's population is estimated to be infected with tubercle *bacilli* and hence at risk of developing active disease. TB is a leading killer of people with HIV. According to the World Health Organization Global TB Report [1], in 2010 there were approximately 8.8 million incident cases of TB globally, of which 1.1 million were among people living with HIV. The disease has been recognized as major public health problem in Ethiopia including Somali regional state and in 2010 there were estimated 220,000 (261/100,000) incident cases of TB, estimated 29,000 deaths (35/100,000) excluding HIV-related mortality [1]. As per Federal Ministry of Health (FMoH) data, TB in Ethiopia was one of the leading causes of morbidity, the fourth main cause of hospital admission,

and the second largest cause of hospital deaths (after malaria) [2]. According to the Somali Regional Health Bureau Report [3], the annual incidence rate during 2008 of smear-positive PTB was 175–250/100,000/year which was higher than the national figure of 165/100,000. The disease is one of the top ten causes of outpatient visit, hospital admission and death in the region. Furthermore, the emergence of multidrug resistant TB (MDR-TB) has become a major public health problem in a number of countries and an obstacle to global TB control [4, 5]. Ethiopia is one of the 27 high burden MDR-TB countries ranking 15th with more than 5000 estimated MDR-TB patients annually [2].

Pastoralists are the seminomadic people whose livelihood largely depends on livestock raising. An estimated 50–100 million pastoralists live in the developing world of which 60% are in sub-Saharan Africa. In the Horn of Africa, pastoralists constitute 70% of the general population, of which 12%

is in Ethiopia [6]. The majority of these pastoralists live in the southeastern and northeastern Somali region of the country having three different livelihood systems, that is, pastoralism, agropastoralism, and urban. Pastoralists and agro-pastoralists both constitute about 85%, while the rest was urban. Due to their mobile lifestyle, pastoralists often stay in border areas and highly volatile and insecure environments that were often beyond the reach of formal health services including TB control programs [7]. Pastoralists in Shinille district of Somali region of Ethiopia were confined to the most arid part of the country. Being geographically isolated in remote rural areas with poor infrastructure and communication, they are considered to be underserved and deprived of all forms of health care and are perceived as of low priority. Work environment, poverty, and lack of awareness are important factors affecting the health seeking behavior and the control strategies. Previously, a study was conducted in the area to explore barriers delaying TB diagnosis among pastoralist TB patients. The study revealed that factors related to sociocultural, perceptions of TB, and pastoralists' limited access to health care are the key factors leading to an apparent delay in diagnosis of pastoralist TB patients [7]. Tuberculosis is still a problem in the area and further high notification rate poses a challenge. Since the perception of pastoralist community in the region, particularly in Shinille district, towards TB has not been well investigated, assessing the baseline information regarding knowledge, attitudes, and practices on TB will offer a good insight about the overall picture of the control activity in the region and thereby assist in the development of a strategy for improving quality of service.

2. Methods

Somali region (state) is the eastern-most of the nine ethnic divisions of Ethiopia. The capital of Somali State is Jijiga. Shinille, the largest of four districts in Shinille Zone which is located in the Somali Region, has a latitude and longitude of $09°41'$N and $41°51'$E with an elevation of 1079 meters above sea level. The region borders are Kenya to the southwest, the Ethiopian regions of Oromia, Somali, and Dire Dawa to the west, Djibouti to the north, and Somalia to the north, east, and south. The region is among the areas of the country sparsely populated with an average population density of about 15 persons per km^2. The region is remote with a mobile nomadic population and inadequate infrastructure. Climatically, it is mostly desert with high average temperatures and low bimodal rainfall. Its economy is weak and reliant predominantly on traditional animal husbandry and marginal farming practices. Shinille district has an estimated total population of 13,132, of whom 6,758 were males and 6,374 were females according to Central Statistical Agency [8]. The two largest ethnic groups reported in the district were the Somali (96.58%) and the Oromo (1.76%), while all other ethnic groups made up the remaining 1.66% of the residents [8]. The major type of activity in population is pastoralism (48%) followed by crop farming (25%) and agropastoralism (17%).

A community-based cross-sectional survey was carried out from February to May 2011. The study population was the heads of pastoralist households with age above 18 years and residing in the study area. As per custom the heads of the family interact first with the society, community, and other visitors and are assumed to have more exposure and knowledge about social and health issues. Household heads having sickness, speaking and hearing problems were exempted from the study. In the absence of the family heads, the other eldest male or female member of the family was selected for the interview. The required sample of 852 household heads was determined using sample size calculation formula for single population proportion [9], with 95% confidence level, and 49.1% assumed prevalence of overall knowledge on TB according to a similar study done on pulmonary tuberculosis (PTB) in Arbaminch area of Ethiopia [10]. The study subjects were selected using cluster sampling technique. For cluster sampling, a design effect of 2 was applied and 10% was added for nonresponse rate accordingly for total sample size calculation. Shinille district has 28 villages and each village is considered as one cluster making a total of 28 clustered villages. Villages were selected randomly to represent the whole population and all households within the selected clusters were included in the sampling. Finally, from each housing unit the household head was selected for the interview. Pastoralists in the region are known to be ethnically and culturally a closely homogeneous group of people, who share one language, religion, and lifestyle. For such a closely homogeneous people by using cluster sampling technique, 852 household heads were deemed an adequate sample size to create the intended quantitative product. In addition because of scattered settlement of the communities on the vast areas of the region it can be expensive to survey. Treating several respondents within a local area as a cluster, finally all participants in the cluster were selected for Interview.

The data were collected by face-to-face interviews using self-structured and pretested questionnaires. The questionnaires were prepared by consulting the literature and modified to fit the local context. The questionnaire was first developed in English and then translated into Somali (local language), and back to English by a different individual to check consistency and conceptual equivalence. Included in the questionnaire were sociodemographic questions (age, sex, education, marital status, occupation, family size, monthly family income, and housing conditions), knowledge on TB causes, symptoms, diagnostic methods, transmission, prevention, treatment, and seriousness of disease, attitudes and practices intended health seeking behaviour, and information sources. Eight trained data collectors and one supervisor having good command on local language were involved in data collection. Prior to data collection, the objective of the study was discussed including practical exercise with data collectors and health education was provided regarding precautionary measures during data collection. An interview guide was also provided to data collectors and supervision was made by one of the authors during data collection process for timely edition of the data and feedback.

One of the authors coordinated the data collection process and rechecked the filled questionnaires. Pretesting of the questionnaire was conducted in *Error woreda* (block) village. During the pretest, the questionnaire was assessed for its clarity, understandability, completeness, reliability, as well as sensitivity of the subject matter. Corrections were made for difficulties and interview time was determined for completing each questionnaire.

The ethical clearance was obtained from the Institutional Review Board of the University of Gondar. Permission was also obtained from Somali Regional State and from administrative bodies of the district including *kebeles* (wards). Verbal consent was obtained from each respondent after explaining the confidentiality and voluntary participation features of the study. Moreover, the study questionnaire was anonymous and interview was conducted in a private setting to maintain privacy of the respondents for sensitive questions. Objectives of the study were explained to the respondents prior to the administration of the interview and confidentiality was maintained by omitting name of the respondents.

Complete data was entered and analyzed using Statistical Package of Social Sciences (SPSS) version 16 for windows statistical program. Results were summarized using descriptive statistics and presented by frequency tables, percentage, and charts. Association was computed between knowledge and sociodemographic variables using bivariate and multivariate analysis techniques. Logistic regression was done to assess the associations of factors with tuberculosis knowledge. The significance of associations are presented using *P* values and the 95% confidence interval of the adjusted odds ratios (AOR).

Overall, knowledge on TB was assessed using questions such as causes of TB, symptoms, diagnostic methods, transmission, prevention, treatment, and seriousness of disease. The responses to these questions were added together and scored for every study participant; the composite score was dichotomized using mean as a cut-off value. A score of one was assigned to correct responses, nil for incorrect/do not know answers. Afterwards, scores above the mean value were categorized under high knowledge and those below the mean value were labelled as having low knowledge on TB. The mean score was taken as the cut-off value and those scored above were categorised in having high TB knowledge. The mean and the median scores were 5.42 and 5.51, respectively. Similarly, attitudes, practices, and intended health seeking behaviour were assessed. Respondents attitude was measured by questionnaire containing two options of agree and disagree. Questions include *were they feel ashamed if some of their relative/family member gets infected with TB, want to keep secrete if they have TB, afraid of TB patients due to their illness, having belief that getting TB is a punishment for sinful act, continue friendship if their friends has TB, willing to provide care to their relative suffering from TB, might allow their daughter/son to marry cured TB patient.*

3. Results and Discussion

A total of 852 respondents aged ≥18 years were selected for this study. Out of this, 2.8% refused to participate while 0.82% could not be available for the interview after two attempts. Lack of interest was the reason for those who refused to participate. Therefore, the data was collected from 821 study subjects out of whom 51.6% were males and 48.4% were females with a response rate of 96.36%.

The highest proportion (30.1%) of the study subjects was within the age group of 25–34 years, and the least proportion (3.5%) was ≥55 years. Majority of the respondents were married (81.0%), while 13.2% were single, and 2.3%, 2.1%, and 1.5% were widowed, separated, and divorced, respectively. More than half of the households (55.2%) had a mean family size of 5. Regarding the occupation of the interviewee, pastoralists were dominant (43.8%), followed by cattle keepers and farmers (34.2%), agro-pastoralists (20.1%), and the rest (1.8%) included merchants, Quran tutors, and shop keepers (Table 1). Regarding pastoralists' education, 62% were illiterate, that is, cannot read and write. Around 34% can read and write, while 3.9% and 0.2% had 1–8 and 9–12 standard education, respectively. All of the study subjects were Muslims and a substantial amount (94.5%) identified themselves with the Somali Ethnic group and the rest (5.5%) with Oromo ethnicity. The median monthly income of the families was between 100 and 300 Birr (Ethiopian currency) approximately equivalent to 5.88–17.65 US$.

The study demonstrated that TB was familiar among pastoralist communities in the study area. The majority (92.8%) of the participants (52.2% males and 47.8% females) had heard about TB (*Kahoo* in the local language), similar to the results from other Ethiopian studies [10, 11]. The common sources of information mentioned by the respondents were radio (38.6%), health service providers (33.2%), and the rest from friends, schools, and relatives (Table 2). As newspapers and televisions were not commonly used in the study area, most of the Somalis had radio listening habit especially the Somali BBC which could be the main source of health information including TB, similar to the study carried out in Nepal [12].

Even though TB is familiar in the study area, there is a wide knowledge gap regarding the causes of the disease among the respondents. Only 10.1% knew bacteria as the medical cause of TB, whereas the majority of the respondents (89.9%) did not know about the cause. The perceived TB causes among 89.9% pastoralists varied from animals to cold air, food shortage, smoking, chewing khat leaves (*Catha edulis forsk*), poverty, hand shaking, sexual intercourse, and even magic (Table 3). Dualeh [13] reported internal injury due to hard work and malnutrition as additional perceived causes of TB. As also documented in other Ethiopian studies, low knowledge regarding medical cause of TB might be due to low education coverage or due to its geographical landscape where many rural and mountainous areas were difficult to access by the health extension workers [11, 14]. Being a pastoralist, and because of the need for child labour, has let the school enrolment rates very low in Somali region having an adult literacy rate for men and women of 15% and 12%, respectively [15]. As limited geographical areas are given to HEWs and accessibility is granted through existing monitoring system, however, due to high mobile nature of the community the accessibility and use of health benefits schemes are always doubtful. Lack of knowledge delays in healthcare seeking behavior, diagnosis and treatment,

TABLE 1: Sociodemographic characteristics of the study population ($n = 821$).

Background Characteristics	Number (%)
Sex	
Male	424 (51.6)
Female	397 (48.4)
Age (years)	
18–24	197 (24.0)
25–34	247 (30.1)
35–44	212 (25.8)
45–54	127 (15.5)
>55	29 (3.5)
Do not know	9 (1.1)
Ethnicity	
Somali	776 (94.5)
Oromo	45 (5.5)
Marital status	
Married	665 (81.0)
Single	108 (13.2)
Separated	12 (1.5)
Divorced	17 (2.1)
Widowed	19 (2.3)
Occupation	
Pastoralist	360 (43.8)
Agro pastoralist	165 (20.1)
Cattle keeping and farming	281 (34.2)
Others*	15 (1.8)
Education	
Cannot read and write	509 (62.0)
Read and write	278 (33.9)
Grade 1–8	32 (3.9)
Grade 9–12	02 (0. 2)
Religion	
Muslim	821 (100)
Household income	
Less than 100 Birr	243 (29.6)
100–300 Birr	424 (51.6)
>300 Birr	77 (9.4)
Refuse to disclose income	77 (9.4)

*merchants, Quran tutors, shop keepers.

TABLE 2: Distributions of respondents by source of information on TB ($n = 821$).

Variables	Frequency (%)
Heard of TB	
Yes	762 (92.8)
No	59 (7.20)
Source of information	
Radio	294 (38.6)
Health service provider	253 (33.2)
Friends/Relatives	163 (21.4)
Schools/Teachers	52 (6.8)

TABLE 3: Knowledge regarding causes, transmission sources, and TB prevention modes ($n = 762$).

Indicators of knowledge	Number (%)
Causes of Tuberculosis	
Cold air	213 (28)
Shortage of food	179 (23.5)
Smoking/chewing	99 (13)
Dust	87 (11.4)
Poverty	79 (10.3)
Bacteria/germ	77 (10.1)
Animals	22 (2.9)
Magic	05 (0.7)
Others*	01 (0.1)
Symptom of TB	
Weight loss	261 (34.3)
Coughing blood	154 (20.2)
Cough lasting >2 weeks	88 (11.5)
Chest pain	75 (9.8)
Vomiting	58 (7.6)
Weakness	57 (7.5)
Loss of appetite	35 (4.6)
Shortness of breath	26 (3.4)
Fever/sweating	02 (0.3)
Do not know	06 (0.8)
Mode of transmission	
By droplet through air	228 (29.9)
Eating utensils	180 (23.6)
Drinking raw milk	142 (18.6)
Hand shaking	87 (11.4)
Sharing towels	74 (9.7)
Sexual intercourse	19 (2.5)
Other**	10 (1.4)
Do not know	22 (2.9)

*Sinful act, **drinking raw animal blood and meat.

resulted in further increase transmission rate, morbidity, mortality, and socioeconomic problems. About 11% and 2.5% of the participants, respectively, believe in hand shaking and sexual intercourse as TB transmission mode (Table 3) and about 4% respondents avoid hand shaking to prevent TB (Table 5). The community misconception regarding hand shaking and sexual intercourse as TB transmission mode may favor wrong attitude development in the society for patients.

Regarding the best method for TB diagnosis, the present study revealed that 37.9% of the participants reported correct sputum examination while the rest (62.1%) mentioned blood diagnosis, skin and urine and stool examination, and X-ray methods (Figure 1). Most (63.7%) of the study participants in

Nepal reported sputum examination as the main TB infection diagnostic method while others mentioned blood and skin examination, physical examination, and X-ray [12].

The studied pastoralists had good knowledge on TB prevention. About 41.3% expressed nose and mouth covering during sneezing and coughing and 21.0% stated BCG

TABLE 4: Percentage distribution of respondents' knowledge regarding TB treatment ($n = 762$).

Variable	Frequency		Total
	Male	Female	
TB is treatable	No (%)	No (%)	No (%)
Yes	389 (51.0)	360 (47.2)	749 (98.3)
No	09 (1.2)	04 (0.5)	13 (1.7)
TB treatment better through			
Modern drug	369 (48.4)	342 (44.9)	711 (93.3)
Traditional	03 (0.4)	05 (0.7)	08 (1.1)
Both	19 (2.5)	11 (1.4)	30 (3.9)
Do not know	07 (0.9)	06 (0.8)	13 (1.7)

TABLE 5: Respondents' knowledge on transmission and prevention of TB.

Indicators of knowledge about TB transmission and prevention	Frequency Number (%)
Who can be infected with TB	
Anybody	361 (47.4)
Poor people	149 (19.6)
Homeless people	101 (13.3)
Alcoholics	65 (8.5)
Drug users	29 (3.8)
People living with HIV	19 (2.5)
Prisoners	04 (0.5)
Do not know	34 (4.4)
Preventive methods	
Covering nose and mouth	315 (41.3)
Through balanced diet	86 (11.3)
BCG vaccination	160 (21.1)
Avoid smoking	125 (16.1)
Avoid drinking alcohol	23 (3.3)
Avoid handshaking	31 (4.1)
Avoid sharing dishes	08 (1.0)
Not sharing bed with others	13 (1.7)
Others*	01 (0.1)

*Early treatment, food, and by avoiding sex.

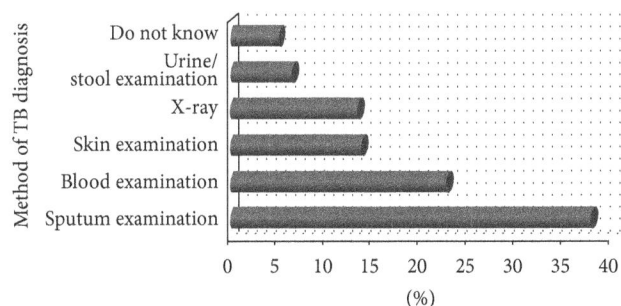

FIGURE 1: Percentage distribution of respondents by knowledge on method of TB diagnosis.

vaccination as preventive methods. Regarding disease treatment, majority of the Shinille pastoralists (98.3%) knew that TB is curable (Table 4) which is in accordance with the study carried out in Afar district, Ethiopia [10]. Majority of the study participants (93.3%) believed that TB treatment is well done with modern medicines. In earlier study from Ethiopia 87.7% informants reported the use of modern drugs as a better option, whereas the rest mentioned both modern drugs and traditional medicines [10].

In accordance with finding from Gondar city of Ethiopia [16], 47.4% of the study participants reported that anybody can be infected with TB while others reported poor, homeless people, alcoholics, drug users, people living with HIV/AIDS, and prisoners could be infected (Table 5). Majority (93.7%) of the pastoralists believed animals to be the source of TB, and

when asked about that, 30.1% responded about sharing same shelter with animals, 25.8% replied about drinking water from the common source and drinking raw milk (18.3%), eating raw meat (13.3%), and drinking raw animal blood (12.5%). Regarding housing conditions and TB, majority (95.3%) of the respondents believed that TB had relation with housing conditions like cooking and sleeping in same room (36.0%), improper ventilation (31.0%), and house cleanliness (33%). Smoking and alcohol consumption have also been cited in other studies conducted in India and Kenya [17, 18]. Respondents' perception of overcrowding of people sleeping in windowless rooms as a risk factor in acquiring infections among the pastoralists in Arusha, Tanzania [19]. In Eastern Ethiopia living in a single room was one of the reported factors that increased the risk of acquiring TB infection [11]. Hence, attention should be given to prevent disease transmission from lack of ventilation since in the study area all family members culturally construct single room house without windows and used it for cooking and sleeping purposes.

The present study showed high proportion of negative attitudes among pastoralist community. The common attitude found was feeling ashamed if relative/family member gets infected with TB (62.2%), keeping it secret if self or family member/relative get TB infection (43.4%), being afraid of TB patients (31.1%), considering the disease as a punishment for sinful act (34.8%), and believing that TB affects breast feeding (46.2%). Almost half of the study participants (49.9%) were not willing to provide care to their relatives suffering with TB, do not allow their children to marry cured TB patient (67.2%),

TABLE 6: Crude and adjusted odds ratio (OR) and 95% confidence intervals (CI) of determinants of TB knowledge.

Predictors	Knowledgeable on TB		Crude OR (95% CI)	Adjusted OR (95% CI)
	High	Low		
Sex				
Male	157	207	1	1
Female*	191	207	0.82 (0.62–1.04)	0.69 (0.47–1.02)
Age (Years)				
18–24*	97	94	1	1
25–34	117	119	0.14 (0.17–1.15)	5.31 (0.33–86.13)
35–44	83	111	0.14 (0.18–1.20)	0.32 (0.09–1.13)
45–54	43	72	0.19 (0.23–1.58)	0.36 (0.11–1.26)
55+	7	11	0.24 (0.03–2.01)	0.50 (0.14–1.74)
Do not know	1	7	0.02 (0.02–2.23)	0.77 (0.21–2.80)
Marital status				
Married*	274	342	1	1
Unmarried	53	50	0.76 (0.49–1.15)	0.57 (0.17–1.94)
Separated	7	4	0.46 (0.13–1.58)	0.69 (0.19–2.51)
Divorced	9	6	0.53 (0.19–1.52)	0.29 (0.04–2.18)
Widowed	5	12	1.92 (0.66–5.52)	0.60 (0.09–3.93)
Occupation				
Pastoralist*	142	197	1	1
Agro pastoralist	62	93	1.08 (0.73–1.59)	1.21 (0.73–2.02)
Cattle keeping and farming	135	119	0.63 (0.46–0.88)	0.45 (0.29–0.69)
Others	9	5	0.40 (0.13–1.22)	0.21 (0.05–1.77)
Ethnicity				
Somali	324	397	1	1
Oromo*	24	17	0.57 (0.30–1.09)	2.24 (0.99–5.07)
Household income				
Less than 100 Birr*	103	122	1	1
100–300 Birr	178	220	1.69 (0.98–2.93)	1.86 (0.93–3.72)
>300 Birr	27	44	1.76 (1.05–2.97)	2.03 (1.06–3.86)
Refuse to answer	40	28	2.33 (1.18–4.59)	3.04 (1.29–7.18)
Family size				
≤five*	112	370	1	1
>five	236	44	0.05 (0.04–0.08)	0.05 (0.03–0.07)

Knowledge score 5.4 (maximum of 8 score) was used as a cut off for comparison.
Variables significantly related ($P < .05$) to knowledge score on univariate analysis were included for multivariate logistic regression analysis. *Reference category.

a man/woman once having TB becomes infertile (36%), and around 26.6% of the informants were not willing to perform religious ceremonies with TB patients on treatment. Some respondents in Andhra Pradesh state of India attributed TB disease to sin, wrath of deities, witchcraft, evil eye, fate, and so forth [20]. In a study in Philippines respondents described TB as being shameful and a *"bad mark on the family"* [21].

The current study revealed that about half of the study participants (50.3%) discuss their problem with doctors/health care provider, while other discussed with pharmacist, parents, spouse, children, and close friends accordingly (Figure 2). The health seeking behaviour revealed that 48.0% and 24.3% of the respondents, respectively, preferred to visit government hospital and health centre if affected with TB (Figure 3) which might be attributed to the current TB control due strategy of Ethiopia where the FMoH creates

awareness about TB through regular advertisement using mass media. The media also advises and encourages TB infected individuals to visit nearby government and private health institution and discuss their problems with health care providers. However, the percentage of TB affected people visiting hospitals is quite low when compared with that of 74.3% reported from Nepal [12].

Regarding the pastoralist daily activities to avoid TB, 22.3% of them kept proper room ventilation, 15.0% do not sleep in the same room with animals, 14.6% do not share bed with sick patients, 13.9% do not drink raw milk, 12.2% do not eat raw meat, and do not share utensils with sick patients (11.0%) (Table 5). The present study found that about 99.5% of the respondents practised hand washing especially after collecting dung and touching the sick animals which is an encouraging fact which must be sustained among the society.

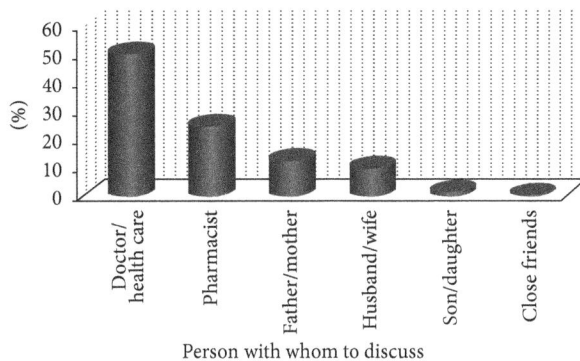

FIGURE 2: Percentage distribution of respondents to discuss their problem on TB infection.

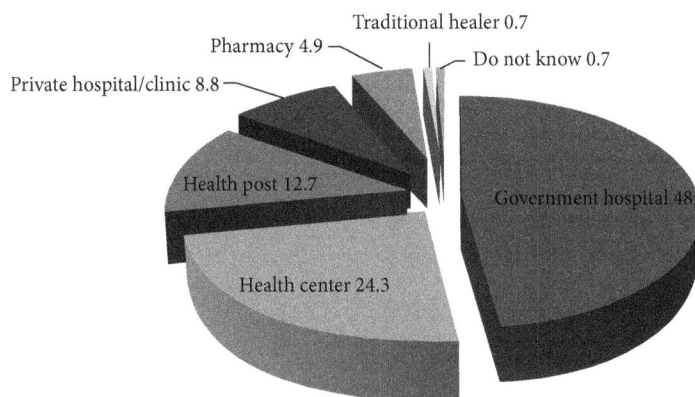

FIGURE 3: Percentage distribution of respondents preference for TB treatment.

The current study revealed that, out of all sociodemographic variables tested, occupation, family size, and household income/month had significance association and become a predictive of overall high TB knowledge. Results from multivariable logistic regression analysis (Table 6) showed that agro-pastoralist, as an occupation, is less likely to be predictive of overall knowledge of TB at (AOR: 1.21, 95% CI: (0.73–2.02)) than pastoralists, which is consistent with the finding of a previous study from Eastern Ethiopia [7] and in pastoral and agro-pastoral communities in Tanzania [19]. This might be because nomadic pastoralists have least access to health and other social services [22, 23]. This study reported that the participants whose household income >300 Birr/month (AOR: 2.03, 95% CI: (1.06–3.86)) were associated with having high knowledge on TB compared to those who had income <300 Birr/month; this might be explained as income increased the chance of getting access to information, education and seeking health care also increased. This study also found that pastoralists having family size of <five become a predictive of high overall knowledge of TB than those having family size >five at (AOR: 0.05, 95% CI: (0.04–0.08)).

4. Conclusion

This study documented familiarity towards TB but observed gaps and low overall knowledge about the disease in the studied pastoral community. Negative attitudes especially discrimination with infected individuals were also revealed. The study participants' practices or activities in avoiding TB and their health seeking behaviour were interesting and should be appreciated by the regional health bureau as it is one of the control strategies for TB. It is vital, therefore, for the regional health bureau to find ways of improving pastoralist's knowledge gap on TB and design strategies to create positive attitude to avoid discrimination of infected individuals with the disease among pastoralist. The regional health bureau should strengthen the available mobile health workers and promote an extensive health education programme to raise the awareness specifically about TB symptoms, means of transmission, prevention, and treatment in relation to the community misconceptions. Training should also be provided to members of pastoralist communities including traditional healers regarding TB control programs. Further research is suggested among pastoralists and control groups and different livelihoods systems in the study area.

Acknowledgments

The support from Somali Regional Health Bureau, Shinille district, and wards officials are acknowledged gratefully.

The authors are thankful to all study participants for their precious time.

References

[1] World Health Organization, *Global Tuberculosis Control: WHO Report*, WHO, Geneva, Switzerland, 2012.

[2] Federal Ministry of Health (FMoH) Ethiopia, *Guidelines for Prevention of Transmission of Tuberculosis in Health Care Facilities, Congregate and Community Setting*, Federal Ministry of Health (FMoH) Ethiopia, Ist edition, 2009.

[3] Somali Regional Health Bureau Report, "Personnel communication and data taken from unpublished report," 2009.

[4] World Health Organization, *Global Tuberculosis Control, Epidemiology Strategy Financing*, WHO, Geneva, Switzerland, 2009.

[5] Government of India, *TB India 2011, RNTCP Status Report*, Central TB Division New Delhi: Ministry of Health and Family Welfare, Government of India, New Delhi, India.

[6] D. Stephen, *Vulnerable Livelihoods in Somali Region*, Institute of Development Studies at the University of Sussex, Brighton, UK, 2006.

[7] A. A. Gele, G. Bjune, and F. Abebe, "Pastoralism and delay in diagnosis of TB in Ethiopia," *BMC Public Health*, vol. 9, article 5, 2009.

[8] Central Statistical Agency, *Population and Housing Census of Ethiopia: Results for Somali Region*, vol. 1, Central Statistical Agency, 2005.

[9] W. W. Daniel, *Biostatistics: A Foundation for Analysis in the Health Science*, pp. 658–659, Willey International, 8th edition, 2005.

[10] L. Mengistu, A. Gobena, M. Gezahegne et al., "Knowledge and perception of pulmonary tuberculosis in pastoral communities in the middle and lower awash valley of afar region, Ethiopia," *BMC Public Health*, vol. 10, article 187, 2010.

[11] M. M. Mesfin, T. W. Tasew, I. G. Tareke, G. W. M. Mulugeta, and M. J. Richard, "Community knowledge, attitudes and practices on pulmonary tuberculosis and their choice of treatment supervisor in Tigray, northern Ethiopia," *Ethiopian Journal of Health Development*, vol. 19, pp. 21–27, 2005.

[12] Government of Nepal, "Knowledge, attitude and practices: Study on tuberculosis among community people," Report of Mahottari District, Ministry of Health and Population and National Tuberculosis Centre, 2009, http://library.elibrary-mohp.gov.np/mohp/collect/mohpcoll/archives/mohp:199/4.dir/doc.pdf.

[13] M. W. Dualeh, "Healthsituation of the drought-affected populations in the Somali National Regional State," 2000, http://www.who.int/disasters/repo/5856.doc.

[14] Austrian Development Cooperation, *Ethiopia Subprogram Health 2004–2006*, Federal Ministry for Foreign Affairs, Addis Ababa, Ethiopia, 2007.

[15] Central Statistical Agency, "Census 2007," 2008, http://www.etharc.org/resources/download/viewcategory/68.

[16] B. Tessema, A. Muche, A. Bekele, D. Reissig, F. Emmrich, and U. Sack, "Treatment outcome of tuberculosis patients at Gondar University Teaching Hospital, Northwest Ethiopia: a five-year retrospective study," *BMC Public Health*, vol. 9, article 371, 2009.

[17] D. M. Nair, A. George, and K. T. Chacko, "Tuberculosis in Bombay: new insights from poor urban patients," *Health Policy and Planning*, vol. 12, no. 1, pp. 77–85, 1997.

[18] R. Liefooghe and J. B. Baliddawa, "From their own perspective. A Kenyan community's perception of tuberculosis," *Tropical Medicine and International Health*, vol. 2, no. 8, pp. 809–821, 1997.

[19] S. Mfinanga, O. Mørkve, R. R. Kazwala et al., "Tribal differences in perception of tuberculosis: a possible role in tuberculosis control in Arusha, Tanzania," *International Journal of Tuberculosis and Lung Disease*, vol. 7, no. 10, pp. 933–941, 2003.

[20] B. Venkatraju and S. Prasad, "Beliefs of patients about the causes of Tuberculosis in rural Andhra Pradesh," *International Journal of Nursing and Midwifery*, vol. 2, no. 2, pp. 21–27, 2010.

[21] M. Nichter, "Illness semantics and international health: the weak lungs/TB complex in the Philippines," *Social Science and Medicine*, vol. 38, no. 5, pp. 649–663, 1994.

[22] A. Sheik-Mohamed and J. P. Velema, "Where health care has no access: the nomadic populations of sub-Saharan Africa," *Tropical Medicine and International Health*, vol. 4, no. 10, pp. 695–707, 1999.

[23] United Nations Development Programme, "Between a rock and hard place: armed violence in African pastoral communities," UNDP Report, 2007, http://www.genevadeclaration.org/fileadmin/docs/regional-publications/Armed-Violence-in-African-Pastoral-Communities.pdf.

8

Maintenance of Sensitivity of the T-SPOT.*TB* Assay after Overnight Storage of Blood Samples, Dar es Salaam, Tanzania

Elizabeth A. Talbot,[1,2] Isaac Maro,[3] Katherine Ferguson,[4] Lisa V. Adams,[1] Lillian Mtei,[3] Mecky Matee,[3] and C. Fordham von Reyn[1]

[1] Dartmouth Medical School, Hanover, NH 03755, USA
[2] Infectious Diseases and International Health Section, 1 Medical Center Drive, Lebanon, NH 03756, USA
[3] Muhimbili University of Health and Allied Sciences, Dar es Salaam, Tanzania
[4] Dartmouth College, Hanover, NH 03755, USA

Correspondence should be addressed to Elizabeth A. Talbot, elizabeth.talbot@dartmouth.edu

Academic Editor: Catharina Boehme

Background. T-SPOT.*TB* is an interferon gamma release assay for detecting *Mycobacterium tuberculosis* infection. The requirement to process within 8 hours is constraining, deters use, and leads to invalid results. Addition of T Cell *Xtend* reagent may allow delayed processing, but has not been extensively field tested. *Design*. Consecutive AFB smear positive adult tuberculosis patients were prospectively recruited in Dar es Salaam, Tanzania. Patients provided a medical history, 1–3 sputum samples for culture and 1 blood sample which was transported to the laboratory under temperature-controlled conditions. After overnight storage, $25\,\mu$L of T Cell *Xtend* reagent was added per mL of blood, and the sample was tested using T-SPOT.*TB*. *Results*. 143 patients were enrolled: 57 patients were excluded because temperature control was not maintained, 19 patients were excluded due to red blood cell contamination, and one did not provide a sputum sample for culture. Among 66 evaluable patients, overall agreement between T-SPOT.*TB* and culture was 95.4% (95%CI; 87.1–99.0%) with Kappa value 0.548. Sensitivity of T-SPOT.*TB* when using T Cell *Xtend* reagent was 96.8% (95%CI; 88.8–99.6%). *Conclusions*. When T Cell *Xtend* reagent is added to specimens held overnight at recommended temperatures, T-SPOT.*TB* is as sensitive as the standard assay in patients with tuberculosis.

1. Introduction

The T-SPOT.*TB* (Oxford Immunotec Ltd, Abingdon, UK) is an interferon gamma release assay (IGRA) for detection of latent *Mycobacterium tuberculosis* infection (LTBI). This assay detects T-lymphocytes specific for *M. tuberculosis* antigens that are absent from *M. bovis* BCG and most environmental mycobacteria [1]. Currently, T-SPOT.*TB* must be performed within 8 hours of sample collection. Logistically, this requires that patients have blood drawn early enough to transport the sample to the laboratory, which must assay samples on the day of receipt. This precludes batching samples, which would save resources and testing supplies. Moreover, in many countries, laboratories are centralized and are not in close proximity to where the blood sample is drawn. Therefore, it is not possible to transport samples to arrive at the receiving laboratory for processing on the same day.

To allow greater test processing flexibility, the manufacturer of T-SPOT.*TB* developed a proprietary reagent called T Cell *Xtend*, which they report can be added to whole blood samples stored at 10–25°C to increase this timeframe up to 32 hours [2].

2. Materials and Methods

The ethical review boards of Dartmouth Medical School (Hanover NH), the National Institute for Medical Research

(Dar es Salaam, Tanzania) and Muhimbili University of Health and Allied Sciences (MUHAS, Dar es Salaam, Tanzania) approved the study. The study was conducted according to the principles of good clinical practice and under the International Conference on Harmonization guidelines.

2.1. Participant Enrolment. All AFB smear positive individuals referred for initiation of TB treatment to one of two National Tuberculosis and Leprosy Programme (NTLP) TB treatment clinics in Dar es Salaam, Tanzania, were approached by a trained study nurse to determine their interest in being included in the study. The study nurse explained the study and answered any questions in the patient's native language. The participants then signed the approved informed consent or, in the presence of a witness, indicated their signature with a fingerprint. All participants provided a medical history, up to three sputum samples and a blood sample for testing by IGRA and were offered HIV testing according to the NTLP guidelines.

2.2. IGRA Testing. A single tube of blood was drawn from each participant. During the initial enrolment period, blood samples were transported to the laboratory under ambient temperature conditions (maximum average temperatures during the enrolment months were 28°C for September and 29°C for October) and, in the latter enrolment period, under temperatures ensured as <25°C by use of a temperature control shipping box (GreenBox Thermal Management System (Thermosafe Brands, Arlington Heights, IL, USA)). The blood samples were then stored overnight in an air conditioned laboratory (<25°C) and tested using T-SPOT.*TB* according to the manufacturer's instructions for use [3]. T Cell *Xtend* reagent was added to each blood sample at 25 μL/mL blood, mixed and incubated for 20 minutes at room temperature before processing. Peripheral blood mononuclear cells (PBMC) were harvested by Ficoll density gradient centrifugation using Leucosep tubes (Oxford Immunotec, Abingdon, UK). The PBMCs were washed, counted using a hemocytometer, and plated at 2.5×10^5 cells per well into a membrane-bottomed plate, coated with anti-interferon gamma antibody. PBMCs were incubated overnight in the presence of the provided TB antigens (ESAT-6 and CFP10) along with controls (positive mitogen control and a nil control). The PBMCs producing interferon gamma were revealed as spots by incubation with an enzyme conjugated secondary antibody for interferon gamma and a colour producing enzyme substrate. Spots were counted, and clinical result was recorded according to the approved algorithm where, compared to the nil control, 6 spots and above are positive and 5 spots and below are negative. Results with a low-mitogen response (<20 spots) or a high-nil control response (>10 spots) were recorded as invalid.

2.3. Mycobacterial Studies. AFB smears were done according to the Ziehl-Neelsen method by trained research personnel. Sputum was cultured for mycobacteria on Lowenstein Jensen slants.

2.4. Statistical Analyses. Sensitivity was calculated as the number of T-SPOT.*TB* positive samples divided by the number of culture positive samples multiplied by 100. 95% confidence limits were calculated. The Kappa statistic was used to measure overall agreement between culture and T-SPOT.*TB* results. Analyses were conducted using Excel.

3. Results

A total of 143 participants were enrolled into the study (Figure 1). The initial 57 blood samples drawn at one clinic were transported and stored at ambient temperatures prior to processing. After processing, it was recognized that these specimens were not reliably kept at temperatures below 25°C (the required temperature per protocol), and therefore these 57 samples were excluded from the final sensitivity analysis. Temperature control measures were instituted for the subsequent collection of samples from an additional 86 participants. Nineteen of these 86 (22.1%) participants were excluded because the laboratorian observed red blood cell contamination in the PBMC layer so the PBMCs could not be accurately counted. One of 86 (1.2%) participants failed to provide a sputum sample for culture and was excluded.

Therefore, 66 results were available for analysis. The participants were all black African and ranged in age from 18–60 years. The majority were male and BCG vaccinated (71% and 77%, resp.); 17 (26%) were HIV-positive, 24 (36%) were HIV-negative, and 25 (38%) declined testing.

Of the 66 T-SPOT.*TB* results, 61 (92.4%) were positive, 4 (6.1%) were negative, and 1 (1.5%) was invalid. The overall agreement between the 65 valid T-SPOT.*TB* and culture results was 95.4% (62/65: 95%CI; 87.1–99.0%) with a Kappa value of 0.548. The sensitivity of the T-SPOT.*TB* assay when run after delayed processing using the T Cell Xtend reagent was 96.8% (60/62: 95%CI; 88.8–99.6%). Among 41 T-SPOT.*TB* results from participants with known HIV status, T-SPOT.*TB* results were positive in 14 (82.4%) of those who were HIV-positive and 23 (95.8%) of those who were HIV-negative (*P* > 0.05). However, limiting to valid results from culture positive patients, the sensitivity of the assay among samples from HIV-positive participants was 92.9% (13/14).

In spite of exclusion because of protocol noncompliance, results from the 57 samples transported at ambient temperature were also analyzed. Of the 57, 40 (70.2%) were positive, 11 (19.3%) were negative, and 6 (10.5%) was invalid. Compared with the results from the 66 samples with temperature control, false negative results among these 57 samples were more common (*P* = 0.05). Results from 19 samples were excluded because of red blood cell contamination showed 14 (73.7%) positive and 5 (26.3%) negative. Compared with the results from 66 samples with temperature control, false negative results among these 19 were statistically significantly more common (*P* = 0.04).

4. Discussion

T-SPOT.*TB* with delayed processing using T Cell *Xtend* among patients with culture-confirmed tuberculosis showed high sensitivity, comparable to that reported for immediate

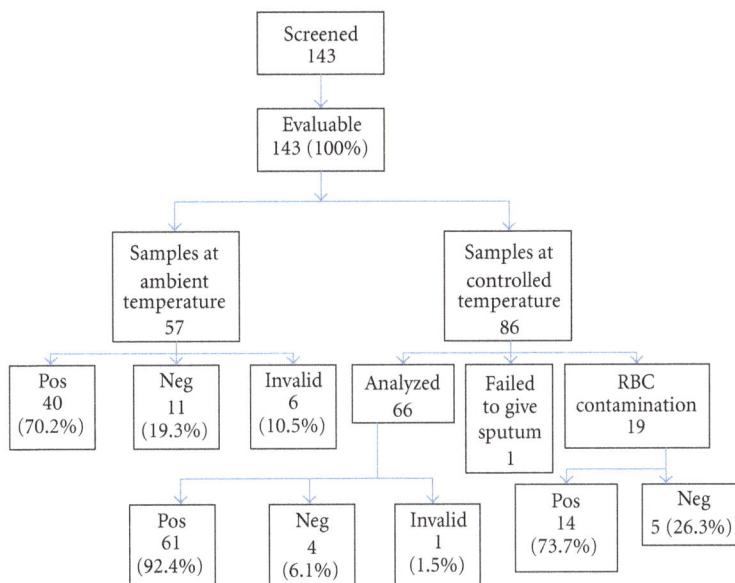

FIGURE 1: Patient flow and testing results using T-SPOT.*TB* and T Cell *Xtend,* Dar es Salaam, Tanzania.

processing. In a recent meta-analysis of 14 studies of T-SPOT.*TB,* (without *Xtend*) in low- and middle-income countries, Metcalfe et al. reported sensitivity of 83% (95% CI, 63–94%) among HIV-positive and -negative tuberculosis patients [4].

This high sensitivity we observed is also consistent with pilot studies with the T Cell *Xtend* reagent completed at three clinical sites including the UK and South Africa [5]. Lenders et al. studied the utility of T Cell *Xtend,* conducting T-SPOT.*TB* assays the same day as collection and approximately one and two days after collection [6]. Spot counts from 66 specimens T-SPOT.*TB* assayed without the T Cell *Xtend* reagent one day after collection were higher than those processed on the day of collection. In contrast, spot counts from 215 specimens assayed two days after collection with the T Cell *Xtend* reagent were similar to those processed on the day of collection. The T Cell *Xtend* reagent reduced the proportion of samples that changed from positive to negative and vice versa (4.54% to 2.83%), but this was not statistically significant [6]. Wang et al. had similar high agreement (98.2%) among 108 specimens of results of immediate T-SPOT.*TB* and T-SPOT.*TB* with the T Cell *Xtend* reagent processed 23–32 hours after collection [7].

In one of our patients, T-SPOT.*TB* was positive and culture was negative (Table 1). This patient was an HIV-infected male, who submitted three sputum specimens which were 3+, 4+ and 1+ AFB smear positive, but all cultures were negative. The T-SPOT.*TB* result was interpreted as positive, given that the Nil control well showed 6 spots, Panel A 6, and Panel B 15. Per the package insert, the test result is positive if Panel A minus Nil control and/or Panel B minus Nil control is 6 spots [3]. It may be that the T-SPOT.*TB* result was falsely positive, or that the culture was falsely negative, perhaps because the patient had received antituberculosis therapy. We do not have follow-up data on the patient to know if they

TABLE 1: Overall agreement between TB culture and T-SPOT.*TB*.

		T-SPOT.*TB*		
		Positive	Negative	Invalid
Culture	Positive	60	2	1*
	Negative	1	2	0

* 1/66 (1.5%) of T-SPOT.TB results was invalid due to a high nil control result.

demonstrated a typical response to antituberculosis therapy, or there was an alternative diagnosis made.

Our samples transported using a validated system for temperature control at or below 25°C showed sensitivity that is equivalent to that reported for the same day T-SPOT.*TB* assay [1, 3]. However, our study clearly illustrates the need to control temperature. In sub-Sahara African settings, a simple solution for shipment over long distances would be required, such as the use of an insulated package system.

Red blood cell contamination also interferes with assay reliability because the presence of large numbers of red blood cells makes accurate counting of the PBMC fraction difficult, and therefore the required number of PBMCs cannot be reliably determined. Red blood cell contamination is more common when a hemocytometer is used (as in this study), and the use of automated instruments that provide a differential count of white blood cells would eliminate this problem.

5. Conclusions

T-SPOT.*TB* can be run on blood samples not contaminated with red blood cells and maintained overnight by the use of T Cell *Xtend* reagent without affecting the sensitivity of the assay. Storage and transport of samples at temperatures

<25°C are critical to obtaining optimum sensitivity, and use of an automated cell counting instrument may correct the reduced sensitivity observed with red blood cell contamination.

Authors' Contributions

E. A. Talbot, L. V. Adams, L. Mtei, and C. F. von Reyn designed the study. E. A. Talbot, I. Maro, K. Ferguson, L. V. Adams, L. Mtei, M. Matee, and C. F. von Reyn participated in the implementation of the trial. E. A. Talbot, L. Mtei, M. Matee, and C. F. von Reyn participated in administration. I. Maro, K. Ferguson, and L. Mtei participated in data collection. E. A. Talbot analyzed the data and wrote the first draft. E. A. Talbot, L. V. Adams, L. Mtei and C. F. von Reyn contributed to the interpretation of the data. All authors reviewed and approved the final paper.

Acknowledgments

The authors would like to express their gratitude to the volunteers who participated in this study. They appreciate the efforts of the clinical research staff: Dr. Ibrahim Mteza, Esther Kayichile, Joyce Wamsele, and Emmanuel Balandya. They also thank Betty Mchaki (DarDar Project) and Wendy Wieland-Alter (Dartmouth Medical School) for their generous laboratory assistance and Miriam Zayumba (DarDar Project) and Susan Tvaroha (Dartmouth College) for assistance with data management. The authors disclose that Oxford Immunotec, the manufacturer of the T-SPOT.*TB* and the T Cell *Xtend* reagent, funded this study and also contributed in on-site study monitoring. Oxford Immunotec did not interpret the findings or write this paper. C. F. von Reyn has been a one-day consultant for Oxford Immunotec on two occasions, and C. F. von Reyn, L. V. Adams, and E. A. Talbot received additional research funding from Oxford Immunotec more than one year prior to this submission. The other authors have no potential conflicts to declare.

References

[1] CDC, "Updated guidelines for using interferon gamma release assays to detect *Mycobacterium tuberculosis* infection—United States, 2010," *Morbidity and Mortality Weekly Report*, vol. 59, no. RR-5, pp. 2–9, 2010.

[2] http://www.oxfordimmunotec.com/XtendpackInsert-english, 2010.

[3] http://www.oxfordimmunotec.com/96-UK, 2010.

[4] J. Z. Metcalfe, C. K. Everett, K. R. Steingart et al., "Interferon-γ release assays for active pulmonary tuberculosis diagnosis in adults in low-and middle-income countries: systematic review and meta-analysis," *Journal of Infectious Diseases*, vol. 204, no. 4, pp. S1120–S1129, 2011.

[5] I. Durrant, J. Radcliffe, and T. Day, "TB testing using T-SPOT.TB after overnight sample storage," *Clinical Microbiology and Infection*, vol. 15, p. pS393, 2009.

[6] L. M. Lenders, R. Meldau, R. N. van Zyl-Smit et al., "Comparison of same day versus delayed enumeration of TB-specific T cell responses," *Journal of Infection*, vol. 60, no. 5, pp. 344–350, 2010.

[7] S. Wang, D. A. Powell, H. N. Nagaraja, J. D. Morris, L. S. Schlesinger, and J. Turner, "Evaluation of a modified interferon-gamma release assay for the diagnosis of latent tuberculosis infection in adult and paediatric populations that enables delayed processing," *Scandinavian Journal of Infectious Diseases*, vol. 42, no. 11-12, pp. 845–850, 2010.

9

Seasonality of Tuberculosis in Delhi, India: A Time Series Analysis

Varun Kumar, Abhay Singh, Mrinmoy Adhikary, Shailaja Daral, Anita Khokhar, and Saudan Singh

Department of Community Medicine, Vardhman Mahavir Medical College and Safdarjung Hospital, New Delhi 110029, India

Correspondence should be addressed to Varun Kumar; drvarunkumar17@gmail.com

Academic Editor: David C. Perlman

Background. It is highly cost effective to detect a seasonal trend in tuberculosis in order to optimize disease control and intervention. Although seasonal variation of tuberculosis has been reported from different parts of the world, no definite and consistent pattern has been observed. Therefore, the study was designed to find the seasonal variation of tuberculosis in Delhi, India. *Methods.* Retrospective record based study was undertaken in a Directly Observed Treatment Short course (DOTS) centre located in the south district of Delhi. Six-year data from January 2007 to December 2012 was analyzed. Expert modeler of SPSS ver. 21 software was used to fit the best suitable model for the time series data. *Results.* Autocorrelation function (ACF) and partial autocorrelation function (PACF) at lag 12 show significant peak suggesting seasonal component of the TB series. Seasonal adjusted factor (SAF) showed peak seasonal variation from March to May. Univariate model by expert modeler in the SPSS showed that Winter's multiplicative model could best predict the time series data with 69.8% variability. The forecast shows declining trend with seasonality. *Conclusion.* A seasonal pattern and declining trend with variable amplitudes of fluctuation were observed in the incidence of tuberculosis.

1. Introduction

Tuberculosis (TB) which can be disseminated widely from active cases through aerosol droplets is an often fatal infectious disease caused by the agent *Mycobacterium tuberculosis*. Despite many efforts to control this disease, TB remains a major public health issue with a high global health burden, particularly with the emergence of multidrug resistant (MDR), extensive drug resistant (XDR), and the recent emergence of total drug resistant (TDR) strains along with coinfection with human immunodeficiency virus (HIV) especially in developing countries [1]. Each year, an estimated 9 million new cases of tuberculosis occur worldwide and responsible for an estimated 1.7 million deaths [2].

While seasonal variation has been widely reported for many respiratory infections in different parts of the world, it is much less documented for TB. There is paucity of data on seasonal variation in pulmonary TB in developing countries, although a number of studies in developed countries have reported peaks in late winter and early spring or summer [3, 4]. Thorpe et al. have found that in Northern India, TB diagnosis peaked between April and June and it reached a nadir between October and December, but in Southern India, no such seasonal variation was found [5].

India bears a disproportionately large burden of the world's tuberculosis rates, as World Health Organization (WHO) statistics for 2011 giving an estimated incidence figure of 2.2 million cases of TB for India out of a global incidence of 8.7 million cases [6]. Since 1998, effective tuberculosis control programs have been rapidly expanding across India allowing for population based analyses with standardized register data.

A study on the economic impact of scaling up of Revised National Tuberculosis Control Program (RNTCP) in India in 2009 shows that on an average each TB case incurs an economic burden of around US$ 12,235 and a health burden of around 4.1 disability adjusted life years (DALYs). Similarly, a death from TB in India incurs an average burden of around US$ 67,305 and around 21.3 DALYs [7]. So the present study was conducted to find if there is any seasonal variability of TB incidence in Delhi, India, and to create the best possible

TABLE 1: Distribution of study subjects according to age and sex ($n = 417$).

Gender	Age (in years)		Total
	≤14	≥15	
Male	11 (2.6)	273 (65.5)	284 (68.1)
Female	7 (1.7)	126 (30.2)	133 (31.9)
Total	18 (4.3)	399 (95.7)	417 (100)

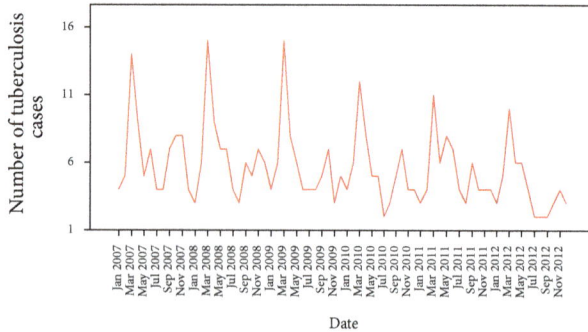

FIGURE 1: Sequence chart of total number of tuberculosis.

univariate model for TB monthly incidence for the last six years with the available time series data.

2. Materials and Methods

The present study was a retrospective record based study undertaken in a Directly Observed Treatment Short course (DOTS) centre of Fatehpur Beri primary health centre located in the south district of Delhi, which caters to a population of 64,000. Three sputum smear examinations were done for acid-fast bacilli (AFB) as per the guidelines of RNTCP. Six-year data from January 2007 to December 2012 were analyzed. The cases were assigned to the month of first positive smear and a total of 417 new smear positive cases of TB were registered during the study period.

Expert modeler of SPSS ver.21 software was used to fit the best suitable model for the time series data. The stationarity of the data was checked by autocorrelation function (ACF) and partial autocorrelation function (PACF). Seasonal adjusted factor (SAF) was used to determine the peak of seasonal variation. The Ljung-Box (modified Box-Pierce) test was used to determine if the model was correctly specified. Forecasting of the incidence of monthly TB cases was also done using the best fit model.

3. Results

According to RNTCP guidelines, 18 (4.3%) were pediatric TB cases and 399 (95.7%) were adults (Table 1).

Figure 1 clearly shows that there has been a steady declining trend in the TB incidence over the study period. The series exhibited a number of peaks; aside from the small scale fluctuations, the significant peak appeared to be separated by

TABLE 2: Monthly tuberculosis incidence during the study period ($n = 417$).

Month	2007	2008	2009	2010	2011	2012
January	4	3	4	4	3	3
February	5	6	6	6	4	5
March	14	15	15	12	11	10
April	9	9	8	8	6	6
May	5	7	6	5	8	6
June	7	7	4	5	7	4
July	4	4	4	2	4	2
August	4	3	4	3	3	2
September	7	6	5	5	6	2
October	8	5	7	7	4	3
November	8	7	3	4	4	4
December	4	6	5	4	4	3
Total	89	78	71	65	64	50

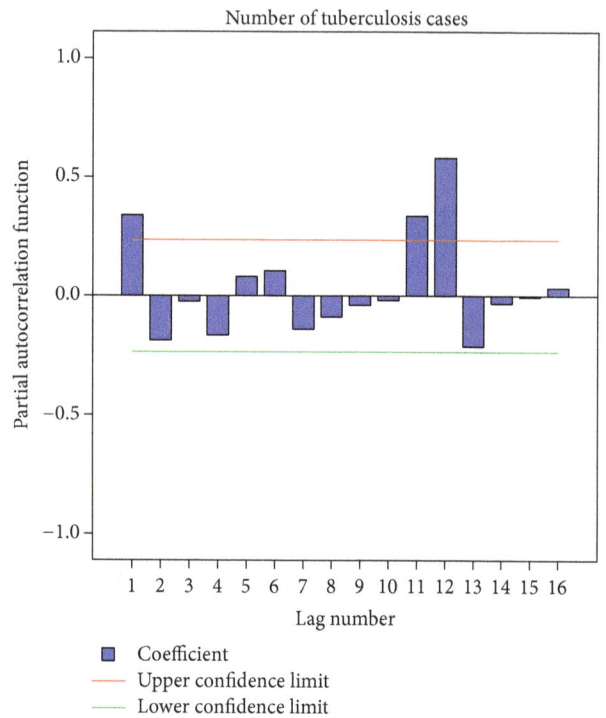

FIGURE 2: Partial autocorrelation plot for tuberculosis cases.

more than a few months. It shows a cyclical seasonal pattern as the peak of newly registered cases follows a similar pattern with an interval of few months between the peaks. Table 2 shows the monthly TB incidence during the study period from January 2007 to December 2012.

The autocorrelation function showed a significant peak at a lag of 12 (autocorrelation = 0.698; Box-Ljung statistics ($P = 0.000$)) suggesting the presence of a seasonal component in the data. Auto correlation function (ACF) showed a significant peak at a lag of 12. Partial autocorrelation function (PACF) also showed a significant peak at a lag of 12 which

TABLE 3: Model statistics for tuberculosis data.

| Model parameter | Stationary R^2 | Ljung-Box statistic | | | Model type |
		Statistics	df	P value	
Tuberculosis monthly incidence	0.698	17.88	15	0.269	Winter's multiplicative model

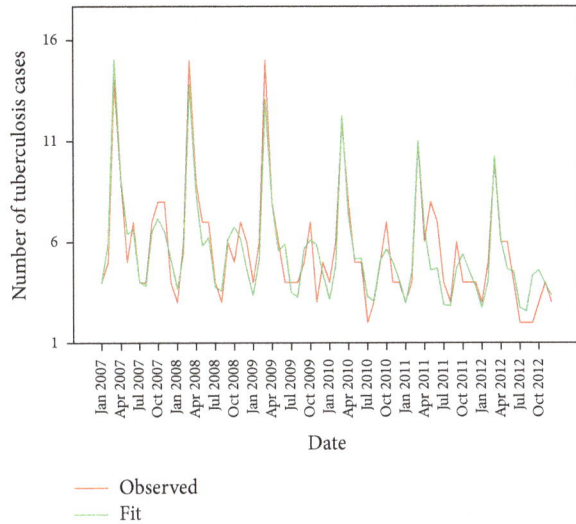

FIGURE 3: Actual (observed) and predicted (fit) values of tuberculosis cases.

TABLE 4: Seasonal adjustment factor (SAF) for tuberculosis cases.

Month	Observed cases	SAF (%)
January	21	59.9
February	32	95.5
March	77	216.4
April	46	132.6
May	37	113.5
June	34	97.2
July	20	58.7
August	19	57.2
September	31	96.8
October	34	105.1
November	30	86.8
December	26	80.4

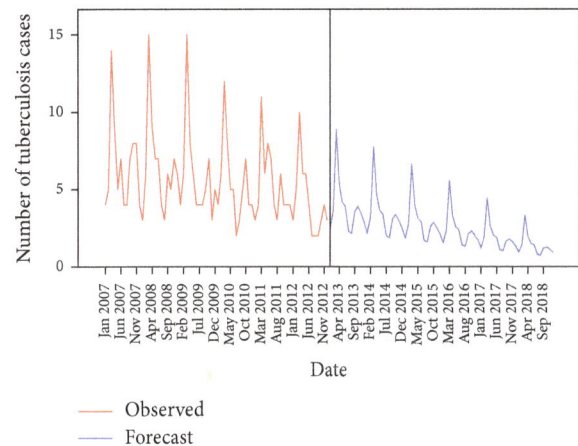

FIGURE 4: Sequence chart for forecasted tuberculosis cases in the near future.

confirmed the presence of a seasonal component in the data (Figure 2).

The time series sequence chart (Figure 1) shows both declining trend and periodic seasonal fluctuations. So the expert modeler of SPSS ver. 21 suggested Winter's multiplicative model as the best fitted mathematical model for this time series data. Figure 3 shows that the observed actual values and the predicted model values matched reasonably well and there was consistency in the trend.

The Ljung-Box (modified Box-Pierce) test indicated that the model was correctly specified (Table 3). The expert modeler detected no outliers in the data.

Although the time series modeler offers a number of different goodness of fit statistics, here stationary R-squared value was used. This statistic provides an estimate of the proportion of the total variation in the series that is explained by the model and is preferable to ordinary R-squared when there is a trend or seasonal pattern, as is the case here. Larger values of stationary R-squared (up to a maximum value of 1) indicate better fit. A value of 0.698 meant that the model could explain 69.8% of the observed variation in the series.

In Winter's multiplicative model, the seasonal adjustments are multiplied by the seasonally adjusted series to obtain the observed values. This adjustment attempts to remove the seasonal effect from a series in order to look at other characteristics of interest that may be "masked" by the seasonal component in effect seasonal components that do not depend on the overall level of the series. Observations without seasonal variation have a seasonal component of 0. Table 4 shows that from the month of March to June

the seasonal adjusted factor (SAF) of TB was more than 0; that is, in these months the registered TB cases were more above the typical months. Among these months, March with SAF = 216.4 had the highest SAF; that is, in this month, the registered TB cases were more than 216.4% above the typical months.

The months of March, April, May, and October have SAF of more than 100. This shows that during these months the number of newly registered TB cases was more than the typical months. This shows that the peak of new TB cases occurs during these months which coincides with the spring season in Delhi.

The same model was used to forecast the monthly tuberculosis incidence for the future from January 2013 to December 2018 and the values are depicted in Figure 4.

The forecasted values also show a declining trend over the years with a peak during the month of March.

4. Discussion

In a previous study conducted in India on assessment of seasonal trends, Thorpe et al. [5] reported that diagnosis of TB peaked between April and June and reached nadir between October and December. Areas in the north India had the highest seasonal variation and low or no seasonality was noted in central and southern regions of India in that study. Seasonal variations have also been reported from various other countries like China [8] and United Kingdom [9]. Since seasons involve variations in various phenomena like temperature, humidity, precipitation, length of daylight, and so forth and also vary by geography and latitude, the presence of seasonal variation and the timing and magnitude of such seasonal variation may depend on some of these factors in ways not yet fully understood. Apart from these reasons, differential access to health care with varying seasons can also be an important factor in new TB case detection. But in the present study, this factor plays a very little role.

The real causes of seasonal patterns of TB remain unknown, but the seasonal trend, with higher incidence rate in winter, may be relevant to the increased periods spent in overcrowded, poorly ventilated housing conditions, these phenomena much more easily seen in winter than during warm seasons. The outside environment determines the amount of time spent indoors and thus the transmissibility of *Mycobacterium tuberculosis* [4]. In the present study, indoor air pollution seems to be a plausible cause for this striking and sustained seasonal pattern in the number of TB cases which can be either primary or reactivated.

A possible link between vitamin D deficiency and impaired host defense to *Mycobacterium tuberculosis* infection leading to primary TB has also been postulated [10]. The relation between exposure to sunlight and risk for active tuberculosis has been increasingly recognized, with the hypothesis being vitamin D deficiency reducing the ability of macrophages to kill intracellular *Mycobacterium tuberculosis* [11]. Delhi is situated in the subtropical region at a latitude level of around 28.2 degree north of equator and plenty of sunlight is expected all-year round except during winter months of December and January.

Another reason for the onset of adult tuberculosis is thought to be due to reactivation, although the mechanism of reactivation and development of overt tuberculosis is not well understood, but it has been attributed to poor nutrition and socioeconomic status [12, 13]. Seasonal changes in the absolute numbers and ratios of T helper and suppressor cells could possibly alter cell mediated immunity, which is crucial to the host response controlling infection with *Mycobacterium tuberculosis*. However, the factors that regulate the seasonal changes in T cell subset numbers or function remain unknown [14].

Based upon the results of this study, we believe that there will be no obvious improvement in the high burden of TB in India in the near future. The results indicate that in the near future, the reported annual TB incidence numbers in India will decrease only slightly. The results of the study can be used for appropriate allocation of resources to target prevention and treatment of tuberculosis. It can also be used to inform travelers on TB risk and screening. Another potential implication of this study's findings are that, given the seasonal variation observed, clinicians, even in locations other than India, should have a higher than usual clinical suspicion for TB (and perhaps a lower threshold to place patients in airborne isolation) in the late winter and spring months.

But the study has its own limitations, with the major one being the lack of clinical data. Since the study is of observational design, the cause and effect relationship could not be established. It is also to be noted that it is a DOTS centre record based study and more sick people are likely to attend tertiary hospital. So it is difficult to predict the variation in the actual population.

5. Conclusion

A seasonal pattern of TB was observed for newly diagnosed smear positive cases with variable amplitudes of fluctuation. These observations are suggestive of the presence of a seasonal disease-modifying factor. This regularity of peak seasonality in TB case detection may prove useful to initiate measures that warrant a better implementation of control measures. This information would be also useful for administration and managers to take extra care to arrange and provide extra facilities during the peak seasons.

References

[1] C. Dye, "Global epidemiology of tuberculosis," *The Lancet*, vol. 367, no. 9514, pp. 938–940, 2006.

[2] World Health Organization, *Global Tuberculosis Control*, World Health Organization, Geneva, Switzerland, 2010.

[3] N. Nagayama and M. Ohmori, "Seasonality in various forms of tuberculosis," *International Journal of Tuberculosis and Lung Disease*, vol. 10, no. 10, pp. 1117–1122, 2006.

[4] M. Ríos, J. M. García, J. A. Sánchez, and D. Pérez, "A statistical analysis of the seasonality in pulmonary tuberculosis," *European Journal of Epidemiology*, vol. 16, no. 5, pp. 483–488, 2000.

[5] L. E. Thorpe, T. R. Frieden, K. F. Laserson, C. Wells, and G. R. Khatri, "Seasonality of tuberculosis in India: is it real and what does it tell us?" *The Lancet*, vol. 364, no. 9445, pp. 1613–1614, 2004.

[6] Tuberculosis facts, *TB Statistics for India*, 2012, http://www.tbfacts.org/tb-statistics-india.html.

[7] Tuberculosis Control in India, *Revised National Tuberculosis Control Program (RNTCP) in India*, http://www.tbcindia.nic.in/pdfs/TB%20India%202013.pdf.

[8] X. X. Li, L. X. Wang, H. Zhang, X. Du, and S. W. Jiang, "Seasonal variations in notification of active tuberculosis cases in China, 2005–2012," *PLoS ONE*, vol. 8, no. 7, Article ID e68102, 2013.

[9] A. S. Douglas, D. P. Strachan, and J. D. Maxwell, "Seasonality of tuberculosis: the reverse of other respiratory diseases in the UK," *Thorax*, vol. 51, no. 9, pp. 944–946, 1996.

[10] P. D. O. Davies, "A possible link between vitamin D deficiency and impaired host defence to *Mycobacterium tuberculosis*," *Tubercle*, vol. 66, no. 4, pp. 301–306, 1985.

[11] A. R. Martineau, S. Nhamoyebonde, T. Oni et al., "Reciprocal seasonal variation in vitamin D status and tuberculosis notifications in Cape Town, South Africa," *Proceedings of the National Academy of Sciences of the United States of America*, vol. 108, no. 47, pp. 19013–19017, 2011.

[12] M. D. Willis, C. A. Winston, C. M. Heilig, K. P. Cain, N. D. Walter, and W. R. Mac Kenzie, "Seasonality of tuberculosis in the United States, 1993–2008," *Clinical Infectious Disease*, vol. 54, pp. 1553–1560, 2012.

[13] D. P. Strachan, K. J. Powell, A. Thaker, F. J. C. Millard, and J. D. Maxwell, "Vegetarian diet as a risk factor for tuberculosis in immigrant south London Asians," *Thorax*, vol. 50, no. 2, pp. 175–180, 1995.

[14] T. G. Paglieroni and P. V. Holland, "Circannual variation in lymphocyte subsets, revisited," *Transfusion*, vol. 34, no. 6, pp. 512–516, 1994.

10

Cytokine Polymorphisms, Their Influence and Levels in Brazilian Patients with Pulmonary Tuberculosis during Antituberculosis Treatment

Eliana Peresi,[1,2] Larissa Ragozo Cardoso Oliveira,[1] Weber Laurentino da Silva,[3]
Érika Alessandra Pellison Nunes da Costa,[1] João Pessoa Araujo Jr.,[4]
Jairo Aparecido Ayres,[5] Maria Rita Parise Fortes,[6] Edward A. Graviss,[7]
Ana Carla Pereira,[3] and Sueli Aparecida Calvi[1]

[1] Tropical Disease Department, Botucatu School of Medicine, UNESP, São Paulo State University, Botucatu, SP, Brazil

[2] Departamento de Doenças Tropicais e Diagnóstico por Imagem, Faculdade de Medicina de Botucatu, UNESP, Rubião Júnior S/N, Botucatu 18618-970, SP, Brazil

[3] Lauro de Souza Lima Institute, Bauru, SP, Brazil

[4] Microbiology and Immunology Department, Bioscience Institute, UNESP, São Paulo State University, Botucatu, SP, Brazil

[5] Nursing Department, Botucatu School of Medicine, UNESP, São Paulo State University, Botucatu, SP, Brazil

[6] Dermatology and Radiotherapy Department, Botucatu School of Medicine, UNESP, São Paulo State University, Botucatu, SP, Brazil

[7] The Methodist Hospital Research Institute, Houston, TX, USA

Correspondence should be addressed to Eliana Peresi; elianaperesi@yahoo.com.br

Academic Editor: Carlo Garzelli

Cytokines play an essential role during active tuberculosis disease and cytokine genes have been described in association with altered cytokine levels. Therefore, the aim of this study was to verify if *IFNG, IL12B, TNF, IL17A, IL10,* and *TGFB1* gene polymorphisms influence the immune response of Brazilian patients with pulmonary tuberculosis (PTB) at different time points of antituberculosis treatment (T1, T2, and T3). Our results showed the following associations: *IFNG* +874 T allele and *IFNG* +2109 A allele with higher IFN-γ levels; *IL12B* +1188 C allele with higher IL-12 levels; *TNF* −308 A allele with higher TNF-α plasma levels in controls and mRNA levels in PTB patients at T1; *IL17A* A allele at rs7747909 with higher IL-17 levels; *IL10* −819 T allele with higher IL-10 levels; and *TGFB1* +29 CC genotype higher TGF-β plasma levels in PTB patients at T2. The present study suggests that *IFNG* +874T/A, *IFNG* +2109A/G, *IL12B* +1188A/C, *IL10* −819C/T, and *TGFB1* +21C/T are associated with differential cytokine levels in pulmonary tuberculosis patients and may play a role in the initiation and maintenance of acquired cellular immunity to tuberculosis and in the outcome of the active disease while on antituberculosis treatment.

1. Introduction

Mycobacterium tuberculosis (*M. tuberculosis*) is an intracellular obligate aerobic pathogen which has a predilection for the lungs [1]. Macrophages initiate phagocytosis of *M. tuberculosis* bacilli and regulate immune responses mediated by proinflammatory cytokines such as TNF-α. Effector T lymphocytes (T cells) and natural killer (NK) cells secrete IFN-γ which activate alveolar macrophages to produce reactive intermediates from nitrogen and oxygen, inhibiting growth and promoting mycobacteria death [2]. IL-12, produced mainly by macrophages and dendritic cells, has a key role in the immune response to *M. tuberculosis*, bridging innate and adaptive immunity. Moreover, IL-12 induces T cells and NK cells to produce proinflammatory cytokines such as IFN-γ and TNF-α while also regulating the production of IL-17 [2, 3]. A synergistic response of IFN-γ, IL-12, TNF-α and IL-17 activates macrophage, stimulating these cells to eliminate the intracellular pathogen, acting as a major effector mechanism of the cellular immune response [4].

Despite the protective effect of Th1 responses against *M. tuberculosis*, certain cytokines, such as TNF-α, are correlated with the immunopathogenesis of the disease [5]. To prevent tissue damage, active tuberculosis is associated with decreased Th1 and increased production and action of suppressing cytokines produced by Th2 and T regulatory (Treg) cells, IL-10, and TGF-β, respectively, which act by deactivating macrophages, modulating proinflammatory cytokines, and reducing the antigen presenting function of T cells [6]. TGF-β also participates in the induction of fibrosis, a hallmark presentation of tuberculosis disease [7].

The dynamics of tuberculosis (TB) disease is complex, as various aspects of the parasite-host interaction contribute to the occurrence and presentation of the outcome. In this scenario there is an important contribution of human genetic susceptibility to disease after exposure to *M. tuberculosis* [8–10]. Cytokines have a key role in the defense against mycobacteria and their genes might be considered candidates for host susceptibility to the onset of active TB disease.

The association between cytokines polymorphisms and human TB susceptibility has been reported in studies with *ex vivo* cytokine production in response to mycobacterial antigens and their correlation with variant genotypes; however few studies have investigated their role in modulating the overall cytokine response during PTB treatment [11–19]. We hypothesized that studying the actual overall immune cytokine pattern of PTB patients could be important to our understanding of active disease and possible establishment of biomarkers of recovery and anti-TB treatment efficiency. Therefore the aim of this study was to verify the influence of *IFNG*, *IL12B*, *TNF*, *IL17A*, *IL10*, and *TGFB1* gene polymorphisms on the overall cytokine response of Brazilian patients with PTB under anti-TB treatment.

2. Material and Methods

2.1. Study Population. The study group enrolled 31 Brazilian patients attending the Infectious and Parasitic Diseases Services at Botucatu Medical School University Hospital, UNESP, Botucatu Teaching Health Centre and Primary Healthcare Units of Botucatu and surrounding region with PTB diagnosis confirmed by sputum smear or culture positivity for *M. tuberculosis* or by clinical-epidemiologic data with laboratory and image exams (radiography or computerized tomography (CT)) compatible with active TB. Patients with PTB concurrent with other active granulomatous diseases or HIV were excluded. All patients diagnosed with PTB received treatment for six months, using the four first-line drugs: isoniazid, ethambutol, pyrazinamide, and rifampicin. For the evaluation of immunologic function, patients' samples were collected based on the anti-TB treatment timeline, defined as T1: after diagnosis and with no more than one month of treatment; T2: with three months of treatment; and T3: with six months of treatment. Patient-specimen distribution for each time point included T1 (n = 5); T2 (n = 1); T3 (n = 2); with two time points T1 and T2 (n = 4); and with the three time

points T1, T2, and T3 (n = 19). For normal controls (C), we studied 20 health care workers from Botucatu Medical School (Botucatu, SP, Brazil), 9 males (mean age 40.4 years), and 11 females (mean age 34.1 years), without clinical complaints and with no history of TB disease, autoimmune disease, and other infectious disease. All controls were BCG vaccinated in childhood and tuberculin skin test (TST) positive (induration ≥ 5 mm). All patients and controls agreed to participate in the study, after study clarification and written informed consent.

2.2. Single Nucleotide Polymorphism (SNP) Genotyping. In the current study seven SNPs were analyzed: *IFNG* +874T/A; *IFNG* +2109A/G; *IL12B* +1188A/C; *TNF* −308G/C; *IL17A* rs7747909; *IL10* −819C/T; and *TGFB1* +29C/T. These polymorphisms were selected after verifying their presence in high frequency (5%) in the Brazilian population.

For the current study, 5 mL of peripheral blood was drawn in an EDTA blood tube (by standard phlebotomy procedures), from PTB patients (n = 31) and controls (n = 20) at base line (T$_0$), and genomic DNA was extracted from leukocytes employing a DNAzol commercial reagent (Invitrogen, Carlsbad, CA, USA), according to the manufacturer's instructions. Quantification and purity of the extracted DNA were determined on a spectrophotometer (NanoDrop 2000 Thermo Fisher Scientific). Amplification of the genomic regions of interest was performed by PCR using 20 to 50 ng of DNA, recombinant Taq DNA polymerase, 0.2 mM of each dNTP (deoxy-nucleotide-adenine, guanine, thymine or cytosine-triphosphate), 0.3 to 1 mM concentration of each of the specific primers, appropriate buffer, and ultrapure water. The *IFNG* +874T/A was genotyped by PCR-ARMS as described by Pravica et al. [20]. The variation at *IFNG* +2109A/G creates a restriction site for the enzyme *AciI* and was genotyped by a previously reported PCR-RFLP method [21]. The *IL12B* +1188 genotyping was performed using a PCR-RFLP method in accordance with García-González et al. [22]. Fluorescence-based TaqMan technology (Applied Biosystems, Foster City, CA, USA) was applied to produce genotypes of *IL17A* and *TGFB1* polymorphisms according to the manufacturer's instructions. The *TNF* −308A/G genotype was defined using a PCR-RFLP method in accordance with Wilson et al. [23].

2.3. Cytokines Gene Expression by Reverse Transcriptase Real Time PCR (RT-qPCR). To evaluate IFN-γ, IL-12, TNF-α, IL-17, IL-10, and TGF-β mRNA expressions, 20 mL of peripheral blood was drawn by a standard procedure in heparinized blood tubes, at a single time point from controls (n = 20) and at three serial time points for PTB patients (n = 31), based on the antituberculosis treatment timeline (T1, T2, and T3), as previously defined. Peripheral blood mononuclear cells (PBMCs) were isolated by a Histopaque gradient separation method [24]. The layer rich in lymphocytes and monocytes was aseptically removed and washed twice with PBS for 15 min at 1500 RPM. The cell suspension was resuspended in 1 mL of PBS and the identification and viability of cells were determined by counting with Turk solution (50 μL aliquots of cell suspension with 50 μL of the dye solution at 5%).

TABLE 1: Primers sequence for qPCR.

Primers	Forward sequence	Reverse sequence
IFN-γ	5'-AAAAGAGTTCCATTATCCGCTACATC-3'	5'-GTTTTGGGTTCTCTCTTGGCTGTTA-3'
IL-12	5'-ACCTCCACCTGCCGAGAAT-3'	5'-CATGGTGGATGCCGTTCA-3'
TNF-α	5'-GGTTTGCTACAACATGGGCTACA-3'	5'-CCCCAGGGACCTCTCTCTAATC-3'
IL-17	5'-TTAGGC ACATGGTGGACAATCGG-3'	5'-ATGACTCCTGGGAAGACCTCA TTG-3'
IL-10	5'-CTTGATGTCTGGGTCTTGGTTCT-3'	5'-GCTGGAGGACTTTAAGGGTTAACCT-3'
TGF-β	5'-AGGGCCAGGACCTTGCTG-3'	5'-CAAGGGCTACCATGCCAACT-3'
β-actin	5'-GCTGGAAGGTGGACAGCGA-3'	5'-GGCATCGTGATGGACTCCG-3'

Total RNA extraction from PBMC (2×10^6 cells/mL) was prepared using Trizol Reagent (Invitrogen, Carlsbad, CA, USA), according to manufacturer's instructions. The relative purity, concentration, and quality of the isolated RNA were determined by spectrophotometry and the ratio of A260–A280 nm exceeded 1.8 for all preparations (NanoDrop1 1000 Spectrophotometer, Thermo Scientific). To ensure complete removal of traces of genomic DNA, 1μg of total RNA was incubated with DNase I (Amp Grade).

First-strand cDNA synthesis was performed with 1μg of total RNA per 60 μL of reaction using Reverse Transcriptase Super Script II (Invitrogen, Carlsbad, CA, USA) and random primers (3μg/μL) (Invitrogen, Carlsbad, CA, USA) according to manufacturer's instructions. Within 5 minutes after RNAse H (Invitrogen, Carlsbad, CA, USA) was added and incubated at 37°C for 20 minutes.

Relative quantification of each target mRNA was performed using a standard curve-based method for relative real-time PCR data processing with a 7300 Real-Time PCR Systems (Applied Biosystems, USA) and Power SYBR Green PCR Master Mix [25]. Primers sets used in the qPCR (amplifying cytokine fragments of mRNA and of the human β-actin mRNA, endogenous mRNA control) are presented in Table 1. Each q-PCR was set in duplicate in a total of 20 mL each, which contained 0.2 mM of each forward and reverse primer, 2 mL of template cDNA, 10 μL qPCR master mix, and 7.2 mL nuclease-free water. In addition, a "no template" control was included in duplicate on each plate to verify that amplicon contamination was absent. PCR conditions were as follows: initial denaturation at 95°C for 10 min and 40 cycles at 95°C for 15 s and 60°C for 60 s, followed by a melting curve. Amplification of specific transcripts was confirmed by melting curve profiles generated at the end of each run. Control samples expression mean received the relative value of 1.0 and concentrations in all other samples were normalized proportionately.

2.4. Plasma Cytokine Levels. Plasma samples were obtained from the same peripheral blood used for the genetic expression of cytokines from controls ($n = 20$) and at three serial time points from patients with PTB, based on the antituberculosis treatment timeline (T1, T2, and T3), as previously defined. Samples were maintained frozen (−80°C) until use and then thawed at room temperature on the day they were used. Quantikine ELISA kits (R & D Systems) were used, according to manufacturer's instructions, to measure IFN-γ,

IL-12, TNF-α, IL-17, IL-10, and TGF-β plasma levels and method sensitivity was in accordance with each kit. Cytokine analysis was not possible in all 31 PTB patients because samples were also used in other experiments; therefore the distribution of individuals among cytokines was IFN-γ ($n = 30$): T1 ($n = 5$); T2 ($n = 1$); T3 ($n = 2$); with two time points T1 and T2 ($n = 4$); with two time points T1 and T3 ($n = 1$); and with the three time points T1, T2, and T3 ($n = 17$); IL-12, IL-17, and IL-10 ($n = 30$): T1 ($n = 7$); T2 ($n = 1$); T3 ($n = 2$); with two time points T1 and T2 ($n = 4$); and with the three time points T1, T2, and T3 ($n = 16$); TNF-α ($n = 30$): T1 ($n = 5$); T2 ($n = 1$); T3 ($n = 2$); with two time points T1 and T2 ($n = 4$); and with the three time points T1, T2, and T3 ($n = 18$); TGF-β ($n = 29$): T1 ($n = 5$); T2 ($n = 1$); T3 ($n = 2$); with two time points T1 and T2 ($n = 4$); and with the three time points T1, T2, and T3 ($n = 17$).

2.5. Statistical Analysis. Comparisons between different genotypes in the control and patient groups were made using Mann-Whitney U Test with two-tail P value. For the analytical comparison between the three time points of the treatment in the PTB case group (T1, T2, and T3), a Friedman test was used to verify which time point differed from the other, a Dunn's multiple comparisons test was applied as a posttest. Results were considered significant when $P < 0.05$. Tests were performed using GraphPad Prism version 5.00 for Windows, GraphPad Software (San Diego, CA, USA), http://www.graphpad.com/.

3. Results

3.1. Demographic Characteristics of PTB Patients. Gender and age distribution among PTB patients was 23 males (mean age of 48.8 years) and 8 females (mean age of 38.9 years) and all patients were BCG (Bacillus Calmette-Guérin) vaccinated in childhood. Despite the large differences of age and sex in controls and PTB patients groups, these variables had no effect on the cytokines expression and plasma levels (data not shown).

PTB patients' diagnosis was confirmed by sputum smear or culture positivity for *M. tuberculosis* ($n = 2$), sputum smear or culture positive for *M. tuberculosis*, and image exams (radiography or CT) compatible with active TB ($n = 19$) or by image exams (radiography or CT) compatible with active TB ($n = 10$) alone with diagnosis confirmation with clinical response after the beginning of the anti-TB treatment.

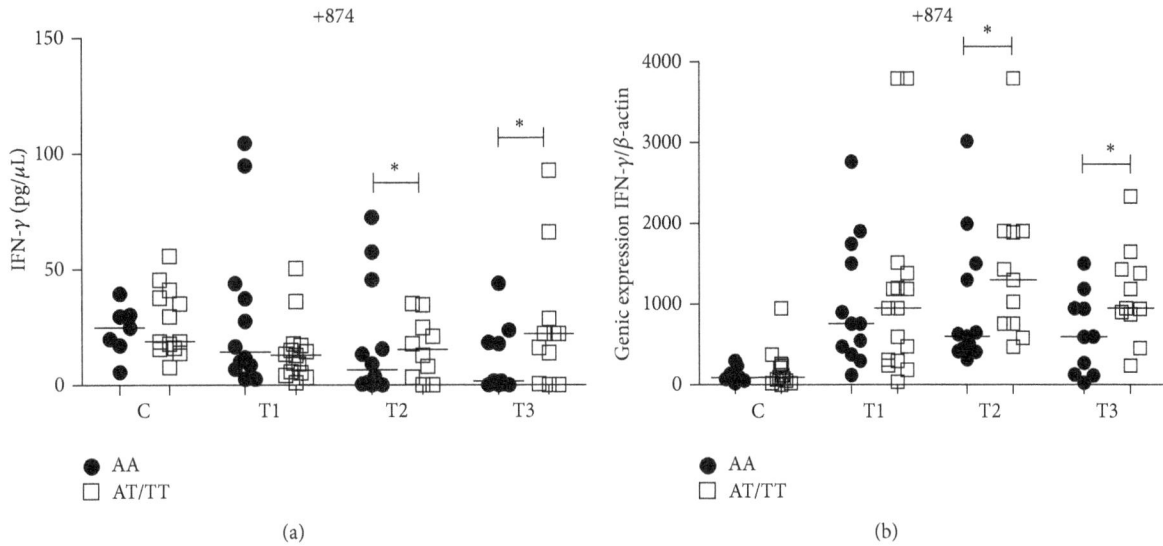

FIGURE 1: Influence of *IFNG* +874T/A gene SNP on IFN-γ plasma levels (a) and mRNA expression (b) in the control group (C) and PTB patients group at three time points of the treatment: T1 (after diagnosis and first month), T2 (three months), and T3 (six months). Data are shown as median levels. $^{*}P < 0.05$.

All patients had respiratory symptoms consistent with dyspnea, cough, and ventilation-dependent pain, and most presented with constitutional symptoms, consistent with weight loss, fever, and weakness at the beginning of the anti-TB treatment (T1). The symptoms were less frequent along treatment timeline (T2) and at the end (T3) all patients were considered recovered. Studies classify pulmonary tuberculosis by its severity as minimal, moderate, or advanced disease, depending on the characteristics of clinical-epidemiologic data and/or image exams (radiography or CT) [16, 19]. In our study medical evaluation of these characteristics showed that all of our patients had a moderate form of active TB disease.

3.2. General Immune Response during Anti-TB Treatment.
In general, when compared to controls, plasma levels of IFN-γ, IL-12, and IL-10 were similar among PTB patients during anti-TB treatment. IL-17 and TGF-β plasma levels were increased among PTB patients only at the beginning of anti-TB treatment (T1) and plasma levels for TNF-α were lower among PTB patients during anti-TB treatment (T1, T2, and T3) (data not shown). When compared to controls, mRNA expression levels of IL-12, TNF-α, and IL-17 were similar among PTB patients during anti-TB treatment (T1, T2, and T3). IFN-γ and IL-10 were increased among PTB patients during anti-TB treatment (T1, T2, and T3) and TGF-β was increased only at the T2 time point among PTB patients (data not shown).

3.3. Influence of IFNG +874T/A and +2109A/G Gene Polymorphisms on IFN-γ Plasma Level and mRNA Expression.
The T allele carriers for *IFNG* +874T/A (AT/TT) in PTB patients were associated with significantly higher plasma and mRNA expression levels of IFN-γ when compared to individuals with AA genotype at T2 ($P = 0.04$; $P = 0.03$, resp.) and T3 ($P = 0.04$; $P = 0.03$) time points of the treatment

(Figures 1(a) and 1(b)). When we compared the three time points, the AA genotype in PTB patients at T1 presented significant higher plasma levels than T2 ($P < 0.05$) and T3 ($P < 0.05$) (Figure 8(a)) and no differences for mRNA expression (Figure 8(b)). T allele carriers at T2 presented with significantly higher mRNA expression levels than at T1 ($P < 0.05$) (Figure 8(b)) and no differences at the IFN-γ plasma level (Figure 8(a)) were seen. There was no influence of this polymorphism on the control group (Figures 1(a) and 1(b)).

Results for the *IFNG* +2109A/G SNP showed that individuals with AA genotype presented higher levels of IFN-γ than the AG genotype in controls ($P < 0.05$) and in PTB patients at T2 ($P = 0.04$) and T3 ($P = 0.02$) (Figure 2(a)). Comparisons between the heterozygous AG genotype of PTB patients time points, using the same individuals, showed that at T1 significantly higher levels of IFN-γ were seen than at T2 ($P < 0.05$) and T3 ($P < 0.05$). There were no differences between treatment time points for PTB patients with the AA genotype (Figure 8(c)). No significant differences in mRNA expression were seen between genotypes in the control group and in PTB patients, although patients with the AA genotype tended to present with higher expression levels when compared to individuals with the AG genotype (Figure 2(b)). There were also no differences between treatment time points of PTB patients for mRNA expression within both genotypes (data not shown). In our study group we did not find individuals with the GG genotype.

3.4. Influence of IL12B +1188A/C Gene Polymorphism on IL-12 Plasma Level and mRNA Expression.
The C allele carriers for *IL12B* +1188 (AC/CC) had significantly higher plasma levels of IL-12 than individuals with the AA genotype in the control group ($P = 0.04$) and at the T2 ($P = 0.03$) time point of PTB patients (Figure 3(a)). IL-12 mRNA expression analysis showed no difference when AA genotype and C allele carriers

(a)

(b)

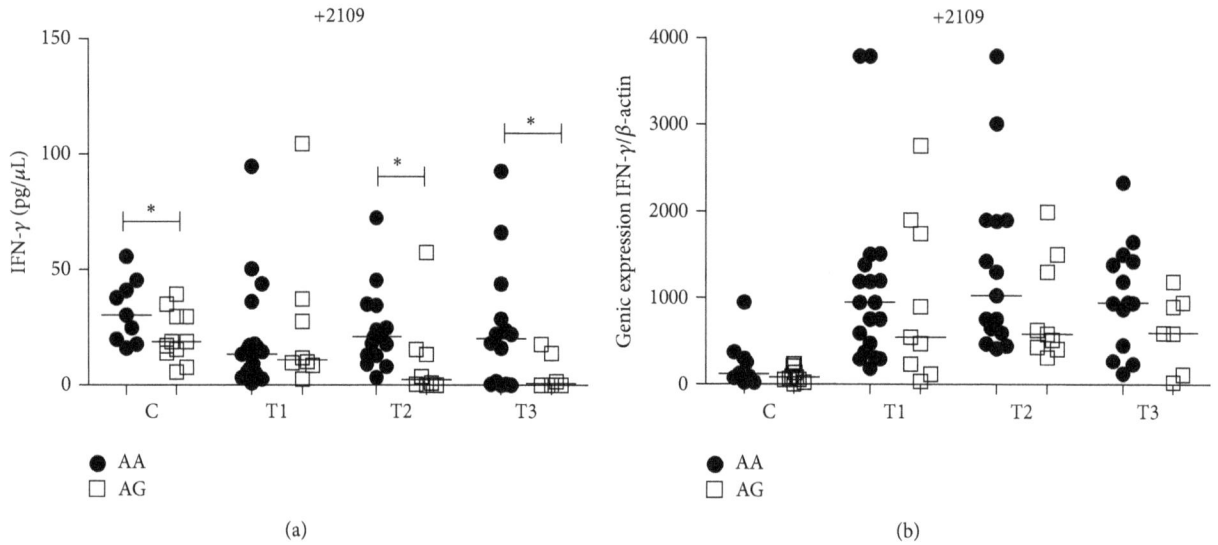

FIGURE 2: Influence of *IFNG* +2109A/G gene SNP on IFN-γ plasma levels (a) and mRNA expression (b) in the control group (C) and PTB patients group at three time points of the treatment: T1 (after diagnosis and first month), T2 (three months), and T3 (six months). Data are shown as median levels. *$P < 0.05$.

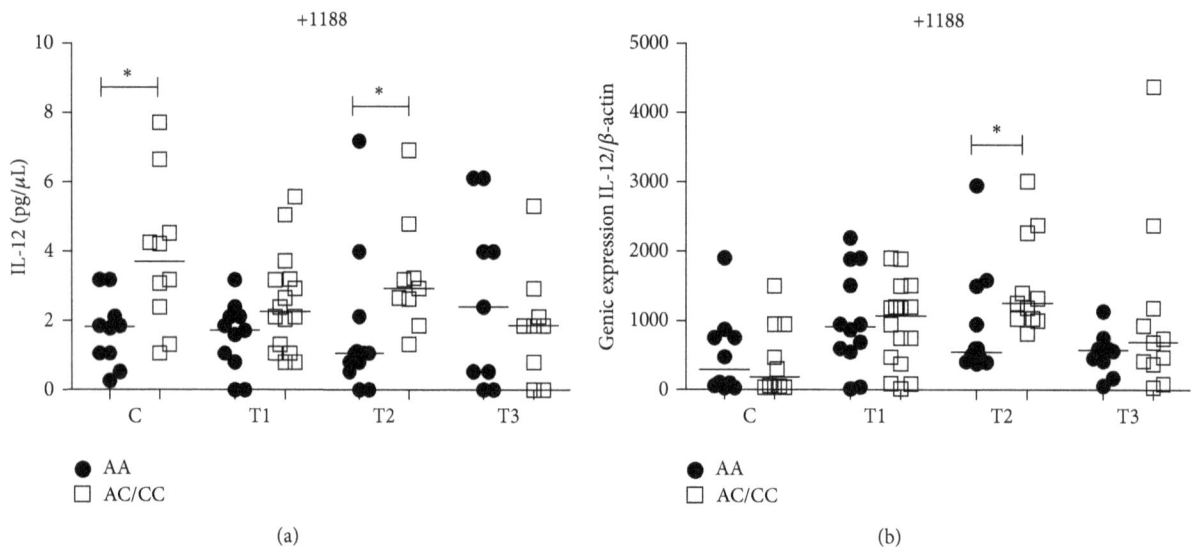

(a)

(b)

FIGURE 3: Influence of *IL12B* +1188A/C gene SNP on IL-12 plasma levels (a) and mRNA expression (b) in the control group (C) and PTB patients group at three time points of the treatment: T1 (after diagnosis and first month), T2 (three months), and T3 (six months). Data are shown as median levels. *$P < 0.05$.

were compared in the control group. However, at the T2 time point for PTB patients, C allele carriers expressed more IL-12 mRNA expression levels than individuals with AA genotype ($P < 0.05$) (Figure 3(b)). There were also no differences between time points of PTB patients for IL-12 plasma and mRNA expression levels within both genotypes (data not shown).

3.5. Influence of TNF −308G/C Gene Polymorphism on TNF-α Plasma Level and mRNA Expression. Control individuals with the AG genotype had significantly higher plasma levels

of TNF-α than those with GG genotype ($P = 0.04$). There was no difference between genotypes in the PTB patients group (Figure 4(a)). The analyses between time points for the GG genotype in PTB patients showed higher levels of TFN-α at T1 when compared with T3 ($P < 0.05$). No differences were seen between time points for the AG genotype PTB patients (Figure 8(d)). The *TNF*-308G/C gene SNP did not influence TNF-α mRNA expression in controls (Figure 4(b)). At T1, PTB patients with the AG genotype had significantly higher mRNA expression levels than those patients with the GG genotype ($P = 0.02$) (Figure 4(b)). There were also no differences between time points of PTB patients for mRNA

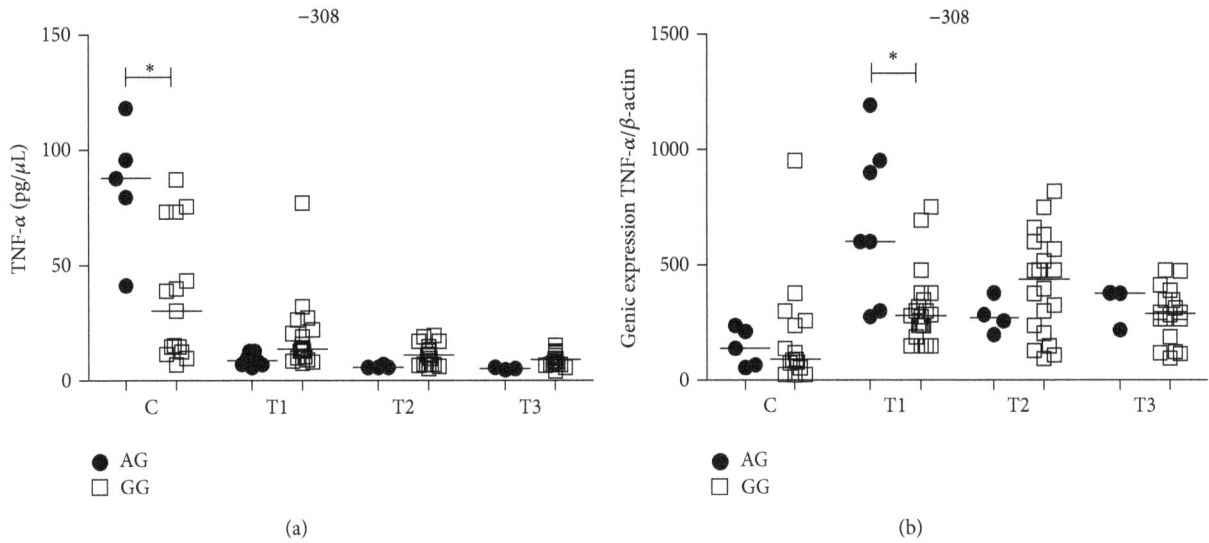

FIGURE 4: Influence of *TNF* −308G/C gene SNP on TNF-α plasma levels (a) and mRNA expression (b) in the control group (C) and PTB patients group at three time points of the treatment: T1 (after diagnosis and first month), T2 (three months), and T3 (six months). Data are shown as median levels. *P < 0.05.

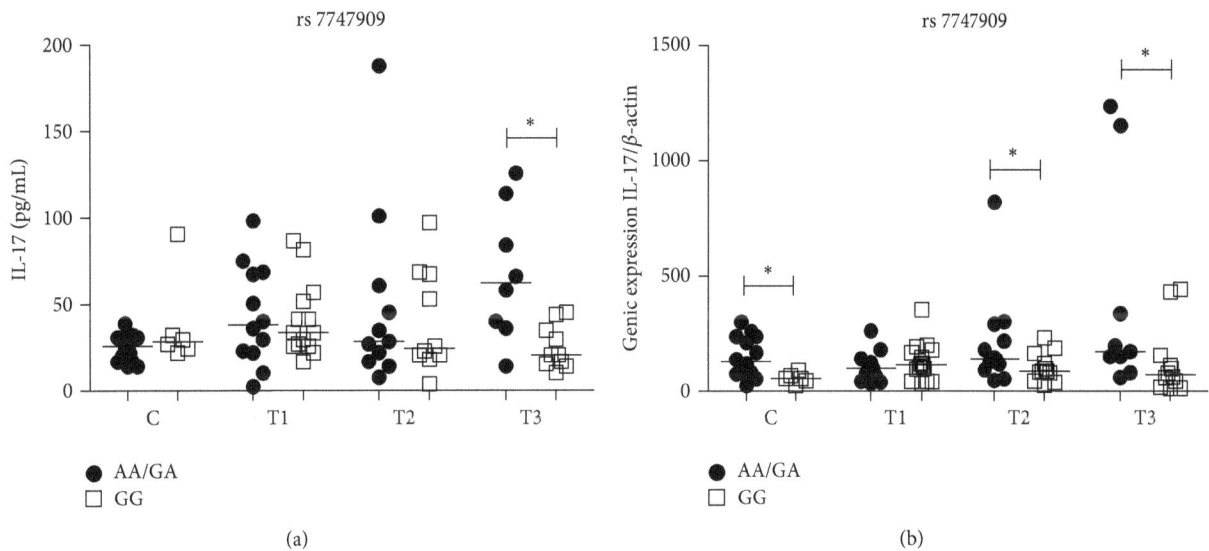

FIGURE 5: Influence of *IL17* SNP rs7747909 on IL-17 plasma levels (a) and mRNA expression (b) in the control group (C) and PTB patients group at three time points of the treatment: T1 (after diagnosis and first month), T2 (three months), and T3 (six months). Data are shown as median levels. *P < 0.05.

expression with either genotype (data not shown). In our study group we did not find individuals carrying the AA genotype.

3.6. Influence of IL17A rs7747909 Gene Polymorphism on IL-17A Plasma Level and mRNA Expression. The marker rs7747909 at *IL17* gene had no influence on IL-17 control plasma levels. PTB patients who were A allele carriers (AA/AG) had significantly higher IL-17 plasma levels only at the T3 time point (P = 0.04) (Figure 5(a)). In controls, the A allele carriers had significantly higher IL-17 mRNA expression levels than individuals with the GG genotype

(P = 0.04). In PTB patients who were A allele carriers we found significantly higher IL-17 mRNA expression levels at the T2 (P < 0.05) and T3 (P = 0.04) time points than patients with the GG genotype (Figure 5(b)). There were no differences between time points of PTB patients for IL-17 plasma and mRNA expression levels within both genotype groups (data not shown).

3.7. Influence of IL10 −819C/T Gene Polymorphism on IL-10 PLasma Level and mRNA Expression. There was no difference in IL-10 plasma levels in the controls between CC genotype and T allele carriers. PTB patients who were carriers

−819

−819

(a)

(b)

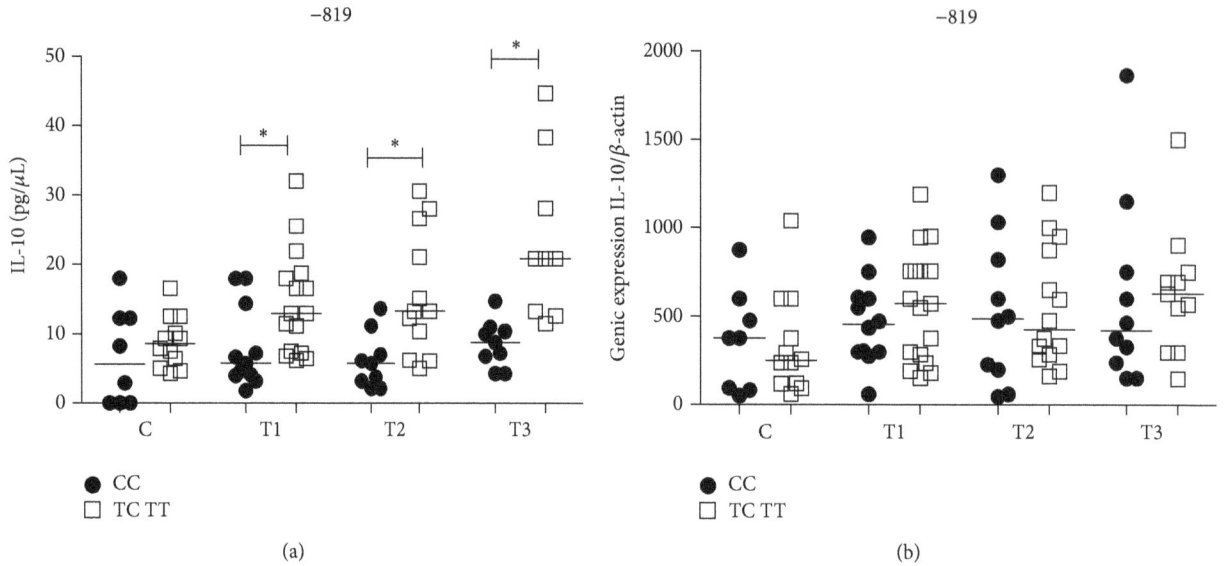

FIGURE 6: Influence of *IL10* −819C/T gene SNP on IL-10 plasma levels (a) and mRNA expression (b) in the control group (C) and PTB patients group at three time points of the treatment: T1 (after diagnosis and first month), T2 (three months), and T3 (six months). Data are shown as median levels $^*P < 0.05$.

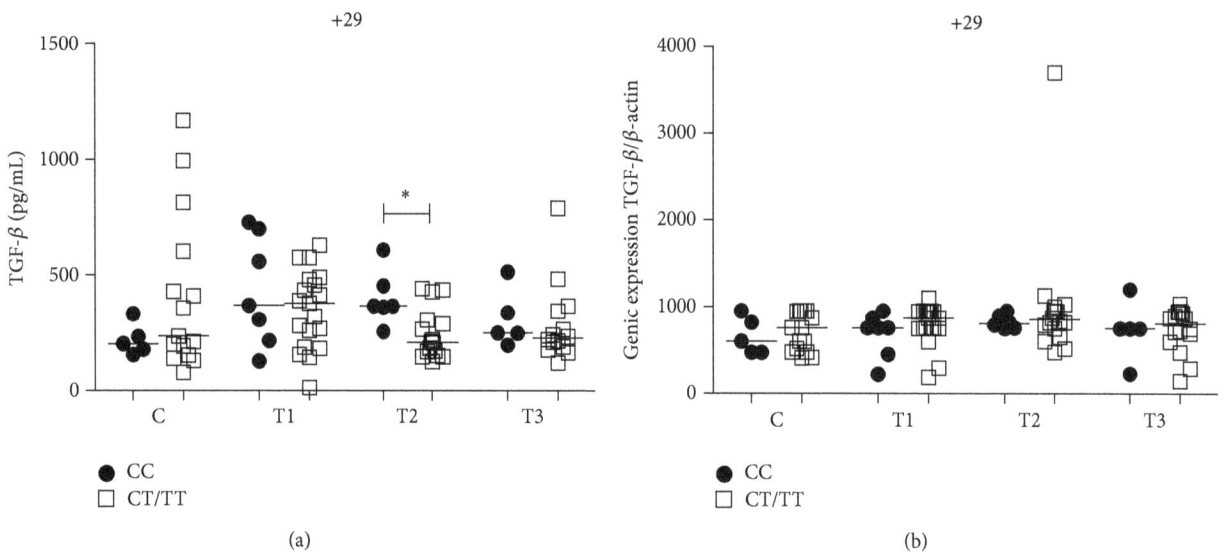

+29

+29

(a)

(b)

FIGURE 7: Influence of *TGFβ1* +29C/T gene SNP on TGF-β plasma levels (a) and mRNA expression (b) in the control group (C) and PTB patients at three time points of the treatment: T1 (after diagnosis and first month), T2 (three months), and T3 (six months). Data are shown as median levels. $^*P < 0.05$.

of the T allele (TC/TT) had significantly higher levels of IL-10 when compared with PTB patients with the CC genotype in all time points of treatment T1 ($P < 0.05$), T2 ($P = 0.03$), and T3 ($P < 0.05$) (Figure 6(a)). IL-10 −819C/T SNP had no influence on IL-10 mRNA expression in the control group and PTB patients when the CC genotype and T allele carriers were compared (Figure 6(b)). There were also no differences between time points in PTB patients for IL-10 plasma and mRNA expression levels within both genotypes (data not shown).

3.8. *Influence of TGFB1 +29C/T Gene Polymorphism on TGF-β Plasma Level and mRNA Expression.* No differences in TGF-β plasma levels were seen in the control group between both genotypes. PTB patients with CC genotype had higher TGF-β plasma levels when compared with T allele carriers only at the T2 time point ($P = 0.02$) (Figure 7(a)). Analyses between time points of PTB patients with CC genotype showed higher TGF-β plasma levels at T1 when compared to T3 ($P < 0.05$) (Figure 8(e)). No differences in mRNA expression were seen in both controls and PTB patients

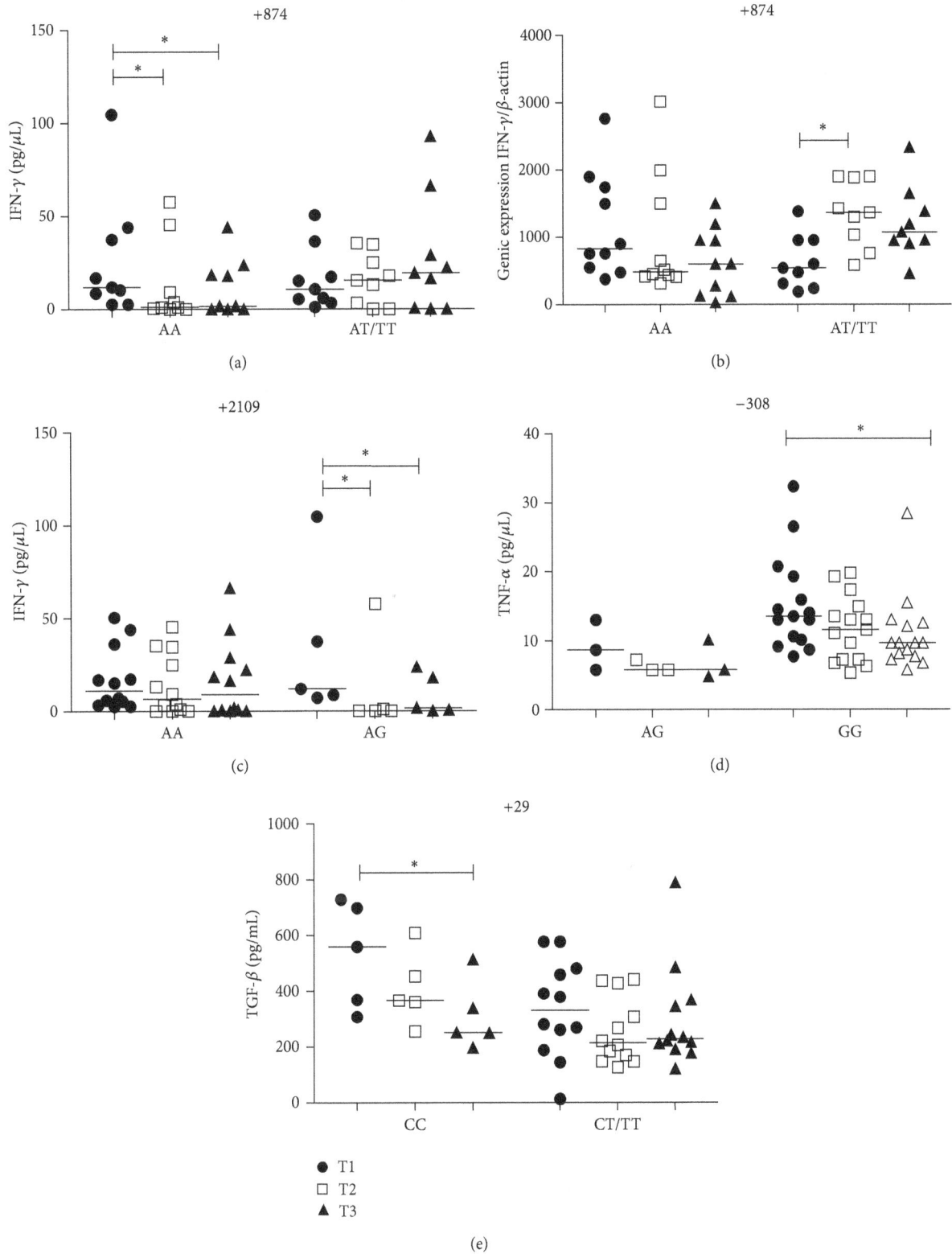

FIGURE 8: Influence of *IFNG* +874T/A gene SNP on IFN-γ plasma levels (a) and mRNA expression (b), *IFNG* +2109A/G gene SNP on IFN-γ plasma levels (c), *TNF* −308G/C gene SNP on TNF-α plasma levels (d), and TGFB1 +29C/T gene SNP on TGF-β plasma levels (e) in PTB patients that have all three time points of the treatment: T1 (after diagnosis and first month), T2 (three months), and T3 (six months). Data are shown as median levels. $^*P < 0.05$.

within both genotypes (Figure 7(b)). There were also no differences between time points of PTB patients for mRNA expression within both genotypes (data not shown).

4. Discussion

It is well known that cytokines play an essential role during the immune response to active TB disease and changes in cytokine levels may lead to abnormal or ineffective immune responses, as seen in human infections caused by *M. tuberculosis* [6]. The genetic component that contributes to susceptibility and progression of PTB most certainly involves an interaction between multiple alleles located on different genes [26]. As a number of cytokine genes have been described in association with altered cytokine levels [13, 20], we evaluated the influence of SNPs at cytokine genes on the overall cytokine response of PTB patients undergoing anti-TB treatment. When pertinent, controls results were considered to indicate an effect of the polymorphism under normal conditions, without the interference of active TB or anti-TB treatment, in other words, an independent genetic effect.

Our results showed that PTB patients who were T allele carriers had higher plasma and mRNA expression levels of IFN-γ at the middle and end of anti-TB treatment. Studies have shown that the *IFNG* +874A/T SNP influences IFN-γ production by providing a binding site for NF-κB and is associated with TB susceptibility [14, 15, 20]. This fact could have functional consequences for the transcription of IFN-γ production [27, 28].

A recent study in Spain showed that the *IFNG* +874 AA genotype had the lowest IFN-γ production in PBMC culture after stimulation with PPD in PTB patients at the time of diagnosis and after completion of therapy [14], which agrees with our results at the end of anti-TB treatment. Still in agreement with our results, 2 additional studies have shown that the homozygous TT genotype of normal and PTB individuals produces higher IFN-γ in response to mycobacterial antigens [15, 16]. In another functional study patients with tuberculosis carrying the genotype +874AA showed significantly lower IFN-γ plasma levels than those with the +874AT and +874TT genotypes [11]. This trend was also seen in the plasma of Indians patients with active PTB [12].

Other studies that evaluated IFN-γ serum levels in HBV infection and IFN-γ production in PBMC cultures in acutely ill patients, cutaneous leishmaniasis, and normal individuals stimulated with LPS (Lipopolysaccharide), PHA (Phytohemagglutinin), or *Mycobacterium leprae* (*M. leprae*) antigens also support our findings of higher IFN-γ levels in PTB patients that were T allele carriers (TA/TT) [29–31]. Another study has shown the relation between an *IFNG* polymorphic microsatellite marker (allele 2) polymorphism and the IFN-γ gene transcription. Since this region shows an absolute correlation with the *IFNG* +874 T allele, this study's findings are in agreement with our results, that showed that the *IFNG* +874 T allele was related to a higher IFN-γ expression from the middle to the end of the anti-TB treatment [20].

Some studies evaluating tuberculosis patients in the initial stages of TB disease using normal controls have found no differences between genotypes of *IFNG* +874 SNP in IFN-γ production, in PBMC cultures of *M. tuberculosis* H37Rv, culture filtrate antigen (CFA) of *M. tuberculosis* nor PHA stimulus [17, 18]. An additional study found no influence of *IFNG* +874 locus on mRNA expression during *Helicobacter pylori* (*H. pylori*) infection [32]. These different findings may be due to ethnic differences in genotypic frequencies among various population studies. This result however is in complete agreement with genetic epidemiologic data that the T allele is associated with protection against TB [33]. This same allele is also associated with resistance to leprosy [34].

Another polymorphism in the *INFG* gene located 2,109 bp downstream from the translation start site in the third intron has been reported to be involved in transcriptional regulation of IFN-γ gene of this polymorphism, although the contribution is still unclear [35, 36]. To our knowledge our study is the first report regarding the functional effect of *INFG* +2109A/G on IFN-γ plasma and mRNA expression levels, as our results showed that controls and PTB patients with the AG genotype had lower plasma levels at the end of the treatment.

IFN-γ is a key cytokine in activation of macrophages for mycobacterial stasis and killing [2]; the persistence of low IFN-γ production from the middle to end of therapy in patients with *IFNG* +874 AA genotype and *INFG* +2109 AG genotype could result in a worse prognosis to the resolution of the active disease and efficiency of the anti-TB treatment and may also underlie their increased risk for reactivation of a latent PTB focus. In agreement with our results, decreased production of IFN-γ in PTB patients when compared with healthy controls have been reported and it may be due to the initial T cell anergy seen in the disease [18, 37–39]. Such an inadequate IFN-γ production may result in failure of macrophage activation, which could lead to active disease progression and could play a role affecting TB diagnostic tests, as *IFG* alleles were associated with microscopy-positive/negative and bacterial culture-positive/negative forms of disease [18, 40].

IL-12 is important in mediating protective immunity against TB. An SNP at 3'UTR region of the *IL12B* gene (+1188A/C) coding for IL-12p40 is known to modulate IL-12p40 levels. The present study showed that *IL12B* +1188 AA genotype is associated with lower IL-12 plasma levels in normal controls and in TB patients after 3 months of anti-TB treatment. Our results agree with another study that evaluated PTB patients and normal controls [17].

Several studies have found that the *IL12B* +1188 C allele is associated with lower IL-12p40 production of PBMC from healthy individuals stimulated with C3 binding glycoprotein, LPS, or PPD [41–43]. Arababadi et al. [30] did not find a significant difference in IL-12 serum level between AA and AC genotypes in occult HBV infection. Discordance between results may be due to differences in ethnicity, diseases, and designs of the studies.

IL-12 production is induced following phagocytosis of *M. tuberculosis* by macrophages and dendritic cells, which leads to development of a Th1 response with production of IFN-γ [1]. Since IL-12p40 is a component of both IL-12p70 and IL-23 and regulates initiation and maintenance of acquired cellular responses to TB, low IL-12p40 levels in AA genotype individuals might have a role in limiting chronic inflammation [44], which could result in more difficulties in resolving active disease and dampen the efficiency of the anti-TB treatment.

TNF-α plays an important role in granuloma formation in tuberculosis [19]. The promoter region of the *TNF* gene is highly polymorphic and our evaluation of the *TNF* −308G/A *locus* showed that normal individuals with the AG genotype had higher TNF-α plasma levels. PTB patients carrying the same genotype tended to have higher levels of TNF-α, though not significant. There are conflicting results regarding the functional effect of the *TNF* −308A/G SNP. Some authors have demonstrated increased TNF-α production related to *TNF* −308 A allele carriers in LPS stimulated PBMC and whole blood cultures of leprosy patients after LPS and *M. leprae* stimulation and of paracoccidioidomycosis patients, while others failed to show any effect of this SNP on TNF-α production after LPS stimulation *in vivo* or *in vitro*, in HCV patients and in tuberculosis patients [19, 44–50].

An *in vitro* expression study has indicated that the *TNF* −308G/A SNP has a direct effect on TNF-α gene regulation, and the A allele at this locus may lead to a higher expression level [51]. Our results agree with this study that demonstrated that PTB patients with the AG genotype at the beginning of anti-TB treatment have higher TNF-α mRNA expression than GG genotype individuals.

Since TNF-α is important for walling off infections and preventing dissemination by granuloma formation, low levels of TNF-α, as seen in our PTB patients, could impair the containment of the *M. tuberculosis* bacilli, leading to difficult resolution of active disease, dampening the efficiency of anti-TB treatment and increasing the reactivation risk, as shown in rheumatoid arthritis patients who were undergoing anti-TNF-α therapy [52, 53].

IL-17 is a potent inflammatory cytokine induced by *M. tuberculosis* infection [54]. To our knowledge this is the first study to verify the functional effect of the *IL17A* rs7747909 polymorphism on IL-17A plasma and mRNA expression levels. Our results showed that A allele carriers (at rs7747909) produce higher plasma levels of IL-17A at the end of therapy and, in general, PTB patients produced higher levels than normal controls.

Although Th17 cells are not as important as Th1 cells in mediating protection against primary *M. tuberculosis* infection, IL-17 appears to be critical to the induction of *M. tuberculosis*-specific memory response and the mediation of protection against challenge infections and during vaccinations [55–57]. Our results suggest that PTB patients have no impairment to IL-17A production.

IL-10 is known to have deactivating properties and undermines human Th1 immunologic responses. About 50% of the observed variability of IL-10 secretion can be explained by genetic factors [58]. Our results showed that *IL10* −819 T allele carriers had higher plasma levels of IL-10 during the 6 months of anti-TB treatment. A previous study evaluating PTB patients showed no influence of this SNP on IL-10 levels

[17]. Additionally, no impact of the *IL10* −819 locus was found on IL-10 serum level of controls and patients with HCV infection or on normal individuals PBMC cultures stimulated with LPS and PPD [13, 48]. A study on patients with leprosy showed that *IL10* −819 T allele carriers produce lower levels of IL-10 when compared with non-T allele carriers [59].

In a recent study evaluating *H. pylori*, patients with SNPs in the promoter region of *IL10* were shown to have higher IL-10 mRNA expression with the GCC haplotype carriers at *IL10* −1082G/A/−819CT//−592C/A and low IL-10 mRNA expression levels in ATA haplotype carriers [32]. In our study the different *IL10* −819 genotypes had no influence on IL-10 mRNA expression.

Published data suggests that IL-10 inhibits synthesis of IFN-γ by T cells and that production of IL-10 has been associated with anergy in tuberculosis [60, 61]. Our results suggest that PTB patients T allele carriers could have more difficulties in building a protective response towards active PTB since they are present with higher levels of IL-10 during anti-TB treatment. These results suggest that in cases with advanced forms of PTB, higher IL-10 production in T allele carries could lead to a worse recovery from active disease and poor anti-TB treatment efficiency.

TGF-β is present in the granulomatous lesions of TB patients [62]. At low concentrations TGF-β is a chemotactic factor for monocytes and acts to induce secretion of IL-1α and TNF-α and, in high concentration, inactivates macrophages, inhibits the expression and function of receptors for IFN-γ, IL-1α, and IL-2, and decreases the production of TNF-α, parallel events related to increase of intracellular mycobacterial growth [63, 64]. Our results showed that PTB patients with the *TGFB1* +21CC genotype have higher TGF-β plasma levels at T2 of the anti-TB treatment. These results are consistent with other studies focused on cancer and myocardial infarction [65–67]. Our results revealed that TGF-β plasma levels were higher at the beginning of the anti-TB treatment in all PTB patients when compared to the controls, which could result in the impairment of the initial protective immune response for the resolution of the active disease and in depressing the efficiency of anti-TB treatment. The fact that PTB patients with the *TGFB1* +21 CC genotype also maintained higher levels of the cytokine at T2 could result in a more persistent active disease.

Our work lacks an association between demographic characteristics and cytokine levels. In addition, the influence of cytokine SNPs on TB outcomes may be driven by a small sample size and by the fact that all patients had a moderate presentation of PTB. We also had differences between the plasma levels patterns and mRNA expression levels patterns of the cytokines evaluated in the controls and TB patients during anti-TB treatment. This fact could be explained by mRNA stability and transcription rate and by factors of translational regulation which could directly affect the expression and production of mediators involved in immune response [68].

The present study suggests that *IFNG* +874T/A, *IFNG* +2109A/G, *IL12* +1188A/C, *IL10* −819C/T, and *TGFB1* +21C/T are associated with different cytokine levels in PTB patients and may play a role in the initiation and maintenance of acquired cellular immunity to TB and in the outcome of the active disease and antituberculosis treatment. As cytokines play a major role in TB immunity, studying the overall cytokine profile determined by the respective functional SNPs and/or other closely linked genes could demonstrate the actual pattern of the cytokine response against the mycobacteria and may provide a better understanding of active TB disease progression and response to the anti-TB treatment and may serve as genetic risk markers of TB susceptibility.

5. Conclusion

In this study we demonstrated that cytokine SNPs can induce different overall cytokine levels in PTB patients during anti-TB treatment and these levels could be important to the outcome of the treatment. Future studies with a larger population and different forms and severity stages of tuberculosis will help to better understand why many individuals are infected by the mycobacterial bacilli but only 10% develop active disease.

Acknowledgment

This study was funded by grants from "Fundação de Amparo à Pesquisa do Estado de São Paulo" (FAPESP), Brazil.

References

[1] A. Raja, "Immunology of tuberculosis," *Indian Journal of Medical Research*, vol. 120, pp. 213–232, 2004.

[2] S. H. E. Kaufmann, "Protection against tuberculosis: cytokines, T cells, and macrophages," *Annals of the Rheumatic Diseases*, vol. 61, no. 2, pp. 1154–1158, 2002.

[3] M. A. Hoeve, N. D. Savage, T. de Boer et al., "Divergent effects of IL-12 and IL-23 on the production of IL-17 by human T cells," *European Journal of Immunology*, vol. 36, pp. 661–670, 2006.

[4] E. Sahiratmadja, B. Alisjahbana, T. de Boer et al., "Dynamic changes in pro- and anti-inflammatory cytokine profiles and gamma interferon receptor signaling integrity correlate with tuberculosis disease activity and response to curative treatment," *Infection and Immunity*, vol. 75, no. 2, pp. 820–829, 2007.

[5] R. van Crevel, T. H. M. Ottenhoff, and J. W. M. van der Meer, "Innate immunity to Mycobacterium tuberculosis," *Clinical Microbiology Reviews*, vol. 15, no. 2, pp. 294–309, 2002.

[6] J. l. Flynn and J. Chan, "Immunology of tuberculosis," *Annual Review of Immunology*, vol. 19, pp. 93–129, 2001.

[7] Z. Toossi and J. J. Ellner, "The role of TGF beta in the pathogenesis of human tuberculosis," *Clinical Immunology and Immunopathology*, vol. 87, pp. 107–114, 1998.

[8] R. Bellamy, "Susceptibility to mycobacterial infections: the importance of host genetics," *Genes & Immunity*, vol. 4, pp. 4–11, 2003.

[9] J. L. Casanova and L. Abel, "Genetic dissection of immunity to mycobacteria: the human model," *Annual Review of Immunology*, vol. 20, pp. 581–620, 2002.

[10] N. Remus, A. Alcais, and L. Abel, "Human genetics of common mycobacterial infections," *Immunologic Research*, vol. 28, pp. 109–129, 2003.

[11] A. C. Vallinoto, E. S. Graça, M. S. Arajo et al., "IFNG +874T/A polymorphism and cytokine plasma levels are associated with susceptibility to *Mycobacterium tuberculosis* infection and clinical manifestation of tuberculosis," *Human Immunology*, vol. 71, no. 7, pp. 692–696, 2010.

[12] Abhimanyu, I. R. Mangangcha, P. Jha et al., "Differential serum cytokine levels are associated with cytokine gene polymorphisms in north Indians with active pulmonary tuberculosis," *Infection, Genetics and Evolution*, vol. 11, no. 5, pp. 1015–1022, 2011.

[13] V. Yilmaz, S. P. Yentour, and G. Saruhan-Direskeneli, "IL-12 and IL-10 polymorphisms and their effects on cytokine production," *Cytokine*, vol. 30, no. 4, pp. 188–194, 2005.

[14] D. López-Maderuelo, F. Arnalich, R. Serantes et al., "Interferon-gamma and interleukin-10 gene polymorphisms in pulmonary tuberculosis," *American Journal of Respiratory and Critical Care Medicine*, vol. 167, no. 7, pp. 970–975, 2003.

[15] N. Sallakci, M. Coskun, Z. Berber et al., "Interferon-γ gene+874T-A polymorphism is associated with tuberculosis and gamma interferon response," *Tuberculosis*, vol. 87, no. 3, pp. 225–230, 2007.

[16] A. Ansari, N. Talat, B. Jamil et al., "Cytokine gene polymorphisms across tuberculosis clinical spectrum in Pakistani patients," *PLoS ONE*, vol. 4, no. 3, Article ID e4778, 2009.

[17] P. Selvaraj, K. Alagarasu, M. Harishankar, M. Vidyarani, D. Nisha Rajeswari, and P. R. Narayanan, "Cytokine gene polymorphisms and cytokine levels in pulmonary tuberculosis," *Cytokine*, vol. 43, no. 1, pp. 26–33, 2008.

[18] M. Vidyarani, P. Selvaraj, S. P. Anand, M. S. Jawahar, A. R. Adhilakshmi, and P. R. Narayanan, "Interferon gamma (IFNγ) & interleukin-4 (IL-4) gene variants & cytokine levels in pulmonary tuberculosis," *Indian Journal of Medical Research*, vol. 124, no. 4, pp. 403–410, 2006.

[19] S. Sharma, J. Rathored, B. Ghosh, and S. K. Sharma, "Genetic polymorphisms in *TNF* genes and tuberculosis in North Indians," *BMC Infectious Diseases*, vol. 10, no. 165, pp. 1–9, 2010.

[20] V. Pravica, C. Perrey, A. Stevens, J. H. Lee, and I. V. Hutchinson, "A single nucleotide polymorphism in the first intron of the human IFN-γ gene: absolute correlation with a polymorphic CA microsatellite marker of high IFN-γ production," *Human Immunology*, vol. 61, no. 9, pp. 863–866, 2000.

[21] S. Henri, F. Stefani, D. Parzy, C. Eboumbou, A. Dessein, and C. Chevillard, "Description of three new polymorphisms in the intronic and 3′ UTR regions of the human interferon gamma gene," *Genes and Immunity*, vol. 3, no. 1, pp. 1–4, 2002.

[22] M. A. García-González, A. Lanas, J. Wu et al., "Lack of association of IL-12 p40 gene polymorphism with peptic ulcer disease," *Human Immunology*, vol. 66, no. 1, pp. 72–76, 2005.

[23] A. G. Wilson, F. S. di Giovine, A. I. F. Blakemore, and G. W. Duff, "Single base polymorphism in the human Tumour Necrosis Factor alpha (TNFα) gene detectable by NcoI restriction of PCR product," *Human Molecular Genetics*, vol. 1, no. 5, p. 353, 1992.

[24] A. Boyum, "Separation of leukocytes from blood and bone marrow. Introduction," *Scandinavian Journal of Clinical & Laboratory Investigation*, vol. 97, article 7, 1968.

[25] A. Larionov, A. Krause, and W. R. Miller, "A standard curve based method for relative real time PCR data processing," *BMC Bioinformatics*, vol. 6, article 62, 2005.

[26] A. Larionov, A. Krause, and W. Miller, "A standard curve based method for relative real time PCR data processing," *BMC Bioinformatics*, vol. 6, article 62, 2005.

[27] A. V. Hill, "The immunogenetics of human infectious diseases," *Annual Review of Immunology*, vol. 16, pp. 593–617, 1998.

[28] T. Heinemeyer, E. Wingender, I. Reuter et al., "Databases on transcriptional regulation: TRANSFAC, TRRD and COMPEL," *Nucleic Acids Research*, vol. 26, pp. 362–367, 1998.

[29] V. Pravica, A. Asderakis, C. Perrey, A. Hajeer, P. J. Sinnott, and I. V. Hutchinson, "In vitro production of IFN-γ correlates with CA repeat polymorphism in the human IFN-γ gene," *European Journal of Immunogenetics*, vol. 26, no. 1, pp. 1–3, 1999.

[30] M. K. Arababadi, A. A. Pourfathollah, A. Jafarzadeh et al., "Non-association of IL-12 +1188 and IFN-γ +874 polymorphisms with cytokines serum level in occult HBV infected patients," *Saudi Journal of Gastroenterology*, vol. 17, no. 1, pp. 30–35, 2011.

[31] U. Vollmer-Conna, B. F. Piraino, B. Cameron et al., "Cytokine polymorphisms have a synergistic effect on severity of the acute sickness response to infection," *Clinical Infectious Diseases*, vol. 47, no. 11, pp. 1418–1425, 2008.

[32] G. I. Matos, C. J. Covas, R. C. Bittar et al., "IFNG +874T/A polymorphism is not associated with American tegumentary leishmaniasis susceptibility but can influence Leishmania induced IFN-gamma production," *BMC Infectious Diseases*, vol. 7, article 33, 2007.

[33] R. Rad, A. Dossumbekova, B. Neu et al., "Cytokine gene polymorphisms influence mucosal cytokine expression, gastric inflammation, and host specific colonisation during *Helicobacter pylori* infection," *Gut*, vol. 53, no. 8, pp. 1082–1089, 2004.

[34] A. G. Pacheco, C. C. Cardoso, and M. O. Moraes, "IFNG +874T/A, IL10 -1082G/A and TNF -308G/A polymorphisms in association with tuberculosis susceptibility: a meta-analysis study," *Human Genetics*, vol. 123, no. 5, pp. 477–484, 2008.

[35] C. C. Cardoso, A. C. Pereira, V. N. Brito-de-Souza et al., "IFNG +874 T>A single nucleotide polymorphism is associated with leprosy among Brazilians," *Human Genetics*, vol. 128, no. 5, pp. 481–490, 2010.

[36] S. Henri, F. Stefani, D. Parzy, C. Eboumbou, A. Dessein, and C. Chevillard, "Description of three new polymorphisms in the intronic and 3′ UTR regions of the human interferon gamma gene," *Genes and Immunity*, vol. 3, no. 1, pp. 1–4, 2002.

[37] M. Liu, B. Cao, H. Zhang, Y. Dai, X. Liu, and C. Xu, "Association of interferon-gamma gene haplotype in the Chinese population with hepatitis B virus infection," *Immunogenetics*, vol. 58, no. 11, pp. 859–864, 2006.

[38] Y. Lin, M. Zhang, F. M. Hofman, J. Gong, and P. F. Barnes, "Absence of a prominent Th2 cytokine response in human tuberculosis," *Infection and Immunity*, vol. 64, no. 4, pp. 1351–1356, 1996.

[39] M. Zhang, Y. Lin, D. V. Iyer, J. Gong, J. S. Abrams, and P. F. Barnes, "T-cell cytokine responses in human infection with *Mycobacterium tuberculosis*," *Infection and Immunity*, vol. 63, no. 8, pp. 3231–3234, 1995.

[40] G. E. Etokebe, L. Bulat-Kardum, M. S. Johansen et al., "Interferon-γ gene (T874A and G2109A) polymorphisms are associated with microscopy-positive tuberculosis," *Scandinavian Journal of Immunology*, vol. 63, no. 2, pp. 136–141, 2006.

[41] M. K. Balcewicz-Sablinska, J. Keane, H. Kornfeld, and H. G. Remold, "Pathogenic *Mycobacterium tuberculosis* evades apoptosis of host macrophages by release of TNF-R2, resulting in inactivation of TNF-α," *Journal of Immunology*, vol. 161, no. 5, pp. 2636–2641, 1998.

[42] A. Davoodi-Semiromi, J. J. Yang, and J. X. She, "IL-12p40 is associated with type 1 diabetes in Caucasian-American families," *Diabetes*, vol. 51, no. 7, pp. 2334–2336, 2002.

[43] S. Stanilova and L. Miteva, "Taq-I polymorphism in 3′UTR of the IL-12 and association with IL-12p40 production from human PBMC," *Genes & Immunity*, vol. 6, pp. 364–366, 2005.

[44] A. M. Cooper, A. Solache, and S. A. Khader, "Interleukin-12 and tuberculosis: an old story revisited," *Current Opinion in Immunology*, vol. 19, pp. 441–447, 2006.

[45] G. Bouma, J. B. A. Crusius, M. Oudkerk Pool et al., "Secretion of tumour necrosis factor α and lymphotoxin α in relation to polymorphisms in the TNF genes and HLA-DR alleles. Relevance for inflammatory bowel disease," *Scandinavian Journal of Immunology*, vol. 43, no. 4, pp. 456–463, 1996.

[46] A. Bozzi, P. P. Pereira, B. S. Reis et al., "Interleukin-10 and tumor necrosis factor-alpha single nucleotide gene polymorphism frequency in paracoccidioidomycosis," *Human Immunology*, vol. 67, no. 11, pp. 931–939, 2006.

[47] C. C. Cardoso, A. C. Pereira, V. N. Brito-de-Souza et al., "TNF -308G > A single nucleotide polymorphism is associated with leprosy among Brazilians: a genetic epidemiology assessment, meta-analysis, and functional study," *The Journal of Infectious Diseases*, vol. 204, no. 8, pp. 1256–1263, 2011.

[48] T. Y. Chen, Y. S. Hsieh, T. T. Wu et al., "Impact of serum levels and gene polymorphism of cytokines on chronic hepatitis C infection," *Translational Research*, vol. 150, no. 2, pp. 116–121, 2007.

[49] E. Louis, D. Franchimont, A. Piron et al., "Tumour necrosis factor (TNF) gene polymorphism influences TNF-α production in lipopolysaccharide (LPS)-stimulated whole blood cell culture in healthy humans," *Clinical and Experimental Immunology*, vol. 113, no. 3, pp. 401–406, 1998.

[50] S. Taudorf, K. S. Krabbe, R. M. G. Berg, K. Møller, B. K. Pedersen, and H. Bruunsgaard, "Common studied polymorphisms do not affect plasma cytokine levels upon endotoxin exposure in humans," *Clinical & Experimental Immunology*, vol. 152, no. 1, pp. 147–152, 2008.

[51] A. G. Wilson, J. A. Symons, T. L. McDowell, H. O. McDevitt, and G. W. Duff, "Effects of a polymorphism in the human tumor necrosis factor alpha promoter on transcriptional activation," *Proceedings of the National Academy of Sciences of the United States of America*, vol. 94, no. 7, pp. 3195–3199, 1997.

[52] M. Feldmann and R. N. Maini, "Anti-TNF-alpha therapy of rheumatoid arthritis: what have we learned?" *Annual Review of Immunology*, vol. 19, pp. 163–196, 2001.

[53] R. Maini, E. W. St Clair, F. Breedveld et al., "Infliximab (chimeric anti-tumour necrosis factor α monoclonal antibody) versus placebo in rheumatoid arthritis patients receiving concomitant methotrexate: a randomised phase III trial," *The Lancet*, vol. 354, no. 9194, pp. 1932–1939, 1999.

[54] S. A. Khader, G. K. Bell, J. E. Pearl et al., "IL-23 and IL-17 in the establishment of protective pulmonary CD4+ T cell responses after vaccination and during *Mycobacterium tuberculosis* challenge," *Nature Immunology*, vol. 8, pp. 369–377, 2007.

[55] S. A. Khader, J. E. Pearl, K. Sakamoto et al., "IL-23 compensates for the absence of IL-12p70 and is essential for the IL-17

response during tuberculosis but is dispensable for protection and antigen-specific IFN-γ responses if IL-12p70 is available," *Journal of Immunology*, vol. 175, no. 2, pp. 788–795, 2005.

[56] M. Umemura, A. Yahagi, S. Hamada et al., "IL-17-mediated regulation of innate and acquired immune response against pulmonary *Mycobacterium bovis* bacille Calmette- Guerin infection," *The Journal of Immunology*, vol. 178, pp. 3786–3796, 2007.

[57] T. M. Wozniak, A. A. Ryan, J. A. Triccas, and W. J. Britton, "Plasmid interleukin-23 (IL-23), but not plasmid IL-27, enhances the protective efficacy of a DNA vaccine against Mycobacterium tuberculosis infection," *Infection and Immunity*, vol. 74, no. 1, pp. 557–565, 2006.

[58] S. H. Opdal, "IL-10 gene polymorphisms in infectious disease and SIDS," *FEMS Immunology and Medical Microbiology*, vol. 42, no. 1, pp. 48–52, 2004.

[59] A. C. Pereira, V. N. Brito-de-Souza, C. C. Cardoso et al., "Genetic, epidemiological and biological analysis of interleukin-10 promoter single-nucleotide polymorphisms suggests a definitive role for -819C/T in leprosy susceptibility," *Genes and Immunity*, vol. 10, no. 2, pp. 174–180, 2009.

[60] V. A. Boussiotis, E. Y. Tsai, E. Yunis et al., "IL-10 producing T cells suppress immune responses in anergic tuberculosis patients," *The Journal of Clinical Investigation*, vol. 105, pp. 1317–1325, 2000.

[61] F. O. Sánchez, J. I. Rodriguez, G. Agudelo, and L. F. Garcia, "Immune responsiveness and lymphokine production in patients with tuberculosis and healthy controls," *Infection and Immunity*, vol. 62, pp. 5673–5678, 1994.

[62] F. Ruscetti, L. Varesio, A. Ochoa, and J. Ortaldo, "Pleiotropic effects of transforming growth factor-β on cells of the immune system," *Annals of the New York Academy of Sciences*, vol. 685, pp. 488–500, 1993.

[63] R. P. Numerof, F. R. Aronson, and J. W. Mier, "IL-2 stimulates the production of IL-1α and IL-1β by human peripheral blood mononuclear cells," *Journal of Immunology*, vol. 141, no. 12, pp. 4250–4257, 1988.

[64] T. M. Lasco, L. Cassone, H. Kamohara, T. Yoshimura, and D. N. McMurray, "Evaluating the role of tumor necrosis factor-alpha in experimental pulmonary tuberculosis in the guinea pig," *Tuberculosis*, vol. 85, pp. 254–258, 2005.

[65] D. J. Grainger, K. Heathcote, M. Chiano et al., "Genetic control of the circulating concentration of transforming growth factor type beta1," *Human Molecular Genetics*, vol. 8, pp. 93–97, 1999.

[66] A. M. Dunning, P. D. Ellis, S. McBride et al., "A transforming growth factorβ1 signal peptide variant increases secretion in vitro and is associated with increased incidence of invasive breast cancer," *Cancer Research*, vol. 63, no. 10, pp. 2610–2615, 2003.

[67] M. Yokota, S. Ichihara, T. L. Lin, N. Nakashima, and Y. Yamada, "Association of a T29 $\rightarrow$ C polymorphism of the transforming growth factor- β1 gene with genetic susceptibility to myocardial infarction in Japanese," *Circulation*, vol. 101, no. 24, pp. 2783–2787, 2000.

[68] J. S. Chang, J. F. Huggett, K. Dheda, L. U. Kim, A. Zumla, and G. A. W. Rook, "Myobacterium tuberculosis induces selective up-regulation of TLRs in the mononuclear leukocytes of patients with active pulmonary tuberculosis," *Journal of Immunology*, vol. 176, no. 5, pp. 3010–3018, 2006.

11

Listening to Those at the Frontline: Patient and Healthcare Personnel Perspectives on Tuberculosis Treatment Barriers and Facilitators in High TB Burden Regions of Argentina

Sarah J. Iribarren,[1,2] **Fernando Rubinstein,**[2] **Vilda Discacciati,**[3] **and Patricia F. Pearce**[4]

[1] School of Nursing, Columbia University, 630 West 168 Street, New York, NY 10032, USA
[2] Institute for Clinical Effectiveness and Healthcare Policy, Dr. Emilio Ravignani 2024, C1414CPT Buenos Aires, Argentina
[3] Division of Family and Community Medicine, Hospital Italiano de Buenos Aires, Juan D. Perón 4190,
  C1181ACH Buenos Aires, Argentina
[4] School of Nursing, Loyola University, 6363 Saint Charles Avenue, Stallings Hall, New Orleans, LA 70118, USA

Correspondence should be addressed to Sarah J. Iribarren; si2277@columbia.edu

Academic Editor: David C. Perlman

Purpose. In Argentina, tuberculosis (TB) control measures have not achieved key treatment targets. The purpose of this study was to identify modes of treatment delivery and explore patient and healthcare personnel perceptions of barriers and facilitators to treatment success. *Methods.* We used semistructured group and individual interviews for this descriptive qualitative study. Eight high burden municipalities were purposively selected. Patients in treatment for active TB ($n = 16$), multidisciplinary TB team members ($n = 26$), and TB program directors ($n = 12$) at local, municipal, regional, and national levels were interviewed. Interviews were recorded, transcribed verbatim, and analyzed using thematic analysis. *Results.* Modes of treatment delivery varied across municipalities and types of healthcare facility and were highly negotiated with patients. Self-administration of treatment was common in hospital-based and some community clinics. Barriers to TB treatment success were concentrated at the system level. This level relied heavily on individual personal commitment, and many system facilitators were operating in isolation or in limited settings. *Conclusions.* We outline experiences and perspectives of the facilitating and challenging factors at the individual, structural, social, and organizational levels. Establishing strong patient-healthcare personnel relationships, responding to patient needs, capitalizing on community resources, and maximizing established decentralized system could mitigate some of the barriers.

1. Introduction

Despite progress in treatment and prevention, tuberculosis (TB) remains a major global public health problem, particularly in low- and middle-income countries [1, 2]. The World Health Organization recommended Directly Observed Treatment, Short-Course (DOTS) strategy includes five key components: securing political commitment, strengthening detection and diagnosis, ensuring drug availability, monitoring outcomes, and providing directly observed therapy (DOT) [3]. Although DOTS has been widely adopted and has contributed to TB control progress, TB case rates in many countries are either stagnant or decreasing more slowly than expected, possibly due to incomplete application of effective

control measures and care [4]. DOTS was implemented in Argentina in 1996, but overall TB treatment success rates have varied little, and there has been no significant improvement over the past 10 years [5].

Treatment success is defined as either the completion of treatment (without bacteriological confirmation) or cure (negative sputum smear at 6 months and at least once prior to 6 months) [6]. In Argentina, success rates have ranged from 48 to 66% for new sputum smear positive over the last 12 years [7], and the last country report (2011/2012) indicates that nearly 45% of new pulmonary TB cases had no final treatment outcome documented [8]. The cause of high rates of loss to follow-up is unclear, other than likely inefficiency in collection of data. Of more than 11,000 new cases identified each year, less than 50% receive treatment by DOT [5]. Specifically in the province of Buenos Aires, with the highest concentration of TB cases, DOT was the reported mode of treatment delivery for only 20% of the documented cases [9]. It is not well understood why DOT is being applied at such low rates or what other modes of treatment delivery are commonly being applied.

Nonadherence to TB therapy can lead to poor health outcomes, such as prolonged infectivity, increase in risk of relapse after treatment, generation and propagation of drug resistance, treatment failure, and increased mortality, all of which pose a serious health risk for individuals and communities [10, 11]. Treatment adherence is considered a primary determinant and a proxy for treatment success, yet not the only requirement for an efficient program [12, 13]. Barriers to treatment completion have been described as an interaction among structural, personal, and organizational factors within a social context [14]. Factors identified as barriers include limited access to healthcare, stigma attached to the disease, quality of medications, drug resistance, and patients' immunity and metabolic capabilities [2, 15].

In Argentina, all TB treatment care, including medication, is provided free of charge in the public sector. The National TB Program (NTP) is responsible for all drug provision and patient monitoring. The National Institute of Respiratory Diseases (ANLIS-Coni) in Argentina recommends an exchange of experiences and methods of success among regions in order to spread successful strategies to other parts of the country [5]. Although investigators in Argentina have reported on TB trends, patterns of resistance, delays in diagnosis and treatment, and outcomes applying DOT [16–21], the experiences and perspectives of patients and healthcare personnel dedicated to TB control have not been previously explored. Qualitative, in-depth inquiry can help to understand a phenomenon to gain insight into the problem and to provide a foundation upon which to identify appropriate solutions [22].

This study served as a foundational study to a prospective cohort trial currently in progress (patient and system factors associated with successful treatment of tuberculosis (1R01AI083229-01)). Specific study aims were to identify modes of treatment delivery and explore perceived barriers to and facilitators of treatment success from the perspective of patients being treated for active TB, multidisciplinary TB team members, and TB program directors at local, municipal, regional, and national levels.

2. Methods

2.1. Study Design.
The study design was descriptive qualitative, using semistructured, face-to-face group and in-depth individual interviews [23, 24]. The theoretical framework to guide research and data analysis was adapted from the treatment adherence model developed by Munro et al. [14]. Factors were organized into the following categories: *individual* (e.g., patient and healthcare worker's individual characteristics, responses, beliefs, or actions); *structural/social* (e.g., factors over which the patient has little control, such

as economic, political, cultural, or environmental factors, discrimination and inequality, gender norms, stigma, or family/community support); and *healthcare services or organizational* (e.g., healthcare center characteristics, system coordination, programs, and data management). The model was selected as an initial organizational and theoretical tool for two reasons: first because treatment adherence is recognized as a major factor in treatment success and second because we believe the model incorporates the complex nature of interactions and levels of factors that influence treatment success. The five key components of DOTS were also considered during analysis [3].

Ethical approval was granted by the Comité de Ética de Protocolos de Investigación (Research Protocol Ethics Committee) of Hospital Italiano, Buenos Aires, Argentina. All participants provided written informed consent.

2.2. Setting and Participants.
The study setting was focused in Health Regions V and VI, located in the province of Buenos Aires. Region V is a large geographic region serving a population of 3.5 million and is comprised of 13 municipalities, each responsible for between 15 and 25 local primary healthcare centers. The region accounted for one-third of the TB cases (incidence 49.2/100,000) within the province of Buenos Aires [25]. Treatment success rates within municipalities in Health Region V range from 33% to 90% (Region V annual report). In Region VI, success rates ranged from 40 to 66%, with an average default (treatment abandonment) rate of 30% over the last 3 years [8].

A sequenced, purposive sampling design was used. Based on historic treatment outcomes and the regional director's recommendation, nine municipalities were selected from Health Regions V and VI. We included municipalities with historically high and low success rates in order to capture perspectives of what factors improved treatment success and what factors appeared to impede it. From within the nine municipalities, patients undergoing TB treatment and their family members ($N = 16$, comprised of 10 patients and six family members) and multidisciplinary healthcare team members ($N = 38$, comprised of TB program directors (national ($n = 1$), regional ($n = 2$), and municipal ($n = 8$) levels), assistant directors ($n = 3$), physicians ($n = 6$), nurses ($n = 5$), social workers ($n = 6$), and community health promoters ($n = 7$)) were interviewed. The district directors reported on average more than 10 years of work experience at the district level, and the other healthcare team members reported from 1 to 17 years. Recruitment of patients and any family members was done by healthcare personnel in the clinics. The healthcare personnel were asked to identify patients undergoing TB treatment or who had abandoned treatment. Patients and family members ranged from 7 to 48 years of age; nine were females. Patients were reimbursed for their time with a $25 USD equivalent voucher for groceries at a local store or provided with basic staple groceries where vouchers were unavailable at the local stores.

2.3. Data Collection and Analysis.
We held nine group interviews. Interviews were conducted separately for provider

(n = 6) and patient/family groups (n = 3). Individual interviews (n = 7) were conducted with providers when they were unable to participate in group interviews or worked independently (e.g., regional and national directors). Interviews were conducted in Spanish, assisted by a semistructured interview guide specifically designed for the study, and moderated by an experienced qualitative researcher (VD). The setting for all interviews was in healthcare centers within the selected municipality or in directors' offices. The semistructured interview guides were developed based on the previously described treatment adherence model [14] and were adapted for patients/families, healthcare teams, and directors. The interview guides focused on program characteristics, general experiences of services, characteristics that favor treatment completion, and challenges and solutions for each group. Field notes were also taken to concurrently highlight themes and to help modify guides to fill gaps where further exploration was needed. The researchers also participated in a day-long regional TB workshop to understand the overall system function.

All interviews were audio-recorded (average = 1 hour, range = 18–127 minutes) and transcribed verbatim in Spanish [26]. Transcripts were uploaded into ATLAS.ti version 6 (GmbH, Berlin, 2009) to assist with data management. Using principles of thematic analysis [23, 24, 27], the transcripts and notes were coded independently by authors SI and VD with an in vivo, open, and selective coding base on the treatment adherence model [14]. Overall coding and analysis were conducted in Spanish and later translated into English (three of the four authors—SI, FR, and VD—are fluent in both languages). Preliminary coding of barriers and facilitators was organized in a matrix from each perspective (patient, healthcare personnel, and directors) at each of the levels (individual, structural/social, and organizational). Then overarching themes from all perspectives were generated for each level. Final analysis with all authors, the report, and thematic generation were conducted in English.

3. Results

We identified varying modes of TB treatment delivery and several perceived barriers and facilitators to TB treatment success. We classified our findings from all participants into individual, structural/social, and organizational factors (Table 1). The modes of treatment delivery varied within healthcare centers and across healthcare facilities and were reported as frequently negotiated. The majority of barriers to treatment success were classified at the organizational/healthcare delivery system level. Interventions considered potential facilitators were not implemented system wide. That is, the degree to which these interventions were implemented was limited to one site or to a few within a municipality. In general, patients and healthcare personnel initially indicated that the system in place *functioned well* but immediately qualified "functioned well" with descriptions of the multiple challenges to TB management and achieving treatment success. We identified that, depending on context, some of the barriers and facilitators were not categorically

fixed (a particular issue can have facilitative characteristics, while simultaneously having barrier characteristics) and thus are fluid in categorical terms. For example, described further below, *DOT* and *feeling better* were both a facilitator and a barrier from the perspectives of both personnel and patients/family members. Direct quotes from patients and healthcare personnel (translated to English from Spanish) are provided as examples to illustrate some of the findings.

3.1. Modes of Treatment Delivery. Most healthcare centers reported providing daily DOT. However, DOT was also reported as being *negotiated* or *tailored* to meet patients' needs. In order to maintain patients who were threatening to default or who were faced with challenges to attend clinic daily and as an incentive for compliance, the number of directly observed days was negotiated, for example, 2-3 days per week, once per week, or twice monthly. One municipality offered only self-administration centralized at one healthcare center. Patients diagnosed and treated at hospitals received treatment by self-administration and were requested to return to the hospital monthly for follow-up visits and for their 1-month supply of medication. Directors and healthcare team members indicated that patients initiating treatment at a hospital would rarely be referred to a healthcare center closer to where they live or patients may be asked and decline this option.

> "There are patients who come to take their medication and there are patients who are given medication weekly and come every week to collect it." [Healthcare personnel, FG]

> "Well, here in Region [number removed] we have supervised treatment starting point...closer to home. The treatment is daily. Sometimes concessions can be made for the issue of distance or because there are healthcare centers that have reduced hours of operations, not like this, which is open 24 hours..." [Municipal director, FG]

3.2. Individual Factors. Individual barriers and facilitators included factors related to individual and healthcare professional TB knowledge, personal experiences and relationships, the treatment regimen and its effects, and individual characteristics of patients or healthcare providers.

3.2.1. Barriers

A Lack of TB Knowledge. Treatment seeking and continuation was described as being impacted by an initial reaction of *fear*, "going to die," fear for family due to loss of work, and stigma related to diagnosis. Fear of TB diagnosis and potential consequences such as social stigma were both augmented and mitigated by knowing someone who had been diagnosed with TB and who had either successfully completed treatment or died from TB. Patients expressed their initial concern about what others in their community would think about them and their families.

TABLE 1: Barriers to and facilitators of successful completion of treatment by category.

	Barriers	Facilitators
Individual	-Drug side effects (e.g., GI upset, bitter taste) -Lack of TB knowledge about the disease and treatment -Fear related to TB (e.g., incurable, loss of work, or discrimination) -Interpretation of feeling better means cured -Comorbidities (e.g., alcoholism, drug addictions) -Personal/family challenges	-Desire to be cured, personal motivation -Personal experience with other TB patients -Strong patient-provider relationship -Personal characteristics of healthcare personnel: committed, compassionate, supportive, able to establish trust (builds rapport with patients and longevity in the community and center), having personal calling to serve others, and able to humanize disease and situation -Interpreting feeling better as cured

Structural/Social	-Access to healthcare centers (e.g., distance, transportation issues, and cost)
	-Poverty, precarious living conditions
	-Low wages for healthcare workers
	-Long treatment course
	-Vulnerable patient populations
	  -Informal employment (e.g., day labor), women with childcare challenges, "health tours," with comorbidities (e.g., addictions, HIV/AIDS), living in poverty, adolescence
	-Discrimination and/or stigmatization
	-Lack of education in communities and schools leading to poor TB awareness and understanding of treatment
	-Perception of low quality of care offered at healthcare center
	-Instability of political commitment/support
	  -Financial subsidy delays and low rates of application due to inadequate dissemination and clarity of policy/regulations
	  -Reassigning positions/frequent staff turnover
	  -Lack of official recognition and monetary compensation of TB positions
		-Dispersed healthcare centers throughout communities/region
		-Free-of-charge medication and services for TB treatment
		-Social support of family and friends, healthcare personnel, volunteer community health promoters

Organization/System/Health Service	-Resistance to use directly observed therapy (DOT) by some healthcare personnel
	-DOT
	-Self-administration standard at hospitals (conflicting messages to patients)
	-Self-administration offered first
	-Low index of suspicion of TB resulting in diagnostic delays
	-Underutilization of decentralized healthcare system
	  -Lack of collaboration/referrals between hospital and healthcare centers
	  -Cases concentrated for treatment at hospital level
	  -Lower treatment success and high rates of abandonment at hospital level
	  -Disparity in size, resources, hours of service, and staff composition at healthcare centers (e.g., short on TB supplies, no computers, and lack of specialists or physicians)
	  -Overburdened staff
	-Inefficiency in collection of data (outcome monitoring)
	  -Patients lost to follow-up, poor tracking
	  -Paper-based healthcare records (no computers at centers)
	  -Lack of centralized surveillance system
	  -Delayed and underreported case outcomes → delayed/incomplete program evaluations (up to 2 years)
	  -Mistrust in accuracy of reported data
		-Subsidy for those who continue/complete treatment
		-Being convinced of DOT effectiveness
		-DOT
		-Decentralized healthcare system
		  -Healthcare centers situated at about every 10–15 blocks
		-Facilitating healthcare center characteristics (limited implementation)
		  -Open 24 hours
		  -Provision of DOT without appointment and through separate door (not having to wait in waiting room)
		  -Use of politically appointed community advocates to find and return patients to treatment
		-Medication availability (not always the case)
		-Established laboratory/diagnostic network considered reliable and available
		-Continuity of healthcare personnel
		-Capacity of TB healthcare team members

"That is to say, people think that it [TB] does not have a cure." [Patient, FG]

"...that there was not a cure, that you would die. This is what one thinks....I realized and at the same time felt bad because he [son] was admitted [to hospital]. I cried all day. What will they say about my son? What am I going to do? On one hand we discriminate ourselves...but later I realized that it wasn't like that." [Family member of patient, FG]

Drug Side Effects. There are many pills to take and there can be side effects. Patients described treatment challenges to continuing treatment due to medication side effects and personal situations.

"Before they [medication] caused nausea. I couldn't eat because all that I ate I threw up and I went to the clinician, but I he couldn't take away the medication because I had to continue. I just wanted to say enough but I knew...I tried to continue. I talked with the clinician and he told me I couldn't abandon the treatment because it [TB] would come back worse." [Patient, FG]

"He didn't want to come any more because the pills made him feel bad, the injections too. He could not take more also because he said it hurt his buttock." [Patient/family member, FG]

Interpretation of feeling better (e.g., weight gain, return of strength, and increased energy) was identified as both a barrier and a facilitator. Patients/family members and healthcare team members described patients as interpreting feeling better as meaning "cured," leading to treatment abandonment even with encouragement to continue from family and healthcare personnel; or patients recognized feeling better as treatment effectiveness and needing to continue treatment.

"Well, he [brother] took everything [medication] and was doing well. After he felt better he stopped, abandoned everything. He thought that he was cured....He said he didn't need it [medication] that he was already better and was not going to continue [treatment]." [Patient/family member, brother died of TB]

3.2.2. Facilitators

Establishing a Strong Patient-Healthcare Personnel Relationship. A key factor contributing to treatment success for both patients and healthcare personnel was establishing a strong patient-healthcare personnel relationship. A strong relationship was considered to facilitate provision of education and be based on respect and the ability to humanize the disease and the situation. Healthcare personnel and patients also need to possess certain individual characteristics. For example, healthcare personnel needed to be committed, compassionate, supportive, and trustworthy and have a personal calling

to serve others. Patients needed to be committed to being cured. There was a perception by some healthcare personnel that if the patient lacked commitment, the problem was with the patient and not the system.

"The most effective way to influence the patient is by having a good doctor-nurse-patient relationship, and they [patients] understand that we are working to better their health and when we suggest something it is for the best." [Healthcare personnel, FG]

"One must use a lot of kindness, in everything but especially this. With this type of disease [TB] we have to provide love, respect, and this at times people do not have. It is fundamental to our work to try to provide consciousness at all levels." [Healthcare personnel, FG]

"It is the determination of the individual and this is what gets you to cure." [Patient, FG]

"The patient that completes DOT also completes treatment in their house. The problem is with the patient, not the system." [Municipal director, individual interview]

3.3. Structural/Social Factors. Structural/social barriers and facilitators included factors related to access to care, TB awareness within the community at large, vulnerable populations, support, stigma, and political commitment to the TB program.

3.3.1. Barriers

Lack of Community TB Education in Communities and Schools. Participants cited a lack of TB awareness in the community at large regarding etiology and treatment and a lack of acknowledgement of the gravity of TB within their communities and specifically within schools. Because of the lack of awareness by communities and healthcare personnel, a low index to suspect TB given certain symptoms was noted, which delayed TB diagnosis. Patients described having symptomatic respiratory complaints that resulted in multiple healthcare visits and misdiagnosis (e.g., pneumonia), and healthcare personnel acknowledged that such misdiagnosis often occurs in some settings. A district coordinator estimated that two to three clinic evaluations occurred for persistent symptoms until TB was suspected and testing provided. In addition, a municipal director reported that lab result notification of 15 days or more further compounded delays in treatment.

"He [son] was vomiting blood. Well, they took him to the hospital the night I was working and when I arrived from work. ...we were sent back. They took him to another hospital [name removed] and we were told the same. They didn't take an X-ray, they didn't do an analysis of the blood, nothing in the emergency...they said since he does drugs." [Mother/prior patient, FG]

"In schools what I see is that TB is not talked about. They talk a lot about HIV, syphilis, sexually transmitted diseases, and maybe TB or pertussis because there was some last year. It [TB] is not taken seriously." [Patient, FG]

"The official agencies put more importance on other things and tuberculosis is a disease which we live with and there needs to be more information." [Municipal director, individual interview]

"…There are little children with facemasks and adults as the whole family is infected and they also are discriminated against…It signals that they are sick, you shouldn't get close, it's contagious. Therefore there is information, and lack of information." [Director, FG]

Vulnerable Populations. Specific populations were perceived as especially vulnerable to treatment success challenges. These populations included those with comorbidities (e.g., drug or alcohol addiction, HIV/AIDS), those for whom employment was informal (e.g., day labor), those considered to be part of a "health tour," adolescents, and those living in poverty in general. Healthcare personnel recognized that loss of work opportunity due to attending daily clinic required for DOT equated to loss of financial ability to care for family. Those considered part of a "health tour" or considered to be outside of the established healthcare system were described as providing false contact information, moving frequently, and coming from neighboring countries to receive treatment and return. This population, in particular, is at high risk for loss to follow-up because of challenges to track and facilitate treatment completion. Adolescents were also considered by healthcare personnel as more challenging than adults to convince to start treatment, specifically those who had dropped out of school, were without stable employment, lacked family support, and were believed to be "unconcerned" about their health in general. Challenges due to poverty were commonly described. Precarious living conditions hindered accessing patients or attempting to track those who had abandoned treatment.

Informal Laborers. "The problem is with the people who at times, because of challenges of work, do not want to come in to take the treatment here [healthcare center] because they say, "I need to continue to work"….They are going to choose a day job and not take the medication." [Healthcare personnel, FG]

Addiction. "The people who we work with don't have means of transportation, are drug addicts, alcoholics. We have average people too but we work a lot with people that do not have means and they suffer because they are drug addicts or alcoholics that begin treatment and then abandon and therefore you have to go find them. It is a manual job, very tiring because it is hard." [Healthcare personnel, FG]

"He [brother] stopped taking the treatment that the doctor from here sent him. Well, he abandoned everything and told me: "Well, I am better." He began to drink and do drugs again." [Patient/family member, FG]

Adolescents. "Family support it seems to me contributes, helps; the level of education as well. I also believe that it is a cultural question. A person who works, who has a family, who has to move ahead, this person will be cured. And the person who is uninterested or is adolescent, a kid who is 20 years old who left school and maybe some days he has a day job and other days he does not, this is the person who is not concerned with continuing treatment, nor is he consistent." [Trained community healthcare worker, FG]

Living in Poverty. "All of this region (…) which is all of this zone, is a region of settlement, region of slums and areas of people who live in very poor standards of living, indigent. You go to places where you find they are almost in caves." [Healthcare personnel, FG]

Staff Turnover. Patients, healthcare personnel, and directors strongly agreed that the stability and consolidation of the healthcare team is vital to achieve treatment success. However, political changes, poor compensation, and/or intent to gain experience and move on were to blame for the high staff turnover rates and the consequent need for staff retraining. New physicians were said to gain experience in more distant healthcare centers and then "move on" when the experience was obtained or when they were offered employment with better compensation. Patients and family members recognized nurses as playing a key role in their care. Nurses were identified as the primary DOT supervisors and treatment coordinators. However, nurses described managing multiple duties (e.g., pharmacy, primary care clinic, and immunization clinic), but without recognition.

"…regarding training, they [healthcare personnel] keep changing, the nurses change, the doctors change." [District director, individual interview]

"The turnover of doctors and nurses leads to these methods [those that work] not being productive." [Healthcare personnel, FG]

Political Commitment Issues. Concerns of political commitment were described as "unofficial" designation of positions in the TB program, varied access to resources, and reassigning staff to different positions after political changes. Healthcare personnel and program directors reported willingness to contribute to TB efforts but in doing so accepted added responsibilities without additional compensation or recognition. The national TB director indicated that his position was only recently designated as an "official" post. Lack of basic resources and varying access to resources at healthcare centers (e.g., no access to computers) were described.

Political changes were highlighted as important because they resulted in reassignment of healthcare personnel to different areas, causing disruption in the flow of delivery of care and requiring training of new staff members. Staffing and resource issues were perceived as compromising established community perception of quality of healthcare services at the local level and confidence, as well as requiring increased efforts and resources to retrain new staff.

3.3.2. Facilitators

Social Support. Social support from family, friends, and healthcare personnel was considered essential to provide emotional and practical support and encouragement.

> "His friends came to my house and were there all day with him. They were with him every minute. They spoke with him, trying to get him to get out of bed and thanks to him and his friends that were with him...they lifted him up...you can say that they were friends. These are true friends. His friend was sick and it didn't matter to him....He came to see him everyday." [Mother of patient talking about son's friend, FG]

Established Infrastructure. The physical establishment of a decentralized healthcare system, although described as being underutilized, was seen as a strength to minimize the challenges of access to TB care. Each municipality managed 15 to 25 local healthcare centers located on average at every 10 to 15 blocks, with some municipalities reporting having healthcare centers that supported more rural populations with challenges of access due to limited public transportation and travel cost. Established and dispersed laboratories were reported by healthcare personnel and directors to be adequately equipped to conduct basic tuberculosis testing.

> "In our country there doesn't exist geographic inaccessibility.....Here it is very rare that there is geographic inaccessibility. You have hospitals, healthcare centers, medical units, all this a part of the imagination—the person knows where to go. I don't know if they know where to go to receive better care but they know where to go.... Abandonment of treatment in Argentina is linked to places of major urban concentration." [Local director, FG]

3.4. Organizational Factors.
Organizational barriers and facilitators included factors related to DOT, interventions with limited implementation, patient tracking, and perception of quality of healthcare services at the local healthcare centers.

3.4.1. Barriers

Resistance to Use/Lack of Belief in DOT. DOT was described as both a facilitator and a barrier. Some patients felt more attended to and that their needs were more quickly addressed, but other participants considered DOT burdensome both to patients and to healthcare services. DOT was described as "intrusive" and "too demanding" and was a likely cause for some patients to return to settings where self-administration was standard. Many of the healthcare personnel and directors stated that there was a belief that those completing treatment by DOT would also complete successfully by self-administration; in contrast, there are patients who, due to challenging situations, will not complete treatment successfully no matter what intervention is used. A major challenge reported by healthcare personnel and directors was trying to convince patients who had initiated self-administration of treatment to transition to DOT once they were transferred to a healthcare center. They believed that, due to customary practices, doubts about the effectiveness of DOT, or issues of feasibility, some providers, particularly at hospitals or in the private sector, offered only self-administration monitored with periodic evaluations. Some healthcare personnel admitted that they themselves first needed to be convinced of the effectiveness of DOT through experience, rather than simply complying with standards. Once convinced, they were better prepared to recommend DOT, and their attitudes towards the strategy spilled over to other personnel and patients. Although convinced, many maintained concerns about feasibility.

> *Patient Perspective of DOT.* "Yes it is difficult [DOT]. It is hard to come in." [Patient, FG]

> "The nurse attends to us, she attends to us very well." [Patient, FG]

> "I don't have a problem coming to the clinic. Besides they attend to me well, the doctor and the nurse." [Patient, FG]

> *Convincing Patients.* "It is to say, practically it is not an obligation, but we try to convince them [patients] to do supervised treatment. Many ask us "why, it is hard for me to come in." What happens is the national program indicates that it has to be supervised treatment or else they don't give us the drugs." [Municipal program director, individual interview]

> *Need to Be Convinced.* "The patient that completes DOT also completes treatment in their house." [District director, FG]

> "...I was here [working in the healthcare system] during the time when treatment was self-administration, period. The idea of treatment changed and I had to be convinced with numbers from where here [one healthcare center] I had patients treated by self-administration and there

[another healthcare center] DOT patients and here was a percentage of abandonment very high and there a percentage of abandonment much lower; therefore I was convinced." [Healthcare personnel, FG]

"…There is a resistance. It is inevitable. The primary resistance is our own until you are convinced that with the direct supervision of treatment, adherence is improved. Once you are convinced, it begins to spill over to everyone else and the patients…" [Healthcare team, FG]

Inefficiency in Data Collection and Management. Data management (e.g., patient notification and tracking) was paper-based, and records were organized and stored idiosyncratically at each healthcare center. None of the healthcare centers visited had access to a computer to manage data (e.g., no electronic medical records or computerized tracking or data management systems). Moreover, the paper-based process varied by healthcare facility. For example, at the healthcare centers where DOT was implemented there was a daily monitoring sheet, and at hospital-based clinics there was a 4× 6 card that documented start dates and dates when a patient came to retrieve the monthly supply of medication. Multiple healthcare personnel reported taking patient records home to create an organized computer-based database to more effectively manage patients.

Patient tracking, referral pathways, and outcome monitoring were reported as discontinuous or fragmented with challenges to assure arrival of transfers to other facilities or to assist in monitoring patient progress. For example, a patient may start treatment in one location, move, and then either continue or abandon treatment or fail to provide information to a new provider to get restarted on a new treatment regimen. An example highlighted was of a patient with MDR-TB who moved to another province and sought treatment. The patient was started on first-line drugs until the prior attending physician phoned later to inquire if the patient had arrived to transfer care of treatment monitoring.

Some healthcare personnel described distrust in the overall accuracy of data reported to the regional or national level. The regional level described high rates of complete treatment outcome reporting. In addition, the challenges to accurate national oversight of TB treatment outcomes were depicted as stemming from known underreporting of cases and outcomes from the private sector. Exacerbating the challenges of oversight and planning were delays of up to 2 years to produce TB reports because of the time required to report and process the paper-based data.

Perception of Low Quality of Care. The decentralized system's potential was recognized as not being maximized. According to the national TB director, TB cases are concentrated in centralized locations, particularly infectious disease specialty hospitals. Healthcare centers were described as varying in size, resource availability, hours of service, and staff composition. Examples provided included having one pulmonologist to attend to patients at multiple healthcare centers, resulting in continuous traveling, days in which centers were without a pulmonologist, and healthcare centers with small, crowded, general waiting rooms where TB patients were required to wait for appointments and to receive treatment. Because of the variability in clinic services and resources across the system, healthcare personnel indicated that there was a perception of a low quality of services provided at the local, smaller healthcare centers by communities and hospital staff. This perception of a low quality of services was thought to contribute to a lack of referrals of patients from a larger facility to a local healthcare center and a general lack of communication among facilities, which was considered another important barrier to patient tracking and treatment completion. Although personnel at local healthcare centers reported attempting to improve communication between centers and hospitals to in turn improve patient referrals, they indicated that these efforts often failed to produce results.

Nonetheless, the participating patients described being satisfied and "cared for" at the local healthcare centers. Healthcare personnel and directors at the healthcare centers felt they were better able to track, follow up, and return defaulters to treatment compared to larger facilities such as the hospitals.

Variability of Services across Healthcare System. "There is one thing very important; every primary healthcare center is a different world. You [researchers] see this one. This is distinct from other centers that are 2 × 2, very small." [Municipal director, individual interview]

"Not having a person, a specialist in a center is an obstacle because the person then has to be transferred to a larger center." [Healthcare personnel, FG]

"There are not enough pulmonologists." "There are not pediatricians." [Healthcare personnel, FG]

"People come to be attended to at the centers with so many children in the waiting room and more during the winter when everything is closed and there is a lack of ventilation." [Healthcare personnel, FG]

Second Class Care. "The healthcare team [at hospital level] do not have confidence in the ability of the health care centers. It is as if they [healthcare centers] are second class. There is this idea that the healthcare centers, because they are peripheral, they are second rate." [Regional director, individual interview]

Lack of Communication among Facilities. "I am trying to incorporate programs at the provincial hospitals but it is difficult because they [hospital personnel] do not want to. We were able to convince one hospital (name removed) to start this year to pass the hospitals statistics because it has a 35% rate of treatment abandonment, *which is why we have currently high rates of tuberculosis and multiresistance. We have lots who [patients] abandon. They [hospital staff] do not notify us; therefore, we cannot go to look for them." [Municipality director, FG]*

"Within this district we have three hospitals (names removed). The hospitals (...) do not refer patients to us. They stay there, they manage them, and it is where we have the highest rates of abandonment because they [hospital staff] do not go out to look for patients [who abandon treatment]." [Healthcare personnel, FG]

Reliance on Personal Commitment. Daily work in the TB program was described as largely based on personal commitment, often "beyond duty," rather than on program structure. Healthcare personnel emphasized that, without their personal commitment, stemming from both personal and external expectations, the program would not accomplish the current results. Examples of personal commitment included use of personal funds to cover expenses for which no resources were assigned and no official budget existed, such as providing breakfast to encourage medication adherence for those who did not have money for proper nutrition, and using personal cars and covering gas expenses to attend community events, make home visits, or travel to healthcare centers for supervision (directors).

"We are the firefighters of medicine risking our life voluntarily." [Municipal director, individual interview]

3.4.2. Facilitators

Individualized Flexible Treatment. As previously described under Modes of Treatment Delivery, flexibility and negotiation with patients to keep them in treatment was seen as a supportive method, an incentive for compliance, and a means to lessen challenges to coming in daily to receive treatment. Although the availability of antituberculosis medication was reported as a problem in the past, healthcare personnel and directors indicated that it was not an issue during the time the interviews were conducted. Additionally, maintaining continuity and stability of healthcare personnel was recognized as an important factor to promote patient and community perception of quality of healthcare services at the local level.

Interventions with Limited Implementation. Interventions limited to one or a few locations were implemented to address some of the identified barriers perceived within their municipality. For example, one of the healthcare centers provided DOT on a walk-in basis (without appointment) and through a separate door around the side of the building. The TB patients were rerouted away from the full waiting rooms. Other program directors reported having a number of healthcare centers open 24 hours a day to facilitate access to treatment for patients. Some municipalities reported utilizing local politically appointed community advocates to locate patients who had abandoned treatment—to go to the patient's

home and encourage the patient to return to treatment if other attempts to return the patient to treatment had failed. They also described training community healthcare promoters to provide information and support and facilitate referrals within their communities. One healthcare center reported training DOT observers (e.g., a night guardsman) to provide DOT to patients outside of hours of attention to facilitate treatment delivery.

"The problem is when they have to go to work. How do they do it? People go far to work and therefore come early. The healthcare center is not open, except those that are open all night which are few...therefore the people leave before and return after [clinic closes]. This is a problem." [Municipal director, individual interview]

Financial Subsidy. Some patients with TB qualify for a government subsidy to offset the financial burden of the disease. The government subsidy was seen by interviewees as an incentive to continue treatment, but healthcare personnel noted that the incentive was undermined by confusing and not well-understood subsidy regulations, leading to low rates of application, and by administrative delays upwards of 6 months following treatment initiation. In addition, it was noted that the subsidy must be initiated by the attending physician, who may not have been the individual who started the paperwork. If the application is not initiated within the first 2 months of treatment, patients lose their opportunity to apply. Regional reports indicated that about 10% of TB patients in Region V were receiving the subsidy. Even though the delay is substantial, it is a marked improvement from the reported historic wait of up to 3 years.

"...people live day by day here. It's not like work will wait six months or nine months when they are better. They are waiting for work....They have to go out and look for money otherwise they do not eat....There is subsidy for tuberculosis that they are paying now, but it arrives at best six months after completing treatment." [Healthcare personnel, FG]

4. Discussion

To our knowledge, this was a first of its kind qualitative study assessing modes of treatment delivery and barriers and facilitators to TB treatment success from multiple perspectives in Argentina. This research served as a foundational evaluation for a study currently in progress to assess patient and system factors associated with successful treatment of tuberculosis. However, evidence from this study may also identify—for both policy makers and healthcare personnel dedicated to TB management—weaknesses within the system and interventions to strengthen the system. Findings highlight that many of the barriers to treatment success were at the system/organizational level, but an interplay of personal and structural/social factors also influenced treatment outcome. Interventions were in place in some districts to counter some of the perceived barriers. The facilitators primarily focused on support (individual and community), flexibility, commitment, and continuity of care.

4.1. Modes of Treatment Delivery. Our findings highlight a potential discrepancy between the reported mode of treatment delivery as DOT and the mode of delivery in practice. We found that DOT was often considered a component of a larger support package and more "flexible" variations were in place to meet patients' needs and situation. Weekly or bimonthly treatment monitoring is, in effect, self-administration. Recent studies have demonstrated that the degree to which treatment is directly supervised can vary between and within countries [28–31]. Reports issued by the government of Argentina also highlight that DOT is not widely implemented in some provinces, especially those with the highest case loads and largest TB burden [5]. The low rates of DOT application could also be related to not all healthcare personnel being convinced that strict DOT was necessary and challenges to convincing patients to start daily DOT at a healthcare center when they had previously received treatment by self-administration from an outpatient hospital-based clinic.

4.2. Individual Factors. Our study highlighted the importance of establishing strong patient-provider relationships to facilitate treatment success, which has been previously described in the literature [14, 31, 32]. However, presumably the development of a strong patient-provider relationship cannot be readily established during self-administration of treatment alone. We found that communication and established relationships with healthcare personnel helped patients combat fear of TB and increased their knowledge of the disease. Stopping treatment due to feeling better has been identified as the cause of nearly 30% of patients abandoning treatment in a study conducted in Zambia [33]. Patients and family members of patients in this study described how challenging it was to convince individuals with TB to continue treatment when they felt better. In this study, most patients were positive about their experiences at their local healthcare centers and were willing to comply with treatment because of an established trust or positive perception of quality of healthcare services at the local level. However, maintaining established community positive perception of quality of healthcare services was described as being undermined by frequent staff turnover or political changes leading to position transfers, both of which affected the continuity of local healthcare teams.

4.3. Structural/Social Factors. Adequate individual and community awareness of TB was considered by patients and healthcare personnel to promote adherence, decrease stigmatization, and improve TB outcomes. Delays in disease detection can result in more advanced and complicated cases. Our findings highlight the need to increase TB knowledge in communities, particularly in schools and among healthcare providers, to address the misconceptions about the disease

and lessen the stigma, as well as decrease diagnostic and treatment delays. What were termed "health tours" by some participants in this study exemplified the challenges to treating and tracking mobile populations. In this study, participants understood that TB was curable. Patients acknowledged that fears were diminished when healthcare personnel informed them about the disease, and healthcare personnel recognized the importance of explicitly informing patients that TB is curable only by completing a full course of treatment. Other researchers have reported similar factors impacting TB treatment success: stigma and fear [34–36], nonsalaried employment, fear of losing employment or the opportunity to work [36, 37], challenges of mobile populations [38], and misconceptions and lack of knowledge about TB and its treatment [14, 39–41].

4.4. Organizational Factors. Adherence to treatment is the responsibility of both the patient and the system; however, the system should facilitate compliance. We identified patient motivation to adhere to treatment and healthcare personnel commitment to the patient as important factors contributing to TB treatment success. Because motivation is difficult to operationalize, and other important influences may be overlooked, Munro et al. [14] warn about attributing personal motivation to treatment adherence. Our findings highlight an organizational reliance on personal commitment of healthcare personnel who: provided food to patients to promote treatment adherence, used personal funds to cover TB treatment-related expenses, and were creating individual databases to better manage and track patient treatment.

The support package, not described as such by participants, included strong patient-healthcare personnel relationships, assistance with applying for financial subsidy, provision of food, and other provider-patient interactions. Patient-centered approaches, individualized support and monitoring of treatment adherence, use of incentives to continue treatment, and interventions to return patients who abandon treatment have been reported in the literature to improve TB outcomes [4, 42–44]. We found that a governmental financial subsidy for patients meeting requirements had been established, but administrative delays in distribution lessened the impact of the subsidy. Providing a subsidy early would help patients who are the most likely to abandon treatment.

Findings from this study suggest strengthening and better utilizing the established decentralized system. Ideally, hospitals in a decentralized system would be utilized for complicated and difficult cases, and healthcare centers would primarily focus on dispersed TB cases. Decentralization of treatment and care has been reported to improve treatment outcomes by minimizing travel cost and distance to access healthcare [45, 46]. In some countries access to health services has been reported to be a major barrier [14, 31, 47, 48]. In this study, in contrast, the healthcare centers were reported to be widely dispersed (estimated at one about every 15–20 blocks) and access to care was not considered the major barrier, although some participants cited having districts with more rural populations. Of more concern was a perceived low quality of healthcare services provided at the smaller community healthcare centers. Many healthcare workers believed the perceived low quality of care led patients to travel further to larger facilities and prevented healthcare personnel from referring patients to local healthcare centers where treatment monitoring could be conducted closer to where the patients lived and where there were fewer cases, making tracking and returning patients who default back to treatment easier. The resulting TB concentration at the larger facilities, where self-administration of treatment was the usual care, was considered a major contributor to patients becoming lost in the system due the difficulties managing, tracking, and returning patients who abandoned treatment. The concentration of cases at larger facilities was, in part, the result of major disparities in the quality of the facilities and services provided at local healthcare centers, fueling the perception of a low quality of healthcare services at the local level and ultimately the underutilization of the established decentralized system. The best methods to strengthen the smaller healthcare centers would need to be identified prior to inundating these centers with TB patient referrals.

4.5. DOTS/DOT. Reflecting on the five DOTS components (securing political commitment, strengthening detection and diagnosis, ensuring drug availability, monitoring outcomes, and providing directly observed therapy (DOT)), a number of our findings highlight persistent operational problems in its implementation. Political commitment to the TB program was questioned with findings, such as lead positions (e.g., the national TB director, regional directors) not officially recognized, standard shifting of personnel with political changes, and varying quality of services offered at the local healthcare centers. With regard to detection and diagnosis, it was recognized that a major barrier was a lack of consideration of potential TB diagnosis (low index of suspicion of TB) by individuals, community, and healthcare professionals, which impacted treatment seeking and delayed diagnosis. Although a regular drug supply was reported at the time of the study, Argentina experienced a medication shortage at the time of the paper's preparation. In Region V, some of the first and second line antituberculosis medications were unavailable for an extended period of time.

Data management was paper-based and was idiosyncratically organized by the healthcare centers. No healthcare center visited had access to a computer to help manage caseloads. This lack of an integrated computerized system to manage patient data may contribute to the high numbers of identified TB cases not having final treatment results (27% according to the latest national TB treatment results from 2009) [49] and monitoring and evaluation delays, which can lead to programmatic failure to respond to poor outcomes. During the duration of the study, an online reporting system, used by regional directors to input paper-based patient data, was being implemented in some provinces, but it was not being used for patient tracking and follow-up at the local level. The impact of the online reporting system has yet to be evaluated. Expanding the current web-based national system to include individual patient tracking and treatment monitoring could decrease the number of cases missing final treatment outcomes and aid healthcare personnel in managing their caseloads.

Lastly, DOT has been alternatively viewed as a supportive model of care and a control model of care that likely decreases responsibility for patient self-care [43]. Our findings suggest that patients who were receiving treatment by DOT believed they were cared for, but many healthcare personnel indicated, in their opinion, that those who completed with DOT would also complete by self-administration. Overall, the DOT strategy was perceived as an effective tool for treatment success, but not sufficient in and of itself. Other factors, such as education, TB knowledge, and socioeconomic situation, were considered more influential. More recently, the effectiveness of DOT has been questioned [37, 42, 43, 50–52]. Instead of a dogmatic approach that insists DOT is the *only* technique to assure effective treatment, DOT is now listed as an example of a *possible* measure to assure and aid in treatment adherence [4]. Congruent with this shift to meet patient-centered needs and offer individualized support, we identified multiple examples of flexible patient-centered approaches such as negotiated number of DOT days, no-wait treatment, training a night guardsman, and 24-hour healthcare centers. Despite the potential benefits, we did not find evidence of patients selecting their own DOT treatment supervisor. Interventions for TB care should be standardized but also allow some flexibility based on the needs of the individual and local healthcare center.

4.6. Limitations. We believe the barriers and facilitators identified in this study provide valuable insights from multiple perspectives into factors impacting TB treatment success in high TB burden regions of Argentina. However, there are some important limitations to mention. Although results may not be generalizable to the entire country, the public healthcare system in other regions of Argentina is governed by similar political and organizational structures. The inclusion of healthcare personnel was through purposive sampling of healthcare municipalities with higher and lower rates of treatment success based on historic records and recommendations of the regional TB director. We interviewed those involved in TB efforts at the selected sites. However, for patient/family participants, we relied on healthcare staff to approach and invite patients to participate. Therefore, we do not know the number of patient/family participants who were invited, declined to participate, or did not show up for the group interviews. Those who agreed to participate in the study may have been those most adherent to their TB treatment. Although we requested that healthcare staff attempt to invite patients who had abandoned treatment, this did not occur. We were, however, able to include testimonies of the family members of such patients and the healthcare professionals who had been responsible for the care of these patients. Unfortunately, some of the audio recordings of the patient/family interviews were difficult for transcriptionists to decipher and sections of recordings were not transcribed, which resulted in fewer direct patient quotes. Lastly, the interviews were focused on healthcare teams at healthcare centers and at the municipal level; therefore, healthcare personnel in hospitals were not interviewed. However, regional directors were able to speak to the process of how patients were managed at the regional hospitals.

5. Conclusions

To make substantive changes in countries where TB treatment success is consistently low and rates of drug resistance are increasing, the investigation and identification of root causes is paramount. Achieving treatment success is inherently multifaceted and cannot be attributed solely to patient characteristics—responsibility lies with the individual and the system. Overall, the healthcare system appeared to rely heavily on personal commitment of both patients and healthcare personnel. Adherence, from patient and healthcare personnel perspectives, was often not a free choice but rather a reflection of behaviors conditioned by the sociocultural and economic context. Identifying the majority of barriers at the organizational level highlighted the importance of strengthening system-level initiatives. Interventions such as quick access to treatment through separate doors, having healthcare facilities open for extended times, and providing incentives or utilizing politically appointed community advocates had limited implementation. Increasing dissemination of TB information to the public and healthcare personnel could help reduce the stigma of TB and thereby decrease delays in diagnosis and treatment. A strengthened political commitment is needed to motivate, distribute, and support competent healthcare personnel throughout the decentralized system, minimize healthcare personnel shifting/turnover during political changes, more quickly allocate treatment subsidies to patients, and improve the accuracy and efficiency of patient monitoring/tracking (e.g., centralized patient tracking system). More uniform staffing and resources across the healthcare services could promote a positive perception of the quality of healthcare services provided at local healthcare centers and improve the utilization of the established decentralized system. Flexible patient-centered care is needed to promote strong patient-healthcare personnel relationships and provide support to patients, especially those concentrated at the larger healthcare facilities receiving treatment by self-administration. Ultimately, recognizing and responding to weaknesses in the healthcare system and tailoring delivery of healthcare to patient needs rather than having patients adapt to the models in existence could impact TB treatment outcomes. Findings can be used to tailor programs to improve TB treatment outcomes in similar settings.

Authors' Contribution

All authors (Sarah J. Iribarren, Fernando Rubinstein, Vilda Discacciati, and Patricia F. Pearce) participated in the conceptualization and design of the study, performed data analysis, and drafted the paper. Vilda Discacciati drafted the interview guides and coordinated and conducted interviews, along with Sarah J. Iribarren and Fernando Rubinstein. All authors (Sarah J. Iribarren, Fernando Rubinstein, Vilda Discacciati, and Patricia F. Pearce) have read and approved the final paper.

Acknowledgments

The authors would like to thank the staff from the Institute for Clinical Effectiveness, Buenos Aires, for providing practical and technical support for this study and the healthcare team members, directors, and the patients and their families for sharing their thoughts and struggles. This study received financial support from the NIH/Fogarty International Clinical Research Scholar program. Dr. Iribarren participated in a year-long mentored research experience, during which this study was completed under the mentorship of Drs. Rubinstein (in Argentina) and Pearce (at home institution in the United States). The authors would also like to thank Christine Pickett for paper editing.

References

[1] P. Das and R. Horton, "Tuberculosis-time to accelerate progress," The Lancet, vol. 375, no. 9728, pp. 1755–1757, 2010.

[2] D. A. Enarsona and N. E. Billo, "Critical evaluation of the Global DOTS Expansion Plan," Bulletin of the World Health Organization, vol. 85, no. 5, pp. 395–398, 2007.

[3] World Health Organization, An Expanded DOTS Framework for Effective Tuberculosis Control, WHO, Geneva, Switzerland, 2002.

[4] Tuberculosis Coalition for Technical Assistance, International Standards for Tuberculosis Care (ISTC). Diagnosis, Treatment, Public Health, The Hague, The Netherlands, 2nd edition, 2009.

[5] Instituto Nacional de Enfermedades Respiratorias E. Coni, Resultado del Tratamiento de los Casos de Tuberculosis, Situación Nacional y por Jurisdicción, Buenos Aires, Argentina, 2010.

[6] World Health Organization, Treatment for Tuberculosis: Guidelines, WHO/HTM/TB, 4th edition, 2009.

[7] World Health Organization, TB Country Profile Argentina, 2010, WHO, Geneva, Switzerland, 2012, http://www.who.int/tb/country/data/profiles/en/.

[8] Instituto Nacional de Enfermedades Respiratorias E. Coni, Notificación de Casos de Tuberculosis en la República Argentina. Período 1980-2012, ANLIS, 2013.

[9] Instituto Nacional de Infermidades Respiritorias E. Coni, Resultados del Tratamiento de Casos de Tuberculosis. Situación Nacional y por Jurisdicción, República Argentina, 2007, 2010.

[10] D. A. Mitchison, "How drug resistance emerges as a result of poor compliance during short course chemotherapy for tuberculosis," International Journal of Tuberculosis and Lung Disease, vol. 2, no. 1, pp. 10–15, 1998.

[11] G. Maartens and R. J. Wilkinson, "Tuberculosis," The Lancet, vol. 370, no. 9604, pp. 2030–2043, 2007.

[12] World Health Organization, Adherence to Long Term Therapies: Evidence for Action, World Health Organization, Geneva, Switzerland, 2003.

[13] World Health Organization, International Standards for Tuberculosis Care: Diagnosis, Treatment and Public Health, T.C.f.T. Assistance, 2006.

[14] S. A. Munro, S. A. Lewin, H. J. Smith, M. E. Engel, A. Fretheim, and J. Volmink, "Patient adherence to tuberculosis treatment: a systematic review of qualitative research," *PLoS Medicine*, vol. 4, no. 7, pp. 1230–1245, 2007.

[15] J. M. Cramm, H. J. Finkenflügel, V. Møller, and A. P. Nieboer, "TB treatment initiation and adherence in a South African community influenced more by perceptions than by knowledge of tuberculosis," *BMC Public Health*, vol. 10, article 72, 2010.

[16] C. Chirico, N. Morcillo, and A. Kuriger, "Is the DOTS strategy a useful tool to fight against Tuberculosis in a median incidence area of Buenos Aires Province?" *International Journal of Tuberculosis & Lung Disease*, 2005.

[17] C. Chirico, A. Kuriger, H. Fernandez, and N. Morcillo, "Evolution of tuberculosis incidence rates in the V sanitary zone of Buenos Aires province during the period 1984–1996," *Medicina*, vol. 59, no. 4, pp. 332–338, 1999.

[18] I. N. de Kantor, O. Latini, and L. Barrera, "Resistance and multiresistance to antitubercular drugs in Argentina and in other Latin American countries," *Medicina*, vol. 58, no. 2, pp. 202–208, 1998.

[19] M. S. Imaz, M. D. Sequeira, A. Aguirre et al., "Bacteriological diagnosis of tuberculosis in Argentina: results of a national survey," *Cadernos de Saude Publica*, vol. 23, no. 4, pp. 885–896, 2007.

[20] D. J. Palmero, M. Ambroggi, A. Brea et al., "Treatment and follow-up of HIV-negative multidrug-resistant tuberculosis patients in an infectious diseases reference hospital, Buenos Aires, Argentina," *International Journal of Tuberculosis and Lung Disease*, vol. 8, no. 6, pp. 778–784, 2004.

[21] E. Zerbini, M. C. Chirico, B. Salvadores, B. Amigot, S. Estrada, and G. Algorry, "Delay in tuberculosis diagnosis and treatment in four provinces of Argentina," *International Journal of Tuberculosis and Lung Disease*, vol. 12, no. 1, pp. 63–68, 2008.

[22] J. W. Creswell, A. C. Klassen, V. L. Plano-Clark, and K. C. Smith, *Best Practices for Mixed Method Research in the Health Sciences*, NIH National Institutes of Health, Washington, DC, USA, 2011.

[23] N. K. Denzin and Y. S. Lincoln, *Handbook of Qualitative Research*, Sage, Thousand Oaks, Calif, USA, 2000.

[24] M. Sandelowski, "Whatever happened to qualitative description?" *Research in Nursing and Health*, vol. 23, no. 4, pp. 334–40, 2000.

[25] C. Chirico, A. Kuriger, M. Etchevarria, L. Casamajor, and N. Morcillo, "Anti-tuberculosis treatment evaluation in Northern districts of Buenos Aires suburbs," *Medicina*, vol. 67, no. 2, pp. 131–135, 2007.

[26] Y. Lincoln and E. Guba, *Naturalistic Inquiry*, Sage Publications, Newbury Park, Calif, USA, 1985.

[27] M. Sandelowski, "What's in a name? Qualitative description revisited," *Research in Nursing and Health*, vol. 33, no. 1, pp. 77–84, 2010.

[28] C. Lienhardt, K. Manneh, V. Bouchier, G. Lahai, P. J. M. Milligan, and K. P. W. J. McAdam, "Factors determining the outcome of treatment of adult smear-positive tuberculosis cases in the Gambia," *The International Journal of Tuberculosis and Lung Disease*, vol. 2, no. 9, pp. 712–718, 1998.

[29] C. Lienhardt and J. A. Ogden, "Tuberculosis control in resource-poor countries: have we reached the limits of the universal paradigm?" *Tropical Medicine and International Health*, vol. 9, no. 7, pp. 833–841, 2004.

[30] K. M. de Cock and R. E. Chaisson, "Will DOTS do it? A reappraisal of tuberculosis control in countries with high rates of HIV infection," *International Journal of Tuberculosis and Lung Disease*, vol. 3, no. 6, pp. 457–465, 1999.

[31] F. Hane, S. Thiam, A. S. Fall et al., "Identifying barriers to effective tuberculosis control in Senegal: an anthropological approach," *International Journal of Tuberculosis and Lung Disease*, vol. 11, no. 5, pp. 539–543, 2007.

[32] J. Ogden, S. Rangan, M. Uplekar et al., "Shifting the paradigm in tuberculosis control: illustrations from India," *International Journal of Tuberculosis and Lung Disease*, vol. 3, no. 10, pp. 855–861, 1999.

[33] F. A. D. Kaona, M. Tuba, S. Siziya, and L. Sikaona, "An assessment of factors contributing to treatment adherence and knowledge of TB transmission among patients on TB treatment," *BMC Public Health*, vol. 4, article 68, 2004.

[34] M. Sagbakken, J. C. Frich, and G. Bjune, "Barriers and enablers in the management of tuberculosis treatment in Addis Ababa, Ethiopia: a qualitative study," *BMC Public Health*, vol. 8, article 11, 2008.

[35] W. Xu, W. Lu, Y. Zhou, L. Zhu, H. Shen, and J. Wang, "Adherence to anti-tuberculosis treatment among pulmonary tuberculosis patients: a qualitative and quantitative study," *BMC Health Services Research*, vol. 9, article 169, 2009.

[36] T. K. Ray, N. Sharma, M. M. Singh, and G. K. Ingle, "Economic burden of tuberculosis in patients attending DOT centres in Delhi," *The Journal of Communicable Diseases*, vol. 37, no. 2, pp. 93–98, 2005.

[37] M. A. Khan, J. D. Walley, S. N. Witter, S. K. Shah, and S. Javeed, "Tuberculosis patient adherence to direct observation: results of a social study in Pakistan," *Health Policy and Planning*, vol. 20, no. 6, pp. 354–365, 2005.

[38] K. W. Kizito, S. Dunkley, M. Kingori, and T. Reid, "Lost to follow up from tuberculosis treatment in an urban informal settlement (Kibera), Nairobi, Kenya: what are the rates and determinants?" *Transactions of the Royal Society of Tropical Medicine & Hygiene*, vol. 105, no. 1, pp. 52–57, 2011.

[39] S. P. Ntshanga, R. Rustomjee, and M. L. H. Mabaso, "Evaluation of directly observed therapy for tuberculosis in KwaZulu-Natal, South Africa," *Transactions of the Royal Society of Tropical Medicine and Hygiene*, vol. 103, no. 6, pp. 571–574, 2009.

[40] M. Sagbakken, J. C. Frich, and G. A. Bjune, "Perception and management of tuberculosis symptoms in Addis Ababa, Ethiopia," *Qualitative Health Research*, vol. 18, no. 10, pp. 1356–1366, 2008.

[41] B. Tekle, D. H. Mariam, and A. Ali, "Defaulting from DOTS and its determinants in three districts of Arsi Zone in Ethiopia," *International Journal of Tuberculosis and Lung Disease*, vol. 6, no. 7, pp. 573–579, 2002.

[42] J. Volmink, P. Matchaba, and P. Garner, "Directly observed therapy and treatment adherence," *The Lancet*, vol. 355, no. 9212, pp. 1345–1350, 2000.

[43] J. C. M. Macq, S. Theobald, J. Dick, and M. Dembele, "An exploration of the concept of directly observed treatment (DOT) for tuberculosis patients: from a uniform to a customised approach," *International Journal of Tuberculosis and Lung Disease*, vol. 7, no. 2, pp. 103–109, 2003.

[44] D. S. Pope and R. E. Chaisson, "TB treatment: as simple as dot?" *The International Journal of Tuberculosis and Lung Disease*, vol. 7, no. 7, pp. 611–615, 2003.

[45] J. K. Kangangi, D. Kibuga, J. Muli et al., "Decentralisation of tuberculosis treatment from the main hospitals to the peripheral health units and in the community within Machakos

District, Kenya," *International Journal of Tuberculosis and Lung Disease*, vol. 7, no. 9, supplement 1, pp. S5–S13, 2003.

[46] T. E. Nyirenda, A. D. Harries, F. Gausi et al., "Decentralisation of tuberculosis services in an urban setting, Lilongwe, Malawi," *International Journal of Tuberculosis and Lung Disease*, vol. 7, no. 9, supplement 1, pp. S21–S28, 2003.

[47] P. C. Hill, W. Stevens, S. Hill et al., "Risk factors for defaulting from tuberculosis treatment: a prospective cohort study of 301 cases in the Gambia," *International Journal of Tuberculosis and Lung Disease*, vol. 9, no. 12, pp. 1349–1354, 2005.

[48] N. Martins, J. Grace, and P. M. Kelly, "An ethnographic study of barriers to and enabling factors for tuberculosis treatment adherence in Timor Leste," *International Journal of Tuberculosis and Lung Disease*, vol. 12, no. 5, pp. 532–537, 2008.

[49] Instituto Nacional de Enfermidades Respiratorias E. Coni, "Evaluation of tuberculosis treatment results in Argentina. National status and by jurisdiction, 2009," 2011, http://www .anlis.gov.ar/inst/iner/archivos/TratamientoTB_2009.pdf.

[50] J. Volmink and P. Garner, "Directly observed therapy for treating tuberculosis," *Cochrane Database of Systematic Reviews*, no. 4, Article ID CD003343, 2007.

[51] T. R. Frieden and J. A. Sbarbaro, "Promoting adherence to treatment for tuberculosis: the importance of direct observation," *World Hospitals and Health Services*, vol. 43, no. 2, pp. 30–33, 2007.

[52] T. M. R. M. de Figueiredo, T. C. S. Villa, L. M. Scatena et al., "Performance of primary healthcare services in tuberculosis control," *Revista de Saude Publica*, vol. 43, no. 5, pp. 825–831, 2009.

12

The Effect of Low CD4+ Lymphocyte Count on the Radiographic Patterns of HIV Patients with Pulmonary Tuberculosis among Nigerians

Christopher Affusim,[1] Vivien Abah,[2] Emeka B. Kesieme,[3] Kester Anyanwu,[1]
Taofik A. T. Salami,[4] and Reuben Eifediyi[5]

[1] Department of Family Medicine, Ambrose Alli University, PMB 8, Ekpoma, Edo state, Nigeria
[2] Department of Family Medicine, University of Benin Teaching Hospital, Benin, Edo State, Nigeria
[3] Department of Surgery, Ambrose Alli University, PMB 8, Ekpoma, Edo state, Nigeria
[4] Department of Internal Medicine, Ambrose Alli University, PMB 8, Ekpoma, Edo state, Nigeria
[5] Department of Obstetrics and Gynaecology, Ambrose Alli University, PMB 8, Ekpoma, Edo state, Nigeria

Correspondence should be addressed to Christopher Affusim; c2ffusimus@yahoo.com

Academic Editor: W. N. Rom

Objective. To assess the radiographic features in patients with Human Immunodeficiency Virus (HIV) complicated by pulmonary tuberculosis (PTB), and the association with CD4 lymphocyte count and sputum smear. *Method.* A prospective study was carried out on 89 HIV positive patients with PTB. The demographics, smoking history, sputum smear result, chest radiographic findings and CD4 lymphocyte count were documented. *Results.* Out of the 89 patients recruited in the study, 41 were males and 48 were females. Eighteen (18) patients had typical radiographic features, 60 patients had atypical radiographic features while only 11 of them had normal radiographic films. Sixty eight (68) patients had CD4 count <200 cells/mm^3, 19 patients had CD4 count between 200–499 cells/mm^3, while only 2 patients had CD4 count from 500 cells/mm^3 upwards. The association between low CD4 count and radiographic finding was statistically significant, (P value < 0.05). Sixty (60) patients had negative sputum smear for Acid and Alcohol Fast Bacilli (AAFB), while the remaining 29 patients had positive smear. The association between low CD4 count and negative smear was statistically significant (P value < 0.05). *Conclusion.* The radiographic pattern and the result of the sputum smear for AAFB has a significant relationship and association with the immune status of patients with Human Immunodeficiency Virus (HIV) complicated by pulmonary tuberculosis.

1. Introduction

Human immunodeficiency virus (HIV) is a potent risk factor for tuberculosis (TB), both through an increase in the reactivation of the latent *Mycobacterium tuberculosis* infection and through an accelerated progression from infection to active disease, by undermining the cell-mediated immunity through depletion of CD4 lymphocytes [1–4].

TB has a great impact on morbidity and mortality in HIV-1 infected individuals than all other opportunistic infections [3]. TB and HIV infections have a synergistic influence on the host immunoregulation. TB can develop at any stage of

immunosuppression regardless of the level of the circulating CD4+ T-lymphocytes [4]. CD4+ lymphocytes count is one of the surrogate markers for evaluating the degree of immunosuppression and HIV disease progression [4].

The levels of circulating CD4+ lymphocytes has a great impact on the radiographic pattern of TB. In HIV infections, TB can produce both typical and atypical radiographic patterns depending on the degree of immunosuppression [5–8]. Atypical radiographic presentations are lower frequency of cavitations, higher frequency of mediastinal lymphadenopathy, lower lung zone infiltrates, and even a normal chest radiograph. Typical presentations include upper lobe fibrosis, bilateral infiltrates, consolidation, and cavitations [6–8]. Thus patients with low CD4 lymphocyte count have more of features of primary TB, while those with a high CD4 count will have features of postprimary TB.

This study was undertaken to determine the effect of low CD4+ lymphocyte count on the radiographic patterns of HIV patients with pulmonary TB among Nigerians. There is dearth of studies on this subject in Nigeria.

2. Materials

2.1. Study Setting. The study was done at University of Benin Teaching Hospital from April to May 2007. This hospital is a government designated centre of excellence for the management of HIV/AIDS. The patients for the study were recruited from the HIV clinic of this hospital. They were confirmed HIV positive patients with pulmonary TB.

2.2. Inclusion Criteria

(1) HIV positive patients with pulmonary TB aged 18 years and above who presented at the clinic within the study period and who had not commenced drug treatment.

(2) All HIV positive patients with pulmonary TB who consented to join in the study.

2.3. Exclusion Criteria

(1) Patients with indeterminate PTB.

(2) Patients with other immunosuppressive diseases like diabetes mellitus, malignancies, and so forth.

3. Method of Data Collection

This was a prospective study done from April to May 2007. Informed consent was obtained from the patients. Information was gathered from the patient's case note. The subject's biodata and the results of the following investigations were collected.

(a) Chest radiograph.

(b) Sputum for acid and alcohol fast bacilli (AAFB).

(c) CD4 cell count.

The chest radiographs were blindly reported by two radiologists who were not aware of the enrolment into the study. The two reached a consensus on radiological findings of a radiograph when there is a disagreement in their evaluation. They evaluated the radiographs for mediastinal lymphadenopathy, infiltrates, cavitations, pleural effusions, and localized or military shadows and also determined the predominantly affected lung zones.

The chest radiograph results were grouped into three namely, those with typical features, those with atypical features, and those with normal films. The sputum smear result was grouped into two namely, those positive for AAFB and those negative for AAFB. The CD4 lymphocyte cell count results was also grouped into three namely, CD4 count <200 cells/mm^3, CD4 count 200–499 cells/mm^3, and CD4 count from 500 cells/mm^3 upwards.

4. Method of Data Analysis

The statistical package for social sciences (SPSS) version 16.0 was used to record and analyse the data. Frequency tables were drawn to show the distribution of data within variables. Contingency tables were drawn to compare two discrete variables. Pearson Chi-square was used to test significance. A P value < 0.05 was considered significant.

5. Case Definition

The diagnosis of PTB/HIV coinfection was based on criteria for diagnosing TB in poor resource settings where there are no facilities and manpower for *mycobacterium tuberculosis* culture: (a) the diagnostic criteria of TB given in the World Health Organisation (WHO) treatment of tuberculosis guideline for national programmes [5]; (b) specificity of clinical criteria in diagnosing TB patient [6, 9].

6. Results

A total of 89 HIV positive patients with pulmonary TB were recruited into the study. Their ages range from 19 years to 65 years. The mean age was 37.73 years. There were 41 males (46.07%) and 48 females (53.93%). Forty-six (46) patients (51.68%) were married, 31 patients (34.83%) were single, and 2 patients (2.25%) were separated from their spouses, while 10 patients (11.23%) had lost their spouses. Five (5) patients (5.62%) had no formal education, 17 patients (19.10%) had tertiary education, and 40 patients (44.94%) had secondary education, while 27 patients (30.34%) had primary education.

More of the patients (74 patients (83.15%)) had never smoked, while a small number (15 patients (16.85%)) had smoked at one time or the other in their lives. Sixty (60) patients (67.42%) had negative sputum smear for acid and alcohol fast bacilli, while 29 patients (32.58%) had positive smear.

The chest X-ray results were as follows: 18 patients (20.22%) had typical chest X-ray features, and 60 patients (67.42%) had atypical features, while the least number 11 patients (12.36%) had normal features. The mean CD4 lymphocyte cell count was 125 cells/mm^3, 68 patients (76.40%) had CD4 count less than 200 cells/mm^3, and 19 patients (21.35%) had CD4 count levels between 200 and 499 cells/mm^3, while 2 patients (2.25%) had CD4 cell count from 500 cells/mm^3 upwards. Table 1 shows the characteristics of the patients studied.

All the 11 patients who had normal chest X-ray findings had CD4 count less than 200 cells/mm^3, while the remaining with CD4 count more than 200 cells/mm^3 had either atypical or typical findings. The association between severe

TABLE 1: Characteristics of the patients in the study.

Characteristics of the patients	Frequency	Percentage
Age	Age range: 19–65 years	
	Mean age: 37.73 years	
Sex	Males: 41	46.07%
	Females: 48	53.93%
Marital status	Married: 46	51.68%
	Single: 31	34.83%
	Separated: 2	2.25%
	Widowed: 10	11.23%
Smoking history	Have smoked: 15	16.85%
	Never smoked: 74	83.15%
Sputum smear	Positive: 29	32.58%
	Negative: 60	67.42%
Chest X-ray	Typical features: 18	20.22%
	Atypical features: 60	67.42%
	Normal features: 11	12.36%
CD4 cell count	<200 cells/mm^3 – 68	76.40%
	200–499 cells/mm^3 – 19	21.35%
	500 cells/mm^3 and above– 2	2.25%

TABLE 2: Relationship between levels of CD4 count and chest X-ray features.

CD4 count	Chest X-ray features		
	Typical	Atypical	Normal
<200	2	55	11
200–499	14	5	0
≥500	2	0	0
Total	18	60	11

P value < 0.05. Relationship is significant.

TABLE 3: Relationship between levels of CD4 count and sputum smear.

CD4 count	Sputum smear	
	Positive	Negative
<200	10	58
200–499	17	2
≥500	2	0
Total	29	60

P value < 0.05. Relationship is significant.

immunosuppression and normal radiograph was statistically significant (P value < 0.05) (Table 2).

Out of all the patients with CD4 less than 100 cells/mm^3, a total of twenty-two (22) patients (24.7%) had CD4 count below 50 cells/mm^3, while sixteen (16) patients (17.98%) had CD4 count between 50 and 100 cells/mm^3. Eighteen (18) of those with CD4 count <50 cells (81.81%) had atypical X-ray features, while fourteen (14) of those with CD4 count 50–100 cells (87.5%) also had atypical X-ray features.

Out of the 60 patients that had negative sputum smears, only 2 of them had CD4 count ≥200 cells/mm^3. The other 58 patients with negative smears had CD4 count <200 cells/mm^3, and the association between severe immunosuppression (CD4 count <200) and negative sputum smear was significant (P value < 0.05) (Table 3).

7. Discussion

Results from the study showed a significant relationship between the CD4 lymphocyte cell count and the radiographic features of HIV positive patients with pulmonary tuberculosis (Table 2). The CD4 count is an indicator of immune status and stage of HIV infection. Severe immunosuppression and CD4 count <200 cells/mm^3 were significantly associated with the presence of mediastinal lymphadenopathy. This is in keeping with other studies worldwide [9–11]. Other features of primary TB (atypical features) like middle and lower lung zone involvement, military pattern, and normal films were also more common in patients with CD4 count <200 cells/mm^3, (Table 2).

Cavity formation and other features of postprimary TB on chest radiograph were found to be common and significantly associated with more immunocompetency (CD4 count ≥200 cells/mm^3). Several other studies on the association between cavity formation and high CD4 count confirm this [11, 12]. Formation of cavities in TB infection requires an adequate delayed type of hypersensitivity reaction and an intact cell-mediated immunity in the host. Typical features (upper lung zone involvement) are seen more often in HIV patients with less immunosuppression than in those with severe immunosuppression. It is not surprising that HIV patients with high CD4 counts will have upper lung zone involvement because TB in the upper lung zone is usually common in HIV negative patients with high CD4 count and thus immunocompetent.

Only 11 out of the 89 patients in the study had normal chest radiographs, and all the 11 patients had CD4 count <200 cells/mm^3. The association between severe immunosuppression and normal radiograph was significant (Table 2). This was supported by another study [13] but was not supported by a study done in USA which found no significant association between CD4 count and normal chest radiograph [11].

The finding of a normal chest radiograph and negative sputum smear microscopy, in HIV patients coinfected with pulmonary TB, poses a great challenge for the diagnosis of pulmonary TB in poor resource countries, where facilities for culture of *mycobacterium tuberculosis* are scanty or nonexistent, and thus diagnosis requires high index of suspicion. More studies are required to confirm if the absence of radiographic findings represents early stages of either primary TB or a reactivation, or one caused by intrathoracic lymphadenopathy unable to be detected by simple radiographic examination [11, 12]. In a cross tabulation between sputum smear and chest X-ray findings, it was found that

TABLE 4: Relationship between sputum smear and chest X-ray features.

Sputum smear	Chest X-ray features		
	Typical	Atypical	Normal
Positive	16	12	1
Negative	2	48	10
Total	18	60	11

P value < 0.05. Relationship is significant.

most of the patients that had atypical chest X-ray features also had negative sputum smears (Table 4). The relationship between these two was significant. This finding confirms that in severe immunosuppression, the usual immune response to TB infection is no longer maintained.

In this study, atypical or primary pattern was common in patients with CD4 count <200 cells/mm^3, while typical or postprimary pattern was commoner in those with CD4 count >200 cells/mm^3 and commonest in those with CD4 count ≥500 cells/mm^3. This was similar to what was found in some other studies [10, 11]. The different radiographic appearances have different pathogenesis, and these were greatly modified by the level of CD4 count (degree of immunosuppression) and cell-mediated immunity.

This study has revealed that various radiographic manifestations of HIV coinfected with pulmonary TB are related to the level of immunosuppression (CD4 count). Physicians need to be aware of this finding, and those in countries with poor resources should have high index of suspicion to be able to make proper diagnosis.

References

[1] TB Advocacy, "World health organisation (WHO) global tuberculosis programme," WHO Fact Sheet No 104, 2002.

[2] E. L. Corbett, C. J. Watt, N. Walker et al., "The growing burden of tuberculosis: global trends and interactions with the HIV epidemic," Archives of Internal Medicine, vol. 163, no. 9, pp. 1009–1021, 2003.

[3] UNAIDS, "Report on the global AIDS epidermic: executive summary," UNAIDS/6, 20E, 2006, http://www.unaids.org/en/HIV_data/2006 Global Report/default.asp.

[4] A. N. Ackah, D. Coulibely, H. Digbeu et al., "Response to treatment, mortality, and CD4 lymphocyte counts in HIV-infected persons with tuberculosis in Abidjan, Cote d'Ivoire," The Lancet, vol. 345, no. 8950, pp. 607–610, 1995.

[5] "Treatment of tuberculosis, guidelines for national programmes," World Health Organisation, Geneva, Switzerland, (document WHO/CDS/TB/2003. 313), 2002.

[6] B. Keshinro and M. Y. Diul, "HIV-TB: epidemiology, clinical features and diagnosis of smear-negative TB," Tropical Doctor, vol. 36, no. 2, pp. 68–71, 2006.

[7] V. K. Kawooya, M. Kawooya, and A. Okwera, "Radiographic appearances in pulmonary tuberculosis in HIV-1 seropositive and seronegative adult patients," East African Medical Journal, vol. 77, no. 6, pp. 303–307, 2000.

[8] E. B. Rizzi, V. Schininà, F. Palmieri, E. Girardi, and C. Bibbolino, "Radiological patterns in HIV-associated pulmonary tuberculosis: comparison between HAART-treated and non-HAART-treated patients," Clinical Radiology, vol. 58, no. 6, pp. 469–473, 2003.

[9] B. Samb, D. Henzel, C. L. Daley et al., "Methods for diagnosing tuberculosis among in-patients in Eastern Africa whose sputum smears are negative," International Journal of Tuberculosis and Lung Disease, vol. 1, no. 1, pp. 25–30, 1997.

[10] J. Murray, P. Sonnenberg, S. C. Shearer, and P. Godfrey-Faussett, "Human immunodeficiency virus and the outcome of treatment for new and recurrent pulmonary tuberculosis in African patients," American Journal of Respiratory and Critical Care Medicine, vol. 159, no. 3, pp. 733–740, 1999.

[11] D. C. Perlman, W. M. El-Sadr, E. T. Nelson et al., "Variation of chest radiographic patterns in pulmonary tuberculosis by degree of human immunodeficiency virus-related immunosuppression," Clinical Infectious Diseases, vol. 25, no. 2, pp. 242–246, 1997.

[12] G. F. Garcia, A. S. Moura, C. S. Ferreira, and M. O. D. C. Rocha, "Clinical and radiographic features of HIV-related pulmonary tuberculosis according to the level of immunosuppression," Revista da Sociedade Brasileira de Medicina Tropical, vol. 40, no. 6, pp. 622–626, 2007.

[13] A. Ahidjo, H. Yusuph, and A. Tahir, "Radiographic features of pulmonary tuberculosis among HIV patients in Maiduguri, Nigeria," Annals of African Medicine, vol. 4, no. 1, pp. 7–9, 2005.

13

An IMS/ATP Assay for the Detection of *Mycobacterium tuberculosis* in Urine

Dawn M. Hunter and Daniel V. Lim

Department of Cell Biology, Microbiology and Molecular Biology, University of South Florida, 4202 E. Fowler Avenue, ISA 2015, Tampa, FL 33620-7115, USA

Correspondence should be addressed to Daniel V. Lim, lim@usf.edu

Academic Editor: Carlo Garzelli

Background. Although sputum smears are the gold standard for diagnosis of tuberculosis, sensitivity in HIV/TB coinfection cases is low, indicating a need for alternative methods. Urine is being increasingly evaluated. *Materials and Methods.* A novel method for detecting *Mycobacterium tuberculosis* (MTB) in synthetic urine using a combined IMS/ATP assay was evaluated. Preliminary work established standard ATP conditions and the sensitivity and specificity of the MTB antibody. Eighty-four blinded samples in four replicate assays were evaluated for the presence of MTB using labeled immunomagnetic beads for capture. Beads were separated, washed, and resuspended in broth and added to a microtiter plate. Bioluminescent output was measured and signal-to-noise ratios were calculated. All samples were plated on Middlebrook 7H10 agar or trypticase soy agar to determine limit of detection and recoveries. *Results and Conclusions.* MTB was distinguished from common bacteriuria isolates and other nontarget bacteria by its ATP results. IMS/ATP successfully detected 19 of 28 samples of MTB in synthetic urine with a limit of detection of 10^4 CFU/ml. Sensitivity and specificity were 67.9% and 82.1%, respectively. This assay offers a possible rapid screening method for HIV-positive patients with suspected coinfection to improve MTB diagnosis.

1. Introduction

There are over 8 million new cases of tuberculosis (TB) annually, with increasing incidence in areas where HIV is prevalent [1]. In 2009, there were 9.4 million new TB cases, with 1.1 million among HIV-positive individuals [2]. Sputum smear microscopy remains the standard for diagnosis. However, sensitivity varies even among HIV-negative patients, with an average sensitivity of less than 60%, and is as low as 20% for patients with HIV/TB coinfection [3]. This is further complicated by an inability to produce sputum among HIV-positive individuals [4–6]. In addition to smear-negative pulmonary TB, HIV-positive individuals tend to have abnormal chest X-rays and clinical presentations, so diagnosis and treatment are often delayed [3, 6, 7]. Furthermore, the sputum procedure is limited in diagnosing extrapulmonary infection, which is more common among patients in this group [3, 8, 9]. The impact of smear-negative disease on diagnostics is significant; even nucleic acid amplification tests such as the Gen-Probe MTD and Roche Amplicor MTB, which have sensitivities greater than 95% in smear-positive cases, have reduced sensitivities of 40–77% in smear-negative cases [3, 10].

Extrapulmonary TB and disseminated disease are more likely with advanced immunosuppression [8, 10]. The kidneys may become involved due to the spread of bacilli through the vascular system from foci in the lung [1, 4]. MTB bacilli can be excreted through the kidneys and detected in the urine of patients who have no symptoms of genitourinary involvement [9, 11]. However, although it has been known since the 1960s that MTB can be found in the urine of patients with pulmonary TB, urine has been a less reliable clinical sample compared to sputum. Urine has not been recommended for routine diagnosis because the sensitivity of urine smear microscopy and the yield of urine cultures have been low; conventional diagnostic methods using urine samples have had "limited clinical usefulness" [4].

However, urine has been increasingly evaluated as a diagnostic sample due to recent developments enabling the detection of mycobacterial DNA and metabolic products in urine, particularly among HIV-infected patients [5, 9, 12–14]. While the number of bacilli in urine varies and excretion is intermittent, the bacillary load for HIV/TB patients with disseminated disease may be high [9, 15]. Mycobacteriuria may be more prevalent than historically believed based on urine culture alone, as recent studies have demonstrated PCR-positive urines with sensitivities up to 66.7% in smear-negative TB [6, 9]. Additionally, urine samples have advantages relative to other biological samples because bacilli can be easily concentrated [15–17], samples are easy to collect, and there are fewer risks associated with handling [4, 6, 9].

More pressing than the need for alternative diagnostic sample types is the need for rapid, easy-to-perform tests that can be used in a point-of-care format [3, 4]. There are several disadvantages to sputum smear microscopy: (1) it is not useful where there is a low bacillary load, (2) it is not useful in cases of extrapulmonary TB, and (3) microscopy can detect other acid-fast bacteria [18]. As already noted, smear-negative TB and extrapulmonary TB are more common in HIV-positive patients. Peripheral laboratories rely on microscopy methods, while no diagnostic tests are currently available at health posts [19]. As noted by the World Health Organization, diagnostic limitations have been a "crucial barrier" to meeting the challenges of HIV-associated TB [20].

Immunomagnetic separation (IMS) has been successfully used to concentrate and recover pathogenic mycobacteria, including MTB [21, 22]. IMS also enables specific target capture and decreases particulate interference in detection assays [23, 24]. ATP bioluminescence assays have demonstrated utility in bacteriuria screening [25, 26], quality control of BCG vaccines [27], and MTB antibiotic susceptibility testing [28]. Combining immunocapture with an ATP-based cell viability assay can provide rapid, specific, semiquantitative detection of live cells [29–31]. The method presented here combines IMS with an ATP-based cell viability assay to provide rapid, specific detection of MTB in urine. The method is easy to perform and could have use in settings where the rate of HIV/TB co-infection is high.

The objectives of this work were to study (1) the sensitivity and specificity of the MTB antibody, (2) the ATP amount released from MTB relative to other organisms using a standard ATP assay, (3) the effect of incubation time and urine pH on IMS/ATP results, and (4) the possible detection of MTB in synthetic urine.

2. Materials and Methods

2.1. Antibodies. Affinity-purified rabbit polyclonal antibody to MTB (BIODESIGN International, Saco, ME) in phosphate-buffered saline (PBS) and affinity-purified goat anti-rabbit antibody conjugated to horseradish peroxidase in PBS (Kirkegaard & Perry Laboratories, Inc., Gaithersburg, MD) were used as detection antibodies in ELISA. Biotin-labeled rabbit polyclonal antibody to MTB in PBS (BIODESIGN International, Saco, ME) was used as the capture antibody in

the IMS/ATP assay. The antibody was immobilized on M280 Streptavidin Dynabeads (Invitrogen, Carlsbad, CA) according to the manufacturer's protocol. Antibody-labeled beads were stored for up to one week at 4°C until use.

2.2. Bacteria. MTB or *Mycobacterium tuberculosis* ATCC 25177 was the target microorganism for all assays. Nontarget microorganisms included common urine isolates [26], other mycobacteria, and *Candida* because of their morphological similarities to MTB. These strains were either ATCC strains or obtained from the University of South Florida Advanced Biosensors Laboratory (ABL) collection and included *Mycobacterium smegmatis* ABL 539, *Mycobacterium avium* ATCC 25921, *Mycobacterium intracellulare* ATCC 13950, *Mycobacterium gordonae* ATCC 14470, *Rhodococcus rhodochrous* ABL 538, *Candida albicans* ABL 537, *Staphylococcus aureus* ATCC 25923, *Staphylococcus epidermidis* ATCC 12228, *Staphylococcus simulans* ATCC 11631, *Enterococcus faecalis* ATCC 19433, *Escherichia coli* K12 ABL 552, *Pseudomonas aeruginosa* ATCC 15442, and *Klebsiella pneumoniae* ATCC 29019. Working stocks of nonmycobacterial strains prepared from frozen cultures were grown for 18 h at 37°C in tryptic soy broth (TSB; BD, Franklin Lakes, NJ). Working stocks of mycobacteria prepared from frozen cultures were grown for two days to three weeks (depending on the strain) at 37°C and 5% CO_2 on Middlebrook 7H10 agar (BD, Franklin Lakes, NJ). All working stocks were maintained at 4°C for up to 30 days. A fresh culture of MTB was incubated on a weekly basis for use in assays. Other bacterial strains used were grown overnight on tryptic soy agar (BD, Franklin Lakes, NJ) at 37°C.

2.3. Sample. Synthetic urine was purchased from Ricca Chemical Company (Arlington, TX). Synthetic urine has been used in a variety of studies, including method validation studies [32–34]. The urine contains urea, sodium chloride, magnesium sulfate heptahydrate, calcium chloride dihydrate, and water. Urine pH was adjusted from ~8.4 to 7.1 ± 0.1 or 5.5 ± 0.1 to determine whether urine pH influenced IMS. Based on these results, urine pH was adjusted to 7.1 ± 0.1 for all blinded assays (described in what follows).

2.4. ELISA. Cells were suspended in 0.01 M PBS with 0.1% Tween-80 (PBST80). Glass beads (0.1 mm, BioSpec Products, Inc., Bartlesville, OK) were added to mycobacterial suspensions to aid in dispersion. Cell suspensions were serially diluted (1 : 10) in PBST80, and consecutive serial dilutions were added to MaxiSorp 96-well microtiter plates (Nalge Nunc International, Rochester, NY) in triplicate (100 µL/well) and incubated for 1 h at 37°C. Plates were washed 3 times with PBS containing 0.05% Tween-20 (PBST), then coated with 100 µL primary antibody in blocking buffer and incubated for 30 minutes at 25°C. Plates were washed again, 100 µL of HRP-labeled secondary antibody in blocking buffer was added to each well, and plates were incubated for 30 min at 25°C. Plates were washed a final time, and peroxidase activity was detected using a QuantaBlu kit (Thermo Fisher, Item 15169) according to manufacturer instructions. Plates were read on a SpectraMax Gemini XS with the following parameters: 340 nm excitation, 470 nm emission, 455 nm cutoff, and PMT set to auto.

Each organism was assayed in duplicate. Signal-to-noise ratios (S : N) for each strain at each concentration were determined by dividing the raw fluorescence by the average background fluorescence. Triplicate S : N from duplicate plates from duplicate plates were averaged and standard deviations were calculated. Average S : N greater than or equal to 2.0 were considered positive.

2.5. Standard ATP Assays.

Cells were suspended in Mueller Hinton II broth (MHII) containing 0.1% Tween-80 (MHII-80) and serially diluted (1 : 10) in MHII-80. Consecutive serial dilutions were added in triplicate (100 μL/well) to Lumitrac 600 microtiter plates (BioExpress, Kaysville, UT). MHII-80 without cells was used to establish background. BacTiter-Glo reagent was added to each well (100 μL/well), contents were mixed briefly on an orbital shaker, and bioluminescent output was measured on a GloMax 96 luminometer (Promega, Madison, WI) at 5, 10, 15, 20, and, in some assays, 40 minutes. S : N for each strain at each concentration were determined by dividing the raw fluorescence by the average background fluorescence.

2.6. IMS/ATP Assays.

Initially, standard IMS/ATP assays were completed using MTB suspended in PBST80. Twenty microliters of antibody-labeled beads were added to each sample, which were then incubated with shaking for 60 minutes at 37°C. Beads were separated from the sample using a magnet, the sample was removed, and beads were washed three times with PBST then resuspended in MHII broth. MHII broth containing only labeled beads was used to establish background. Samples (100 μL per well) were added to Lumitrac 600 plates followed by 100 μL per well of BacTiter-Glo reagent. Contents of the plates were mixed briefly on an orbital shaker, incubated for 5 min at 25°C, and read at 5, 10, 15, and 20 minutes using a GloMax 96 luminometer with no delay and 1 sec integration. Sample S : N were determined by dividing the raw fluorescence by the average background fluorescence.

Subsequently, the IMS/ATP assay was evaluated using MTB suspended in synthetic urine. The procedure was the same except sample incubation time was 30–60 min at 37°C to determine the impact of incubation time on IMS/ATP results. For the final set of IMS/ATP assays in synthetic urine, sample incubation time was 30 min, and samples were blinded and number coded. For all blinded samples, four replicate wells at each concentration were averaged for each time point. Sample codes were revealed after assay completion and analysis.

2.7. Statistical Analysis.

To evaluate the effect of urine pH and incubation time, paired t-tests were performed comparing S : N at each concentration from 10^3 to 10^6 CFU/mL at each pH or for each incubation time (SigmaPlot 11, Systast Software, Inc., Chicago, IL). Differences in means were considered statistically significant for $P \leq 0.05$ (95% confidence level).

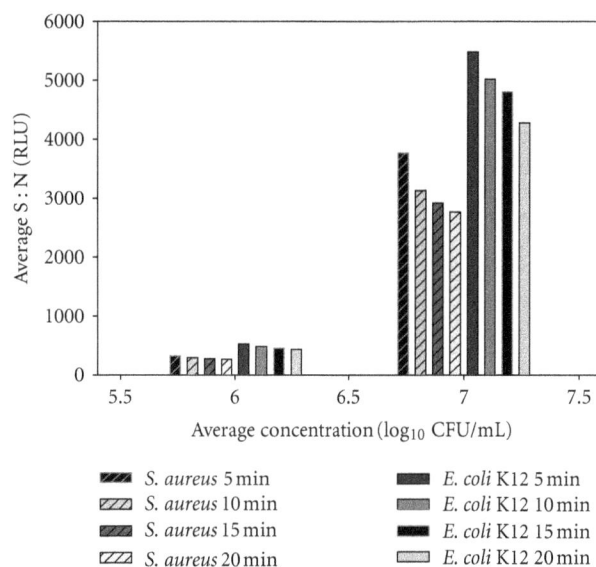

FIGURE 1: Standard ATP assay results for *S. aureus* and *E. coli* K12 at 10^6 and 10^7 CFU/mL. Organisms were suspended and serially diluted in Mueller Hinton II broth containing 0.1% Tween-80 and evaluated using the BacTiter-Glo basic ATP assay.

3. Results and Discussion

3.1. ELISA.

The detection limit of MTB by ELISA was approximately 10^5 CFU/mL. Some cross-reactivity with *M. smegmatis*, *E. coli* K12, *K. pneumoniae*, and *P. aeruginosa* was noted, but S : N for these strains ranged from 2.5 to 3.4 RLU, slightly above the positive cutoff of 2 RLU. There was increased cross-reactivity for these strains at concentrations near 10^7 CFU/mL; therefore, the assay would be utilized for screening purposes rather than confirmation due to the potential for false positives. Also, the relatively high detection limit of the assay would not positively identify low bacillary load samples. However, with the standard practice of centrifugation, filtration, and/or pooling of urine samples combined with IMS, the numbers of tubercle bacilli could be in the detectable range.

3.2. Standard ATP Assays.

Generally, Gram-positive and Gram-negative bacteria exhibited decreasing signal over time as ATP was consumed (Figure 1). In contrast, organisms with a thicker cell wall, including the mycobacteria and *Candida*, exhibited increasing signal over time due to the additional time required to break down the cell walls to release ATP (Figure 2). The increase in signal is a distinguishing feature of mycobacteria and *Candida* that could allow differentiation from other common organisms associated with bacteriuria, namely, *E. coli* and mixed Gram-positive cocci [26]. It was also routinely observed that MTB had a modest increase in signal relative to other mycobacteria. The signal at 20 min was 0.96–1.06 times higher than the signal at 5 min for MTB, whereas the signal at 20 min for *M. smegmatis*, *M. gordonae*, and *M. intracellulare* was 1.65–3.26, 1.19–1.80, and 1.20–1.55 times higher, respectively, than the signal at 5 min. The signal for *C. albicans* at 20 min was 2.8–3.2 times higher

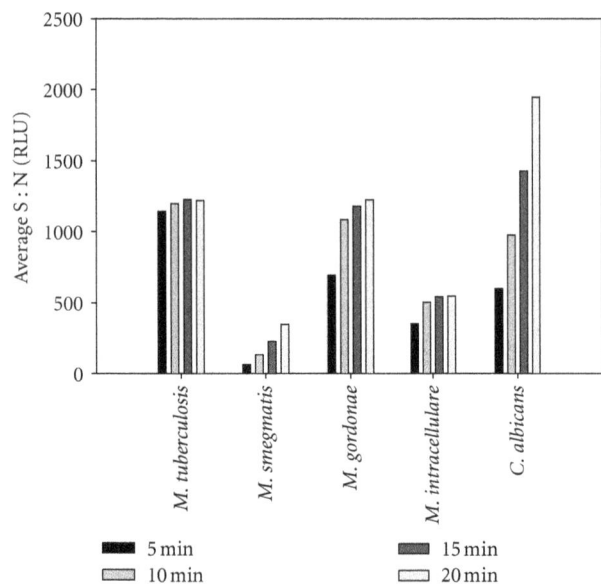

FIGURE 2: Standard ATP assay results for various mycobacteria and *Candida albicans* at approximately 10^6 CFU/ml. Organisms were suspended and serially diluted in Mueller Hinton II broth containing 0.1% Tween-80 and evaluated using the BacTiter-Glo basic ATP assay.

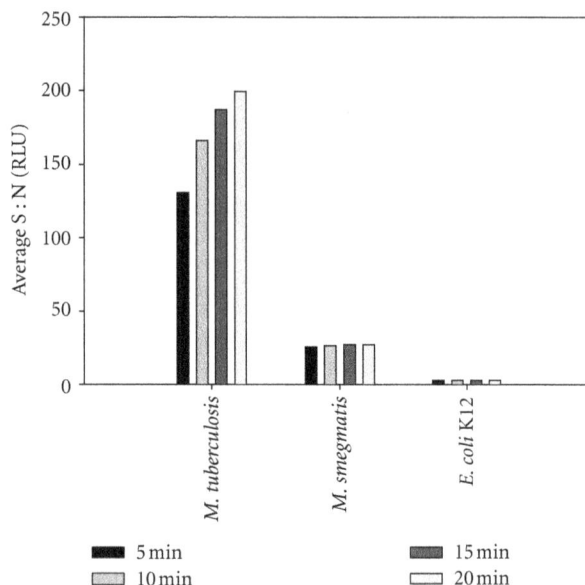

FIGURE 3: IMS/ATP assay at approximately 10^6 CFU/ml in PBS containing 0.1% Tween-80.

than the signal at 5 min. The modest increase in MTB signal could enable differentiation between MTB and other mycobacteria or *C. albicans* in a screening assay. It should be noted, however, that these results may not mirror real-world samples. *C. albicans* was grown for 18 h and used immediately, whereas the mycobacteria were grown for 2 days (*M. smegmatis*) up to 3 weeks (MTB), so the metabolic activity of the mycobacteria varied in comparison and could have been lower due to differences in growth phase.

Furthermore, only evaluating samples for a change in S : N over time would lead to misidentification of samples because of noted cross-reactivity in ELISA and similar increases in S : N for other mycobacteria and *C. albicans*. The standard ATP results for MTB revealed that, generally, at least one time point after the first time point (T1) will be greater than T1 and that the average S : N over all four time points should be greater than T1 due to the increases in S : N. Therefore, data for the blinded assays were evaluated on two factors: (1) whether the S : N at any time point after T1 was greater than T1 and (2) whether the average S : N over all four time points divided by T1 was greater than 1. For this analysis, because MTB demonstrated increasing S : N over time, factor (2) was only evaluated if there was an increase in S : N after T1; otherwise, the sample was considered negative.

3.3. IMS/ATP Assays

3.3.1. Initial Assays. IMS/ATP parameters were established through preliminary assays. Standard IMS assays in PBST80 revealed a clear affinity of the MTB antibody for MTB over nontargets using IMS (Figure 3), which is significant given the cross-reactivity observed in ELISA. Additionally, side-by-side IMS/ATP assays performed using urine at pH 5.5 ± 0.1

and 7.1 ± 0.1 revealed that there was no significant difference among S : N and that S : N were in the same log for the same concentration regardless of pH. Recoveries as determined by total viable counts were also similar (data not shown). Based on these data coupled with normal human urine normally being close to pH 7 [35], all subsequent assays were performed at pH 7.1 ± 0.1.

There was no significant difference in mean S : N for either 30 or 60 min incubation time, with mean S : N for MTB being slightly higher with 30 min incubation, while mean S : N for *E. coli* K12 were slightly higher with a 60 min incubation. Increased incubation time may increase the potential for nontarget binding while failing to improve detection of the target. Therefore, a 30 min incubation period was implemented for all subsequent assays. There were several advantages to this approach: (1) antibody-antigen binding is rapid and strong, and a 60 min incubation period may be unnecessary, (2) a short incubation period would not increase the metabolic activity or enhance ATP levels for slow-growing MTB as would be expected with an organism that has a shorter generation time, and (3) overall assay time was reduced.

3.3.2. Blinded Assays. One blinded assay including 20 samples (4 MTB and 16 nontargets) was performed to evaluate the sample analysis described in Section 3.2. All four MTB samples were identified using this analysis. In addition, a cutoff for factor (2) was identified based on the results for the nontargets. The mean for average S : N/T1 was 0.95 ± 0.2, making the upper limit for negative samples 0.97. Therefore, if samples met factor (1), they were considered positive for average S : N/T1 ≥ 0.98. Four replicate assays were completed using this analysis. The results for MTB are reported in Table 1.

TABLE 1: Summary results for detection of MTB in synthetic urine—blinded assays.

Replicate	Conc. (CFU/mL)	S:N at T1	S:N at any time point > T1	Average S:N (T1–T4)	Average S:N/T1	Send for confirmation
1	10^5	17.60	X	20.40	1.16	Yes
	10^5	12.69	X	18.45	1.45	Yes
	10^5	15.81	X	18.11	1.15	Yes
	10^4	2.14		2.07	0.97	No
	10^4	1.64	X	1.72	1.05	Yes
	10^4	2.30	X	4.09	1.78	Yes
	10^3	1.02		0.98	0.96	No
2	10^6	9.86	X	9.75	0.99	Yes
	10^6	12.99	X	12.83	0.99	Yes
	10^6	11.27	X	11.44	1.01	Yes
	10^5	4.00		3.76	0.94	No
	10^5	2.71		2.65	0.98	No
	10^5	3.61	X	3.58	0.99	Yes
	10^4	12.47	X	12.24	0.98	Yes
	10^4	15.43		15.05	0.98	No
3	10^6	4.45	X	4.60	1.03	Yes
	10^6	3.83		3.74	0.98	No
	10^6	3.72	X	3.75	1.01	Yes
	10^5	1.64	X	1.64	1.01	Yes
	10^5	1.16		1.11	0.95	No
	10^5	1.23		1.19	0.97	No
	10^4	1.11	X	1.09	0.98	Yes
	10^4	1.12		1.09	0.97	No
4	10^6	1.71	X	1.93	1.13	Yes
	10^6	8.57	X	14.65	1.71	Yes
	10^6	1.39	X	1.40	1.01	Yes
	10^6	5.62	X	7.20	1.28	Yes
	10^5	1.65	X	1.67	1.01	Yes

TABLE 2: Summary results for false positives in the blinded assays.

Organism	Replicate	Conc. (CFU/mL)	S:N at T1	S:N at any time point > T1	Average S:N (T1–T4)	Average S:N/T1	Send for confirmation
M. smegmatis	1	10^6	23.80	X	57.50	2.42	Yes
	2	10^6	4.29	X	4.52	1.05	Yes
	2	10^6	3.98	X	4.26	1.07	Yes
M. intracellulare	3	10^6	1.56	X	1.56	1.00	Yes
C. albicans	3	10^6	347.1	X	378.0	1.09	Yes
	3	10^6	264.2	X	392.4	1.49	Yes
	3	10^5	44.76	X	48.48	1.08	Yes
	4	10^5	15.81	X	28.14	1.78	Yes
	4	10^5	19.03	X	32.6	1.71	Yes
	4	10^4	1.75	X	2.92	1.67	Yes
K. pneumoniae	3	10^6	1.09	X	1.05	0.96	No
E. faecalis	3	10^6	7.95	X	7.73	0.97	No
	4	10^6	13.54	X	12.87	0.95	No

TABLE 3: Mean S : N for detection of *M. tuberculosis* by IMS/ATP. Data is averaged from the four replicates reported.

Mean concentration (CFU/mL)		$2.82E + 06$	$2.82E + 05$	$2.82E + 04$
Mean S : N	5 min	8.74	2.16	1.16
	10 min	10.01	2.25	1.15
	15 min	11.26	2.39	1.13
	20 min	12.46	2.43	1.11

Overall, 19 of 28 MTB samples were flagged for confirmation, resulting in a sensitivity of 67.9%. This is much higher than the approximately 20% sensitivity typical of sputum smear microscopy in HIV-positive patients with suspected TB [26] and is on a par with alternative diagnostic tests like the LAM ELISA, which has a reported sensitivity of 67–85% in HIV-positive patients [5]. All 19 flagged samples exhibited an increase in S : N for at least one time point after T1, and all yielded an average S : N/T1 of 0.98 or greater. None of the samples considered negative exhibited an increase in S : N for any time point after T1, and this result was not restricted by concentration. One of one sample at 10^3 CFU/mL, three of seven at 10^4, four of ten at 10^5, and one of ten at 10^6 were negative by this analysis. The variability in results could have been impacted by several factors, including the age of the cultures, whose metabolic activity may have been significantly lower than what would be observed for bacteria isolated from an active infection, as well as the use of spiked, synthetic urine. It would be important to evaluate this method using actual clinical samples to determine whether these factors have, in fact, influenced the results.

The specificity of the assay was 82.1%, with 10 false-positives out of 56 total samples (Table 2). All of the false-positives met both factors of the analysis—they exhibited an increase in S : N at any time point after T1, and they yielded an (average S : N/T1) > 1.0 in all instances. Two organisms—*K. pneumoniae* and *E. faecalis*—satisfied factor (1) in three instances, but none satisfied factor (2), and thus were considered negative. As for *M. smegmatis*, the false positive was not surprising given the cross-reactivity noted at 10^6 CFU/mL in ELISA. However, *M. smegmatis* is rarely found in urine and not at the concentrations evaluated [36, 37]. Therefore, *M. smegmatis* was not evaluated in replicates 3 and 4.

Two observations can be made for *C. albicans*. First, standard ATP assays revealed that *C. albicans* generally yields higher overall signals and greater increases relative to MTB. This is evident from the S : N at T1 (Table 2), as well as the results for average S : N/T1 relative to MTB. The mean average S : N/T1 for *C. albicans* was 1.47 versus 1.14 for positive MTB samples. Second, *C. albicans* is not as commonly isolated from urine specimens as other organisms, so it is less likely to pose a problem with real-world samples. Yeasts comprised only 4 of 178 samples (0.02%) in one study of microorganisms isolated from 400 urine specimens [26].

Finally, the only other organism to result in a false-positive was *M. intracellulare*. This result is significant since

M. intracellulare is part of the *M. avium* complex known to be an opportunistic pathogen of immunocompromised patients [38]. While only one of seven *M. intracellulare* samples and none of five *M. avium* samples resulted in a false-positive, it would be important to evaluate these organisms further in future assays.

The mean S : N across replicates for a given concentration were consistent, with S : N at 10^4 and 10^5 CFU/mL in the same log (Table 3). An increase in S : N over time was observed for the two highest concentrations but not for the samples at 10^4 CFU/mL, which may explain the inconsistent detection of this concentration in individual assays.

The described IMS/ATP assay could have utility as a screening assay in reference or peripheral laboratories where HIV/TB co-infection rates are high. The assay is rapid, takes less than 1 h to complete, and requires minimal reagents and equipment. Even with potential cross-reactivity, the assay has merit, because the objective is to screen, rather than confirm. This novel assay is potentially useful as a diagnostic, screening assay for the detection of MTB in HIV-positive patients.

Acknowledgments

This research was supported by the U.S. Army Research, Development and Engineering Command. The authors would like to thank Kelly Leach for assistance with sample preparation, Stephaney Leskinen for editing, and Azliyati Azizan for guidance during this project.

References

[1] J. B. Eastwood, C. M. Corbishley, and J. M. Grange, "Tuberculosis and the kidney," *Journal of the American Society of Nephrology*, vol. 12, no. 6, pp. 1307–1314, 2001.

[2] World Health Organization, *Global Tuberculosis Control: Fact Sheet*, World Health Organization, Geneva, Switzerland, 2010.

[3] M. D. Perkins and J. Cunningham, "Facing the crisis: improving the diagnosis of tuberculosis in the HIV era," *Journal of Infectious Diseases*, vol. 196, supplement 1, pp. S15–S27, 2007.

[4] J. Peter, C. Green, M. Hoelscher, P. Mwaba, A. Zumla, and K. Dheda, "Urine for the diagnosis of tuberculosis: current approaches, clinical applicability, and new developments," *Current Opinion in Pulmonary Medicine*, vol. 16, no. 3, pp. 262–270, 2010.

[5] M. Shah, N. A. Martinson, R. E. Chaisson, D. J. Martin, E. Variava, and S. E. Dorman, "Quantitative analysis of a urine-based assay for detection of lipoarabinomannan in patients with tuberculosis," *Journal of Clinical Microbiology*, vol. 48, no. 8, pp. 2972–2974, 2010.

[6] G. Torrea, P. van de Perre, M. Ouedraogo et al., "PCR-based detection of the *Mycobacterium tuberculosis* complex in urine of HIV-infected and uninfected pulmonary and extra-pulmonary tuberculosis patients in Burkina Faso," *Journal of Medical Microbiology*, vol. 54, no. 1, pp. 39–44, 2005.

[7] H. Getahun, M. Harrington, R. O'Brien, and P. Nunn, "Diagnosis of smear-negative pulmonary tuberculosis in people with HIV infection or AIDS in resource-constrained settings: informing urgent policy changes," *The Lancet*, vol. 369, no. 9578, pp. 2042–2049, 2007.

[8] M. P. Golden and H. R. Vikram, "Extrapulmonary tuberculosis: An overview," *American Family Physician*, vol. 72, no. 9, pp. 1761–1768, 2005.

[9] K. Gopinath and S. Singh, "Urine as an adjunct specimen for the diagnosis of active pulmonary tuberculosis," *International Journal of Infectious Diseases*, vol. 13, no. 3, pp. 374–379, 2009.

[10] D. V. Havlir and P. F. Barnes, "Tuberculosis in patients with human immunodeficiency virus infection," *The New England Journal of Medicine*, vol. 340, no. 5, p. 367, 1999.

[11] E. Mortier, J. Pouchot, L. Girard, Y. Boussougant, and P. Vinceneux, "Assessment of urine analysis for the diagnosis of tuberculosis," *British Medical Journal*, vol. 312, no. 7022, pp. 27–28, 1996.

[12] A. Aceti, S. Zanetti, M. S. Mura et al., "Identification of HIV patients with active pulmonary tuberculosis using urine based polymerase chain reaction assay," *Thorax*, vol. 54, no. 2, pp. 145–146, 1999.

[13] C. C. Boehme, P. Nabeta, D. Hillemann et al., "Rapid molecular detection of tuberculosis and rifampin resistance," *The New England Journal of Medicine*, vol. 363, no. 11, pp. 1005–1015, 2010.

[14] V. Choudhry and R. Saxena, "Detection of *Mycobacterium tuberculosis* antigens in urinary proteins of tuberculosis patients," *European Journal of Clinical Microbiology and Infectious Diseases*, vol. 21, no. 1, pp. 1–5, 2002.

[15] S. K. Chadha and R. P. Sahi, "Urinary tract involvement in pulmonary tuberculosis," *Indian Journal of Tuberculosis*, vol. 18, no. 2, pp. 54–57, 1971.

[16] V. K. Challu, B. Mahadev, R. Rajalakshmi, and K. Chaudhuri, "Recovery of tubercle bacilli from urine of pulmonary tuberculosis patients and its comparison with the corresponding sputum isolates," *Indian Journal of Tuberculosis*, vol. 36, no. 2, pp. 107–111, 1989.

[17] N. Selvakumar, A. M. Reetha, S. P. Vanajakumar et al., "Mycobacteriuria in pulmonary tuberculosis patients in Madras, South India," *Indian Journal of Tuberculosis*, vol. 40, pp. 43–45, 1993.

[18] J. Syed, "Tuberculosis diagnostic pipeline," TAG 2010 Pipeline Report, HIV i-Base HIV Treatment Bulletin, 2010, http://i-base.info/htb/13614.

[19] Stop TB Partnership, "TB diagnostics pipeline," 2007, TB Diagnostics Working Group, http://www.stoptb.org/.

[20] World Health Organization, "TB diagnostics and laboratory strengthening," 2011, http://www.who.int/tb/laboratory/en/.

[21] E. Liandris, M. Gazouli, M. Andreadou, L. A. Sechi, V. Rosu, and J. Ikonomopolous, "Detection of pathogenic mycobacteria based on functionalized quantum dots coupled with immunomagnetic separation," *PLoS One*, vol. 6, no. 5, Article ID e20026, 2011.

[22] G. H. Mazurek, V. Reddy, D. Murphy, and T. Ansari, "Detection of *Mycobacterium tuberculosis* in cerebrospinal fluid following immunomagnetic enrichment," *Journal of Clinical Microbiology*, vol. 34, no. 2, pp. 450–453, 1996.

[23] A. N. Sharpe, "Separation and concentration of samples," in *Detecting Pathogens in Food*, T. A. McMeekin, Ed., pp. 52–68, CRC Press, Boca Raton, Fla, USA, 2003.

[24] K. A. Stevens and L. A. Jaykus, "Bacterial separation and concentration from complex sample matrices: a review," *Critical Reviews in Microbiology*, vol. 30, no. 1, pp. 7–24, 2004.

[25] R. B. Schifman, M. Wieden, J. Brooker et al., "Bacteriuria screening by direct bioluminescence assay of ATP," *Antimicrobial Agents and Chemotherapy*, vol. 20, no. 4, pp. 644–648, 1984.

[26] W. D. Welch, L. Thompson, M. Layman, and P. M. Southern Jr., "Evaluation of two bioluminescence-measuring instruments, the turner design and lumac systems, for the rapid screening of urine specimens," *Journal of Clinical Microbiology*, vol. 20, no. 6, pp. 1165–1170, 1984.

[27] D. S. Askgaard, A. Gottschau, K. Knudsen, and J. Bennedsen, "Firefly luciferase assay of adenosine triphosphate as a tool of quantitation of the viability of BCG vaccines," *Biologicals*, vol. 23, no. 1, pp. 55–60, 1995.

[28] L. E. Nilsson, S. E. Hoffner, and S. Ansehn, "Rapid susceptibility testing of *Mycobacterium tuberculosis* by bioluminescence assay of mycobacterial ATP," *Antimicrobial Agents and Chemotherapy*, vol. 32, no. 8, pp. 1208–1212, 1988.

[29] R. N. Bushon, A. M. Brady, C. A. Likirdopulos, and J. V. Cireddu, "Rapid detection of *Escherichia coli* and enterococci in recreational water using an immunomagnetic separation/adenosine triphosphate technique," *Journal of Applied Microbiology*, vol. 106, no. 2, pp. 432–441, 2009.

[30] D. M. Hunter, S. D. Leskinen, S. Magaña, S. M. Schlemmer, and D. V. Lim, "Dead-end ultrafiltration concentration and IMS/ATP-bioluminescence detection of *Escherichia coli* O157:H7 in recreational water and produce wash," *Journal of Microbiological Methods*, vol. 87, no. 3, pp. 338–342, 2011.

[31] J. Lee and R. A. Deininger, "Detection of *E. coli* in beach water within 1 hour using immunomagnetic separation and ATP bioluminescence," *Luminescence*, vol. 19, no. 1, pp. 31–36, 2004.

[32] A. Dalhoff, W. Stubbings, and S. Schubert, "Comparative *in vitro* activities of the novel antibacterial finafloxacin against selected Gram-positive and Gram-negative bacteria tested in Mueller-Hinton broth and synthetic urine," *Antimicrobial Agents and Chemotherapy*, vol. 55, no. 4, pp. 1814–1818, 2011.

[33] L. L. Swaim, R. C. Johnson, Y. Zhou, C. Sandlin, and J. R. Barr, "Quantification of organophosphorus nerve agent metabolites using a reduced-volume, high-throughput sample processing format and liquid chromatography-tandem mass spectrometry," *Journal of Analytical Toxicology*, vol. 32, no. 9, pp. 774–777, 2008.

[34] P. Uppuluri, H. Dinakaran, D. P. Thomas, A. K. Chaturvedi, and J. L. Lopez-Ribot, "Characteristics of *Candida albicans* biofilms grown in a synthetic urine medium," *Journal of Clinical Microbiology*, vol. 47, no. 12, pp. 4078–4083, 2009.

[35] MedlinePlus, 2011, Urine pH. *MedlinePlus*, a service of the U.S. National Library of Medicine through the National Institutes of Health, http://www.nlm.nih.gov/medlineplus/ency/article/003583.htm.

[36] V. M. Bapat, A. M. Bal, R. S. Bhuta, and D. R. Salvi, "Mycobacteriuria—whether a forerunner of manifest tuberculosis?" *Journal of Association of Physicians of India*, vol. 54, pp. 588–590, 2006.

[37] C. H. Collins, J. M. Grange, and M. D. Yates, *Organization and Practice in Tuberculosis Bacteriology*, Butterworths, London, UK, 1985.

[38] C. B. Inderlied, C. A. Kemper, and L. E. M. Bermudez, "The *Mycobacterium avium* complex," *Clinical Microbiology Reviews*, vol. 6, no. 3, pp. 266–310, 1993.

14

Prevalence of Tuberculosis, Drug Susceptibility Testing, and Genotyping of Mycobacterial Isolates from Pulmonary Tuberculosis Patients in Dessie, Ethiopia

Minwuyelet Maru,[1] **Solomon H. Mariam,**[1,2] **Tekle Airgecho,**[1]
Endalamaw Gadissa,[1] **and Abraham Aseffa**[1]

[1]*Armauer Hansen Research Institute, P.O. Box 1005, Jimma Road, Addis Ababa, Ethiopia*
[2]*Aklilu Lemma Institute of Pathobiology, Addis Ababa University, P.O. Box 1176, Addis Ababa, Ethiopia*

Correspondence should be addressed to Solomon H. Mariam; solomon.habtemariam@aau.edu.et

Academic Editor: Vincent Jarlier

Due to their initially seemingly high cost, timely diagnosis and effective treatment of tuberculosis (TB) are usually hampered by lack or shortage of resources in many high TB burden countries. However, the benefits of effective treatment can eventually outweigh those of empirical treatment. Here, a cross-sectional study was conducted on samples from smear-positive new and retreatment TB patients. Data on sociodemographic and HIV status were collected. Samples were cultured for identification, conventional drug sensitivity testing, and molecular typing by deletion typing and spoligotyping. The results showed the youth were disproportionately affected. New cases were being treated following general treatment guidelines only. Monoresistance or multiple drug resistance was found in 16.5% of new patients. Spoligotyping showed that there were 44 patterns with families H3 and T1 (lineage 4) and CAS-Delhi (lineage 3) being dominant. Some rare patterns from lineage 7 were also found. Spoligotype pattern, HIV positivity, and previous treatment were not associated with drug resistance. That the vast majority of the patients were new cases and young and the large number of these patients with mono- or multiple drug resistance indicate that most TB cases are due to recent transmissions and that urgent actions are needed to curb the transmissions.

1. Introduction

The latest World Health Organization (WHO) reports show that there were 9.0 million new tuberculosis (TB) cases and 1.5 million tuberculosis (TB) deaths, leaving TB as the second leading cause of death from an infectious disease worldwide, after the human immunodeficiency virus (HIV) [1]. Coinfection with the HIV fuels the global TB crisis, and successful TB treatment is further complicated and hampered by the existence of multidrug-resistant (MDR) TB and extensively drug-resistant (XDR) TB (MDR TB plus additional resistance to a fluoroquinolone and an injectable second-line drug). Nearly half a million cases of MDR TB emerge every year worldwide, of which ~50,000 are also XDR TB [2]. The WHO report states that "progress towards targets for diagnosis and treatment of MDR TB is far off-track," with less than 25% of MDR TB cases detected in most MDR TB-burdened countries [3]. The estimated TB cases and TB deaths in children were 6% and 8% of the global totals, respectively, in 2012 [3].

Globally, drug susceptible TB is reported to be decreasing, but MDR and XDR TB are on the rise mainly due to the excessively large number of MDR TB cases being left undiagnosed, untreated, or inappropriately treated each year [4–6]. Thus, the WHO declared MDR TB a public health crisis in 2012. This indicates selection of the more severe forms of TB at a global scale and subsequent transmissions generating primary MDR. An increase in MDR and XDR TB and increase in childhood TB (i.e., recent transmissions) are strong indicators that there is schism in the TB control programs.

Inappropriate drug regimen, patient defaulting, previous antituberculosis treatment, delays in diagnosis and initiation of effective treatment, and primary infection with MDR TB strains are among the risk factors leading to MDR/XDR TB [7]. The global burden of MDR TB cases between 1994 and 2009 ranged from 0 to 28% in new cases and from 0 to 61% in previously treated cases [8, 9]. Since the TB *Bacillus* is not delimited by geographic boundaries and people have become increasingly more mobile, TB strains, including those that harbor drug resistance, spread globally. During the last couple of decades, epidemiological studies of TB globally have been facilitated following the introduction of several genotyping methods, with applications including distinction whether recurrent TB is due to reactivation, exogenous reinfection or mixed infection, classification of clinical isolates into phylogenetic lineages and strain levels, determination of the population structures, development of drugs and vaccines, and whencombined with drug susceptibility testing (DST) and epidemiologic data, transmission of MDR and XDR strains [10, 11].

According to the WHO report, Ethiopia had an estimated incidence of 223, prevalence of 212, and TB deaths of 32 per 100,000 [1]. Ethiopia had one of the lowest estimated rates of MDR TB in both new and retreatment cases (1.6% and 12%, resp.) among 27 high-burden countries. This report also showed that only 1% of new bacteriologically confirmed TB cases and only 4.4% of retreatment cases had DST coverage.

Prevalence of TB as well as levels of drug resistance and treatment success reported from other areas of Ethiopia varied greatly as shown by some recent reports [12–15]. The objectives of this study were (i) to study the prevalence of TB in the study area (Dessie, Ethiopia), (ii) to characterize the species of mycobacteria causing pulmonary TB among new and retreatment cases, (iii) to determine the drug susceptibility patterns of the mycobacterial isolates, (iv) to type the mycobacterial isolates molecularly, and (v) to assess the efficacy of treatment. These objectives emanated from the lack of information regarding the TB situation in the study area.

2. Materials and Methods

2.1. The Study Site and Duration of the Study. This study was conducted in Dessie, northeast Ethiopia, on samples obtained from pulmonary TB (PTB) patients at one government and two private hospitals and three health centers. These patients were obtained while they were seeking health care at their own times. There were no culture and DST capabilities but facilities for microscopic examination of acid-fast Bacilli and radiological examination were available. Sputum samples were collected from PTB patients from October 1, 2012, to September 30, 2013.

2.2. Study Design. A cross-sectional study was conducted on samples from smear-positive newly diagnosed and retreatment PTB patients, age ≥10 years. Surveys focusing on sociodemographic data were done using prestructured questionnaire.

Morning sputum samples were collected using universal sputum collection tubes and immediately stored at −20°C following WHO guidelines [16] until they were transported to the laboratory at the Armauer Hansen Research Institute (AHRI). Then, sputum samples were first decontaminated and concentrated following Petroff's method [17]. Each specimen was inoculated into two Lowenstein-Jensen slants, one containing 0.6% glycerol and the other 0.6% sodium pyruvate.

2.3. Drug Susceptibility Testing. DST was performed for isoniazid (INH), rifampicin (RMP), ethambutol (EMB), and streptomycin (STR) (Sigma, St. Louis, USA) using modified proportion Middlebrook 7H10 agar method [18]. Briefly, twenty-four well plates were used for the DST. Each well contained 2.5 mL complete medium supplemented with 10% OADC and 0.5% glycerol. Drugs were added at the following concentrations: INH 0.064, 0.125, 0.2, and 1.0 μg/mL; RMP at 1.0 μg/mL; EMB at 4.0, 5.0, and 8.0 μg/mL; and STR at 2.0 μg/mL. Mycobacterial suspensions for inoculation into wells were prepared by taking representative sample of 5–10 mg from primary culture with a sterile loop (diameter 0.7 mm and internal diameter of 3 mm) (Becton Dickinson, France) which delivers 0.01 mL. Then, it was placed in a spherical, flat-bottomed tube containing glass beads and drops of distilled water added slowly with continuous shaking to adjust the turbidity of the bacterial suspension to that of a McFarland standard 1. Two drug-free wells, one containing a 1 : 100 dilution of the bacterial suspension and another containing undiluted bacterial suspension, were included as controls. Inoculated plates were incubated within a 37°C incubator. Plates were read at 21–28 days. The MIC breakpoints were 0.2 μg/mL, 1 μg/mL, 5 μg/mL, and 2 μg/mL for INH, RMP, EMB, and STR, respectively.

2.4. DNA Extraction and Molecular Typing. To obtain DNA for typing, two loops of colonies from LJ slants were resuspended in 50 μL distilled water and heat-killed at 80°C for one hour. The fluid portion excluding debris was transferred to a new tube.

To differentiate *M. tuberculosis* from other species of mycobacteria, PCR targeting region of difference 9 (RD9) was conducted [19]. Spoligotyping [20] was performed to determine the presence or absence of the 43 spacers. SPOTCLUST [21] was used to generate octal codes. SITVITWEB [10] was utilized to assign SITs (spoligotype international types) and families for the isolates.

Data were analyzed by SPSS software version 20 (IBM, USA). The presence or absence of association between drug resistance and spoligotype, HIV status, and treatments history was assessed. A *P* value less than 0.05 was considered statistically significant.

2.5. Quality Control. M. tuberculosis H37Rv (ATCC 27294) and *M. bovis* (AF 61/2122/97) were included for quality control in DST, RD9 deletion typing, and spoligotyping. Laboratory procedures were done following standard operational procedures.

3. Results

3.1. Sociodemographic and Clinical Data. A total of 144 smear-positive PTB patients ≥ 10 years of age, consisting of 128 (88.9%) new cases and 16 (11.1%) retreatment cases, were enrolled in this study. The mean length of stay before seeking health care was 6.49 ± 6.1 weeks (range 2–48 weeks). Sixty-four (44.4%) were females and 80 (55.6%) were males (see Table S1, in Supplementary Material available online at http://dx.doi.org/10.1155/2015/215015). The median age of the patients was 27.5 years (range 10–78 years). Twenty-five (17.4%) of all patients were HIV-positive (consisting of 20 new cases (7 males and 13 females) and 5 retreatment cases (3 males and 2 females)) (Table S1, Supplementary Material). Of these, 17/25 (68%) were urban dwellers with 7/17 (41.2%) being males and 10/17 (58.8%) being females. The rest (8/25, 32%) were rural dwellers with 3/8 (37.5%) and 5/8 (62.5%) being males and females, respectively. With the caveat that the sample size is small, we deduce that, overall, HIV positivity was higher in both urban and rural dweller females (15/64, 23.4%) than in males (10/80, 12.5%).

When stratified by age group, a staggering > 67.4% (97/144) were between 10 and 30 years of age, with 31/97 (32%) and 66/97 (68%) being in the age groups 10–20 and 21–30, respectively. Four patients in each of these two age groups were retreatment cases while 89/97 (91.7%) were new cases. Fifty-three (54.6%) of the 97 patients were males while 44 (45.4%) were females. Overall, the TB patients were split 50 : 50 between urban and rural residency. However, in the age groups 10–20 and ≥41 years, the rural PTB patients outnumbered the urban PTB patients by 2 : 1 (data not shown).

Among the 144 patients, there were 32 (22.2%) who were 31–40 years of age (with 24 new cases and 8 retreatment cases). Of these, 18 were males (12 rural and 6 urban residents) and 14 were females (7 rural and 7 urban residents). The rest (15, 10.4%) were 41–78 years old and all were new cases, with 11 (73%) of them being rural residents.

Of the 144 patient samples, 26 samples (from 25 new cases and 1 retreatment case) failed to grow in culture and DST and spoligotyping were performed on 118 (103 new cases and 15 retreatment cases) samples.

3.2. Drug Resistance. Of 103 new cases, 86 were susceptible to the four drugs and 17 showed resistance to one or more drugs. Of 15 retreatment cases, 11 were susceptible to all four drugs and 4 were resistant to one or more drugs, including 2 MDR cases. Overall, 21 patients from both cases showed various patterns of drug resistance (Table 1). RMP monoresistance was observed in neither HIV-positive nor HIV-negative TB patients.

In the age group ≤ 30 years, 4 patients had INH monoresistant TB, 2 each had STR or EMB monoresistant TB, and 3 had TB resistant to both INH and STR, all in new cases (Table S2, Supplementary Material). There were 8 patients that were retreatment cases in that age group; however, they did not exhibit resistance to any drug (Table S3, Supplementary Material).

Among the 24 new cases aged 31–40 years, 1 was resistant to INH alone, 1 was resistant to STR alone, and 4 were

TABLE 1: Number of drug susceptible or resistant isolates in new and retreatment TB patients.

Drug(s)	New cases		Retreatment cases	
	Susceptible	Resistant	Susceptible	Resistant
INH	91	5 (0 : 5)*	11	1
RMP	103	0	13	0
STM	93	3 (0 : 3)*	14	0
EMB	101	2 (0 : 2)*	14	0
INH + RMP	91	0	11	1
INH + STM	88	7 (1 : 6)*	11	0
INH + EMB	89	0	11	1
INH + RMP + STM	88	0	11	1
INH + RMP + EMB	89	0	11	0
INH + RMP + STM + EMB	86	0	11	0

*Ratio of HIV+ to HIV− patients that exhibited the drug resistance. All resistant retreatment cases except the INH-EMB resistant were HIV−.

resistant to both INH and STR (Table S2, Supplementary Material), while DST could not be performed for 3 other new cases because of culture negativity. The other 15 new cases aged 31–40 years were all sensitive to the four tested drugs. Among the 8 retreatment cases in that age group, 3 were fully sensitive to all four drugs, 1 was resistant to INH alone, 1 was resistant to both INH and EMB, and 2 were MDR cases, while 1 was culture negative (Table S3, Supplementary Material). No drug resistance was observed in the 12 of 15 patients (with positive cultures) above 40 years of age (all of them new cases) (Table S2, Supplementary Material).

Cultures were negative for 8 (7 new cases and 1 retreatment case) of the 25 HIV-positive patients. In the remaining 17 HIV-positive patients, drug resistance was observed in only 2, indicating there was no association between HIV positivity and drug resistance. The larger HIV-negative subgroup, on the contrary, consisted of most (19/21) patients with resistance to one or more drugs (including 2 retreatment MDR TB cases). Likewise, no association was observed between any resistance to first-line drugs and previous treatment. Most resistance was seen against INH, either alone or in combination (Table 1); however, there was no association of any resistance to INH with gender, HIV status, TB case, or age (Table 2). Though the sample size is small, MDR TB appeared to be strongly associated with previous history of treatment (P < 0.01) and lineage 3 *M. tuberculosis* (Table S3, Supplementary Material, and Table 3). Of all patients that were resistant to one or more drugs (21 in total), 17 (81%) were in new cases. Seventeen of 21 (81%) cases resistant to one or more drugs were new cases, but none of them exhibited MDR TB.

3.3. Molecular Typing. RD9 deletion typing indicated that all of the 118 isolates were *M. tuberculosis* (data not shown).

The spoligotype patterns of patient isolates with their octal designations, spoligotype international types (SITs), lineages, and family are shown in Table 4. There were a total

TABLE 2: The risk of any resistance to INH by gender, HIV status, previous anti-TB treatment, and age group assessed using the Chi square test.

Variable	Any resistance to INH		OR (95% CI)	P value
	Susceptible (%)	Resistant (%)		
Sex			0.67 (0.22–1.94)	0.47
Male	54 (84.4)	10 (15.6)		
Female	48 (88.8)	6 (11.2)		
HIV status			0.82 (0.17–4.02)	0.81
Positive	15 (88.2)	2 (11.8)		
Negative	87 (86.1)	14 (13.9)		
Previous history of anti-TB treatment			0.36 (0.10–1.32)	0.11
Yes	11 (73.3)	4 (26.7)		
No	91 (88.3)	12 (11.7)		
Age				0.58
10–15	4 (100)	0 (0)		
16–30	67 (90.5)	7 (9.4)		
31–45	22 (70.9)	9 (29.0)		
>45	9 (100)	0 (0)		
Total	97 (82.2)	21 (17.8)		

TABLE 3: Association of INH resistance or multidrug resistance with lineages.

	Lineage 3	Lineage 4	Lineage 7	P value
INH				0.96
Susceptible	28	66	6	
Resistant	5	10	1	
Total	33	76	7	
MDR				0.07
Yes	2	0	0	
No	31	76	7	
Total	33	76	7	

of 44 different patterns. Families H3 (with 18.2%), T1 (with 15.9%), and CAS-Delhi (with 13.6%) represented the majority with clustered isolates in this study. SIT 25 (lineage 3) and SIT 53 (lineage 4) accounted for the largest number of isolates with 17.8% and 16.95%, respectively. The patterns obtained showed that lineage 4 was the most dominant with 78 isolates in 30 diverse patterns, followed by lineage 3 with 33 isolates in 11 diverse patterns and lineage 7 with 7 isolates in 3 diverse patterns. SIT 53 (with 20 clustered isolates), SIT 25 (with 21 clustered isolates), and SIT 343 (with 5 clustered isolates) were the most frequent in lineages 4, 3, and 7, respectively.

There were 14 isolates belonging to the T superfamily (7T1, 4T3, 2T, and 1T3-ETH). CAS1-Delhi and CAS-Kili were represented by 6 isolates and 1 isolate, respectively. The H3 clade had 6 isolates. LAM9 and LAM10 were represented by 3 isolates and 1 isolate, respectively, and Manu2 and X1 clades were represented by 1 isolate each. Ten unknown or orphan patterns not found in SITVITWEB were found in this work. All except one were represented by 1 isolate and could be called orphans according to the SITVIT designation [10].

Some patterns within lineage 7 rarely represented in the database are also reported in this study.

4. Discussion

This study was conducted to assess the molecular diversity and drug susceptibility pattern of mycobacterial isolates as well as prevalence of TB in a sample of patients in Dessie, Ethiopia. Sociodemographic characteristics, HIV status, and previous TB treatment were compared to type of strains and drug susceptibility patterns. Several issues of outstanding clinical relevance that either corroborate previous findings from Ethiopia or pinpoint major gap of knowledge that require further studies are associated with this study.

A high percentage (17/103 (16.5%)) of new cases harbored resistance to one or more of the tested drugs (most of which were only little short of being MDR). Since these cases are not generally suspects for MDR or any resistance because they are new cases [1, 22], they remain undiagnosed and are treated empirically with the standard first-line drugs without any prior DST (assuming the capacity for DST is in place). Thus, treatment efficacy is destined to be ineffective because of the undetected resistance to those one or more drugs, as also shown by other studies (e.g., [23, 24]). Such empirical treatments of patients with undetected resistance with single or mixed infections may lead to more severe forms of drug resistance, including MDR TB [25, 26]. Studies show that MDR TB can evolve into XDR TB over time and during treatment (and from XDR to pan-resistant) [27–30]. Furthermore, there is a high risk of transmission of this primary resistance to new individuals. It is also likely we could have found more resistance in the 25 other new case samples, were they not culture negative.

In addition, most of the active cases of tuberculosis were found to be children and young adults. This is a serious concern for future TB control. Tuberculosis affecting people

TABLE 4: Spoligotype pattern of *M. tuberculosis* isolates from pulmonary tuberculosis patients of Dessie and its surroundings, Ethiopia.

Number	Spoligotype pattern	Octal code	SIT	Family	Frequency (%)	Linage
0		7777747776071	451 (H37Rv)			4
1		7777777776071	53	T1	20 (25.6)	4
2		7770003776071	149	T3-ETH	10 (12.8)	4
3		7777777760731	52	T2	7 (8.9)	4
4		7773737760771	37	T3	6 (7.69)	4
5		7777777520771	121	H3	3 (3.8)	4
6		7777777720771	50	H3	3	4
7		7777743760771	61	LAM10	3	4
8		7777567776071	302	X1	2 (2.56)	4
9		7377377720771	871	H3	2	4
10		7377373720771	Unknown	H3	2	4
11		6177777760771	751	T1	1 (1.28)	4
12		0077777760771	Orphan	T	1	4
13		3777377660760	**1889**	**T1**	**1**	**4**
14		7177777760771	Orphan	T1	1	4
15		7773777760671	358	T1	1	4
16		7767373760771	565	T3	1	4
17		7767373760771	Orphan	T1	1	4
18		7777607760771	42	LAM9	1	4
19		7777607760761	**1074**	**LAM9**	**1**	**4**
20		7777407760771	**1800**	**LAM9**	**1**	**4**
21		7777377760731	1077	Ambiguous: T4	1	4
22		7777577760731	584	T2	1	4
23		7667767760771	Orphan	T1	1	4
24		7777777720671	168	H3	1	4
25		7777777720471	**747**	**H3**	**1**	**4**
26		6775677420731	Orphan	H3	1	4
27		7777777420771	777	H3	1	4

TABLE 4: Continued.

Number	Spoligotype pattern	Octal code	SIT	Family	Frequency (%)	Linage
28		777777777760711	78	T	1	4
29		757000377760771	Orphan	T3	1	4
30		177000377760771	Orphan	T3	1	4
31		703777740003171	25	CAS1-Delhi	21 (63.6)	3
32		703777740000000000	1264	CAS1-Delhi	3 (9.09)	3
33		703777740002171	1787	CAS1-Delhi	1 (3.03)	3
34		703777740003571	289	CAS1-Delhi	1	3
35		703777740000771	357	CAS1-Delhi	1	3
36		703777740003771	26	CAS1-Delhi	1	3
37		703377400001771	21	CAS1-Kili	1	3
38		777777470000000000	Orphan		1	3
39		777737770000771	2306		**1**	**3**
40		703777747177771	Orphan		1	3
41		777777777763771	54	Manu2	1	3
42		700000007175771	343		5 (71.4)	7
43		700000007177771	910		1 (14.28)	7
44		700000004177771	1729		1	7
Total					118	

of all ages is a concern, but it is even more so when the vast majority of the patients are new cases, children, and the youth (especially in a country with a population age structure that is pyramidal). Children are more prone to exposure, infection, and progression to disease than are adults. The success of control of all forms of TB will be jeopardized unless TB in children is controlled, since they will serve as future reservoirs from which further amplification will occur [31]. A recent study from northwest Ethiopia showed that 82% of PTB patients were both new cases and below 40 years of age and 4.2% of these cases were MDR [32]. A recent report from a nationwide study also indicated that 55% of TB cases in a majority of newly diagnosed cases were in the young age groups (15–34 years) [33]. These findings are indicative of the overall prevalence of TB in the general population that is disproportionately affecting the young population that are due to ongoing or recent transmissions of TB rather than reactivation of latent infections. Recent transmissions contribute to the majority of TB cases in both low and high incidence countries [34, 35] and, in high incidence countries, most such transmissions are believed to occur outside of households [35, 36]. Thus, some transmissions or epidemiological links can be difficult to trace.

Moreover, the findings of high rates of retreatment cases that are drug susceptible as well as of new cases that are drug-resistant (as described above) are serious concerns that raise questions on the efficacy of treatment and TB transmission control strategies, respectively. In the 11 retreatment cases that were susceptible to all 4 drugs (4 of them HIV-positive and most of them of young age), neither mixed infection with both susceptible and resistant strains in the first episodes nor the presence of clonal populations (that are invariably susceptible to the drugs) serves as explanations for the occurrence of the second episodes. Subtherapeutic drug levels are known to cause treatment failure even with treatment adherence, but the ensuing drug resistance that usually follows [37–39] was not seen in these patients, at least until this study. Reinfection with drug susceptible strains appears to be the most likely explanation. Since we did not have serially collected samples from these patients, we were unable to genotype the isolates from both episodes, although this analysis may not always delineate reinfection from relapse [40]. Drug susceptible TB in retreatment TB patients has been reported from Ethiopia before [13, 41, 42]. For example, one of these studies [13] reported that 27% of culture-positive retreatment cases were susceptible to all 4 first-line drugs tested. However, these studies apparently regarded such form of TB as unimportant and gave no emphasis on it except mentioning in passing. Further studies are needed on the reason(s) for drug susceptible TB in previously treated patients as this area of research has not been addressed before in the Ethiopian context. This study [13] also reported an alarmingly high level (46%) of MDR TB in retreatment cases from a specialized TB referral hospital, which is a huge increase from that reported previously [1].

In most resource-poor countries, new case MDR TB patients are identified only after first-line therapy fails, by which time these patients could have further disseminated the disease [8, 43]. This calls for a paradigm shift and

points to both the necessity for reevaluation of the belief that associates being new case with a drug susceptible case and the need for strain genotype-based individually tailored drug regimen. The concept of primary resistance is not new, but it is obviously overshadowed by this belief. Delayed initiation of effective therapy, inappropriate therapy, and absence of transmission control are reasons for amplification of primary resistance [44, 45]. Assuming each infectious case can transmit it to 10–15 persons/year [46], the magnitude of the problem cannot be underestimated.

The importance of individualized drug regimen for treatment of MDR and XDR TB cases is highlighted by diversity in strain genotype and/or by treatment failure following compliance to treatment that is based on general treatment guidelines [28, 47, 48]. Moreover, the phenomenon of cross-resistance (e.g., to both the first-line drug INH and the second-line drug ethionamide due to a missense mutation in the *inhA* promoter) [49, 50] renders both antibiotics ineffective (ethionamide is a component of the drug regimen for both MDR and XDR TB patients in Ethiopia [1, 22]). This makes identifying the specific molecular mechanism of resistance to INH important. The same can be said for the aminoglycosides, for example, for both kanamycin and STR [51] and amikacin, kanamycin, and capreomycin [52–54]. In this study, 11 isolates were STR resistant (including 3 monoresistance cases, 1 MDR case, and 7 INH-STR double resistance cases), most (10/11) of which were in new cases. Another study [41] also reported high STR resistance from a region in which this study site is a part. Further information is needed for the reasons for this high level of STR resistance.

Regulations and measures for better infection control in all hospitals and other hot spots in communities (by proper ventilation, avoiding congregated settings, raising public TB awareness, etc.) should be instituted [55]. It is critical that all public and private parties involved in the management and treatment of TB work in concert and streamline their activities [8]. Rapid DST capabilities for all cases are critically needed. However, until those capabilities are built, the spectrum of drug resistance circulating in the communities must be known if standard drug regimens will continue to be used. Regular follow-up of $CD4^+$ levels of HIV-TB patients with mono- or multiple drug resistance is advisable. Collection and storage of isolates from each patient as well as complete treatment record keeping are strongly recommended for use in retrospective studies and further analyses and to monitor progress of therapy. These measures should be applied together; one or the other alone, or even all but one, will not suffice. These recommendations have been passed on to clinicians and authorities with jurisdiction over the study area.

This study has some limitations. These include unavailability of treatment records for all patients, the use of only one DST method and inability to test drug resistance for more first- and second-line drugs, and the limited genotyping data. Finally, the study period was limited to one year.

In conclusion, this study provided important findings and recommendations that can be incorporated into the current practices in the control of TB in the study area and other areas with similar situations. The high rates of TB in the vulnerable children and the youth require immediate attention for proper protective measures, along with further enhancement of case detections. The finding that more than 80% of the patients with resistance to one or more drugs were new cases and that the vast majority were also ≤30 years of age is a strong indicator of recent transmissions with primary resistant infections. Available reports on resistance are usually for MDR and XDR cases and these usually focus on retreatment cases. This work reports very high (16.5%) monodrug and multiple drug resistance involving first-line drugs in new cases. Undetected resistance represents a hidden danger fueling more drug resistance. Even with accurate diagnosis and effective treatment in place, unless ongoing transmission is aggressively dealt with, the gains from the former are likely to be elusive.

Acknowledgments

The authors thank the hospitals, health centers, and the TB patients for their assistance and participation in this study. This work was supported by funds from the AHRI core budget. Additional funding was provided by Addis Ababa University.

References

[1] World Health Organization, *Global Tuberculosis Report 2014*, World Health Organization, Geneva, Switzerland, 2014.

[2] World Health Organization, "Drug-resistant TB surveillance & response supplement," Global Tuberculosis Report, 2014.

[3] World Health Organization, *Global Tuberculosis Report 2013*, World Health Organization, Geneva, Switzerland, 2013.

[4] E. M. Streicher, B. Müller, V. Chihota et al., "Emergence and treatment of multidrug resistant (MDR) and extensively drug-resistant (XDR) tuberculosis in South Africa," *Infection, Genetics and Evolution*, vol. 12, no. 4, pp. 686–694, 2012.

[5] B. Müller, S. Borrell, G. Rose, and S. Gagneux, "The heterogeneous evolution of multidrug-resistant *Mycobacterium tuberculosis*," *Trends in Genetics*, vol. 29, no. 3, pp. 160–169, 2013.

[6] I. Abubakar, M. Zignol, D. Falzon et al., "Drug-resistant tuberculosis: time for visionary political leadership," *The Lancet Infectious Diseases*, vol. 13, no. 6, pp. 529–539, 2013.

[7] J. R. Andrews, N. S. Shah, D. Weissman, A. P. Moll, G. Friedland, and N. R. Gandhi, "Predictors of multidrug-and extensively drug-resistant tuberculosis in a high HIV prevalence community," *PLoS ONE*, vol. 5, no. 12, Article ID e15735, 2010.

[8] E. Nathanson, P. Nunn, M. Uplekar et al., "MDR tuberculosis—critical steps for prevention and control," *The New England Journal of Medicine*, vol. 363, no. 11, pp. 1050–1058, 2010.

[9] World Health Organization, *Multidrug and Extensively Drug-Resistant TB (M/XDR-TB): 2010 Global Report on Surveillance and Response*, World Health Organization, Geneva, Switzerland, 2010, http://whqlibdoc.who.int/publications/2010/9789241599191_eng.pdf.

[10] C. Demay, B. Liens, T. Burguière et al., "SITVITWEB—a publicly available international multimarker database for studying *Mycobacterium tuberculosis* genetic diversity and molecular epidemiology," *Infection, Genetics and Evolution*, vol. 12, no. 4, pp. 755–766, 2012.

[11] T. Weniger, J. Krawczyk, P. Supply, D. Harmsen, and S. Niemann, "Online tools for polyphasic analysis of *Mycobacterium tuberculosis* complex genotyping data: now and next," *Infection, Genetics and Evolution*, vol. 12, no. 4, pp. 748–754, 2012.

[12] B. Tessema, A. Muche, A. Bekele, D. Reissig, F. Emmrich, and U. Sack, "Treatment outcome of tuberculosis patients at Gondar University Teaching Hospital, Northwest Ethiopia. A five-year retrospective study," *BMC Public Health*, vol. 9, article 371, 2009.

[13] D. Abate, B. Taye, M. Abseno, and S. Biadgilign, "Epidemiology of anti-tuberculosis drug resistance patterns and trends in tuberculosis referral hospital in Addis Ababa, Ethiopia," *BMC Research Notes*, vol. 5, article 462, 2012.

[14] B. Seyoum, M. Demissie, A. Worku, S. Bekele, and A. Aseffa, "Prevalence and drug resistance patterns of *Mycobacterium tuberculosis* among new smear positive pulmonary tuberculosis patients in Eastern Ethiopia," *Tuberculosis Research and Treatment*, vol. 2014, Article ID 753492, 7 pages, 2014.

[15] S. D. Hamusse, M. Demissie, D. Teshome, and B. Lindtjørn, "Fifteen-year trend in treatment outcomes among patients with pulmonary smear-positive tuberculosis and its determinants in Arsi Zone, Central Ethiopia," *Global Health Action*, vol. 7, 2014.

[16] World Health Organization, *Guideline for Surveillance of Drug Resistance in Tuberculosis*, World Health Organization, Geneva, Switzerland, 4th edition, 2009.

[17] P. Kent and G. Kubica, *Public Health Mycobacteriology: A Guide for the Level III Laboratory*, U. S. Department of Health and Human Services, Centers for Disease Control, Atlanta, Ga, USA, 1985.

[18] B. van Klingeren, M. Dessens-Kroon, T. van der Laan, K. Kremer, and D. van Soolingen, "Drug susceptibility testing of *Mycobacterium tuberculosis* complex by use of a high-throughput, reproducible, absolute concentration method," *Journal of Clinical Microbiology*, vol. 45, no. 8, pp. 2662–2668, 2007.

[19] L. M. Parsons, R. Brosch, S. T. Cole et al., "Rapid and simple approach for identification of *Mycobacterium tuberculosis* complex isolates by PCR-based genomic deletion analysis," *Journal of Clinical Microbiology*, vol. 40, no. 7, pp. 2339–2345, 2002.

[20] J. Kamerbeek, L. Schouls, A. Kolk et al., "Simultaneous detection and strain differentiation of *Mycobacterium tuberculosis* for diagnosis and epidemiology," *Journal of Clinical Microbiology*, vol. 35, no. 4, pp. 907–914, 1997.

[21] I. Vitol, J. Driscoll, B. Kreiswirth, N. Kurepina, and K. P. Bennett, "Identifying *Mycobacterium tuberculosis* complex strain families using spoligotypes," *Infection, Genetics and Evolution*, vol. 6, no. 6, pp. 491–504, 2006.

[22] Ministry of Health, *Guidelines for Clinical and Programmatic Management of TB, Leprosy and TB/HIV in Ethiopia*, Ministry of Health, Addis Ababa, Ethiopia, 2012.

[23] J. A. Caminero, G. Sotgiu, A. Zumla, and G. B. Migliori, "Best drug treatment for multidrug-resistant and extensively drug-resistant tuberculosis," *The Lancet Infectious Diseases*, vol. 10, no. 9, pp. 621–629, 2010.

[24] B. Müller, V. N. Chihota, M. Pillay et al., "Programmatically selected multidrug-resistant strains drive the emergence of extensively drug-resistant tuberculosis in South Africa," *PLoS ONE*, vol. 8, no. 8, Article ID e70919, 2013.

[25] S. M. Hingley-Wilson, R. Casey, D. Connell et al., "Undetected multidrug-resistant tuberculosis amplified by first-line therapy in mixed infection," *Emerging Infectious Diseases*, vol. 19, no. 7, pp. 1138–1141, 2013.

[26] T. C. Rodwell, F. Valafar, J. Douglas et al., "Predicting extensively drug-resistant *Mycobacterium tuberculosis* phenotypes with genetic mutations," *Journal of Clinical Microbiology*, vol. 52, no. 3, pp. 781–789, 2014.

[27] F. A. Post, P. A. Willcox, B. Mathema et al., "Genetic polymorphism in *Mycobacterium tuberculosis* isolates from patients with chronic multidrug-resistant tuberculosis," *Journal of Infectious Diseases*, vol. 190, no. 1, pp. 99–106, 2004.

[28] A. D. Calver, A. A. Falmer, M. Murray et al., "Emergence of increased resistance and extensively drug-resistant tuberculosis despite treatment adherence, South Africa," *Emerging Infectious Diseases*, vol. 16, no. 2, pp. 264–271, 2010.

[29] R. R. Kempker, A. S. Rabin, K. Nikolaishvili et al., "Additional drug resistance in *Mycobacterium tuberculosis* isolates from resected cavities among patients with multidrug-resistant or extensively drug-resistant pulmonary tuberculosis," *Clinical Infectious Diseases*, vol. 54, no. 6, pp. e51–e54, 2012.

[30] K. Stoffels, C. Allix-Béguec, G. Groenen et al., "From multidrug- to extensively drug-resistant tuberculosis: upward trends as seen from a 15-Year nationwide study," *PLoS ONE*, vol. 8, no. 5, Article ID e63128, 2013.

[31] D. Shingadia and J. A. Seddon, "Epidemiology and disease burden of tuberculosis in children: a global perspective," *Infection and Drug Resistance*, vol. 7, pp. 153–165, 2014.

[32] B. Tessema, J. Beer, M. Merker et al., "Molecular epidemiology and transmission dynamics of *Mycobacterium tuberculosis* in Northwest Ethiopia: new phylogenetic lineages found in Northwest Ethiopia," *BMC Infectious Diseases*, vol. 13, no. 1, article 131, 2013.

[33] A. H. Kebede, Z. Alebachew, F. Tsegaye et al., "The first population-based national tuberculosis prevalence survey in Ethiopia, 2010-2011," *The International Journal of Tuberculosis and Lung Disease*, vol. 18, no. 6, pp. 635–639, 2014.

[34] G. D. van der Spuy, R. M. Warren, M. Richardson, N. Beyers, M. A. Behr, and P. D. van Helden, "Use of genetic distance as a measure of ongoing transmission of *Mycobacterium tuberculosis*," *Journal of Clinical Microbiology*, vol. 41, no. 12, pp. 5640–5644, 2003.

[35] S. Verver, R. M. Warren, Z. Munch et al., "Proportion of tuberculosis transmission that takes place in households in a high-incidence area," *The Lancet*, vol. 363, no. 9404, pp. 212–214, 2004.

[36] T. Kompala, S. V. Shenoi, and G. Friedland, "Transmission of tuberculosis in resource-limited settings," *Current HIV/AIDS Reports*, vol. 10, no. 3, pp. 264–272, 2013.

[37] J. Reynolds and S. K. Heysell, "Understanding pharmacokinetics to improve tuberculosis treatment outcome," *Expert Opinion on Drug Metabolism and Toxicology*, vol. 10, no. 6, pp. 813–823, 2014.

[38] J. G. Pasipanodya, H. McIlleron, A. Burger, P. A. Wash, P. Smith, and T. Gumbo, "Serum drug concentrations predictive of pulmonary tuberculosis outcomes," *Journal of Infectious Diseases*, vol. 208, no. 9, pp. 1464–1473, 2013.

[39] J. G. Pasipanodya, S. Srivastava, and T. Gumbo, "Meta-analysis of clinical studies supports the pharmacokinetic variability hypothesis for acquired drug resistance and failure of antituberculosis therapy," *Clinical Infectious Diseases*, vol. 55, no. 2, pp. 169–177, 2012.

[40] T. Cohen, P. D. van Helden, D. Wilson et al., "Mixed-strain *Mycobacterium tuberculosis* infections and the implications for tuberculosis treatment and control," *Clinical Microbiology Reviews*, vol. 25, no. 4, pp. 708–719, 2012.

[41] S. A. Yimer, M. Agonafir, Y. Derese, Y. Sani, G. A. Bjune, and C. Holm-Hansen, "Primary drug resistance to anti-tuberculosis drugs in major towns of Amhara region, Ethiopia," *APMIS*, vol. 120, no. 6, pp. 503–509, 2012.

[42] B. Tessema, J. Beer, F. Emmrich, U. Sack, and A. C. Rodloff, "Analysis of gene mutations associated with isoniazid, rifampicin and ethambutol resistance among *Mycobacterium tuberculosis* isolates from Ethiopia," *BMC Infectious Diseases*, vol. 12, article 37, 2012.

[43] S. Basu, G. H. Frledland, J. Medlock et al., "Averting epidemics of extensively drug-resistant tuberculosis," *Proceedings of the National Academy of Sciences of the United States of America*, vol. 106, no. 18, pp. 7672–7677, 2009.

[44] N. R. Gandhi, D. Weissman, P. Moodley et al., "Nosocomial transmission of extensively drug-resistant tuberculosis in a rural hospital in South Africa," *Journal of Infectious Diseases*, vol. 207, no. 1, pp. 9–17, 2013.

[45] H. S. Cox, C. McDermid, V. Azevedo et al., "Epidemic levels of drug resistant tuberculosis (MDR and XDR-TB) in a high HIV prevalence setting in Khayelitsha, South Africa," *PLoS ONE*, vol. 5, no. 11, Article ID e13901, 2010.

[46] World Health Organization, *Tuberculosis*, World Health Organization, 2015, http://www.who.int/mediacentre/factsheets/fs104/en/.

[47] J. E. M. de Steenwinkel, M. T. Ten Kate, G. J. de Knegt et al., "Consequences of noncompliance for therapy efficacy and emergence of resistance in murine tuberculosis caused by the Beijing genotype of *Mycobacterium tuberculosis*," *Antimicrobial Agents and Chemotherapy*, vol. 56, no. 9, pp. 4937–4944, 2012.

[48] M. Klopper, R. M. Warren, C. Hayes et al., "Emergence and spread of extensively and totally drug-resistant tuberculosis, South Africa," *Emerging Infectious Diseases*, vol. 19, no. 3, pp. 449–455, 2013.

[49] A. Banerjee, E. Dubnau, A. Quemard et al., "*inhA*, a gene encoding a target for isoniazid and ethionamide in *Mycobacterium tuberculosis*," *Science*, vol. 263, no. 5144, pp. 227–230, 1994.

[50] B. Müller, E. M. Streicher, K. G. P. Hoek et al., "*inhA* promoter mutations: a gateway to extensively drug-resistant tuberculosis in South Africa?" *International Journal of Tuberculosis and Lung Disease*, vol. 15, no. 3, pp. 344–351, 2011.

[51] A. Z. Reeves, P. J. Campbell, R. Sultana et al., "Aminoglycoside cross-resistance in *Mycobacterium tuberculosis* due to mutations in the 5′ untranslated region of *whiB7*," *Antimicrobial Agents and Chemotherapy*, vol. 57, no. 4, pp. 1857–1865, 2013.

[52] S. B. Georghiou, M. Magana, R. S. Garfein, D. G. Catanzaro, A. Catanzaro, and T. C. Rodwell, "Evaluation of genetic mutations associated with *Mycobacterium tuberculosis* resistance to

amikacin, kanamycin and capreomycin: a systematic review," *PLoS ONE*, vol. 7, no. 3, Article ID e33275, 2012.

[53] L. E. Via, S.-N. Cho, S. Hwang et al., "Polymorphisms associated with resistance and cross-resistance to aminoglycosides and capreomycin in *Mycobacterium tuberculosis* isolates from south Korean patients with drug-resistant tuberculosis," *Journal of Clinical Microbiology*, vol. 48, no. 2, pp. 402–411, 2010.

[54] L. Jugheli, N. Bzekalava, P. de Rijk, K. Fissette, F. Portaels, and L. Rigouts, "High level of cross-resistance between kanamycin, amikacin, and capreomycin among *Mycobacterium tuberculosis* isolates from Georgia and a close relation with mutations in the *rrs* gene," *Antimicrobial Agents and Chemotherapy*, vol. 53, no. 12, pp. 5064–5068, 2009.

[55] World Health Organization, *WHO Policy on TB Infection Control in Health-Care Facilities, Congregate Settings and Households*, WHO/HTM/TB/2009.419, World Health Organization, Geneva, Switzerland, 2009.

15

Performance of Clinical Algorithms for Smear-Negative Tuberculosis in HIV-Infected Persons in Ho Chi Minh City, Vietnam

Duc T. M. Nguyen,[1] Hung Q. Nguyen,[2] R. Palmer Beasley,[3] Charles E. Ford,[4] Lu-Yu Hwang,[3] and Edward A. Graviss[3,5]

[1] Department of Pediatrics, University of British Columbia and BC Children's Hospital, 4480 Oak Street, A4-198 AD, Vancouver, BC, Canada V6H 3V4
[2] Department E (HIV Infection), Hospital for Tropical Diseases (HTD), Ho Chi Minh City, Vietnam
[3] Division of Epidemiology, Human Genetics & Environmental Sciences, University of Texas School of Public Health (UTSPH), Houston, TX 77030, USA
[4] Division of Biostatistics, University of Texas School of Public Health (UTSPH), Houston, TX 77030, USA
[5] Department of Pathology and Genomic Medicine, The Methodist Hospital Research Institute (THMRI), Houston, TX 77030, USA

Correspondence should be addressed to Duc T. M. Nguyen, duc.nguyen@cw.bc.ca and Edward A. Graviss, eagraviss@tmhs.org

Academic Editor: Carlo Garzelli

Background. Tuberculosis (TB) disease diagnosis in Vietnam relies on symptom screening, chest radiography (CXR), and acid fast bacilli (AFB) sputum smear which have a poor sensitivity in HIV patients. We evaluated the performance of clinical algorithms in screening and diagnosing AFB smear-negative TB in HIV patients. *Methods.* We enrolled 399 HIV-positive patients seeking care at a HIV clinic in Ho Chi Minh City (HCMC), Vietnam. Participants' demographics, medical history, common TB symptoms, CXR, and laboratory tests were collected. *Results.* Of 399 HIV patients, 390 had initial AFB-negative smears and 22/390 patients had positive cultures. Symptom screening missed 54% (12/22) of smear-negative pulmonary TB (PTB) cases. Multivariate analysis found CD4+ cell level and CXR were significant PTB predictors. An algorithm combining four TB symptoms and TST presented a high sensitivity (100%), but poorly specific (24%) diagnostic performance for smear-negative PTB. *Conclusion.* Up to 54% of PTB cases in the HIV-infected population may be missed in the routine screening and diagnostic procedures used in Vietnam. Symptom screening was a poor overall diagnostic measure in detecting smear-negative TB in HIV patients. Our study results suggest that routine sputum cultures should be implemented to achieve a more accurate diagnosis of TB in HIV patients.

1. Introduction

HIV-infected patients with tuberculosis (TB) coinfection may present with atypical manifestations of pulmonary TB (PTB) and a higher rate of negative sputum smears for acid fast bacilli (AFB) [1–3]. Though being less infectious than AFB smear-positive PTB, AFB smear-negative PTB is still a potentially important source of TB transmission and predicts a worse prognosis for HIV-infected patients [4–6]. Therefore, early and accurate diagnosis of sputum smear-negative PTB for HIV-infected patients is urgently important for not only

improving the patient's life expectancy, but also preventing disease transmission to the general population.

The diagnosis of TB disease in developing countries like Vietnam relies mainly on symptom screening, chest radiography (CXR), and AFB sputum smear, which have a poor sensitivity in HIV-positive patients [3, 7]. Sputum culture is not routinely available for smear-negative patients, especially at district-level public health institutions [7]. Moreover, current data on the performance of clinical, radiographic, and laboratory characteristics in predicting

AFB smear-negative PTB for HIV-infected patients are still limited and inconsistent [6, 8].

This reasoning led us to evaluate the diagnostic performance of available clinical, radiographic, and laboratory factors in diagnosing AFB smear-negative PTB for HIV-infected patients at a district-level HIV clinic in Ho Chi Minh City (HCMC), Vietnam. Data obtained from this study will help develop a standard algorithm for AFB smear-negative PTB in areas where both HIV and TB are prevalent and provide the basis for future studies on more accurate and rapid tools for TB diagnosis.

2. Material and Methods

2.1. Enrollment. This study was conducted at the An Hoa Clinic, a neighborhood HIV clinic located in District 6, HCMC, Vietnam. An Hoa Clinic is where approximately 65% of District 6's HIV patients come for screening of opportunistic infections and receiving antiretroviral therapy (ART) [9, 10].

To our knowledge, this was the first study to investigate the prevalence of AFB smear-negative PTB in HIV-infected patients in Vietnam. As there was no preliminary published data for calculating power or sample size, we used a convenient sample size calculation for this pilot study. In this cross-sectional study, 399 HIV-infected subjects were consecutively enrolled from August 2009 through June 2010. Inclusion criteria included: (a) District 6 residents, (b) age ≥ 15 years, (c) had not been treated for TB during the past year, and (d) laboratory-confirmed HIV infection.

2.2. Data Collection. This study was part of the "Tuberculosis in HIV-infected individuals in Ho Chi Minh City, Vietnam" project and the detailed methodology has been described elsewhere [11]. Briefly, written informed consent was obtained for all study participants before subjects were interviewed. A standardized data collection form was used to gather information on participants' demographics, medical history, TB symptoms, and laboratory results.

After interview, participants were referred to the Pham Ngoc Thach Hospital for Tuberculosis and Lung Diseases (PNT) in District 5, HCMC for chest radiography (CXR), tuberculin skin test (TST), AFB sputum smears and cultures, and CD4+ cell count.

CXR was conventionally performed on posterior-anterior view (PA) using large films and read by a trained blinded radiologist. The radiologist reviewed radiographs for TB-specific presentations such as cavitations, military tuberculosis, consolidation, infiltrates, nodules, fibrosis, pleuritis, and adenopathy. CXRs with TB-specific presentations were classified as abnormal CXR suggestive for TB disease (TB-CXR).

TST was placed on the volar surface of participants' forearm by intradermally injecting 5 tuberculin units of purified protein derivative (PPD-Hanoi, Vietnam) [12]. Results were read after 48–72 hours of placement. An induration of at least 5 mm was classified as positive [13]. CD4+ cell level in participants' plasma was recorded in cell/mm^3.

Two sputum specimens were collected for each participant as per World Health Organization (WHO)'s guidelines [14], one at home and the other at the PNT Hospital in the early morning. Sputum specimens were decontaminated by NaOH-NALC 2% solution before being aliquoted for smear examination and culture [15]. Direct sputum microscopic examination was performed for acid fast bacilli (AFB) using the Ziehl-Neelsen method as per the Vietnamese National TB Program Guidelines [7]. Sputum smear results were categorized as smear-negative, when both smears were negative for AFB, or smear-positive, when at least one smear was positive for AFB. Sputum cultures were also performed on the Löwenstein-Jensen medium for *Mycobacterium tuberculosis* (MTB). We applied one sputum culture per patient as per the routine procedure at the PNT hospital. The cultures were consistently performed on the second specimens which were collected at the hospital. MTB was differentiated from mycobacteria other than tuberculosis (MOTT) by the niacin accumulation test. A subject was classified as a pulmonary TB (PTB) case when he/she had a sputum culture positive for MTB [16].

MTB isolates were assessed for the susceptibility to rifampin, isoniazid, streptomycin, and ethambutol by the Canetti-Grosset proportion method [17]. Resistant TB was defined as isolate resistant to at least one anti-TB drug. MDR-TB was defined as an isolate resistant to rifampin and isoniazid [16].

2.3. Ethics. This study was approved by the Institutional Review Boards (IRBs) of The Methodist Hospital Research Institute (TMHRI) and HCMC Provincial AIDS Committee (PAC).

2.4. Data Analysis. As the main objective of this study was to evaluate the performance of potential predictors in diagnosing smear-negative, culture-positive PTB, the data set used in this analysis included only HIV-infected patients having sputum smears negative for AFB. Univariate odds ratios (OR) with 95% confidence intervals (CI) were calculated to evaluate the possible association between smear-negative PTB and different variables in terms of demographics, clinical symptoms, chest radiography, and laboratory test results. All variables evaluated in univariate analysis were then included in a multivariate regression model to identify potential predictors for PTB by calculating adjusted ORs with 95% confidence intervals (CI). We calculated the sensitivity, specificity, positive predictive value (PPV), negative predictive value (NPV), positive likelihood ratio (LR+), negative likelihood ratio (LR−), and area under the receiver operating characteristic (ROC) curve to evaluate the diagnostic performance of the common (and available) TB symptoms, CXR, TST, CD4+ cell level, and various combinations among them [18, 19]. All statistical analyses in this study were performed with STATA version 10.1 (StataCorp LP College Station, TX). A P value < 0.05 was considered statistical significant.

TABLE 1: Potential predictors for pulmonary tuberculosis in 390 HIV-infected persons having sputum smears negative for acid fast bacilli.

Characteristics	All patients (N = 390)	PTB (n = 22)	No PTB (n = 368)	Unadjusted OR (95% CI)	Adjusted OR[a] (95% CI)
Men	277 (71.0)	20 (90.9)	257 (69.8)	4.32 (0.99, 18.79)	6.82 (0.65, 72.24)
Median age, years (IQR)	30 (27–34)	31 (28–34)	30 (27–34)	0.98 (0.91, 1.06)	0.95 (0.86, 1.04)
Median household, person (IQR)	6 (4–7)	6 (5–8)	6 (4–7)	1.06 (0.94, 1.18)	1.08 (0.95, 1.23)
Incarcerated history	63 (16.2)	6 (27.3)	57 (15.5)	2.05 (0.76, 5.45)	0.91 (0.29, 2.90)
Smoker	308 (79.0)	20 (90.9)	288 (78.3)	2.78 (0.64, 12.14)	0.40 (0.03, 4.67)
Alcoholism	168 (43.1)	9 (40.9)	159 (43.2)	0.91 (0.38, 2.18)	0.78 (0.28, 2.18)
Intravenous drug users	248 (63.6)	17 (77.3)	231 (62.8)	2.02 (0.73, 5.59)	1.24 (0.32, 4.80)
TB treatment history	173 (44.4)	10 (45.5)	163 (44.3)	1.05 (0.44, 2.49)	0.89 (0.27, 2.92)
Receiving ART	225 (57.7)	11 (50.0)	214 (58.2)	0.72 (0.30, 1.70)	0.58 (0.18, 1.83)
Cough	101 (25.9)	6 (27.3)	95 (25.8)	1.08 (0.41, 2.83)	0.59 (0.16, 2.20)
Fever	24 (6.2)	4 (18.9)	20 (5.4)	**3.87 (1.20, 12.50)***	3.33 (0.71, 15.66)
Weight loss	78 (20.0)	6 (27.3)	72 (19.6)	1.54 (0.58, 4.08)	1.61 (0.40, 6.44)
Sweats	11 (2.8)	1 (4.6)	10 (2.7)	1.71 (0.21, 13.95)	0.57 (0.04, 7.62)
Loss of appetite	38 (9.7)	4 (18.2)	34 (9.2)	2.18 (0.70, 6.82)	2.14 (0.47, 9.67)
Chills	34 (8.7)	5 (22.7)	29 (7.9)	**3.44 (1.18, 9.99)***	1.84 (0.41, 8.19)
Fatigue	61 (15.6)	6 (27.3)	55 (14.9)	2.13 (0.80, 5.69)	0.74 (0.18, 3.05)
Positive TST	220 (56.4)	16 (72.7)	204 (55.4)	2.14 (0.82, 5.60)	2.36 (0.76, 7.33)
CD4+ cell/μL <200	84 (21.5)	10 (45.5)	74 (20.1)	**3.31 (1.38, 7.96)****	**3.35 (1.20, 9.37)***
TB-CXR	122 (31.3)	14 (63.6)	108 (29.4)	**4.21 (1.72, 10.33)****	**4.38 (1.52, 12.61)****

[a] Adjusted in the multivariate model.
TB-CXR: abnormal radiograph suggestive of tuberculosis.
PTB: pulmonary tuberculosis due to *Mycobacterium tuberculosis*.
OR: odds ratio.
CI: confidence interval.
IQR: interquartile range.
* P value < 0.05.
** P value < 0.01.

3. Results

3.1. Study Population. A total of 639 HIV-infected patients who registered as District 6 residents and sought care at the An Hoa Clinic during the study timeframe were screened for eligibility by the study staff. There were 120 patients ineligible by the inclusion criteria and 83 patients eligible, but refused to participate. Most of the ineligible patients were currently receiving or had recently received ($\leq$ 1 year) TB treatment. Among 436 HIV-patients eligible by the inclusion criteria who agreed to participate in the study, 37 patients were excluded due to incomplete procedures (6 withdrew before having the interview, 26 attended the interview then withdrew without having any test done, 4 missed CXR, and 1 missed sputum culture result). Of 399 HIV-infected patients completing all study procedures, 9 (2.3%) were sputum AFB smear-positive and were excluded. The data of 390 (97.7%) patients with sputum smear-negative results were analyzed further. Among these smear-negative patients, the frequency of sputum culture results positive for MTB, MOTT, and negative were 22 (5.6%), 1 (0.3), and 367 (94.1%), respectively (Figure 1).

Of 390 AFB smear-negative HIV-infected patients, the majority were men (277/390 (71%, 95% CI 67–76%)) and a substantial proportion of the study sample was made up of injecting drug users (248/390 (63.6%, 95% CI 61.3–70.9%)).

Among four common TB symptoms (cough, fever, weight loss, and night sweats, [20] cough and weight loss were reported by participants at the highest frequency, 25.9% (101/390, 95% CI 21.5–30.3%) and 20% (78/390, 95% CI 2.0–24.0%), respectively. One-fifth (21.5%) of participants had CD4+ cell level below 200/mm^3 and one-third (31.3%) had chest radiograph classified as TB-CXR (Table 1).

3.2. Correlation of Demographic, Clinical, and Laboratory Characteristics with Tuberculosis. Our univariate analysis found that AFB smear-negative pulmonary TB was significantly associated with fever, chills, CD4+ cell level < 200/mm^3, and TB-CXR. A multivariate regression model was developed from significant and clinically important covariates. The Hosmer-Lemeshow goodness-of-fit statistic for this model had a P value = 0.69, which indicated that the model fit well with the data [19]. This multivariate model had good discrimination with the area under the ROC curve (sensitivity versus 1 − specificity) of 0.83. Multivariate regression analysis found that only the CD4+ cell level below 200/mm^3 and TB-CXR were significantly associated with AFB smear-negative PTB (P value < 0.01). Demographic characteristics, medical history, and common TB symptoms presented no significant association with AFB smear-negative PTB (Table 1).

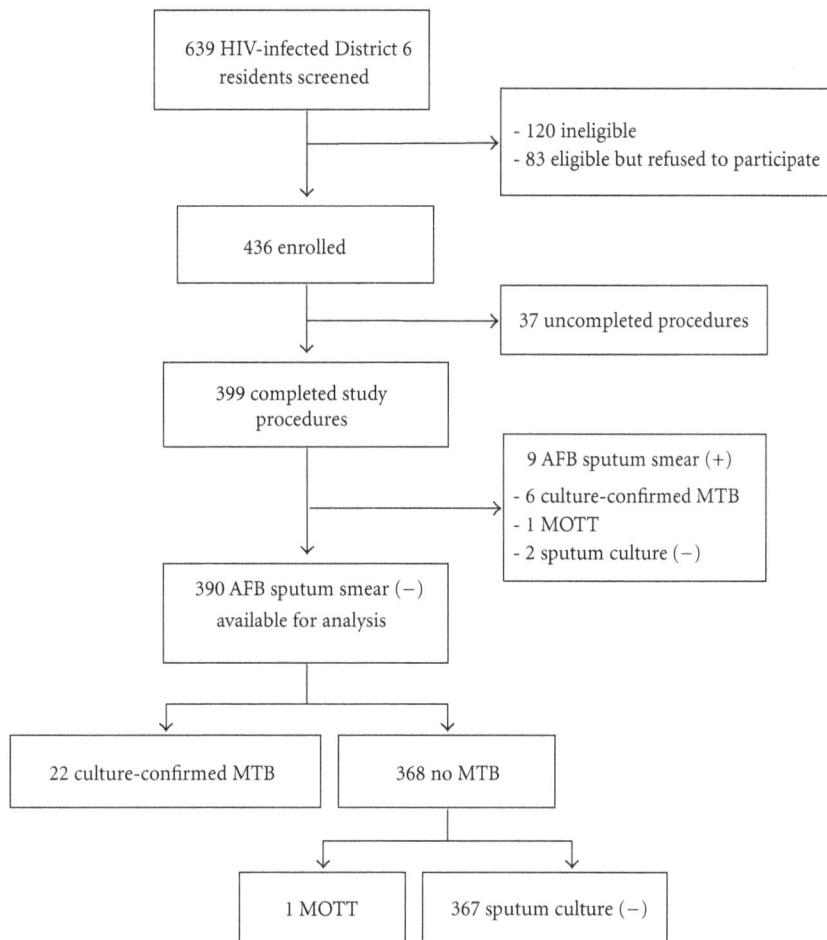

FIGURE 1: Patient enrollment flow chart. AFB-positive: having at least one AFB-positive sputum smear. AFB-negative: having both AFB-negative sputum smears.

3.3. Performance of Symptom-Based Algorithm in Screening AFB Smear-Negative TB. Among 390 HIV-infected patients, a total of 143 patients were positively screened by the algorithm of four common TB symptoms (cough, fever, night sweat, and weight loss). Table 2 presents the poor performance of different combinations of clinical predictors in screening AFB smear-negative individuals. The combination of four TB common symptoms could identify only 10/22 (46%, 95% CI 24.1–66.8%) TB cases with a positive likelihood ratio of 1.25 and a negative likelihood ratio of 0.85. Although the combination of symptoms and TST had 100% sensitivity (22/22 PTB cases identified), this algorithm was not a good predictor for ruling out PTB with a positive likelihood ratio of 1.32 and a specificity of 24%.

4. Discussion

Like other developing countries, the diagnosis of pulmonary tuberculosis in Vietnam relies mainly on clinical screening, CXR, and sputum smear examination. While recommended by the World Health Organization (WHO) for diagnosis of AFB smear-negative TB in HIV-infected patients, sputum culture is still not routinely available at the district-level

HIV clinics in Vietnam [14]. Although some authors have suggested clinical symptoms can be significant predictors of smear-negative PTB, neither clinical symptoms nor TST were significantly associated with smear-negative PTB in our population [6]. Among available potential predictors, our data found only a decrease CD4+ cell level below $200/mm^3$ and an abnormal CXR (TB-CXR) as being significant predictors for PTB in HIV-infected patients having sputum AFB-negative smears.

Consistent with previous studies, our data failed to identify neither any single symptom nor combination of symptoms which could be a sensitive predictor for smear-negative, culture-confirmed PTB [6, 8]. Recently, the WHO has recommended using combination of cough, fever, weight loss, and night sweats as the initial screening tool to exclude active TB cases before initiating preventing treatment for persons living with HIV in most resource-constrained settings [20]. However, our data showed that symptom screening may miss up to 54% of AFB smear-negative PTB cases among HIV-infected patients (sensitivity = 46% and negative likelihood ratio = 0.85). We also found 12 (3%) new smear-negative PTB cases, which would be missed by the current routine diagnostic tools (Table 1). Therefore,

TABLE 2: Performance of different algorithms in screening TB for 390 HIV-infected patients having sputum smear negative to AFB.

Combination of predictors	Sensitivity	Specificity	PPV	NPV	LR+	LR−	Area under ROC curve*
Combination of three clinical predictors							
Cough or fever or night sweats	8/22 (36)	266/368 (72)	8/102 (7)	266/280 (95)	1.31	0.88	0.54
Cough or night sweat or weight loss	9/22 (41)	236/368 (64)	9/141 (6)	236/249 (95)	1.14	0.92	0.52
Fever or night sweats or weight loss	8/22 (36)	285/368 (78)	8/91 (9)	285/299 (95)	1.61	0.82	0.57
Combination of four clinical predictors							
Cough or fever or night sweats or weight loss	10/22 (46)	235/368 (64)	10/143 (7)	235/247 (95)	1.25	0.85	0.55
Combination of four clinical predictors and TST							
Symptoms or TST	22/22 (100)	89/368 (24)	22/301 (7)	89/89 (100)	1.32	0	0.62

*ROC curve: receiver operating characteristic curve.
PPV: positive predictive value. NPV: negative predictive value.
LR+: positive likelihood ratio, calculated by sensitivity ÷ (1 − specificity).
LR−: negative likelihood ratio calculated by (1 − sensitivity) ÷ specificity [18].
Sensitivity, specificity, PPV, and NPV are reported as proportion (%).
CXR: chest radiography.
Cough: lasting ≥2 weeks in the past 4 weeks.
Fever: lasting ≥2 weeks in the past 4 weeks.
Night sweats: lasting ≥2 weeks in the past 4 weeks.
Weight loss: lasting ≥2 weeks in the past 4 weeks.

results from this study confirm the need of routinely applying sputum culture for HIV-infected patients in Vietnam [21]. In public health settings where the sputum culture is not available, chest radiography in addition to the CD4+ cell level below 200/mm³ could be feasible but poor diagnostic tools for AFB smear-negative PTB in HIV-infected individuals.

Among 22 AFB smear-negative PTB cases, 7 (32%) were classified as resistant to TB; of which, 5 cases were resistant to streptomycin, 1 case was resistant to streptomycin and isoniazid, and 1 MDR-TB case which was resistant to streptomycin, rifampin, isoniazid, and ethambutol (data not shown). Although this important issue still needs to be investigated further with a larger study, these findings strongly suggest the need for rapid and accurate diagnostic tools for detecting resistant TB cases in HIV patients having AFB-negative sputum smears. GeneXpert MTB/RIF, a rapid assay endorsed by the WHO [20], which can simultaneously identify MTB and its susceptibility to the most common first-line anti-TB drug—rifampin, would be a feasible choice and should be evaluated in the HIV-infected population in Vietnam.

A similar study to our study in a setting of high TB prevalence suggested that smear-negative PTB cases were more likely to be confirmed by sputum culture as MOTT than in smear-positive PTB cases [6]. Our study found only two MOTT cases, which were equally distributed in the two groups of smear status-one in each. However, our sample size may not be powerful enough to evaluate the association between MOTT and AFB negative smear status. Further studies with larger sample sizes should be conducted to investigate thoroughly this important issue. As MOTT and MTB have distinct prognoses and therapy [22], a better understanding on their diagnostic characteristics would be useful in developing clinical algorithms for their differential diagnosis, especially in low-resource settings.

Our study has some notable limitations. First, the study was conducted at a single clinic. However, as the majority (65%) of An Hoa Clinic's patients were District 6 residents, the clinic received most of the HIV-infected patients residing in the District [23], and the study subjects were consecutively enrolled from patients having AFB-negative sputum smears, our study sample should represent the district's smear-negative HIV-infected population. Second, our study used only one sputum culture for each patient as we followed the routine procedure often used in Vietnam. This single culture procedure may obviously underestimate the real number of PTB cases [24]. Third, the Löwenstein-Jensen sputum culture technique used in our study may miss some PTB cases [24]. Liquid-based culture technique such as the WHO approved MGIT should be deployed as a more rapid and accurate alternative for Löwenstein-Jensen technique where local resources allowed [24, 25]. The possible use of available nucleic acid amplification tests (NAATs) should also be considered to help enhance the detection of smear-negative tuberculosis [26].

In conclusion, diagnosis of smear-negative PTB in HIV-infected patients is a real challenge for clinicians at district-level HIV clinics in Vietnam where the sputum culture is not available. Our data showed the poor clinical performance of symptoms screening for AFB smear-negative PTB and confirmed the urgency of routinely applying sputum culture for HIV-infected individuals to improve the detection of not only smear-negative PTB but also TB disease in general. Where the sputum culture is not available, the algorithm of CXR plus CD4+ cell count could be a feasible but poor diagnostic tool. As no published data is available regarding MOTT in Vietnam, the issue of differentiation between MOTT and MTB should be further investigated. Future studies on more affordable, rapid, and accurate tests for TB infection would also be necessary to timely provide specific treatment for patients in need, reduce mortality, and minimize TB transmission to the general population.

Acknowledgments

The authors acknowledge the contribution of the study team from the following institutions in the process of data collection and laboratory testing: The HCMC AIDS Committee; the An Hoa Clinic, Distinct 6 Health Center; and the Pham Ngoc Thach Hospital's Laboratories and Imaging Diagnostic Department. The project was funded in part by the Baylor-UT Houston Center for AIDS Research (CFAR) Core Support Grant no. AI36211 from the National Institute of Allergy and Infectious Diseases (NIAID), Research Grant no. D43TW007669 from the Fogarty International Center (FIC), National Institutes of Health (NIH), and supported in part by a Grant from the Vietnam Education Foundation (VEF). The content is solely the responsibility of the authors and does not necessarily represent the official views of the CFAR, VEF, FIC, PAC, or the NIH. Dr. Beasley is recognized posthumously.

References

[1] C. D. Wells, J. P. Cegielski, L. J. Nelson et al., "HIV infection and multidrug-resistant tuberculosis—the perfect storm," *Journal of Infectious Diseases*, vol. 196, supplement 1, pp. S86–S107, 2007.

[2] P. Monkongdee, K. D. McCarthy, K. P. Cain et al., "Yield of acid-fast smear and mycobacterial culture for tuberculosis diagnosis in people with human immunodeficiency virus," *American Journal of Respiratory and Critical Care Medicine*, vol. 180, no. 9, pp. 903–908, 2009.

[3] K. P. Cain, K. D. McCarthy, C. M. Heilig et al., "An algorithm for tuberculosis screening and diagnosis in people with HIV," *New England Journal of Medicine*, vol. 362, no. 8, pp. 707–716, 2010.

[4] M. A. Behr, S. A. Warren, H. Salamon et al., "Transmission of *Mycobacterium tuberculosis* from patients smear-negative for acid-fast bacilli," *The Lancet*, vol. 353, no. 9151, pp. 444–449, 1999.

[5] N. J. Hargreaves, O. Kadzakumanja, C. J. M. Whitty, F. M. L. Salaniponi, A. D. Harries, and S. B. Squire, "'Smear-negative' pulmonary tuberculosis in a DOTS programme: poor outcomes in an area of high HIV seroprevalence," *International Journal of Tuberculosis and Lung Disease*, vol. 5, no. 9, pp. 847–854, 2001.

[6] A. Tamhane, P. Chheng, T. Dobbs, S. Mak, B. Sar, and M. E. Kimerling, "Predictors of smear-negative pulmonary tuberculosis in HIV-infected patients, Battambang, Cambodia," *International Journal of Tuberculosis and Lung Disease*, vol. 13, no. 3, pp. 347–354, 2009.

[7] Vietnamese Ministry of Health, Guidelines for Diagnosis and Treatment of Tuberculosis 03/24/2009.

[8] J. L. Davis, W. Worodria, H. Kisembo et al., "Clinical and radiographic factors do not accurately diagnose smear-negative tuberculosis in HIV-infected inpatients in Uganda: a cross-sectional study," *PLoS One*, vol. 5, no. 3, article e9859, 2010.

[9] People Committee of District 6, HCMC. District 6 Official Website 2010, http://www.quan6.hochiminhcity.gov.vn/pages/gioi-thieu-tong-quat.aspx.

[10] Q. H. Nguyen, "An Hoa Clinic's annul report to the HCMC Provincial AIDS Committee 2009," 2009.

[11] D. T. M. Nguyen, N. Q. Hung, and L. T. Giang, "Improving the diagnosis of pulmonary tuberculosis in HIV-infected individuals in Ho Chi Minh City, Vietnam," *The International Journal of Tuberculosis and Lung Disease*, vol. 15, no. 11, pp. 1528–1535, 2011.

[12] World Health Organization (WHO), "The WHO standard tuberculin test," WHO/TB/Technical Guide 3, 1963.

[13] Centers for Disease Control and Prevention (CDC), Tuberculin Skin Testing 2010 07/01.

[14] World Health Organization (WHO), "Improving the diagnosis and treatment of smear-negative pulmonary and extrapulmonary tuberculosis among adults and adolescents," 2007.

[15] D. T. M. Ha, N. T. N. Lan, V. S. Kiet et al., "Diagnosis of pulmonary tuberculosis in HIV-positive patients by microscopic observation drug susceptibility assay," *Journal of Clinical Microbiology*, vol. 48, no. 12, pp. 4573–4579, 2010.

[16] Centers for Disease Control and Prevention (CDC), Tuberculosis (TB) 2009 06/01/2009.

[17] G. Canetti, S. Froman, J. Grosset et al., "Mycobacteria: laboratory methods for testing drug sensitivity and resistance," *Bulletin of the World Health Organization*, vol. 29, pp. 565–578, 1963.

[18] D. A. Grimes and K. F. Schulz, "Refining clinical diagnosis with likelihood ratios," *The Lancet*, vol. 365, no. 9469, pp. 1500–1505, 2005.

[19] D. Hosmer and S. Lemeshow, *Model-Building Strategies and Methods for Logistic Regression. Applied logistic regression*, John Wiley & Son, New York, NY, USA, 2nd edition, 2000.

[20] World Health Organization (WHO), Department of HIV/AIDS Stop, TB Department, "Guidelines for intensified tuberculosis case-finding and isoniazid preventive therapy for people living with HIV in resource-constrained settings," WHO Guidelines 2010.

[21] World Health Organization (WHO), *Strategic and Technical Advisory Group for Tuberculosis*, 2008.

[22] D. E. Griffith, T. Aksamit, B. A. Brown-Elliott et al., "An official ATS/IDSA statement: diagnosis, treatment, and prevention of nontuberculous mycobacterial diseases," *American Journal of Respiratory and Critical Care Medicine*, vol. 175, no. 4, pp. 367–416, 2007.

[23] Q. H. Nguyen, "An overview of 2 Years of ARV Treatment 9/2005—8/2007," Updated In 7/2007.

[24] P. Monkongdee, K. D. McCarthy, K. P. Cain et al., "Yield of acid-fast smear and mycobacterial culture for tuberculosis diagnosis in people with human immunodeficiency virus," *American Journal of Respiratory and Critical Care Medicine*, vol. 180, no. 9, pp. 903–908, 2009.

[25] World Health Organization (WHO), "Strategic and technical advisory group for tuberculosis," Report on Conclusion and Recomendations, 2007.

[26] J. L. Davis, L. Huang, W. Worodria et al., "Nucleic acid amplification tests for diagnosis of smear-negative TB in a high HIV-prevalence setting: a prospective cohort study," *PLoS One*, vol. 6, no. 1, article e16321, 2011.

16

Tuberculin Skin Tests versus Interferon-Gamma Release Assays in Tuberculosis Screening among Immigrant Visa Applicants

Stella O. Chuke,[1,2] Nguyen Thi Ngoc Yen,[3] Kayla F. Laserson,[2,4] Nguyen Huu Phuoc,[3] Nguyen An Trinh,[3] Duong Thi Cam Nhung,[3] Vo Thi Chi Mai,[3] An Dang Qui,[3] Hoang Hoa Hai,[3] Le Thien Huong Loan,[3] Warren G. Jones,[5,6] William C. Whitworth,[2] J. Jina Shah,[7,8,9] John A. Painter,[7] Gerald H. Mazurek,[2] and Susan A. Maloney[4,7]

[1] Northrop Grumman Information Systems Sector, 2800 Century Parkway NE, Atlanta, GA 30345, USA

[2] Division of Tuberculosis Elimination, Centers for Disease Control and Prevention (CDC), Mail Stop E-10, 1600 Clifton Road NE, Atlanta, GA 30333, USA

[3] Cho Ray Hospital, 201B Nguyen Chi Thanh Street, District 5, Ho Chi Minh City, Vietnam

[4] Center for Global Health, CDC, Mail Stop D-68, 1600 Clifton Road NE, Atlanta, GA 30333, USA

[5] International Organization for Migration (IOM), 1B Pham Ngoc Thach District 1, Ho Chi Minh City, Vietnam

[6] International Organization for Migration (IOM), P.O. Box 55040, Westlands, Nairobi 00200, Kenya

[7] Division of Global Migration and Quarantine, CDC, Mail Stop E-03, 1600 Clifton Road NE, Atlanta, GA 30333, USA

[8] Department of Family & Community Medicine, University of California, San Francisco, 500 Parnassus Avenue, MU 3E, San Francisco, CA 94143, USA

[9] Genentech, Inc., 1 DNA Way, South San Francisco, CA 94080, USA

Correspondence should be addressed to Gerald H. Mazurek; gym6@cdc.gov

Academic Editor: Juraj Ivanyi

Objective. Use of tuberculin skin tests (TSTs) and interferon gamma release assays (IGRAs) as part of tuberculosis (TB) screening among immigrants from high TB-burden countries has not been fully evaluated. *Methods.* Prevalence of *Mycobacterium tuberculosis* infection (MTBI) based on TST, or the QuantiFERON-TB Gold test (QFT-G), was determined among immigrant applicants in Vietnam bound for the United States (US); factors associated with test results and discordance were assessed; predictive values of TST and QFT-G for identifying chest radiographs (CXRs) consistent with TB were calculated. *Results.* Of 1,246 immigrant visa applicants studied, 57.9% were TST positive, 28.3% were QFT-G positive, and test agreement was 59.4%. Increasing age was associated with positive TST results, positive QFT-G results, TST-positive but QFT-G-negative discordance, and abnormal CXRs consistent with TB. Positive predictive values of TST and QFT-G for an abnormal CXR were 25.9% and 25.6%, respectively. *Conclusion.* The estimated prevalence of MTBI among US-bound visa applicants in Vietnam based on TST was twice that based on QFT-G, and 14 times higher than a TST-based estimate of MTBI prevalence reported for the general US population in 2000. QFT-G was not better than TST at predicting abnormal CXRs consistent with TB.

1. Introduction

Tuberculosis (TB) is the single leading cause of death from a curable infectious disease [1], with a global death toll of 1.4 million persons in 2011 [2]. The global incidence of TB has increased from approximately 1.2 million in 1995 [3] to an estimate of 8.7 million in 2011 [2]. About one-third of the world's population is infected with the causative organism, *Mycobacterium tuberculosis* (MTB) [4]. Without intervention, 5 to 10% of those latently infected with MTB are expected to develop active and infectious TB during their lifetime [5].

Global migration has had an increasingly important effect on the epidemiology of TB in the United States and other countries. Although the overall number of new TB cases is decreasing in the US, there has been a significant increase in the proportion of US TB cases in persons born outside the US, with foreign-born persons accounting for 57% of new TB cases in 2006 [6] and 62% in 2011 [7]. To decrease the risk of TB transmission and to improve TB diagnosis and treatment outcomes, immigrant visa applicants are screened for infectious TB [8–11]. For visa applicants ≥15 years of age residing outside the US, medical evaluation includes screening with a chest radiograph (CXR), followed by sputum examination if the CXR is suggestive of TB [12]. For visa applicants already residing within the US and for those outside the US who are <15 years of age, medical evaluation includes screening with either a tuberculin skin test (TST) or an interferon gamma release assay (IGRA), followed by a CXR if either test is positive [12]. However, the utility of TSTs and IGRAs among immigrants and refugees from high TB-burden countries, such as Vietnam, has not been fully evaluated.

Employing recently developed IGRAs may facilitate TB screening. IGRAs such as the QuantiFERON-TB test (QFT) and the QuantiFERON-TB Gold test (QFT-G) were developed as aids for diagnosing MTB infection (MTBI) which includes both latent TB infection (LTBI) and infection manifesting as active TB disease [13]. IGRAs may be completed with a single patient visit, may be less subjective, and may be performed more rapidly than TST [13]. QFT uses tuberculin purified protein derivative (PPD) as the TB antigen and includes an *M. avium* PPD as a control for reactivity to nontuberculous mycobacteria (NTM) [14]. QFT-G assesses reactivity to two MTB proteins, early secretory antigenic target 6 (ESAT-6) and culture filtrate protein 10 (CFP-10) [13]. ESAT-6 and CFP-10 are absent from all bacille Calmette-Guerin (BCG) vaccine strains and most NTM [15]. QFT-G may be more specific than TST and QFT because of less cross-reactivity with BCG and NTM [16]. The QuantiFERON-TB Gold In-Tube test (QFT-GIT) was introduced after this study was initiated and QFT-GIT was conceptualized in part as a result of this study. QFT-GIT facilitates testing by including antigens or control reagents in special tubes used to collect blood for the test [13].

In 2011, immigrants from Vietnam accounted for 5% of US TB cases and 8% of TB cases among foreign-born US residents [7]. Despite meeting WHO targets of 70% smear-positive case detection and 85% cure rates in 1996, Vietnam remains a high TB burden country with an estimated prevalence of 323 cases per 100, 000 persons in 2011 [2]. This high burden of disease increases the risk of TB transmission in Vietnam [17, 18] and in other developed nations to which immigrants may be resettling [19]. Vietnam has maintained its policy of BCG vaccination of children at birth since 1924 [20–22] and coverage is high (93.7% by a 2007 estimate) [22].

The objectives of this study conducted among immigrant visa applicants in Vietnam were to (1) determine the prevalence of MTBI based on TST and QFT-G; (2) assess the association of various factors (including *M. avium* reactivity

as measured by QFT) with TST and QFT-G results and discordance; and (3) compare the predictive values of TST and QFT-G at identifying CXRs consistent with TB.

2. Methods

This study was part of a larger study examining the efficacy of TB screening among immigrant visa applicants [23, 24] and included a systematic sample of adult immigrant visa applicants. Subjects were recruited on Wednesdays from among adults (age ≥ 18 years) presenting for immigrant medical examinations (MEs) at Cho Ray Hospital in Ho Chi Minh City, Vietnam, from June 12, 2002, to March 12, 2003. MEs are performed in clinics at this hospital five days a week. Wednesday was chosen as the day to recruit because of convenience. MEs are performed according to the 1991 technical instructions published by CDC [10]. All subjects provided written consent. The study was approved by human subject protection committees at CDC, Cho Ray Hospital, Pasteur Institute, and Pham Ngoc Thach National Tuberculosis and Lung Disease Center.

Information relating to nativity, gender, medical history, findings on physical examination, HIV test results, and CXR findings was abstracted from standardized ME forms. Subjects were asked for additional information related to prior TB disease or treatment, TB exposure, TB symptoms, and BCG vaccination. Each subject was examined for the presence of a BCG scar. Subjects with CXR findings consistent with TB were asked to provide sputum on 3 consecutive days. Uncentrifuged sputa were examined for AFB using both Auramine O fluorescence and Ziehl-Neelsen staining methods [25]. Sputa from subjects were decontaminated and digested with oxalic acid (due to pseudomonas in the town water supply) and cultured for mycobacteria using the BACTEC 460 system (Becton, Dickinson and Company, Franklin Lakes, NJ) and Lowenstein-Jensen slants as previously described [24].

Blood samples for QFT and QFT-G were obtained before PPD injections. TSTs were administered by the Mantoux method using 0.1 mL (5 TU) of Tubersol PPD (Connaught Laboratories Inc., Toronto, ON). TST induration was measured 48 to 72 hours after PPD injection by trained health care workers who were blinded to QFT and QFT-G results. Indurations ≥10 mm were interpreted as positive. QFT and QFT-G were performed and interpreted as previously described [26] by staff blinded to results of other tests. TB response by QFT-G was the larger of the interferon gamma responses to CFP-10 or ESAT-6. CXRs were interpreted by panel physicians who were blinded to TST, QFT, and QFT-G results but were aware of other clinical findings.

2.1. Statistical Methods. Demographic, clinical, and laboratory data from each subject were entered into a Microsoft Access Database (Microsoft Corp., Redmond, WA). All data analyses were performed using SPSS (version 15.0; SPSS Inc., Chicago, IL). *M. avium* reactivity was coded as "positive" when QFT results were "Negative for *M. tuberculosis* infection with *M. avium* reactivity" as defined previously [26]; otherwise it was coded as "negative." CXRs were coded as "positive" if findings were consistent with TB according to published criteria [27]. CXRs were coded as "negative" if they were normal or showed only abnormalities that were not consistent with TB (e.g., fractured rib or cardiac enlargement).

Prevalence of MTBI was calculated among those who had TST, QFT, QFT-G, and CXRs completed. Test agreement, positive predictive value (PPV), and negative predictive value (NPV) were calculated among subjects with determinate QFT-G results who had TST and CXR completed. Agreement beyond chance was assessed using Cohen's Kappa coefficient (κ) with a $\kappa > 0.75$ representing excellent agreement, 0.40–0.75 representing fair to good agreement, and <0.40 representing poor agreement [28]. PPVs or NPVs were compared using a predictive value statistic that utilized the Wald procedure [29]. The McNemar test was used to compare estimates of prevalence [30]. Tests for significance were 2-sided and considered statistically significant at a P value of < 0.05. Discordance between TST and QFT-G was classified as "TST positive but QFT-G negative," or "TST negative but QFT-G positive." Discordance between CXR and TST and between CXR and QFT-G was classified in a similar manner.

Univariate and multivariate logistic regressions were used to assess association of the subject characteristics listed in Table 1 with test results and with test discordance. Multivariate models were created using factors with P values < 0.2 in univariate analysis and <0.05 in stepwise logistic regression until the best fitting, parsimonious model was identified. Model fit was evaluated using the Hosmer-Lemeshow test [31]. No interactions between subject characteristics were considered to be of interest *a priori*.

3. Results

As depicted in Figure 1, of the 1,276 subjects in the systematic sample who consented, 30 (2.4%) were excluded because QFT-G was not completed. Characteristics of those excluded (data not shown) did not differ statistically from characteristics of the remaining 1,246 subjects who had QFT-G, TST, and CXR completed (Table 1). As summarized in Table 1, CXR findings for 272 (21.8%) subjects were consistent with TB; 362 (29.1%) subjects had *M. avium* reactivity by QFT; 721 (57.9%) subjects had positive TST results with induration ≥ 10 mm; 352 (28.3%) subjects had positive QFT-G results and 83 (6.7%) subjects had indeterminate QFT-G results. Positive TST results were more prevalent than positive QFT-G results, and both were more prevalent than positive CXRs (all P values ≤ 0.001). Of the 272 subjects with CXRs consistent with TB, 110 (40%) provided sputum and 12 had AFB seen on smear. Culture results were available for 67 subjects and 16 had positive cultures for *M. tuberculosis*. None of the 16 subjects with positive cultures for *M. tuberculosis* had a prior history of TB; all had a positive TST; and 7 (43.8%) had a positive QFT-G.

Mean, median, and interquartile range for TB response values stratified by QFT-G interpretation are shown in Table 2. TB responses were within 0.25 IU/mL of the 0.35 IU/mL cutoff for 70 (19.9%) of 352 QFT-G interpreted as positive and 192 (23.7%) of 811 QFT-G interpreted as negative.

As shown in Table 3, positive CXR results were associated with increased age, male sex, and abnormal chest examination; positive TST results (i.e., induration ≥ 10 mm) were associated with increased age, male sex, and prior BCG vaccination (assessed by self-report or by scar); and positive QFT-G results were associated with increased age. *M. avium* reactivity was inversely associated with positive TST results and positive QFT-G results. Seven subjects had prior TB, all of whom had CXRs consistent with TB, 6 (85.7%) of whom had a positive TST, and 2 (28.6%) had a positive QFT-G. "Prior TB" was not included as a variable in our final multivariate models because all seven subjects with prior TB had CXR findings consistent with TB disease and this prevented convergence of the model, or "Prior TB" was not associated with TST or QFT-G results in univariate analyses (P values > 0.2).

Indeterminate QFT-G results were not associated with any subject characteristics examined but were inversely associated with *M. avium* reactivity with an odds ratio of 0.35 (95% CI: 0.19–0.68). Further analysis showed that TST induration ≥ 15 mm was not associated with BCG vaccination ($P = 0.46$), but associations with age ($P < 0.01$) and male sex ($P = 0.03$) remained significant in our multivariate model and induration ≥ 15 mm also remained inversely associated with *M. avium* reactivity ($P < 0.01$).

When limited to subjects with determinate QFT-G results (all of whom had TST and CXR completed), overall agreement between TST and QFT-G, between CXR and TST, and between CXR and QFT-G was 59.4%, 50.1%, and 63.4%, respectively, (Table 4) and agreement beyond chance was poor. The PPVs of TST and QFT-G for a positive CXR were 25.9% (95% CI: 22.6%–29.2%) and 25.6% (95% CI: 21.0%–30.1%), respectively. The NPVs of TST and QFT-G for a negative CXR were 83.8% (95% CI: 80.5%–87.1%) and 79.8% (95% CI: 77.0%–85.6%), respectively. While PPVs for TST and QFT-G were similar ($P = 0.87$), the NPV for TST was greater than the NPV for QFT-G ($P < 0.01$).

As shown in Table 5, there were 398 (34.2%) subjects with positive TST but negative QFT-G results, and this discordance was associated with increased age, male sex, and prior BCG vaccination. There were 74 (6.4%) subjects with negative TST but positive QFT-G results and none of the subject characteristics examined were associated with this discordance.

As shown in Table 6, there were 79 (6.8%) subjects with positive CXR but negative TST results, and this discordance was associated with increased age and other major medical conditions. There were 501 (43.1%) subjects with negative CXR but positive TST results. This discordance was associated with increased age, male sex, and BCG vaccination and inversely associated with *M. avium* reactivity.

As shown in Table 7, there were 164 (14.1%) subjects with positive CXR but negative QFT-G results, and this discordance was associated with increased age, history of TB disease, and abnormal chest examination. There were 262 (22.5%) subjects with negative CXR but positive QFT-G results and this discordance was inversely associated with age.

Table 1: Subject characteristics and test results of US-bound immigrant visa applicants in Vietnam.

Characteristics	
Subjects evaluated:	$N = 1246$
Age in years:	
Mean/median	38.5/37.5
Minimum/maximum	18.0/86.0
Sex: number (%)	
Female	842 (67.6)
Male	404 (32.4)
Country of birth: n (%)	
Vietnam	1235 (99.1)
Other (China or Cambodia)	11 (0.9)
Prior history of TB	7 (0.6)
Reported prior contact with a TB patient: n (%)	
Any contact	96 (7.7)
Household contact	93 (7.5)
TB symptoms*: n (%)	3 (0.2)
Other major medical conditions**: n (%)	17 (1.4)
BCG vaccination status***: n (%)	
Not vaccinated	735 (59.0)
Vaccinated	511 (41.0)
HIV test results: n (%)	
Negative	1239 (99.4)
Positive	7 (0.6)
Chest examination: n (%)	
Normal	1239 (99.4)
Abnormal	7 (0.6)
Chest radiograph: n (%)	
Normal or not consistent with TB****	974 (78.2)
Findings consistent with TB	272 (21.8)
TST results: n (%)	
<5 mm	278 (22.3)
5 to 9 mm	247 (19.8)
10 to 14 mm	403 (32.3)
≥15 mm	318 (25.5)
QFT results: n (%)	
Negative for MTB infection without *M. avium* reactivity	234 (18.8)
Negative for MTB infection with *M. avium* reactivity	362 (29.1)
Positive for MTB infection	564 (45.3)
Indeterminate	86 (6.9)
QFT-G results: n (%)	
Negative	811 (65.1)
Positive	352 (28.3)
Indeterminate	83 (6.7)

n: number in subset of N; TB: tuberculosis; BCG: bacille Calmitte-Guérin; HIV: human immunodeficiency virus; MTB: *Mycobacteria tuberculosis*; TST: tuberculin skin test; QFT: QuantiFERON-TB test; QFT-G: QuantiFERON-TB Gold test.
*TB Symptoms included cough, dyspnea, fever, unintended weight loss, and hemoptysis.
**Other major medical conditions included diabetes, renal failure, silicosis, gastrectomy, and malignancies.
***Reported BCG status based on interview. All subjects reporting BCG vaccination also had scars compatible with vaccination history.
****Chest radiographs were normal for 967 subjects while 7 subjects had abnormal chest radiographs with lesions not consistent with TB (e.g., fractured rib or cardiac enlargement).

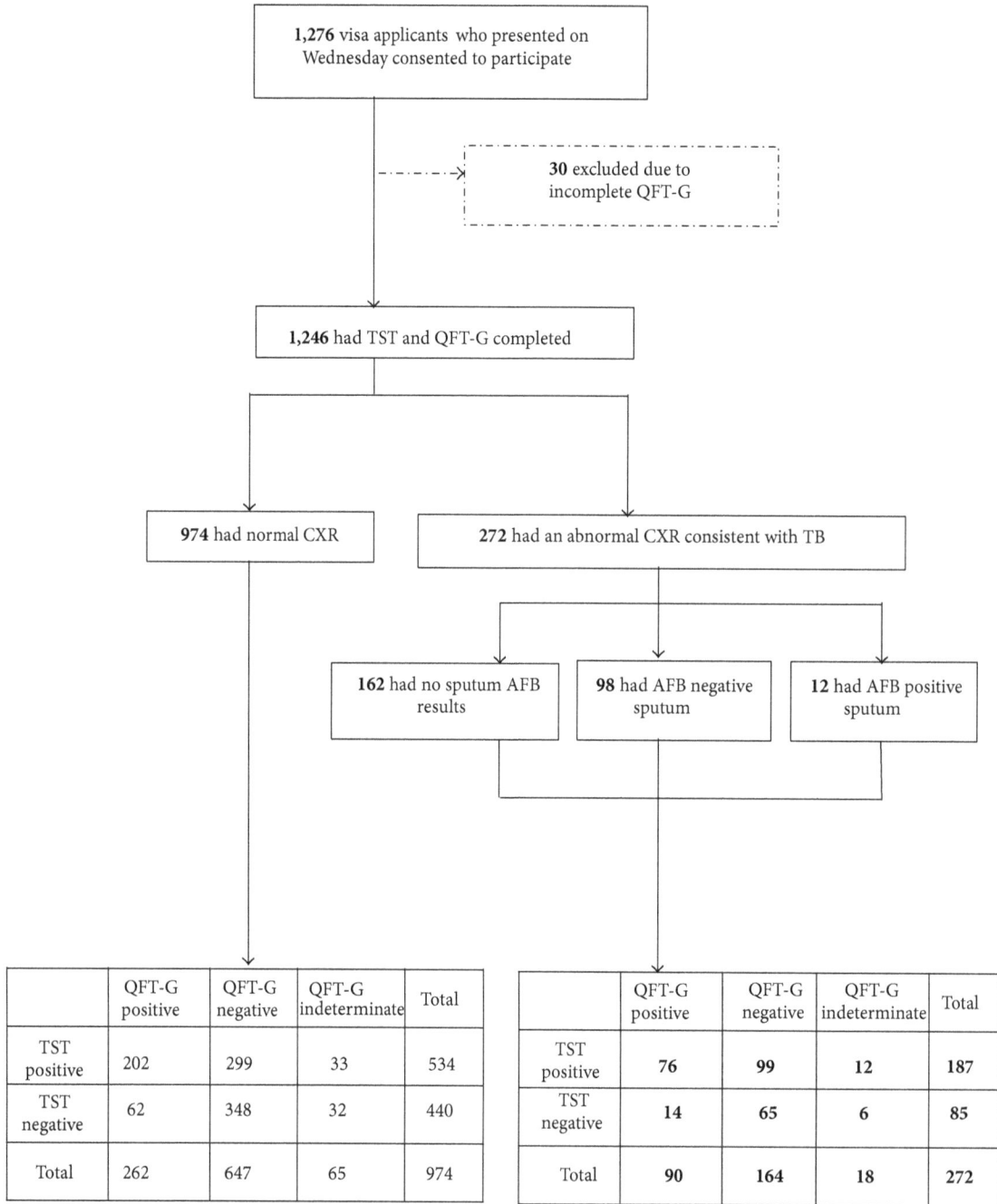

FIGURE 1: Participation diagram. Immigrant visa applicants who presented to Cho Ray Hospital on Wednesdays were asked to participate. QFT-G: QuantiFERON-TB Gold test; TST: tuberculin skin test; CXR: chest radiograph; TB: tuberculosis; AFB: acid fast bacillus.

4. Discussion

Our study demonstrates high MTBI prevalence among US-bound immigrant applicants as compared to the general US population. Of the 1,246 immigrant applicants included in our systematic sample from June 12, 2002, to March 12, 2003, 58% had a positive TST and 28% had a positive QFT-G. Both of these measures of MTBI prevalence are higher than the 4.2% prevalence reported among the general US population

in 2000 based on TST [32]. The prevalence of MTBI among visa immigrant applicants based on the TST is 14 times higher than the prevalence in the general US population using the same test. The prevalence among immigrant applicants based on QFT-G is 7 times higher than the TST-based estimate in the general US population. Estimates among other segments of the Vietnamese population also suggest high rates of MTBI. TST was positive in 61.1% of healthcare workers in Hanoi, Vietnam [33]. In 2005-2006, 6 to 7% of school children

TABLE 2: Mean, median, and interquartile range for TB response.

	Negative QFT-G	Positive QFT-G
Count	811	352
Mean (IU/mL)	0.05	3.91
Median (IU/mL)	0.30	1.53
Interquartile range (IU/mL)	0.10	3.60

QFT-G: QuantiFERON-TB Gold test.

6 to 9 years of age in Ho Chi Minh Province had TST reactions ≥ 15 mm [34]. As there is no diagnostic gold standard for documenting most MTBIs (including LTBI, culture-negative pulmonary TB, and most extrapulmonary TB), the true prevalence of MTBI is unknown.

TB screening of immigrant visa applicants overseas relies heavily on CXRs [10, 11]. All adult immigrant applicants residing outside the US are required to have a CXR and are not required to have a test for MTBI. In contrast, immigrant applicants already residing in the US are screened for MTBI with a TST or IGRA, and those with evidence of MTBI are required to have a CXR. Those with CXR findings compatible with TB are evaluated further for infectious TB by sputum AFB smear and/or culture. Screening by CXR is intended to identify applicants with infectious TB and has been effective [35]. Our study demonstrated that substantially fewer adult immigrant applicants had evidence of TB on CXR (22%) than had a positive TST (58%) or a positive QFT-G (28%). Thus, the current screening algorithm may leave a substantial number of immigrant applicants with LTBI undetected, untreated, and at increased risk of subsequently developing TB. In addition, people with extrapulmonary TB may have a normal CXR, [11, 24] and these persons may be missed using the current screening algorithm that relies on CXR.

Characteristics associated with a positive TST, QFT-G, or CXR (i.e., an abnormal CXR consistent with TB) were different (Table 3). Of the multiple subject characteristics associated with positive test results, only one (increased age) was associated with positive results by all three tests. The association with age suggests accumulating MTBI. Alternatively, older persons may have lived when TB was more prevalent and the association with age may represent a cohort effect. For CXR, this may also reflect cumulative scarring, disease, or infection due to other organisms or illness, but the associations with age persisted after adjustment for other factors.

Agreement between TST and QFT-G, CXR and TST, and CXR and QFT-G was poor (Table 4). Various subject characteristics are associated with the different types of discordance (Tables 5, 6, and 7). Some discordance may reflect the accumulation or presence of CXR lesions due to illnesses other than TB, as suggested by associations of discordance with age, other major medical conditions, and abnormal chest exams (Tables 6 and 7). Poor agreement between TST and QFT-G has been described in other studies [16, 36–39]. TST positive but QFT-G negative discordance has been attributed to false-positive TST results following BCG vaccination [36, 40] or NTM exposure [38] and false-negative

IGRA results [16, 37, 41–43]. TST negative but QFT-G positive discordance has been associated with immune suppression with lower TST sensitivity [26, 44], false-positive QFT-G results as described among low risk healthcare workers [45], or unexplained [42] as seen with the present study (Table 5).

BCG may contribute to false-positive TST results because it produces many of the antigens produced by MTB and that are present in the tuberculin PPD. However, BCG does not produce the antigens used in QFT-G (i.e., ESAT-6 and CFP-10) [15]. BCG is an attenuated *M. bovis* strain so that vaccination and infection do not typically cause disease or CXR lesions. In our study, BCG vaccination was associated with (1) positive TST results, (2) TST positive but QFT-G negative discordance, and (3) CXR negative but TST positive discordance (using a 10 mm cutoff). These findings support the hypothesis that some TST reactions ≥ 10 mm may be due to BCG vaccination. They appear to disagree with conclusions of others that induration ≥ 10 mm is unlikely due to BCG administered at infancy and more than 10 years prior to the TST [46] because BCG is given only at birth in Vietnam [21] and the youngest subject enrolled in our study was 18 years of age. Further analysis of our data showed that TST induration ≥ 15 mm was not associated with BCG vaccination. This suggests that, in our study population, TST induration < 15 mm (including those with induration of 10 to 15 mm) may be due to BCG vaccination, but induration ≥ 15 is more likely due to MTBI than to BCG. Prior BCG vaccination does not account for all TST positive but QFT-G negative discordance since almost half (46%) of the TST results ≥ 15 mm were in subjects who were not vaccinated. Additionally, this type of discordance was associated with age and it is unlikely that the degree of discordance due to BCG would increase with age.

We hypothesized that NTM infection might cause false-positive TST results and contribute to TST positive but QFT-G negative discordance. However, *M. avium* reactivity was not associated with TST positive but QFT-G negative discordance. Additionally, positive TST results and positive QFT-G results were less common among participants with *M. avium* reactivity as measured by QFT (Table 3). One possibility is that *M. avium* responsiveness may offer some protection against MTB infection. This is in contrast to findings in the US where *M. avium* reactivity was associated with TST induration ≥ 10 mm and with TST positive but QFT-G negative discordance, but not with positive QFT-G results [16]. These findings were attributed to cross-reactivity with *M. avium* causing false-positive TST reactions.

We observed an association between male sex and (1) positive TST results, (2) CXR findings consistent with TB, (3) TST positive but QFT-G negative discordance, and (4) negative CXR but positive TST results. Male predominance among those infected with MTB and those with TB disease has been described previously and may be due to gender differences in occupational or social MTB exposure [17, 47, 48]. Smoking may increase TB risk and smoking among Vietnamese males is common but among females is rare [49, 50]. These findings and the observation that almost half (46%) of the TST results ≥ 15 mm were QFT-G negative suggest that some of the discordance is due to false-negative QFT-G results as suggested previously [16, 37, 41–43].

TABLE 3: Subject characteristics associated with chest radiographs consistent with tuberculosis; TST induration ≥ 10 mm; or positive QFT-G results.

Characteristic	N	CXR consistent with tuberculosis		TST induration ≥ 10 mm		Positive QFT-G	
		n	aOR* (95% CI)	n	aOR* (95% CI)	n	aOR* (95% CI)
Total	1,246	272		721		352	
Age group							
18–20 years	139	9 (6.5%)	1.0	49 (35.3%)	1.0	25 (18.0%)	1.0
21–30 years	293	19 (6.5%)	1.01 (0.44–2.32)	143 (48.8%)	**2.17 (1.40–3.35)**	77 (26.3%)	**1.66 (1.002–2.759)**
31–40 years	294	36 (12.2%)	2.06 (0.96–4.42)	199 (67.7%)	**4.14 (2.67–6.43)**	89 (30.3%)	**1.97 (1.19–3.25)**
41–50 years	268	80 (29.9%)	**5.87 (2.84–12.15)**	171 (63.8%)	**3.49 (2.24–5.46)**	91 (34.0%)	**2.29 (1.39–3.79)**
51–64 years	207	99 (47.8%)	**12.94 (6.23–26.89)**	137 (66.2%)	**4.22 (2.61–6.81)**	60 (29.0%)	**1.81 (1.07–3.07)**
≥65 years	45	24 (64.4%)	**25.12 (10.06–62.70)**	22 (48.9%)	1.92 (0.95–3.92)	10 (22.2%)	1.26 (0.55–2.89)
Sex							
Female	842	148 (17.6%)	1.0	439 (52.1%)	1.0	226 (26.8%)	
Male	404	124 (30.7%)	**1.69 (1.24–2.29)**	282 (69.8%)	**2.09 (1.60–2.73)**	126 (31.2%)	N.S. and NIM
BCG status							
Not vaccinated	735	191 (26.0%)		398 (54.1%)	1.0	215 (29.3%)	
Vaccinated	511	81 (58.8%)	N.S. and NIM	323 (63.2%)	**1.62 (1.25–2.09)**	137 (26.8%)	
Chest exam							
Normal	1239	266 (21.5%)	1.0	718 (57.9%)		351 (28.3%)	
Abnormal	7	6 (85.7%)	**31.23 (3.04–320.68)**	3 (42.9%)	N.S. and NIM	1 (14.3%)	N.S. and NIM
M. avium reactivity							
No	884	217 (24.5%)		550 (62.2%)	1.0	268 (30.3%)	1.0
Yes	362	55 (15.2%)	N.S. and NIM	171 (47.2%)	**0.59 (0.46–0.77)**	84 (23.2%)	**0.71 (0.53–0.95)**

CXR: chest radiographs; TST: tuberculin skin test; QFT-G: QuantiFERON-TB Gold test; n: number in subset of N; aOR: adjusted odd ratio; 95% CI: 95% confidence interval; N.S.: not significant; NIM: not in model; BCG: bacille Calette-Guérin; TB: tuberculosis; QFT: QuantiFERON-TB test.
*Multivariate models were created using factors with P values ≤0.2 in univariate analysis and <0.05 in stepwise logistic regression until the best fitting, parsimonious model was identified. Model fit was evaluated using the Hosmer-Lemeshow test. Negative and indeterminate QFT-G results were coded as "not positive." The variable "Prior TB" was not included in the model because all 7 subjects with prior TB had CXR findings consistent with TB disease and its inclusion prevented convergence of the model. **Bold font** indicates statistically significant adjusted odds ratios (aORs).

TABLE 4: Agreement* of TST versus QFT-G, CXR versus TST, and CXR versus QFT-G.

	TST versus QFT-G	CXR versus TST	CXR versus QFT-G
Positive/positive results; n (%)	278 (23.9)	175 (15.0)	90 (7.7)
Negative/negative results; n (%)	413 (35.5)	408 (35.1)	647 (55.6)
Positive/negative results; n (%)	398 (34.2)	79 (6.8)	164 (14.1)
Negative/positive results; n (%)	74 (6.4)	501 (43.1)	262 (22.5)
Agreement; % (95% CI)	59.4 (56.6–62.2)	50.1 (47.2–52.9)	63.4 (60.6–66.2)
Kappa coefficient; κ (95% CI)	0.24 (0.19–0.28)	0.09 (0.05–0.13)	0.058 (0.001–0.115)

CXR: chest radiographs; TST: tuberculin skin test; QFT-G: QuantiFERON-TB Gold test; n: number in subset of N; 95% CI: 95% confidence interval.
*Agreement was assessed among 1,163 subjects; data from 83 subjects with indeterminate QFT-G results were excluded from analysis.

Neither TST nor QFT-G performed well as predictors of an abnormal CXR consistent with TB in this population. The PPVs of both TST and QFT-G for an abnormal CXR were extremely low (25.9% and 25.6%, resp.), which may not be surprising because we expect that a large number of those with a normal CXR may have LTBI that has not progressed to TB disease. The NPVs of TST and QFT-G were also less than optimal (83.8% and 79.8%, resp.), possibly because many CXR abnormalities are not due to TB. Of more importance is the accuracy of these tests for active TB disease. Too few culture results were available to reliably assess the sensitivity of TST or QFT-G for culture-confirmed TB in our systematic

sample. A review of studies comparing TST and QFT-G among people with active TB reports a pooled sensitivity of 77% and 78%, respectively [51].

We recognize several limitations with this study. First, while immigrant applicants from all regions of Vietnam are evaluated at the Cho Ray Hospital Clinic, it is unknown if the prevalence of MTBI in the general Vietnamese population is similar to the prevalence among immigrant applicants. Second, selection bias could have occurred due to our restriction of enrollment to applicants presenting on Wednesday. However, none of our experiences or data suggested an enrollment bias. Third, recall bias may limit studies that

TABLE 5: Subject characteristics associated with TST and QFT-G discordance.

Characteristic	N	TST positive but QFT-G negative		TST negative but QFT-G positive	
		n	aOR* (95% CI)	n	aOR* (95% CI)
Total	1,163**	398		74	
Age group in years					
18–20 yrs	130	27 (20.8%)	1.0	7 (5.4%)	N.S. and NIM
21–30 yrs	270	80 (29.6%)	**1.86 (1.12–3.09)**	25 (9.3%)	
31–40 yrs	279	116 (41.6%)	**2.81 (1.72–4.61)**	16 (5.7%)	
41–50 yrs	252	85 (33.7%)	**2.16 (1.30–3.59)**	14 (5.7%)	
51–64 yrs	189	76 (40.2%)	**3.17 (1.86–5.39)**	10 (5.3%)	
≥65 yrs	43	14 (32.6%)	**2.27 (1.03–4.99)**	2 (4.7%)	
Sex					
Female	781	239 (30.6%)	1.0	56 (7.2%)	N.S. and NIM
Male	382	159 (41.6%)	**1.62 (1.24–2.10)**	18 (4.7%)	
BCG status					
Not vaccinated	684	203 (29.7%)	1.0	44 (6.4%)	N.S. and NIM
Vaccinated	479	195 (40.7%)	**1. 79 (1.38–2.34)**	30 (6.3%)	

TST: tuberculin skin test; QFT-G: QuantiFERON-TB Gold test; n: number in subset of N; aOR: adjusted odd ratio; 95% CI: 95% confidence interval; N.S.: not significant; NIM: not in model; BCG: bacille Calmitte-Guérin; QFT: QuantiFERON-TB test.
*Multivariate models were created using factors with P values ≤0.2 in univariate analysis and <0.05 in stepwise logistic regression until the best fitting, parsimonious model was identified. Model fit was evaluated using the Hosmer-Lemeshow test. **Bold font** indicates statistically significant aORs.
**Data from 83 subjects with indeterminate QFT-G results were excluded from analysis.

TABLE 6: Subject characteristics associated with CXR and TST discordance.

Characteristic	N	CXR positive but TST negative		CXR negative but TST positive	
		n	aOR* (95% CI)	n	aOR* (95% CI)
Total	1163**	79		501	
Age group in years					
18–20 yrs	130	6 (4.6%)	1.0	42 (32.3%)	1.0
21–30 yrs	270	3 (1.1%)	**0.23 (0.06–0.94)**	120 (44.4%)	**1.90 (1.22–2.98)**
31–40 yrs	279	7 (2.5%)	0.53 (0.17–1.59)	161 (57.7%)	**2.91 (1.87–4.53)**
41–50 yrs	252	19 (7.5%)	1.59 (0.62–4.11)	103 (40.9%)	1.54 (0.98–2.42)
51–64 yrs	189	32 (16.9%)	**3.88 (1.57–9.62)**	69 (36.5%)	1.38 (0.85–2.25)
≥65 yrs	43	12 (27.9%)	**6.76 (2.31–19.79)**	6 (14.0%)	0.39 (0.15–1.004)
Sex					
Female	781	51 (6.5%)		324 (41.5%)	1.0
Male	382	28 (7.3%)	N.S. and NIM	177 (46.3%)	**1.33 (1.03–1.73)**
Other major medical conditions					
No	1146	72 (6.3%)	1.0	497 (43.4%)	
Yes	17	7 (41.2%)	**4.52 (1.58–12.96)**	4 (23.5%)	N.S. and NIM
BCG status					
Not vaccinated	684	58 (8.5%)		253 (37.0%)	1.0
Vaccinated	479	21 (4.4%)	N.S. and NIM	248 (51.8%)	**1.61 (1.25–2.07)**
M. avium reactivity					
No	812	58 (7.1%)		369 (45.4%)	1.0
Yes	351	21 (6.0%)	N.S. and NIM	132 (37.5%)	**0.71 (0.54–0.93)**

CXR: chest radiograph; TST: tuberculin skin test; n: number in subset of N; aOR: adjusted odd ratio; 95% CI: 95% confidence interval; N.S.: not significant; NIM: not in model; BCG: bacille Calmitte-Guérin; QFT: QuantiFERON-TB test.
*Multivariate models were created using factors with P values ≤0.2 in univariate analysis and <0.05 in stepwise logistic regression until the best fitting, parsimonious model was identified. Model fit was evaluated using the Hosmer-Lemeshow test. **Bold font** indicates statistically significant adjusted odds ratios (aORs).
**Data from 83 subjects with indeterminate QFT-G results were excluded from analysis.

TABLE 7: Subject characteristics associated with CXR and QFT-G discordance.

Characteristic	N	CXR positive but QFT-G negative		CXR negative but QFT-G positive	
		n	aOR* (95% CI)	n	aOR* (95% CI)
Total	1163**	164		262	
Age group in years					
18–20 yrs	130	8 (6.2%)	1.0	24 (18.5%)	1.0
21–30 yrs	270	7 (2.6%)	0.36 (0.12–1.02)	69 (25.6%)	1.52 (0.90–2.55)
31–40 yrs	279	18 (6.5%)	1.02 (0.43–2.43)	72 (25.8%)	1.54 (0.92–2.58)
41–50 yrs	252	47 (18.7%)	**3.16 (1.44–6.95)**	60 (23.8%)	1.38 (0.82–2.34)
51–64 yrs	189	64 (33.9%)	**7.60 (3.49–16.53)**	35 (18.5%)	1.004 (0.565–1.784)
≥65 yrs	43	20 (14.1%)	**13.26 (5.22–33.72)**	2 (4.7%)	**0.215 (0.05–0.95)**
Prior TB					
No	1157	160 (13.8%)	1.0	262 (22.7%)	
Yes	6	4 (66.7%)	**16.26 (2.42–109.33)**	0 (0.0%)	N.S. and NIM
Chest exam					
Normal	1157	160 (13.8%)	1.0	262 (22.7%)	
Abnormal	6	4 (66.7%)	**20.81 (2.76–156.68)**	0 (0.0%)	N.S. and NIM

CXR: chest radiograph; QFT-G: QuantiFERON-TB Gold; n: number in subset of N; aOR: adjusted Odd Ratio; 95% CI: 95% confidence interval; TB: tuberculosis; N.S.: Not Significant; NIM: Not in model.
*Multivariate models were created using factors with P-values ≤0.2 in univariate analysis and <0.05 in stepwise logistic regression until the best fitting, parsimonious model was identified. Model fit was evaluated using the Hosmer-Lemeshow test. **Bold font** indicates statistically significant adjusted odds ratios (aORs).
**Data from 83 subjects with indeterminate QFT-G results were excluded from analysis.

rely on questionnaires, especially when asking about BCG vaccination. In Vietnam, with universal BCG vaccination and estimated vaccination coverage of 93.7%, we might have expected higher reported BCG vaccination rates than the 41% that we found among the study participants. On the other hand, our findings might be related to the specific visa applicant pool we evaluated (in terms of such variables as birth place/province within Vietnam, mobility, age, or socioeconomic strata); our study collected information on the presence of BCG scars as well, and we found that for every individual with a positive BCG vaccination history, there was a corresponding scar seen on physical examination. If we assumed that BCG vaccination was universal (but masked by recall bias linked to absence of a visible scar) and removed BCG from our models, the magnitude of the adjusted odds ratios for the remaining variables (e.g., age, sex, and *M. avium* reactivity) changed little and there was no addition or loss of variables with significance (data not shown). QFT and QFT-G have been supplanted by the newer QuantiFERON-TB Gold In-Tube test (QFT-GIT). Similar study outcomes would be expected with QFT-GIT as compared to QFT-G because of similar sensitivity and specificity [51]. Availability of QFT for this study allowed assessment of *M. avium* reactivity which could no longer be done with a commercial assay.

In conclusion, the estimated prevalence of MTBI among US-bound visa applicants in Vietnam based on TST was twice that based on QFT-G and 14 times higher than a TST-based estimate of MTBI prevalence reported for the general US population at approximately the same time. QFT-G was not better than TST at predicting abnormal CXRs consistent with TB.

Disclosure

The Centers for Disease Control and Prevention (CDC) provided funding for this study. CDC reviewed the study design, data collection methods, and analysis plans prior to approval. CDC cleared the paper for publication according to established guidelines. Cellestis Ltd. (VIC, Australia) provided antigens and ELISA kits that were used to measure interferon gamma concentrations. No outside funders had a role in the analysis, decision to publish, or preparation of the paper.

Disclaimer

The contents of this document are the sole responsibility of the authors and do not necessarily represent the views of the Centers for Disease Control and Prevention. Mention of trade commercial products does not imply endorsement by the US Government.

Authors' Contribution

Susan A. Maloney, Kayla F. Laserson, J. Jina Shah, and Gerald H. Mazurek conceived and designed the study and experiments. Le Thien Huong Loan, Nguyen Thi Ngoc Yen, Vo Thi Chi Mai, An Dang Qui, Nguyen Huu Phuoc,

Nguyen An Trinh, Duong Thi Cam Nhung, Warren G. Jones, Gerald H. Mazurek, Susan A. Maloney, and Kayla F. Laserson performed or supervised the experiments or data collection. Stella O. Chuke, Le Thien Huong Loan, William C. Whitworth, and Gerald H. Mazurek analyzed the data. Stella O. Chuke, Gerald H. Mazurek, William C. Whitworth, John A. Painter, Kayla F. Laserson, and Susan A. Maloney wrote the paper with input from all authors.

Acknowledgments

The authors thank the volunteers who participated in this study. They also thank Carla A. Winston, John M. Williamson, and William K. Y. Pan for advice on statistical methods; Brandon H. Campbell for assistance with data management; Eugene McCray and Drew L. Posey for explanation of the technical instructions for panel physicians; and Jay K. Varma, Truong Van Viet, Tran Thi Tin, Truong Xuan Lien, Nguyen Thi Thu, Nguyen Thi Ngoc Lan, Martin S. Cetron, and Tomas O'Rourke for their contribution to this study.

References

[1] C. Dye, "Global epidemiology of tuberculosis," *The Lancet*, vol. 367, no. 9514, pp. 938–940, 2006.

[2] World Health Organization, "Global Tuberculosis Control: WHO Report 2012," 2012, http://www.who.int/tb/publications/global_report/en/index.html.

[3] World Health Organization, "Global Tuberculosis Control. WHO Report 1997," 1997, http://www.who.int/tb/publications/1997/en/index.html.

[4] M. C. Raviglione, D. E. Snider Jr., and A. Kochi, "Global epidemiology of tuberculosis: morbidity and mortality of a worldwide epidemic," *Journal of the American Medical Association*, vol. 273, no. 3, pp. 220–226, 1995.

[5] Centers for Disease Control and Prevention, "Targeted tuberculin testing and treatment of latent tuberculosis infection," *MMWR: Morbidity and Mortality Weekly Report*, vol. 49, pp. 1–51, 2000.

[6] K. P. Cain, S. R. Benoit, C. A. Winston, and W. R. Mac Kenzie, "Tuberculosis among foreign-born persons in the United States," *Journal of the American Medical Association*, vol. 300, no. 4, pp. 405–412, 2008.

[7] Centers for Disease Control and Prevention, "Reported Tuberculosis in the United States, 2011," 2012, http://www.cdc.gov/tb/statistics/reports/2011/pdf/report2011.pdf.

[8] Centers for Disease Control and Prevention, "Tuberculosis among foreign-born persons entering the United States. Recommendations of the Advisory Committee for Elimination of Tuberculosis," *MMWR Recommendations and Reports*, vol. 39, pp. 1–21, 1990.

[9] Y. Liu, M. S. Weinberg, L. S. Ortega, J. A. Painter, and S. A. Maloney, "Overseas screening for tuberculosis in U.S.-bound immigrants and refugees," *The New England Journal of Medicine*, vol. 360, no. 23, pp. 2406–2415, 2009.

[10] Centers for Disease Control and Prevention, "1991 Technical Instructions for panel physicians for medical examination of aliens," 1992, http://www.cdc.gov/immigrantrefugeehealth/exams/ti/panel/technical-instructions/panel-physicians/tuberculosis.html.

[11] Centers for Disease Control and Prevention, "2007 Tuberculosis Screening and Treatment Technical Instructions for Panel Physicians," 2009, http://www.cdc.gov/immigrantrefugeehealth/pdf/tuberculosis-ti-2009.pdf.

[12] Centers for Disease Control and Prevention, "Tuberculosis Technical Instructions for Civil Physicians: 2008 Tuberculosis Component of Technical Instructions for the Medical Examination of Aliens in the United States," 2008.

[13] G. H. Mazurek, J. Jereb, A. Vernon, P. LoBue, S. Goldberg, and K. Castros, "Updated guidelines for using interferon gamma release assays to detect Mycobacterium tuberculosis infection. United States, 2010," *Morbidity and Mortality Weekly Report*, vol. 59, no. 5, pp. 1–25, 2010.

[14] G. H. Mazurek and M. E. Villarino, "Guidelines for using the QuantiFERON-TB test for diagnosing latent Mycobacterium tuberculosis infection. Centers for Disease Control and Prevention," *MMWR Recommendations and Reports*, vol. 52, no. 2, pp. 15–18, 2003.

[15] P. Andersen, M. E. Munk, J. M. Pollock, and T. M. Doherty, "Specific immune-based diagnosis of tuberculosis," *The Lancet*, vol. 356, no. 9235, pp. 1099–1104, 2000.

[16] G. H. Mazurek, M. J. Zajdowicz, A. L. Hankinson et al., "Detection of *Mycobacterium tuberculosis* infection in United States Navy recruits using the tuberculin skin test or whole-blood interferon-γ release assays," *Clinical Infectious Diseases*, vol. 45, no. 7, pp. 826–836, 2007.

[17] T. Horie, L. T. Lien, L. A. Tuan et al., "A survey of tuberculosis prevalence in Hanoi, Vietnam," *International Journal of Tuberculosis and Lung Disease*, vol. 11, no. 5, pp. 562–566, 2007.

[18] T. N. Buu, D. van Soolingen, M. N. T. Huyen et al., "Tuberculosis acquired outside of households, rural Vietnam," *Emerging Infectious Diseases*, vol. 16, no. 9, pp. 1466–1468, 2010.

[19] H. M. El Sahly, G. J. Adams, H. Soini, L. Teeter, J. M. Musser, and E. A. Graviss, "Epidemiologic differences between United States- and foreign-born tuberculosis patients in Houston, Texas," *Journal of Infectious Diseases*, vol. 183, no. 3, pp. 461–468, 2001.

[20] J. Bablet, "La prémunition antituberculeuse des nouveau nés par ingestion de BCG en Cochinchine (1924-1925)," *Archives Des Instituts Pasteur D'Indochine*, vol. 2, pp. 208–212, 1925.

[21] N. T. Huong, B. D. Duong, N. V. Co et al., "Tuberculosis epidemiology in six provinces of Vietnam after the introduction of the DOTS strategy," *International Journal of Tuberculosis and Lung Disease*, vol. 10, no. 9, pp. 963–969, 2006.

[22] A. Zwerlingand and M. Pai, "The BCG World Atlas: A database of Global BCG vaccination Policy and Practice," 2011, http://www.bcgatlas.org/.

[23] K. F. Laserson, N. T. N. Yen, C. G. Thornton et al., "Improved sensitivity of sputum smear microscopy after processing specimens with C18-carboxypropylbetaine to detect acid-fast bacilli: a study of United States-bound immigrants from Vietnam," *Journal of Clinical Microbiology*, vol. 43, no. 7, pp. 3460–3462, 2005.

[24] S. A. Maloney, K. L. Fielding, K. F. Laserson et al., "Assessing the performance of overseas tuberculosis screening programs: a study among US-bound immigrants in Vietnam," *Archives of Internal Medicine*, vol. 166, no. 2, pp. 234–240, 2006.

[25] P. T. Kent and G. P. Kubica, *Public Health Mycobacteriology: A Guide for the Level III Laboratory*, 1985.

[26] G. H. Mazurek, S. E. Weis, P. K. Moonan et al., "Prospective comparison of the tuberculin skin test and 2 whole-blood

interferon-γ release assays in persons with suspected tuberculosis," *Clinical Infectious Diseases*, vol. 45, no. 7, pp. 837–845, 2007.

[27] The American Thoracic Society and Centers for Disease Control, "Diagnostic standards and classification of tuberculosis in adults and children," *The American Journal of Respiratory and Critical Care Medicine*, vol. 161, pp. 1376–1395, 2000.

[28] J. L. Fleiss, "The measurement of interrater agreement," in *Statistical Methods For Rates and Proportions*, R. A. Bradley, J. S. Hunter, D. G. Kendal, and G. S. Watson, Eds., pp. 212–236, John Wiley and Sons, New York, NY, USA, 1981.

[29] W. Leisenring, T. Alonzo, and M. S. Pepe, "Comparisons of predictive values of binary medical diagnostic tests for paired designs," *Biometrics*, vol. 56, no. 2, pp. 345–351, 2000.

[30] A. Trajman and R. R. Luiz, "McNemar χ^2 test revisited: comparing sensitivity and specificity of diagnostic examinations," *Scandinavian Journal of Clinical and Laboratory Investigation*, vol. 68, no. 1, pp. 77–80, 2008.

[31] D. W. Hosmer and S. Lemeshow, *Applied Logistic Regression*, John Wiley and Sons, New York, NY, USA, 1989.

[32] D. E. Bennett, J. M. Courval, I. Onorato et al., "Prevalence of tuberculosis infection in the United States population: the national health and nutrition examination survey, 1999-2000," *The American Journal of Respiratory and Critical Care Medicine*, vol. 177, no. 3, pp. 348–355, 2008.

[33] L. T. Lien, N. T. L. Hang, N. Kobayashi et al., "Prevalence and risk factors for tuberculosis infection among hospital workers in Hanoi, Viet Nam," *PLoS ONE*, vol. 4, no. 8, Article ID e6798, 2009.

[34] T. N. Buu, H. T. Quy, N. C. Qui, N. T. N. Lan, D. N. Sy, and F. G. J. Cobelens, "Decrease in risk of tuberculosis infection despite increase in tuberculosis among young adults in urban Vietnam," *International Journal of Tuberculosis and Lung Disease*, vol. 14, no. 3, pp. 289–295, 2010.

[35] P. Lowenthal, J. Westenhouse, M. Moore, D. L. Posey, J. P. Watt, and J. Flood, "Reduced importation of tuberculosis after the implementation of an enhanced pre-immigration screening protocol," *International Journal of Tuberculosis and Lung Disease*, vol. 15, no. 6, pp. 761–766, 2011.

[36] Y. A. Kang, H. W. Lee, H. I. Yoon et al., "Discrepancy between the tuberculin skin test and the whole-blood interferon γ assay for the diagnosis of latent tuberculosis infection in an intermediate tuberculosis-burden country," *Journal of the American Medical Association*, vol. 293, no. 22, pp. 2756–2761, 2005.

[37] H. Mahomed, E. J. Hughes, T. Hawkridge et al., "Comparison of Mantoux skin test with three generations of a whole blood IFN-γ assay for tuberculosis infection," *International Journal of Tuberculosis and Lung Disease*, vol. 10, no. 3, pp. 310–316, 2006.

[38] A. K. Detjen, T. Keil, S. Roll et al., "Interferon-γ release assays improve the diagnosis of tuberculosis and nontuberculous mycobacterial disease in children in a country with a low incidence of tuberculosis," *Clinical Infectious Diseases*, vol. 45, no. 3, pp. 322–328, 2007.

[39] S. V. Kik, W. P. J. Franken, S. M. Arend et al., "Interferon-gamma release assays in immigrant contacts and effect of remote exposure to *Mycobacterium tuberculosis*," *International Journal of Tuberculosis and Lung Disease*, vol. 13, no. 7, pp. 820–828, 2009.

[40] A. Nienhaus, A. Schablon, and R. Diel, "Interferon-gamma release assay for the diagnosis of latent TB infection: analysis of discordant results, when compared to the tuberculin skin test," *PLoS ONE*, vol. 3, no. 7, Article ID e2665, 2008.

[41] S. O'Neal, K. Hedberg, A. Markum, and S. Schafer, "Discordant tuberculin skin and interferon-gamma tests during contact investigations: a dilemma for tuberculosis controllers," *International Journal of Tuberculosis and Lung Disease*, vol. 13, no. 5, pp. 662–664, 2009.

[42] M. Pai, S. Kalantri, and D. Menzies, "Discordance between tuberculin skin test and interferon-gamma assays [1]," *International Journal of Tuberculosis and Lung Disease*, vol. 10, no. 8, pp. 942–943, 2006.

[43] N. R. Pollock, A. Campos-Neto, S. Kashino et al., "Discordant QuantiFERON-TB gold test results among US healthcare workers with increased risk of latent tuberculosis infection: a problem or solution?" *Infection Control and Hospital Epidemiology*, vol. 29, no. 9, pp. 878–886, 2008.

[44] J. Y. Lee, H. J. Choi, I.-N. Park et al., "Comparison of two commercial interferon-γ assays for diagnosing *Mycobacterium tuberculosis* infection," *European Respiratory Journal*, vol. 28, no. 1, pp. 24–30, 2006.

[45] M. Ahmad and G. R. Pesola, "False-positive QuantiFERON gold tests," *Chest*, vol. 138, p. 84, 2014.

[46] M. Farhat, C. Greenaway, M. Pai, and D. Menzies, "False-positive tuberculin skin tests: what is the absolute effect of BCG and non-tuberculous mycobacteria?" *International Journal of Tuberculosis and Lung Disease*, vol. 10, no. 11, pp. 1192–1204, 2006.

[47] P. Hudelson, "Gender differentials in tuberculosis: the role of socio-economic and cultural factors," *Tubercle and Lung Disease*, vol. 77, no. 5, pp. 391–400, 1996.

[48] R. W. Sutter and E. Haefliger, "Tuberculosis morbidity and infection in Vietnamese in Southeast Asian refugee camps," *The American Review of Respiratory Disease*, vol. 141, no. 6, pp. 1483–1486, 1990.

[49] A. J. Plant, R. E. Watkins, B. Gushulak et al., "Predictors of tuberculin reactivity among prospective Vietnamese migrants: the effect of smoking," *Epidemiology and Infection*, vol. 128, no. 1, pp. 37–45, 2002.

[50] R. E. Watkins and A. J. Plant, "Does smoking explain sex differences in the global tuberculosis epidemic?" *Epidemiology and Infection*, vol. 134, no. 2, pp. 333–339, 2006.

[51] M. Pai, A. Zwerling, and D. Menzies, "Systematic review: T-cell-based assays for the diagnosis of latent tuberculosis infection: an update," *Annals of Internal Medicine*, vol. 149, no. 3, pp. 177–184, 2008.

17

Multiplex Analysis of Pro- or Anti-Inflammatory Serum Cytokines and Chemokines in relation to Gender and Age among Tanzanian Tuberculous Lymphadenitis Patients

Tehmina Mustafa,[1,2] **Karl Albert Brokstad,**[3] **Sayoki G. Mfinanga,**[4] **and Harald G. Wiker**[5]

[1]*Centre for International Health, Department of Global Public Health and Primary Care, University of Bergen, 5021 Bergen, Norway*
[2]*Department of Thoracic Medicine, Haukeland University Hospital, 5021 Bergen, Norway*
[3]*Broegelmann Research Laboratory, Department of Clinical Science, University of Bergen, 5021 Bergen, Norway*
[4]*National Institute for Medical Research, Muhimbili, Tanzania*
[5]*The Gade Research Group for Infection and Immunity, Department of Clinical Science, University of Bergen, 5021 Bergen, Norway*

Correspondence should be addressed to Tehmina Mustafa; tehmina.mustafa@cih.uib.no

Academic Editor: Paul R. Klatser

Objectives. Tuberculous lymphadenitis is the most common form of extrapulmonary tuberculosis (TB) with a female and paediatric preponderance, postulated to be due to differences in the immune response. The aim of this study was to analyze the differences in the serum cytokine levels of tuberculous lymphadenitis patients with respect to age and gender. *Methods.* A multiplex bead-based enzyme-linked immunosorbent assay was used to measure IFN-γ, TNF-α, GM-CSF, IL-1β, IL-2, IL-4, IL-5, IL-6, IL-8, IL-10, IL-12, IL-15, and IL-17 levels in sera of patients ($n = 86$) and healthy controls ($n = 23$). *Results.* Levels of IFN-γ, TNF-α, GM-CSF, IL-1β, IL-2, IL-4, and IL-6 were higher in adult patients than in controls, while those of IL-12 were lower ($P < 0.05$). Children had lower levels of TNF-α, GM-CSF, and IL-5 and higher levels of IL-2 compared with adult patients ($P < 0.05$). The male adult patients had higher levels of IL-17 and lower levels of IL-12 compared with female adult patients ($P < 0.05$). *Conclusion.* There were significant differences in the levels of circulating cytokines with respect to gender and age. Children had generally lower levels of cytokines as compared to adults, which could make them more susceptible. Findings do not support that female preponderance is due to differences in immune response.

1. Introduction

Extrapulmonary tuberculosis (TB) constitutes about 15 to 20% of all cases of TB. The true rate may be even higher due to incomplete reporting in many developing countries. The annual global incidence of EPTB has been increasing in last decades due to the changing TB control practices, spread of Human Immune Deficiency Virus (HIV), and the population growth. Lymphadenitis is the most common form of extrapulmonary TB with a female and paediatric preponderance [1–4]. Children belong to the category of relatively susceptible individuals to develop TB. The mechanisms by which women and children become more susceptible to develop TB lymphadenitis are not fully understood. TB lymphadenitis is usually a self-contained disease and there

is a granulomatous immune response in the lymph nodes which is considered to be a correlate of protective immunity. Formation of granulomas is achieved by cell-mediated immunity orchestrated by a complex interplay of cytokines and chemokines [5]. However, despite an effective cell-mediated immunity, eradication of the pathogen is not achieved and the disease runs a chronic course [6]. Mechanisms involved in the regulation of immune responses in TB lymphadenitis are not clear, and the knowledge of systemic levels of different cytokines is limited. Few studies have sought to determine the cytokine balance at the systemic level in a small number of patients with TB lymphadenitis by using the *ex vivo* cytokine production capacity of isolated peripheral blood mononuclear cells or CD4[+] T cells after stimulation [7, 8]. The *ex vivo* stimulated production of cytokines does not necessarily

TABLE 1: The characteristics of the study population.

	Adults ($n = 61$)	Children ($n = 25$)
Age in years	Median 28, range 16–75	Median 9, range 2–14
Males (n)	27	10
Females (n)	34	15
Culture positive (n)	13/61[*]	3/23[*]
HIV positive (n)	5/44[*]	0/12[*]
BCG vaccinated (n)	45/57[*]	21/25[*]

n = number of cases; [*]denominator denotes the number of cases where results were available.

provide insight into the actual status of the cytokine network *in vivo*. Indeed, in patients with severe bacterial infections much of the observed organ injury is considered to be related to enhanced *in vivo* production of proinflammatory cytokines, while peripheral blood mononuclear cells isolated from those patients produce significantly less cytokines upon stimulation as compared to cells from healthy controls [9]. We therefore decided to investigate unstimulated serum samples from TB lymphadenitis patients. The aim was to compare the immune response among TB lymphadenitis patients with respect to gender and age. A cytokine panel which best represented the spectrum of immune process involved in TB was analysed by multiplex bead-based enzyme-linked immunosorbent assay. This included the Th1 (INF-γ, TNF-α) versus Th2 (IL-4, IL-5) balance, T-cell stimulation (IL-2, IL-12), macrophage activation (IL-1β), granuloma formation (IL-8), limitation of inflammation (IL-10), and other inflammatory cytokines and chemokines (IL-6, GM-CSF, IL-15, and IL-17).

2. Material and Methods

2.1. Patients. This study was conducted using a serum bank from patients diagnosed with TB lymphadenitis. These patients were recruited in an epidemiological study from four districts: Babati, Karatu, Hanang, and Mbulu of the Karatu region, Tanzania [10]. These patients were small-scale farmers, cattle-keepers, and nomads. The characteristics of the study population are provided in Table 1.

Diagnosis of TB lymphadenitis was based on strong clinical evidence according to the National Tuberculosis and Leprosy Control Programme clinical guidelines [11], that is, history of TB exposure, history of chronic relapsing fever, weight loss, and cervical swelling not responding to the common antibiotics. This was followed by the decision by a clinician to treat with a full course of anti-TB chemotherapy. The majority of patients presented with swelling in the neck. Other symptoms such as fever, pain, and weight loss were infrequent. About 50% of patients gave a history of TB in the family. History of previous TB treatment was given by about 1% of patients. Cervical lymph nodes were the main lymph nodes affected, enlarged in about 89% of the cases, while the axillary, inguinal, and mesenteric lymph nodes were

involved in a small proportion of cases [10]. In only 1% of patients there was concomitant pulmonary TB, and in 99% of patients no pulmonary or another extrapulmonary spread than lymphadenitis was observed.

Sera from 23 healthy Tanzanian blood donors aged between 18 and 70 were used as controls. These sera were obtained from the blood bank at Muhimbili Medical Centre, Dar es Salaam, Tanzania [12]. Skin tests or IGRA test for mycobacterial infection was not performed in the study subjects. BCG vaccination status was determined by history of vaccination and the presence of vaccination scar.

2.2. Ethics Statement. Ethical clearance was obtained from the National Medical Research Coordinating Committee in Tanzania. The project was discussed with and was exempted from ethical clearance in Norway as the principal investigator and the patient material were from Tanzania. All the participants provided their consent to participate in this study. In case of minors, consent was obtained from the parents. The consent was verbal as the study participants were from rural Tanzania and could not read or write. This consent form was approved by the ethics committee. The normal control sera used in the study were obtained from the biobank left after the completion of another study on the blood donors from Tanzania [12]. These sera were stored at the University of Bergen and permission to use these in this study was obtained from the responsible persons in Tanzania and Norway.

2.3. Collection and Storage of Blood Serum. Blood was drawn from the patients using standardized phlebotomy procedures. Handling and processing were similar for all patients. Blood samples were collected without anticoagulant into 10 mL BD vacutainer Z (Becton Dickinson & Company, NJ, USA) and allowed to coagulate for 20 to 30 minutes at room temperature. The sera were separated and transferred to NUNC tubes (NUNC/Thermo Fischer, Roskilde, Denmark) and stored at −20°C. The NUNC tubes were labelled with identification numbers to ensure the confidentiality of the results. The samples were later shipped to the University of Bergen, Norway, where they were aliquoted and stored at −20°C.

2.4. Culture and HIV Test Procedures. Open biopsy specimens were taken from all patients before starting any anti-TB chemotherapy. The specimens were divided into two, one for culture and another for histology. The specimen for culture was placed in a universal container and stored in a deep freezer. These frozen biopsy specimens were processed for culture using aseptic techniques in a safety cabinet. All specimens were decontaminated, digested by standard procedures, and inoculated onto Lowenstein-Jensen egg medium under 37°C incubation for at least eight weeks.

For HIV testing, pre- and posttest counselling were conducted, and patients were assured that the results would be handled confidentially. HIV testing was performed using single Behringer ELISA tests (Dade, Behring Marburg GmbH, Emil-von-Behring Marburg, Germany). Positive cases were repeated with Wellcozyme HIV Recombinant

TABLE 2: Serum cytokine levels in the adult and paediatric patients with tuberculous lymphadenitis and healthy controls.

Cytokine (pg/mL)	Adult patients ($n = 61$) Median (range)	Healthy controls ($n = 23$) Median (range)	P value*	Pediatric patients ($n = 25$) Median (range)	P value**
IFN-γ	0.0 (0–42.8)	0.0 (0–1.5)	0.001	0.0 (0–40.4)	0.268
TNF-α	8.4 (0–352.5)	2.5 (0–51.7)	0.005	3.2 (0–33.4)	0.015
GM-CSF	35.2 (0–506.9)	0.0 (0–379.2)	0.007	0.0 (0–147.9)	0.023
IL-1β	48.7 (0–6305.4)	0.0 (0–933.2)	0.004	4.0 (0–610.5)	0.338
IL-2	0.0 (0–28.2)	0.3 (0–16.3)	0.038	1.0 (0–105.6)	0.003
IL-4	0.0 (0–18.5)	0.0 (0–4.3)	0.002	0.0 (0–5.4)	0.208
IL-5	1.0 (0–10.0)	0.5 (0–12.5)	0.559	0.0 (0–1.5)	0.001
IL-6	47.4 (0–25781.5)	0.0 (0–9355.1)	0.000	44.1 (0–587.4)	0.244
IL-8	370.4 (0–386578.0)	65.9 (1.6–2888.2)	0.071	68.2 (0–3551.4)	0.195
IL-10	0.0 (0–29.3)	0.0 (0–36.2)	0.560	0.0 (0–9.9)	0.233
IL-12	0.0 (0–37.8)	2.7 (0–15.3)	0.000	0.0 (0–9.5)	0.701
IL-15	0.0 (0–61.4)	0.0 (0–12.7)	0.812	0.6 (0–53.3)	0.385
IL-17	0.0 (0–133.7)	0	0.282	0	0.262

*P value for difference between adult patients and healthy controls and **P value for difference between adult and pediatric patients.

(Murex Biotech, UK). Tests were conducted according to the manufacturer's protocol. Mycobacterial cultures were conducted at the Central Tuberculosis Reference Laboratory (CTRL) at NIMR Muhimbili Medical Centre, and HIV testing at National Reference Laboratory, at Muhimbili University of Health and Allied Sciences, Tanzania.

2.5. Multiplex Cytokine Bead-Based Enzyme-Linked Immunosorbent Assay (ELISA). To detect cytokines in the sera, a human cytokine thirteen-plex antibody bead assay (Biosource, Camarillo, CA, USA) was used according to the manufacturer's instructions with a Luminex 100 System. IFN-γ, TNF-α, GM-CSF, IL-1β, IL-2, IL-4, IL-5, IL-6, IL-8, IL-10, IL-12, IL-15, and IL-17 were quantified (pg/mL). A standard curve was created from threefold dilution series of premixed standards. The assay was performed in a 96-well filter bottom plate supplied with the kit. Premixed beads coated with the target antibodies were added to each well, followed by the 50 μL of incubation buffer. 100 μL/well of the assay diluent was subsequently added. Premixed standards and samples were then added to the wells and incubated for 2 hours. Subsequently premixed biotinylated detector antibody was added to each well and incubated for 1 hour, followed by incubation with Streptavidin-RPE for 30 minutes. All steps were performed at room temperature, and the samples and reagents were kept in the dark during the procedure. Between each step the plates were washed twice and each incubation step was performed on a rotating platform (600 rpm).

2.6. Data Management and Statistical Analysis. Statistical analysis was conducted using SPSS for Windows. A non-parametric Mann-Whitney test was used for two group comparisons. Spearman's rank correlation was performed to determine the relationship between two variables. P values less than 0.05 were considered significant.

3. Results

3.1. Cytokines/Chemokines in Adult Patients. Table 2 shows the cytokine levels in the adult TB lymphadenitis patients and healthy blood donors from Tanzania. Serum levels of IFN-γ, TNF-α, GM-CSF, IL-1β, IL-2, IL-4, and IL-6 were higher in the patients compared with healthy controls, while IL-12 levels were lower. Serum levels of IL-5, IL-8, IL-10, IL-15, and IL-17 were not statistically different in the two groups. There was a large variation in the amount of different cytokines in the sera of both patients and controls. Table 3 shows the correlations between various cytokines and chemokines. There was a positive correlation among IFN-γ, TNF-α, GM-CSF, IL-1β, IL-6, and IL-8. Th1 cytokines IFN-γ and TNF-α also correlated positively with the anti-inflammatory cytokine IL-10.

3.2. Differences in the Cytokine/Chemokines between Adults and Children. The levels of cytokines were generally lower in children as compared to adults with exception of IL-2 which was higher (Table 2). However, the statistically significant differences were only observed between serum levels of TNF-α, GM-CSF, and IL-5 and IL-2. There was a significant positive correlation among IFN-γ, TNF-α, GM-CSF, IL-6, and IL-8. Unlike the adult population, a negative correlation was observed between IL-5 and IL-12 and no significant positive correlation was observed between IFN-γ and TNF-α with anti-inflammatory IL-10 (Table 4).

3.3. Difference in Cytokines/Chemokines between Male and Female Adult Patients. The female adults had significantly lower levels of IL-17 and higher levels of IL-12 compared with the male adult patients (Table 5).

3.4. Relation of Cytokine/Chemokine Levels with Mycobacterial Culture. As detection of mycobacteria by culture reflects

Table 3: Relationship between the serum levels of cytokines in adult patients with tuberculous lymphadenitis ($n = 61$) based on Spearman's rank correlation. The values shown are the correlation coefficients.

	TNF-α	GM-CSF	IL-1β	IL-2	IL-4	IL-5	IL-6	IL-8	IL-10	IL-12	IL-15	IL-17
IFN-γ	.729**	.741**	.723**	.058	.018	.252*	.732**	.551**	.335**	−.193	−.025	.178
TNF-α		.828**	.724**	.081	.055	.217	.674**	.577**	.315*	−.035	.119	−.103
GM-CSF			.723**	.062	−.012	.230	.794**	.651**	.210	−.063	.075	−.051
IL-1β				.213	.312*	.287*	.687**	.539**	.275*	−.109	.208	.154
IL-2					.150	.275*	.076	−.028	.181	.183	.454**	.086
IL-4						.061	−.012	.068	.034	−.207	.037	.251
IL-5							.138	.261*	.241	.022	.188	−.134
IL-6								.597**	.066	−.038	−.050	.050
IL-8									.123	−.011	−.057	.076
IL-10										−.043	.068	.218
IL-12											.459**	−.171
IL-15												.011

**Correlation is significant at the 0.01 level (2-tailed). *Correlation is significant at the 0.05 level (2-tailed).

Table 4: Relationship between the serum levels of cytokines in children with tuberculous lymphadenitis ($n = 25$) based on Spearman's rank correlation. The values shown are the correlation coefficients.

	TNF-α	GM-CSF	IL-1β	IL-2	IL-4	IL-5	IL-6	IL-8	IL-10	IL-12	IL-15
IFN-γ	.566**	.716**	.369	−.244	.389	.274	.440*	.497*	.151	−.200	−.111
TNF-α		.802**	.611**	.028	.213	.303	.528**	.648**	.108	−.047	.291
GM-CSF			.726**	.039	.442*	.527**	.758**	.875**	.026	−.191	.154
IL-1				.336	.490*	.646**	.596**	.671**	−.176	−.114	.424*
IL-2					−.226	−.039	.122	.150	−.133	.256	.448*
IL-4						.745**	.341	.376	.008	−.391	−.076
IL-5							.401*	.469*	.070	−.538**	−.038
IL-6								.842**	−.190	−.282	.072
IL-8									−.068	−.115	.194
IL-10										−.259	−.474*
IL-12											.530**

**Correlation is significant at the 0.01 level (2-tailed). *Correlation is significant at the 0.05 level (2-tailed).

Table 5: Differences in the serum cytokine levels in the adult Tanzanian patients based on gender and mycobacterial culture from lymph nodes.

Cytokine (pg/mL)	Male ($n = 27$) Median (range)	Female ($n = 34$) Median (range)	P value*	Culture positive ($n = 13$) Median (range)	Culture negative ($n = 48$) Median (range)	P value**
IFN-γ	0.0 (0–42.8)	0.0 (0–30.9)	0.98	0.0 (0–22.4)	0.0 (0–42.8)	0.383
TNF-α	3.2 (0–352.5)	11.8 (0–73)	0.15	8.4 (0.5–352.5)	12.4 (0–72.9)	0.874
GM-CSF	35.2 (0–507)	55.1 (0–457)	0.96	35.2 (0–506.9)	34.5 (0–457.7)	0.864
IL-1β	72.6 (0–1338)	5.7 (0–6305)	0.51	0.0 (0–1338.8)	66.5 (0–6305.4)	0.746
IL-2	0.0 (0–28)	0.0 (0–19.8)	0.31	0.0 (0–28.2)	0.0 (0–19.8)	0.193
IL-4	0 (0–9.5)	0 (0–18)	0.30	0.0 (0–6.8)	0.0 (0–18.5)	0.360
IL-5	1.5 (0–10)	0.75 (0–6.4)	0.16	1.0 (0–8.1)	1.0 (0–10.0)	0.465
IL-6	46.4 (0–18979)	55.5 (0–25781)	0.80	46.4 (0–18979.1)	55.6 (0–25781.5)	0.825
IL-8	362 (0–27670)	419 (0–386577)	0.70	638.2 (0–27670.3)	366.4 (0–386578.0)	0.486
IL-10	0.0 (0–29)	0.0 (0–22)	0.96	0.0 (0–29.3)	0.0 (0–22.8)	0.513
IL-12	0 (0–20.7)	0.1 (0–37)	0.03	0.3 (0–20.7)	0.0 (0–37.8)	0.029
IL-15	0.0 (0–61)	0.0 (0–25)	0.77	0.6 (0–21.1)	0.0 (0–61.4)	0.223
IL-17	0 (0–134)	0	0.04	0.0 (0–26.1)	0.0 (0–133.7)	0.638

*P value for difference between males and females and **P value for difference between culture positive and culture negative TB patients.

the lesions with higher bacillary load, a comparison was made between he culture-positive and culture-negative cases to see how this difference is reflected in the immune response. Among the adult patients, 13 (21%) cases were culture-positive and these cases had higher level of IL-12 compared with culture-negative cases (Table 5). IL-12 correlated positively only with IL-15 in culture-positive patients. The levels of the other cytokines were not statistically different. Among children culture results were available for 23 cases and 3 (13%) cases were culture-positive. The levels of cytokines were not statistically different between the two groups. When the adult and paediatric patients were combined, the difference in culture-positive and culture-negative cases was similar to that in the adult patients.

4. Discussion

Pathogenic mycobacteria are known to stimulate the immune response in such a way that the eradication of the pathogen is not fully achieved and the inappropriately simulated immune response leads to tissue destruction and the progression of disease rather than achieving the eradication of infection [5, 13–15]. In this study there were higher levels of the proinflammatory cytokines IFN-γ, IL-2, and TNF-α, and the chemokines GM-CSF, IL-1β, and IL-6 among TB cases as compared to controls. The levels of the anti-inflammatory cytokines IL-10 and IL-5 which are expected to balance the proinflammatory cytokines were not different between TB cases and controls. These findings imply that a relative lack of anti-inflammatory cytokines and thereby reduced inhibition of immune response to *M. tuberculosis* may be responsible for disease progression.

Lower levels of TNF-α and GM-CSF in sera from children compared with adults may indicate that the immune response in children may not be as effective as that in adults to control TB as both GM-CSF and TNF-α have been associated with increased resistance to mycobacterial infection [16, 17]. This may explain an increased preponderance of TB lymphadenitis among children. A recent study has indeed shown that healthy children generally secrete lower levels of cytokines as compared to adults [18]. One weakness of the study is that we do not have control sera from age-matched healthy children. Therefore, the serum levels of pediatric patients were not compared with the controls.

A higher female preponderance for TB lymphadenitis in adults has been suggested to be due to differences in the immune response [2, 19]. In this study the female patients had lower levels of IL-17 and higher levels of IL-12 compared with adult male patients. Production of IL-17 is shown to be negatively regulated by IL-12 in human T cells [20]. Recent findings suggest a role for IL-17-producing Th17 cells in TB with an early but transient Th17 burst which apparently contributes to protection whereas long lasting Th17 activity causes pathology [21–23]. The balance between IL17 and IL12 may partially explain the increased susceptibility of females as compared to males. However due to large dispersion in the data and several observations below the detection limit of the assay, it is difficult to make any firm conclusion. Further studies are required to understand the significance of these differences.

In this study, IL-12 p40 concentrations were lower in patients with active TB than in healthy controls. Paradoxically, patients with positive cultures had significantly higher IL-12 serum levels than culture-negative TB patients. Considering the essential role of IL-12 in a protective immune response to TB and that positive cultures are associated with a higher mycobacterial burden, it is difficult to explain this finding. IL-12 correlated positively only with IL-15 in all patients and in culture-positive patients. These two cytokines have been shown to activate natural killer cell function [24]. However no difference in the levels of other cytokines/chemokines between culture positive and negative patients suggests that TB lymphadenitis severity may result mainly from the immune response rather than the bacterial load in the tissues.

5. Conclusion

As compared with the controls, TB lymphadenitis patients secreted more proinflammatory cytokines and chemokines, except IL-12, while the levels of the anti-inflammatory cytokines were not different suggesting the role of inappropriate immune stimulation in the disease pathogenesis. There were significant differences in the levels of circulating cytokines with respect to gender and age. Children had generally lower levels of cytokines as compared to adults, and significantly lower levels of TNF-α and GM-CSF indicate that the immune response in children may not be as effective as that in adults which could make them more susceptible to TB. Female patients had lower levels of IL-17 and higher levels of IL-12 compared with male patients; however these findings do not support that female preponderance is due to differences in immune response.

Disclosure

The study sponsors had no involvement in the study design, the collection, analysis, and interpretation of data; in the writing of the paper; and in the decision to submit the paper for publication.

Acknowledgments

The authors thank Dr. Said Aboud at the Muhimbili University College of Health Sciences and the late Professor Roald Matre at the Department of Microbiology and Immunology (the Norwegian Council for Higher Education's Programme for Development, Research and Education (NUFU), Project no. 44003 PRO 42.2.91), University of Bergen, for the provision of control sera. They also thank Professor Odd Mørkve and Dr. Anne Ma Dyrhol Riise for constructive review of the paper. This study was supported by funds from the University of Bergen and from Helse-Vest, the Norwegian health-related research funding agency.

References

[1] M. C. Dandapat, B. M. Mishra, S. P. Dash, and P. K. Kar, "Peripheral lymph node tuberculosis: a review of 80 cases," *British Journal of Surgery*, vol. 77, no. 8, pp. 911–912, 1990.

[2] M. R. Purohit, T. Mustafa, O. Mørkve, and L. Sviland, "Gender differences in the clinical diagnosis of tuberculous lymphadenitis-a hospital-based study from Central India," *International Journal of Infectious Diseases*, vol. 13, no. 5, pp. 600–605, 2009.

[3] E. D. Carrol, J. E. Clark, and A. J. Cant, "Non-pulmonary tuberculosis," *Paediatric Respiratory Reviews*, vol. 2, no. 2, pp. 113–119, 2001.

[4] A. Polesky, W. Grove, and G. Bhatia, "Peripheral tuberculous lymphadenitis: epidemiology, diagnosis, treatment, and outcome," *Medicine*, vol. 84, no. 6, pp. 350–362, 2005.

[5] M. P. Etna, E. Giacomini, M. Severa, and E. M. Coccia, "Pro- and anti-inflammatory cytokines in tuberculosis: a two-edged sword in TB pathogenesis," *Seminars in Immunology*, vol. 26, no. 6, pp. 543–551, 2014.

[6] J. M. Tufariello, J. Chan, and J. L. Flynn, "Latent tuberculosis: mechanisms of host and bacillus that contribute to persistent infection," *Lancet Infectious Diseases*, vol. 3, no. 9, pp. 578–590, 2003.

[7] R. Hussain, Z. Toossi, R. Hasan, B. Jamil, G. Dawood, and J. J. Ellner, "Immune response profile in patients with active tuberculosis in a BCG vaccinated area," *Southeast Asian Journal of Tropical Medicine and Public Health*, vol. 28, no. 4, pp. 764–773, 1997.

[8] M. L. Wilsher, C. Hagan, R. Prestidge, A. U. Wells, and G. Murison, "Human in vitro immune responses to *Mycobacterium tuberculosis*," *Tubercle and Lung Disease*, vol. 79, no. 6, pp. 371–377, 1999.

[9] C. Munoz, J. Carlet, C. Fitting, B. Misset, J.-P. Bleriot, and J.-M. Cavaillon, "Dysregulation of in vitro cytokine production by monocytes during sepsis," *The Journal of Clinical Investigation*, vol. 88, no. 5, pp. 1747–1754, 1991.

[10] S. G. M. Mfinanga, O. Morkve, R. R. Kazwala et al., "Mycobacterial adenitis: role of *Mycobacterium bovis*, non-tuberculous mycobacteria, HIV infection, and risk factors in Arusha, Tanzania," *East African Medical Journal*, vol. 81, no. 4, pp. 171–178, 2004.

[11] D. o. P. M. Ministry of Health, *National Tuberculosis, and Leprosy Control Program, Tanzania, Annual Reports 1979–2001*, Ministry of Health, D. o. P. M., 2005.

[12] S. Aboud, E. F. Lyamuya, E. K. Kristoffersen, and R. Matre, "Immunity to tetanus in male adults in Dar es Salaam, Tanzania," *East African Medical Journal*, vol. 79, no. 2, pp. 73–76, 2002.

[13] T. Mustafa, G. Bjune, R. Jonsson, R. H. Pando, and R. Nilsen, "Increased expression of fas ligand in human tuberculosis and leprosy lesions: a potential novel mechanism of immune evasion in mycobacterial infection," *Scandinavian Journal of Immunology*, vol. 54, no. 6, pp. 630–639, 2001.

[14] T. Mustafa, S. J. Mogga, S. G. Mfinanga, O. Mørkve, and L. Sviland, "Immunohistochemical analysis of cytokines and apoptosis in tuberculous lymphadenitis," *Immunology*, vol. 117, no. 4, pp. 454–462, 2006.

[15] T. Mustafa, H. G. Wiker, O. Mørkve, and L. Sviland, "Reduced apoptosis and increased inflammatory cytokines in granulomas caused by tuberculous compared to non-tuberculous mycobacteria: role of MPT64 antigen in apoptosis and immune

response," *Clinical and Experimental Immunology*, vol. 150, no. 1, pp. 105–113, 2007.

[16] M. Denis and E. Ghadirian, "Granulocyte-macrophage colony-stimulating factor restricts growth of tubercle bacilli in human macrophages," *Immunology Letters*, vol. 24, no. 3, pp. 203–206, 1990.

[17] V. Kindler, A.-P. Sappino, G. E. Grau, P.-F. Piguet, and P. Vassalli, "The inducing role of tumor necrosis factor in the development of bactericidal granulomas during BCG infection," *Cell*, vol. 56, no. 5, pp. 731–740, 1989.

[18] N. O. Nielsen, B. Soborg, M. Børresen, M. Andersson, and A. Koch, "Cytokine responses in relation to age, gender, body mass index, *Mycobacterium tuberculosis* infection, and otitis media among inuit in greenland," *American Journal of Human Biology*, vol. 25, no. 1, pp. 20–28, 2013.

[19] G. H. Bothamley, "Sex and gender in the pathogenesis of infectious tuberculosis: a perspective from immunology, microbiology and human genetic," in *Gender and Tuberculosis*, V. K. T. A. W. A. Diwan, Ed., NHV Report, pp. 41–53, The Nordic School of Public Health, Gothenburg, Sweden, 1998.

[20] M. A. Hoeve, N. D. L. Savage, T. de Boer et al., "Divergent effects of IL-12 and IL-23 on the production of IL-17 by human T cells," *European Journal of Immunology*, vol. 36, no. 3, pp. 661–670, 2006.

[21] A. Cruz, A. G. Fraga, J. J. Fountain et al., "Pathological role of interleukin 17 in mice subjected to repeated BCG vaccination after infection with *Mycobacterium tuberculosis*," *The Journal of Experimental Medicine*, vol. 207, no. 8, pp. 1609–1616, 2010.

[22] S. A. Khader, G. K. Bell, J. E. Pearl et al., "IL-23 and IL-17 in the establishment of protective pulmonary CD4$^+$ T cell responses after vaccination and during *Mycobacterium tuberculosis* challenge," *Nature Immunology*, vol. 8, no. 4, pp. 369–377, 2007.

[23] T. Korn, E. Bettelli, M. Oukka, and V. K. Kuchroo, "IL-17 and Th17 cells," *Annual Review of Immunology*, vol. 27, pp. 485–517, 2009.

[24] N. N. Sotiriadou, S. A. Perez, A. D. Gritzapis et al., "Beneficial effect of short-term exposure of human NK cells to IL15/IL12 and IL15/IL18 on cell apoptosis and function," *Cellular Immunology*, vol. 234, no. 1, pp. 67–75, 2005.

18

The Use of Xpert MTB/Rif for Active Case Finding among TB Contacts in North West Province, South Africa

Limakatso Lebina,[1] Nigel Fuller,[2] Tolu Osoba,[2] Lesley Scott,[3] Katlego Motlhaoleng,[1] Modiehi Rakgokong,[1] Pattamukkil Abraham,[1] Ebrahim Variava,[4] and Neil Alexander Martinson[1,5]

[1]*Perinatal HIV Research Unit, University of Witwatersrand, Johannesburg 2000, South Africa*
[2]*Public Health, School of Medicine, University of Liverpool, Liverpool L69 7ZX, UK*
[3]*Department of Molecular Medicine and Hematology, University of the Witwatersrand, Johannesburg 2000, South Africa*
[4]*Department of Internal Medicine, Klerksdorp/Tshepong Hospital Complex, North West Department of Health and University of the Witwatersrand, Johannesburg 2000, South Africa*
[5]*DST/NRF Centre of Excellence for Biomedical TB Research, University of the Witwatersrand, Johannesburg 2000, South Africa*

Correspondence should be addressed to Limakatso Lebina; lebinal@phru.co.za

Academic Editor: Brian Eley

Introduction. Tuberculosis is a major cause of morbidity and mortality especially in high HIV burden settings. Active case finding is one strategy to potentially reduce TB disease burden. Xpert MTB/Rif has recently been recommended for diagnosis of TB. *Methods.* Pragmatic randomized trial to compare diagnosis rate and turnaround time for laboratory testing for Xpert MTB/Rif with TB microscopy and culture in household contacts of patients recently diagnosed with TB. *Results.* 2464 household contacts enrolled into the study from 768 active TB index cases. 1068 (44%) were unable to give sputum, but 24 of these were already on TB treatment. 863 (53%) participants sputum samples were tested with smear and culture and 2.7% (23/863; CI. 1.62–3.78) were diagnosed with active TB. Xpert MTB/Rif was used in 515 (21%) participants; active TB was diagnosed in 1.6% (8/515; CI: 0.52–2.68). *Discussion and Conclusions.* Additional 31 cases were diagnosed with contact tracing of household members. When Xpert MTB/Rif is compared with culture, there is no significant difference in diagnostic yield.

1. Introduction

Despite recent reports of global reductions in annual TB incidence, tuberculosis (TB) remains a major public health problem with 9 million new TB cases diagnosed globally in 2013 [1]; TB is responsible for 2.4% of all deaths and is second after HIV as the leading infectious cause of mortality [2]. 78% of TB cases among HIV-infected individuals live in Africa [1]. In South Africa the TB burden is particularly severe; in 2011 annual TB incidence was 993/100,000 [3], when the estimated population HIV seroprevalence was 11% [4].

The WHO recommends active case finding for close contacts of a person with TB disease as one of the strategies for early diagnosis for TB and curbing transmission [1]. Typically, symptom screening is used to identify presumptive TB, which requires further investigation, and then using laboratory-based mycobacterial identification or chest X-rays to confirm or rule out the diagnosis is standard in many countries [5, 6]. Poor access to sensitive tests for TB such as mycobacterial culture and the prolonged duration to obtain both positive and negative culture results lead to limited use, particularly in developing countries where cost and limited laboratory infrastructure are barriers [5, 7]. Xpert MTB/Rif (Cepheid Sunnyvale, CA), a rapid point-of-care molecular test for TB that has sensitivity four times that of microscopy and can detect rifampicin resistance, was endorsed by the World Health Organization for use in endemic areas for TB diagnosis [8, 9].

Most studies of Xpert MTB/Rif have included presumptive TB as a source of both cases and noncases. Our prior experience has been that substantial proportions of contacts are found to have culture positive sputum, despite reporting no symptoms, and would therefore not be investigated further. The use of Xpert MTB/Rif in community screening or TB contact tracing for active TB cases, including those who are not presumptive TB, has not been reported on.

2. Methods

2.1. The Setting. Matlosana district is in the North West province. It is 160 km west of Johannesburg and has an estimated population of 500 000 people. It consists of Klerksdorp as the major town and three (Stilfontein, Orkney, and Hartbeesfontein) other gold mine towns. There are four townships (residential areas formerly designated for Blacks) around each of the towns, namely, Jouberton, Khuma, Kanana, and Tigane. The Matlosana Health district is serviced by one regional hospital and 16 community clinics.

2.2. Sampling. We conducted a pragmatic randomized trial of the use of Xpert MTB/Rif and TB microscopy and culture in diagnosing TB among household contacts of patients recently diagnosed with TB within a large implementation science program, done between 31/01/2011 and 07/06/2012. Xpert MTB/Rif was only introduced in the study in the last 7 months. The randomization into receiving smear, microscopy, and culture or GeneXpert was done by one of the administrators at the head office. The team leader would call while doing home visits to find out how the specific households were to be randomized. The Block Stratified Randomization Windows version 6.0 was used to assign each household to GeneXpert or standard smear microscopy and culture using the participant study numbers.

Both adults and children who had standard clinical diagnosis of TB in the last three months were considered eligible for enrollment in the massive active case finding study. A standard clinical diagnosis of TB included anyone with bacteriological/laboratory confirmation of TB or who had been started on TB treatment on the basis of clinical features or anyone who died in the hospital prior to getting TB treatment but had clinical features suggestive of TB. The index patient had to have been living in the Matlosana district for at least six months prior to enrollment. Index patients were approached to provide written informed consent for collection of their sociodemographic data and for the study team to make a household visit when other household contacts would be screened for TB. At households, each household member provided written consent with assent and parental/guardian coconsent for younger household members. The household members were enrolled if they slept in that house more than 2 nights a week or ate more than four meals a week or shared a living space for a cumulative 8 hours per week. Block randomization was used to assign each household to have their sputum assessed either by Xpert MTB/Rif or by the study standard of smear microscopy and liquid mycobacterial growth indicator tube (MGIT) culture (SLC).

The study team either interviewed or reviewed hospital or clinic records of the index patient to collect data on duration of symptoms; date of admission and date of discharge or death; the basis of the TB diagnosis; and their HIV status.

During household visits contacts had a TB symptom screen according to WHO guidelines; spot sputum TB collected; HIV testing (finger prick-rapid test or laboratory saliva based oral test, Orasure); CD4 count test for HIV-infected individuals; and weight and height measurements. Participants with abnormal results were referred to their local clinics for further treatment.

Specimens of fresh sputum for SLC were sent to a central laboratory for testing. At the central laboratory, the specimen was decontaminated, auramine stained, and examined with fluorescence microscopy for detection of acid-fast bacilli (AFB and MGIT). MGIT-positive specimens received another Ziel Neelsen (ZN) stain to confirm the presence of mycobacterium. If the ZN stain was positive, the mycobacterium would undergo genotyping using HAIN test to confirm that it is *Mycobacterium tuberculosis* and whether it is resistant to any drugs. Trained personnel at four local clinics analyzed sputum for Xpert MTB/Rif. Specimens of fresh sputum were tested in GX IV Xpert (four cartridges) to analyze sputum samples for TB.

Data were analyzed using Statistical Analysis Software (SAS) version 9.2 to compare the two groups of the household contacts pragmatically randomized into receiving SLC and those that received Xpert testing. We report characteristics of index cases and household contacts. Categorical data frequencies and percentages were calculated with their 95% confidence interval (CI) and proportions were compared using the Chi-square test. Odds ratios were determined by univariate analysis and unadjusted odds ratio estimated after controlling for other risk factors. The active case finding study received local ethics approvals from the University of Witwatersrand and the regional hospital's and provincial research committees. Delayed procurement of Xpert in two clinics resulted in some contacts that were pragmatically randomized for Xpert MTB/Rif actually receiving SLC. Moreover, if sputum volumes were low or sputum was delivered too late in the afternoon they were also sent for SLC.

3. Results

In total, 768 households of 768 index TB cases were visited during the ten months (September 2011 to June 2012) when household members were pragmatically randomized to receive either SLC or Xpert MTB/Rif. Index TB cases were recruited from the local clinics (411; 53.5%) and 357 (46.5%) were in-patients from the hospital (Table 1). The vast majority of index cases were HIV-infected, 81% (623/768); 75.8% (582/768) had CD4 count results, of which 69.6% (405/582) were less than 250 cells/mm^3. Specimens from 9 (2.5%) index patients were found to have multidrug resistant TB (MDRTB); all were from Tshepong hospital (Table 2).

The median number of household members was 2 (IQR 1–3; range 2–13) per household, and 2464 household members were enrolled; 9 were not included in analysis due to incomplete data. Among household contacts, 1086 (44%) were unable to provide a sputum specimen for TB screening tests and 863 (35%) participants' sputa were submitted to the laboratory for SLC while 515 (21%) of participants received Xpert MTB/Rif testing. Those who were not able to provide

TABLE 1: Comparison of household contacts characteristics and results following randomization to SLC or Xpert MTB/Rif test.

Variable	Sputum SLC screened	Sputum Xpert MTB/Rif screened	P values (calculated from X^2)
Households	393/768 (51.2%)	198/768 (25.8%)	<0.0001*
Index patient, *hospital*	177/357 (49.6%)	92/357 (25.8%)	<0.0001*
Jouberton township	315/863 (36.5%)	241/515 (46.8%)	0.0002*
Gender, *female*	524/863 (60.7%)	318/515 (61.7%)	0.7046^
HIV positive	200/863 (23.2%)	90/515 (17.5%)	0.0120*
Positive TB symptom screen	74/863 (8.6%)	40/515 (7.7%)	0.5985^
Smokers	146/863 (16.9%)	76/515 (14.8%)	0.2912^
Alcohol use	235/863 (27.2%)	122/515 (23.7%)	0.1466^
BMI < 18.5	305/863 (35.3%)	209/515 (40.5%)	0.0516^
Diabetes (>10 mmol/L)	12/863 (1.4%)	6/515 (1.2%)	0.7214^
New cases of TB	23/863 (2.7%)	8/515 (1.6%)	0.1782^

*Significant; ^not significant.

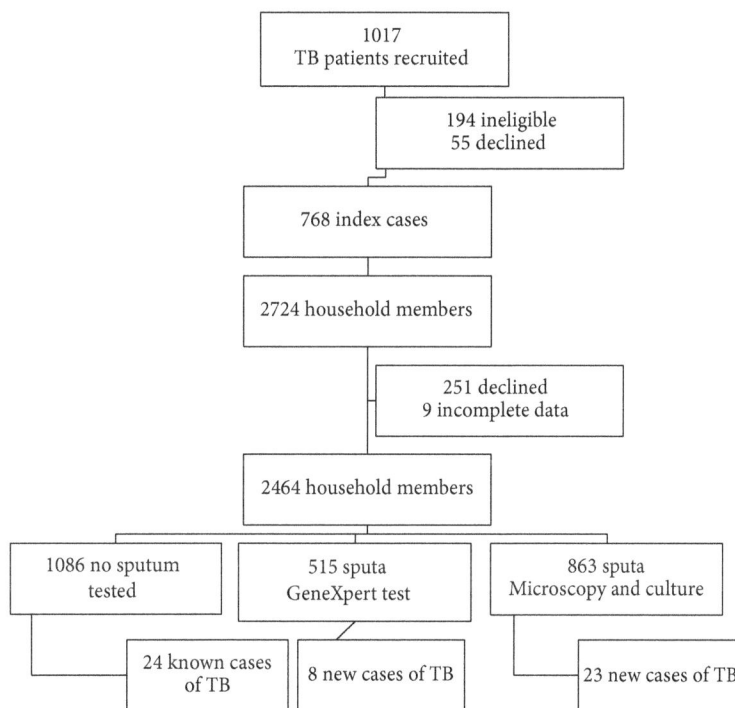

FIGURE 1: Flowchart of results of the study to determine if the use of GeneXpert is comparable to SLC in diagnosing TB among household contacts in active case finding.

specimens included children, household members already on TB treatment, and those with an unproductive cough.

Overall, based on Xpert MTB/Rif, SLC, and medical history, 55/2464 (2.2%; CI: 1.62–2.78) household members were found to have TB. A total of 24 household members were already on TB treatment based on their medical records. Therefore, 31 additional household members were diagnosed with TB by study team (1.26%; CI: 0.82–1.7). The prevalence of undiagnosed TB among the group that received SLC was 2.7% (23/863; CI: 1.62–3.78), while in Xpert MTB/Rif group it was 1.6% (8/515; CI: 0.52–2.68) (X^2 = 1.81; P value = 0.18) (Figure 1). All patients newly diagnosed with TB were referred to their local clinics for initiation of TB treatment.

In sputum samples submitted for SLC, 0.5% (4/863; CI: 0.01–0.91) cases of TB were diagnosed on smear alone (and confirmed on culture), and the turnaround time (laboratory testing) for smear was 2 days. Of all sputum cultures 9.4% (81/863; 7.5–11.4) of these were detected as positive by the MGIT but considered contaminated as the Ziehl Neelsen confirmation was negative in 19.8% (16/81; CI: 11.1–28.5). Further testing of the 65 sputum samples by HAIN MTBDR Plus (genotyping) confirmed *Mycobacterium tuberculosis* (MTB) in 23 cases and the other 42 cases were mycobacterium other than tuberculosis (MOTT) or contaminated. 13% (3/23; CI: −0.7–26.7) were MDRTB; 1 was resistant to only isoniazid and 1 resistant to only rifampicin.

TABLE 2: Characteristics of household members.

Variables	Sputum SLC screened	Sputum Xpert MTB/Rif screened	No sputum provided for testing
		Number (%); median (IQR)	
Population	863 (35%)	515 (21%)	1086 (44%)
Median age years	27 (16–48)	23 (13–45)	10 (4–24)
<15 years	172 (19.9%)	146 (28.3%)	649 (59.8%)
15–45 years	451 (52.2%)	234 (45.6%)	332 (30.5%)
>45 years	238 (27.6%)	117 (22.7%)	105 (9.7%)
Missing	2 (0.2%)	18 (3.5%)	
Gender			
Males	327 (37.9%)	184 (35.9%)	492 (45.3%)
Females	524 (60.7%)	318 (61.7%)	594 (54.7%)
Missing	12 (1.4%)	13 (2.5%)	
Township			
Jouberton	315 (36.5%)	241 (46.8%)	381 (35.1%)
Kanana	306 (35.5%)	92 (17.9%)	427 (39.3%)
Khuma	77 (8.9%)	63 (12.2%)	105 (9.7%)
Tigane	103 (11.9%)	98 (19.0%)	125 (11.5%)
Others	62 (7.2%)	20 (4.1%)	48 (4.4%)
HIV status			
HIV negative	576 (66.7%)	334 (64.8%)	696 (64.1%)
HIV positive	200 (23.2%)	90 (17.5%)	118 (10.9%)
Unknown	87 (10.1%)	91 (17.7%)	272 (25%)
Recent CD4 count			
Number done	66	9	13
Median	394 (276; 551)	377 (184; 503)	446 (265; 635)
Below 350	25/66 (37.9%)	4/9 (44.4%)	5/13 (38.5%)
Symptom screen			
Cough	59 (6.8%)	30 (5.8%)	38 (3.5%)
Productive Cough	37 (4.3%)	23 (4.5%)	19 (1.7%)
Weight loss	21 (2.4%)	9 (1.8%)	15 (1.4%)
Night sweats	12 (1.4%)	9 (1.8%)	9 (0.8%)
Unwell	13 (1.5%)	6 (1.2%)	9 (0.8%)
Smoking history			
None	705 (81.7%)	422 (81.9%)	948 (87.3%)
Yes	146 (16.9%)	76 (14.8%)	106 (9.8%)
Missing data	12 (1.4%)	17 (3.3%)	32 (2.9%)
Alcohol use			
None	616 (71.4%)	377 (73.2%)	899 (82.8%)
Yes	235 (27.2%)	122 (23.7%)	155 (14.3%)
Missing data	12 (1.4%)	16 (3.1%)	32 (2.9%)
Body mass index			
<18.5	305 (35.3%)	209 (40.6%)	633 (58.3%)
18.5–24.9	319 (37%)	161 (31.3%)	262 (24.1%)
25–29.9	111 (12.9%)	53 (10.3%)	60 (5.5%)
>30	107 (12.4%)	72 (14.0%)	75 (6.9%)
Missing data	21 (2.4%)	20 (3.9%)	56 (5.2%)
Blood glucose			
Normal	793 (91.9%)	415 (80.5%)	1021 (94.0%)
High (>10 mmol/L)	12 (1.4%)	6 (1.2%)	9 (0.8%)
Not tested	58 (6.7%)	94 (18.3%)	56 (5.2%)

Of the 515 samples tested by Xpert MTB/Rif, 93.2% (480/515; CI: 91–95.4) had no MTB detected, 1.6% (8/515; CI: 0.52–2.68) had MTB detected, and 5.2% (27/515; CI: 3.3–7.1) had errors or invalid results. Of the specimens in which MTB was detected, 12.5% (1/8; CI: −10.4–35.4) had rifampicin resistance detected. The error rate of results on Xpert MTB/Rif testing was 3.5% (18/515; CI: 1.9–5.1).

The majority (75.4%; 163/216; CI: 69.8–81.2) of participants that had data (n = 216) on the days to positivity required 15 or more days for testing to be completed on MGIT.

The TB symptoms screen was positive in 6.6% (162/2464) of the participants, with cough being the commonest symptom observed in 127 (127/162–78.4%). In the 2464 TB contacts household members that were screened, about half were symptom negative and unable to provide sputum for TB tests. There was no significant difference in positive TB screen between the Xpert MTB/Rif tested (7,7%; 40/515) and the SLC tested participants (8,6%; 74/863), P value 0.5985.

The overall HIV prevalence among household contacts was 16.6% (408/2464; CI: 15.1–18.1). Almost half of the participants who were unable to provide sputum had BMI below 18.5, but the same group also had about two-thirds (59.8%; 649/1086) of the participants under the age of 15 years. Only 21.6% (88/408) participants that were HIV positive had recent CD4 count results available, and 8.3% (34/408) CD4 count results were below 350 cells/mm^3.

68.6% (1542/2247) of the participants with unknown HIV status preferred rapid HIV tests to Orasure. 77% (1730/2247) of participants who did not know their HIV status were HIV-tested; 204/1730 (11.8%) newly diagnosed HIV-infected individuals were identified and referred for further care. The risk factors for undiagnosed TB identified were HIV positive status (adjusted OR: 4.99; CI: 2.15–11.59), positive TB symptoms screen (adjusted OR: 3.13; CI: 1.2–8.17), and diabetes (adjusted OR: 3.12; CI: −0.36–26.87). However, the data on smoking did not show it to be a significant risk factor with an OR of 1.16 (CI: 0.46–2.89) in univariate analysis and an adjusted OR of 0.77 (CI: 0.22–2.76). Smokers and males also appear to have a slightly higher risk of having undiagnosed TB, but it is not significant. However when adjusting for other potentially confounding factors, male gender (OR: 2.27) and diabetes (OR: 3.12) are other additional factors with a significant risk.

4. Discussion

This study comparing the use of Xpert MTB/Rif and SLC in diagnosing TB among household contacts found that TB microscopy and culture diagnosed more cases of TB, but the difference in proportions was not statistically significant (P = 0.18). The overall undiagnosed TB prevalence in household contacts of patients recently diagnosed with TB was 1.3%.

An additional 31 cases of TB (1.3%; 31/2464; CI: 0.85–1.75) were diagnosed. This yield of new TB cases is lower than the 6% (169/2843; CI: 5–7) that was diagnosed in the same community, in another study that was comparing the prevalence of TB among household contacts with an active TB patient and random households with no known active TB case [10]. However the yield is still higher than the 0.4% (4/983; CI: 0.01–0.8) that was diagnosed in random households [10]. This

also confirms that contact tracing that is targeted at community members considered to be at high risk of TB like household contacts yields more new TB cases compared to community wide approach that had a yield of 0.02% [11]. The lower diagnostic yield of Xpert MTB/Rif compared to microscopy and culture (8/515; 1.6%; CI: 0.5–2.7 versus 23/863; 2.7%; CI: 1.6–3.8) was similar to that observed in the screening of mine workers for TB in which Xpert MTB/Rif diagnosed 2.1% while culture diagnosed 2.7% [12]. The differences in diagnostic yield by Xpert MTB/Rif or culture were not statically significant in this study and in that done by Dorman et al. [13].

The major advantage of Xpert MTB/Rif is that it reduces mean time of laboratory testing for TB from 16 days of culture to two hours [14]. Although the costs of Xpert MTB/Rif are higher or comparable to culture in some settings [15] the cost benefits of the quick turnaround time for results and reduced number of visits prior to diagnosis and early initiation of treatment make it cost-effective [16, 17].

The overall (newly diagnosed and known cases on treatment) prevalence of TB among household contacts was 2.2% (55/2464; CI: 1.6–2.8). This prevalence rate is higher than the country level estimate of TB prevalence of 768/100,000 (0.77%) in 2011 [3]. There were 3 cases (3/23; 13%; CI: 0.7–26.7) of confirmed multidrug resistant (MDR) TB diagnosed on culture among the newly diagnosed TB cases, and this is higher than the national level of 1.8% MDR cases in new TB cases [1]. This could have been influenced by the 9 cases (9/768; 1.2%; CI: 0.4–2.0) of the index cases being MDR TB cases.

The error rate of results on Xpert MTB/Rif testing was 3.5% (18/515; CI: 1.9–5.1). This is similar to the error or invalid results rate of 5% observed by Van Rie et al. [7]. There were a total of 42 sputum specimens (44/863; 4.7%; CI: 3.3–6.1) that tested positive on culture, which were later confirmed as mycobacterium other than tuberculosis (MOTT), and 16 (16/863; 1.9%; CI: 1.0–2.8) contaminated. The active case finding study in a mobile HIV service had 16% (162/1011; CI: 13.7–18.3) and 4.7% (47/1011; CI: 3.3–5.9) as MOTT [18].

The HIV prevalence in TB household contacts was 16% (408/2464; CI: 15.1–18.1), which is higher than the regional (North West province) estimated HIV prevalence of 11.3% [19]. Since the 1980s, HIV has been identified as a major risk factor for developing TB, and other risk factors include malnutrition, poor socioeconomic conditions, and smoking [5]. There was no data collected on nutritional status or socioeconomic status in this study to inform if these were other risk factors. The noncommunicable diseases associated with high risk of TB are diabetes mellitus and chronic tobacco-related lung disease and regular screening is recommended to exclude subclinical TB [14]. A positive TB symptom screen being a risk factor for undiagnosed TB is in keeping with the literature. The WHO has recommended symptom screen for TB as part of routine care and active case finding [20] but symptom screen has been shown to be less sensitive in HIV positive people [21–23]. TB contacts under the age of five years have been reported to be at even a higher risk of undiagnosed TB [12]. There were few children under the age of five years, but review of contacts below 15 years did not appear to be a significant risk factor. The major risk factors for undiagnosed TB in household contacts are HIV positive status (OR: 5.1) and positive symptom screen (OR: 4.9).

5. Conclusion

There is no significant difference in the diagnostic yield of Xpert MTB/Rif compared to microscopy and culture. Contact tracing and active case finding for household TB contacts diagnose additional cases of TB. In communities that have a high prevalence of HIV and TB home-based screening for TB and HIV provides early diagnosis of diseases and referral for the appropriate care. A large Xpert MTB/Rif and culture comparison study among household contacts in which participants receive both tests is required to establish whether Xpert MTB/Rif sensitivity compares with culture in screening for TB.

Competing Interests

The authors declare that they have no competing interests.

References

[1] World Health Organization, "Global Tuberculosis Report 2014," WHO report 2014, http://apps.who.int/iris/bitstream/10665/137094/1/9789241564809_eng.pdf.

[2] World Health Organization, "The Top Ten Causes of Death," Fact Sheet 310, World Health Organization, Geneva, Switzerland, 2013, http://www.who.int/mediacentre/factsheets/fs310/en/index.html.

[3] World Health Organization, "South Africa tuberculosis profile," WHO Report, World Health Organization, Geneva, Switzerland, 2012, http://www.who.int/tb/country/data/profiles/en/.

[4] UNAIDS, "South Africa HIV and AIDS Estimates—2011," UNAIDS 2012 Report, http://www.unaids.org/en/regionscountries/countries/southafrica/.

[5] M. S. Jassal and W. R. Bishai, "Epidemiology and challenges to the elimination of global tuberculosis," Clinical Infectious Diseases, vol. 50, supplement 3, pp. S156–S164, 2010.

[6] J. E. Golub, C. I. Mohan, G. W. Comstock, and R. E. Chaisson, "Active case finding of tuberculosis: historical perspective and future prospects," The International Journal of Tuberculosis and Lung Disease, vol. 9, no. 11, pp. 1183–1203, 2005.

[7] A. Van Rie, L. Page-Shipp, L. Scott, I. Sanne, and W. Stevens, "Xpert® MTB/RIF for point-of-care diagnosis of TB in high-HIV burden, resource-limited countries: hype or hope?" Expert Review of Molecular Diagnostics, vol. 10, no. 7, pp. 937–946, 2010.

[8] S. D. Lawn and M. P. Nicol, "Xpert® MTB/RIF assay: development, evaluation and implementation of a new rapid molecular diagnostic for tuberculosis and rifampicin resistance," Future Microbiology, vol. 6, no. 9, pp. 1067–1082, 2011.

[9] World Health Organization, Tuberculosis Diagnostics Automated DNA Test. WHO Endorsement and Recommendations, World Health Organization, Geneva, Switzerland, 2010, http://www.who.int/tb/features_archive/xpert_factsheet.pdf.

[10] A. E. Shapiro, E. Variava, M. H. Rakgokong et al., "Community-based targeted case finding for tuberculosis and HIV in household contacts of patients with tuberculosis in South Africa," American Journal of Respiratory and Critical Care Medicine, vol. 185, no. 10, pp. 1110–1116, 2012.

[11] R. M. Pronyk, B. Joshi, R. J. Hargreaves et al., "Active case finding: understanding the burden of tuberculosis in rural South Africa," International Journal of Tuberculosis and Lung Disease, vol. 5, no. 7, pp. 611–618, 2001.

[12] D. Thind, S. Charalambous, A. Tongman, G. Churchyard, and A. D. Grant, "An evaluation of 'Ribolola': a household tuberculosis contact tracing programme in North West Province, South Africa," The International Journal of Tuberculosis and Lung Disease, vol. 16, no. 12, pp. 1643–1648, 2012.

[13] S. E. Dorman, V. N. Chihota, J. J. Lewis et al., "Performance characteristics of the cepheid Xpert MTB/RIF test in a tuberculosis prevalence survey," PLoS ONE, vol. 7, no. 8, Article ID e43307, 2012.

[14] C. C. Boehme, M. P. Nicol, P. Nabeta et al., "Feasibility, diagnostic accuracy, and effectiveness of decentralised use of the Xpert MTB/RIF test for diagnosis of tuberculosis and multidrug resistance: a multicentre implementation study," The Lancet, vol. 377, no. 9776, pp. 1495–1505, 2011.

[15] G. Meyer-Rath, K. Schnippel, L. Long et al., "The impact and cost of scaling up genexpert MTB/RIF in South Africa," PLoS ONE, vol. 7, no. 5, Article ID e36966, 2012.

[16] A. Vassall, S. van Kampen, H. Sohn et al., "Rapid diagnosis of tuberculosis with the Xpert MTB/RIF assay in high burden countries: a cost-effectiveness analysis," PLoS Medicine, vol. 8, no. 11, Article ID e1001120, 2011.

[17] G. Theron, A. Pooran, J. Peter et al., "Do adjunct tuberculosis tests, when combined with Xpert MTB/RIF, improve accuracy and the cost of diagnosis in a resource-poor setting?" European Respiratory Journal, vol. 40, no. 1, pp. 161–168, 2012.

[18] K. Kranzer, S. D. Lawn, G. Meyer-Rath et al., "Feasibility, yield, and cost of active tuberculosis case finding linked to a mobile hiv service in cape town, south africa: a cross-sectional study," PLoS Medicine, vol. 9, no. 8, Article ID e1001281, 2012.

[19] Human Science Research Council (HSRC), "South African National HIV prevalence, incidence, behaviour and communication survey," HSRC 2008 Report, 2009.

[20] A. Zumla, M. Raviglione, R. Hafner, and C. F. Von Reyn, "Tuberculosis," The New England Journal of Medicine, vol. 368, no. 8, pp. 745–755, 2013.

[21] World Health Organization, Recommendations for Investigating Contacts of Persons with Infectious Tuberculosis in Low- and Middle Income Countries, World Health Organization, Geneva, Switzerland, 2013.

[22] G. Chamie, A. Luetkemeyer, E. Charlebois, and D. V. Havlir, "Tuberculosis as part of the natural history of HIV infection in developing countries," Clinical Infectious Diseases, vol. 50, supplement 3, pp. S245–S254, 2010.

[23] C. J. Hoffmann, E. Variava, M. Rakgokong et al., "High prevalence of pulmonary tuberculosis but low sensitivity of symptom screening among HIV-infected pregnant women in South Africa," PLoS ONE, vol. 8, no. 4, Article ID e62211, 2013.

19

Drug Resistance Pattern of MTB Isolates from PTB Patients

Rajani Ranganath,[1] **Vijay G. S. Kumar,**[2] **Ravi Ranganath,**[3]
Gangadhar Goud,[4] **and Veerabhadra Javali**[5]

[1] *Department of Microbiology, Navodaya Medical College and Research Centre, Raichur, Karnataka, India*
[2] *Department of Microbiology, JSS Medical College and Research Centre, Mysore, Karnataka 570 015, India*
[3] *Usha Kidney Care, Bellary, Karnataka 583103, India*
[4] *Department of Community Medicine, VIMS, Bellary, Karnataka 583104, India*
[5] *Department of Orthopaedics, Navodaya Medical College and Research Centre, Raichur, Tamil Nadu 641043, India*

Correspondence should be addressed to Rajani Ranganath; simpletone82@gmail.com

Academic Editor: Jacques Grosset

Background. TB is a global pandemic disease. All TB control programs were not successful due to the emergence of multidrug resistance in *M. tuberculosis* strains. Objective of the present study was to detect the rate of MDR-MTB in this part of India. *Methods.* One hundred and thirty clinical MTB strains isolated from patients on treatment and confirmed as MTB by MPT64 antigen detection were tested for drug susceptibility against Streptomycin, INH, Rifampicin, and Ethambutol by MBBact automated system. *Result.* Thirty-two were MDRs (25.61%). 31.2%, 28%, 17.6%, and 21.6% were resistant to INH, RIF, Ethambutol, and Streptomycin, respectively. Resistance to either INH or Rifampicin was 20.8% and 13.88%, respectively. Combined INH and Rifampicin resistance was seen in 18.05% isolates. *Conclusion.* Drug resistance rate is high in patients treated previously and who have been irregular on treatment.

1. Introduction

Tuberculosis (TB) is the second leading cause of death from an infectious disease worldwide after human immunodeficiency virus (HIV). Inspite of free supply of drugs, 1.4 million TB deaths occurred worldwide in 2011. Recently, World Health Organization has estimated that 3.7% of new TB cases are MDRs. MDR-TB global average rate is 20%. About 9% of these cases also are resistant to at least one injectable second line antitubercular drugs. These strains are called extensively drug resistant (XDR) TB cases [1]. During the middle of twentieth century, tuberculosis rate in Europe and North America decreased to an extent that it was thought as totally eradicated. Health care providers started to announce that TB is eradicated. TB sanatoriums were closed. But M. tuberculosis bounced back in 1980s with a vengeance and has spread all over the world. Unholy nexus between TB and HIV has further increased not only TB rate but also mortality. Drug resistance (DR) in MTB is a manmade problem. Defaulting by the patient, poor quality of drugs and lack of awareness have

contributed to the present grim situation of TB management. In 1993, increasing reports of MDRTB were noted from USA [2] and WHO declared TB as global emergency [3].

WHO's millennium development goal to reduce TB by 2015 has failed. Drug resistance in MTB is manmade and is a consequence of suboptimal regimens and treatment interruptions [4]. MTB strains exhibiting resistance to INH and Rifampicin, the two main first line drugs, are designated as MDRTB strains. These MDR strains require prolonged treatment using second line drugs which are highly toxic and less effective [5, 6]. WHO and International Union against TB and Lung diseases (IUATLD) initiated a global TB surveillance program in 1990 to take stock of global prevalence of drug resistant TB opened global surveillance centres as state referral laboratories (TB SRLs) [7]. The responsibility of these centres was MDRTB case DATA collection Drug resistance in MTB is of two types, primary or Innate resistance and secondary or Acquired resistance. Acquired drug resistance is due to many reasons, defaulting by the patient is one reason. Presence of primary resistance and acquired resistance in MTB strains is an indicator of TB control program efficacy (of the past and the ongoing). Distribution and rate of MDR and XDR-TB are not uniform. They vary in different places, regions, and countries. This is the first study attempting to detect in vitro drug resistance pattern of MTB isolates covering a population of ten millions using MBBacT automated culture and DST system.

2. Materials and Methods

2.1. Study Setting. This study was done at JSS teaching hospital, Mysore, Karnataka, which is a referral centre for carrying out DST, from April 2011 to May 2012.

2.2. Study Population. 130 sputum smear positive cases aged 20 years and above were included and cases below the age of 20 years and sputum smear negative cases were excluded. All these 130 cases were previously treated for TB and then referred to JSS centre for mycobacterium culture and DST. These mainly included patients who had been treated at this centre or other health centres from neighboring states implementing directly observed treatment under supervision (DOTS) strategy or patients who are referred by private practitioners. Most of private practitioners do not follow RNTCP guidelines for DST and hence patients who had relapsed or defaulted (with a history of previous treatment) or who had remained sputum positive after ≥5 mths of ATT were referred for DST. About 104 (80%) of the cases were failures, 13 (10%) were relapse, and remaining 13 (10%) were treatment after default. Sputum samples were collected from patients before starting retreatment.

Early morning expectorated sputum samples were collected in sterile containers on two successive days. Smears were made from the collected samples and stained by Ziehl Neelsen (ZN) staining. The smears were screened for acid fast bacilli (AFB) and positive smears were graded as per Revised National Tuberculosis Control Programme (RNTCP) guidelines [8].

2.3. Processing of Sputum Specimens by Modified Petroff's Method. 5 mL of sputum specimen was transferred to centrifuge tube and double the volume of sterile 4% sodium hydroxide (NAOH) was added aseptically. It was mixed well and placed in incubator at 37°C for 15 mins. After 20 mins, centrifuge tube was removed from incubator and 15 mL of sterile distilled water (SDW) was added. It was then centrifuged at 3000 ×g for 15 mins. Supernatant fluid was discarded slowly into a container with 5% phenol solution. Pellet was washed with SDW at 3000 ×g for 15 min and supernatant was discarded. Sediment was later used to inoculate into MBBacT culture bottle.

2.4. MBBacT Automated System. Principle: if microorganisms are present in the test sample, CO_2 is produced as organisms metabolize substrates in culture medium. Colour of gas permeable sensor installed at the bottom of each culture bottle changed to light green/yellow.

2.5. MP Culture Bottle. It contains 10 mL of media and an internal sensor that detects CO_2 as an indicator of microbial growth.

2.6. MBBacT Antibiotic Supplement Kit. It consists of antibiotic supplement and reconstitution fluid. antibiotic supplement was reconstituted with 10 mL of Reconstitution fluid before use. Once reconstituted, it had a shelf life of 7 days. Reconstitution fluid contains components which ensure optimal growth of *Mycobacteria* present in sputum samples. MBBacT culture bottles and antibiotic supplement kit was stored under refrigeration (2–8°C) and was equilibrated to room temperature (30 mins) before use.

2.7. Inoculation. MP culture bottle was disinfected with alcohol pad and was allowed to dry. Aseptically 0.5 mL of reconstituted antibiotic supplement was added to each of culture bottle. Pink tint in medium indicated that reconstitution fluid has been added successfully. 0.5 mL of NAOH decontaminated sputum sample was inoculated and loaded into instrument.

2.8. Interpretation. When instrument indicated a positive bottle by flagging, ZN smear was done to detect AFB. If *nonmycobacterial* organisms were seen on grams stain, entire bottle contents were reprocessed through another decontamination procedure and inoculated into a new culture bottle or discarded and another specimen for culture was obtained. Bottles flagged negative only after 42 days. Inoculated MBBacT culture bottles were autoclaved before disposal.

2.9. Identification of MTB. Identification of MTB was done by MPT64 immunochromatographic antigen detection test, manufactured by SD Bioline, South Korea [9].

2.10. SD Bioline TB Ag MPT64. Mouse monoclonal anti-MPT64 was immobilized on the nitrocellulose membrane as the capture material (test line). Colloidal gold particles were used for antigen capture and detected in a sandwich type assay. Presence of only control band indicates negative result. Presence of 2 coloured bands within the result window, no matter which band appears first, indicates a positive result. If the control band is not visible, test is invalid [9].

2.11. DST in MBBacT. Processing for AST: proportion method was used for determining DST as per RNTCP guidelines [8]. MTB H37Rv strain was used as control strain. Six process bottles were required for each MBBacT positive sample. Four bottles were labeled as S, I, R, E (Streptomycin, Isoniazid, Rifampicin, and Ethambutol). One bottle was labeled as Direct Control (DC) and other as Proportional Control (PC). 0.5 mL of restoring fluid (contains nutrients to enhance the growth of *mycobacteria*) was added to all six bottles aseptically. 0.5 mL of corresponding antibiotics were added to the process bottles labeled as S, I, R, and E aseptically. 0.5 mL of sterile distilled was added in Direct Control and Proportional Control aseptically.

Source of inoculum: 0.5 mL of flagged MBBacT positive culture bottle was called seed bottle. This "seed" bottle was taken for AST processing.

All drugs were in chemically pure powder form and were stored at −20°C in desiccators as recommended by manufacturer (HiMedia). Drug concentrations used were INH 0.2 mg/L, RIF 40 mg/L, EMB 2 mg/L, and SM 3 mg/L and were dissolved in deionized water. All stock solutions were sterilized by membrane filtration through 0.22 μm pore sizes and stored at −80°C in small aliquots. The frozen drug solutions were used immediately after thawing and the remaining was discarded and never stored in freezer again. Working solution was prepared freshly from the stock solution.

2.12. Preparation of Inoculum for Drug Containing Bottles and Direct Control. Seed bottle was vortexed to break the clumps. 3 mL of inoculum from this bottle was withdrawn into a sterile bijou bottle with 2-3 mm glass beads. It was vortexed to break the clumps and was standardized to 1Mac Farland. 0.5 mL of the standardized inoculum was added to the process bottles labeled as S, I, R, and E and Direct Control aseptically.

2.13. Preparation of Inoculum for Proportional Control. 0.1 mL of inoculum was taken from positive MBBacT bottle and added to 9.9 mL of sterile distilled water (1/100 dilution). 0.5 mL of inoculum from this was added to the Proportional Control bottle aseptically. Bottles were loaded into MBBacT.

2.14. Reading and Interpretation of Results. When the instrument indicated a positive bottle, bottles were removed according to the procedure. The test was invalid if the DC and PC were not flagged positive within 15 days. If flagged positive within 2 days or less, then contamination or a fast growing AFB was suspected so that the bottles were subcultured and the tests were repeated if required. If DC and PC were determined positive within 1 day of each other then it indicated that 1/100 dilution was not done properly.

If the antibiotic containing bottles were flagged positive after the PC bottle, then the test organism was considered as susceptible provided with DC bottle flagged positive. If the antibiotic containing bottles were flagged positive before the PC bottle, then the test organism was considered as resistant provided with DC bottle flagged positive.

Data entry and analysis were performed using SPSS version 17. Chi square and percentages were applied wherever necessary. P value < 0.05 was considered as statistically significant. The research proposal was cleared by medical faculty ethical review committee.

3. Results

Out of 130 sputum smear positive cases, 78 (60%) were male and 52 (40%) were female. Among 130 isolates, 1 (0.76%) was contaminated and 1 (0.76%) did not yield growth of *mycobacterium*. Average turnaround time for culture by MBBacT method was 5 to 7 days. All remaining 128 isolates were identified as MTB by MPT64 antigen detection test and

TABLE 1: Sensitivity pattern of MTB to four antitubercular (ATT) drugs.

Name of the drug	No. of sensitive strains (%)	No. of resistant strains (%)
Isoniazid (INH)	86 (68.8)	39 (31.2)
Rifampicin (RIF)	90 (72)	35 (28)
Ethambutol (EMB)	103 (82.4)	22 (17.6)
Streptomycin (SM)	98 (78.4)	27 (21.6)
Resistance to any drug	—	72 (57.6)

TABLE 2: Resistance pattern of 72 drug resistant strains of MTB to four ATT drugs.

Number of drugs	Name of drugs	No. of resistant strains (%)	Total (%)
1 drug	Isoniazid (INH)	15 (20.8)	31 (25.61)
	Rifampicin (RIF)	10 (13.88)	
	Ethambutol (EMB)	4 (5.55)	
	Streptomycin (SM)	2 (2.77)	
2 drugs	INH + RIF	13 (18.05)	22 (18.18)
	INH + SM	4 (5.55)	
	INH + EMB	3 (4.16)	
	EMB + SM	2 (2.77)	
3 drugs	INH + RIF + SM	9 (12.5)	14 (11.57)
	INH + RIF + EMB	5 (6.94)	
4 drugs	INH + RIF + SM + EMB	5 (6.94)	5 (4.13)
MDR-TB		32 (25.61)	

were put up for DST against SIRE drugs. DST results were invalid in 3 out of 128 isolates.

Table 1: among remaining 125 isolates, 72 (57.6%) were resistant to one or more drugs. Resistance to INH, RIF, EMB, and SM was found to be 31.2%, 28%, 17.6%, and 21.6%, respectively (P < 0.05, CI 95%).

Table 2 shows the resistance pattern of 72 drug resistant isolates. Single drug resistance was observed in 31 (25.61%), any two drug resistance in 22 (18.18%), any three drug resistance in 14 (11.57%), and all four drug resistance was found in 5 (4.13%). MDR was found in 32 (25.61%). Among monoresistance INH 15 (20.8%) was found to be the highest proportion, followed by RIF 10 (13.88%), and in polyresistant strains, the highest proportion was found in INH + RIF combination 13 (18.05%) (P value < 0.05, CI 95%).

4. Discussion

Drug resistant tuberculosis is either acquired due to poor management of treatment or transmission from infectious drug resistant TB patients. As found in many other studies history of antitubercular treatment has been consistently associated with risk of MDR-TB [9].

Overall MDR rate observed in this study is 32 (25.61%). Our findings are concordant with other studies reported from Chandigarh (27.6%) [10], Tamil Nadu state (25%) [11],

Mumbai (25.25%) [12], and Gujarat (30.2%) [13]. But higher rates were observed in Dehradun (57.22%) [14] and Delhi 53.6% [15] and the lowest rates were seen in Sewagram Wardha (9.2–9.6%) [16, 17]. High rate of MDRTB in our setting is understandable, as this is a referral centre for mycobacterial culture and DST and therefore receives a large number of samples from chronic patients.

The highest resistance is seen in Isoniazid (31.2%) which is the most popular drug followed by Rifampicin (28%), Streptomycin (21.6%), and Ethambutol (17.6%). Similar resistance pattern was reported by Vijay et al. in Bangalore to INH (27.4%), RIF (15.5%), SM (23%), and EMB (6.6%) [18]. Resistance pattern reported by Sethi et al. from Chandigarh in previously treated patients to INH (46.9%), RIF (27.6), SM (22.22%), and EMB (10%) [10]. Resistance reported by Lina et al. from Mumbai in previously treated patients shows INH (30.41%), RIF (58.55%), SM (46.95%), and EMB (3.67%) [12].

Resistance to INH was found to be 31.2% in this study. Similar findings were reported by Vijay et al. from Bangalore (27.4%) [18] and Dam et al. from Delhi (20.18%) [19]. Still higher rates of INH resistance were reported by Paramasivan et al. from Tamil Nadu (81%) [20], Sethi et al. from Chandigarh (46.9%) [10], and Gopi et al. from Raichur (52.3%) [21]. This high resistance may be because of poor compliance by the patients and its widespread use in treatment of tuberculosis.

Rifampicin resistance in our study is 28%. Resistance for RIF is considered as surrogate marker for detection of MDR-TB. Similar findings were reported by Paramasivan et al. from Tamil Nadu (25%) [11], Sethi et al. from Chandigarh (27.6%) [10], and Jain et al. from New Delhi (33.3%) [17]. Still higher rates of RIF resistance are reported by Rawat et al. from Uttarakhand (57.22%), [14], Janmeja and Raj from Haryana (49%) [22], and Paramasivan et al. from Raichur (100%) [20]. Reason for this high resistance may be due to irregular use in other conditions like leprosy, pyrexia of unknown origin (PUO), and leishmaniasis.

In this study drug resistance against streptomycin was found to be 21.6%, which is in concordance with reports by Vijay et al. from Bangalore (23%) [18] and Rawat et al. from Uttarakhand (22.22%) [14]. Resistance of 17.6% was noted against Ethambutol in our study. Similar corroborative resistance pattern was seen in studies from Negi et al. from Delhi (20.65%) [23] and Rawat et al. from Uttarakhand (10%) [14].

In this study INH monoresistance (20.8%) was found to be high. Our results are concordant with reports by Sethi et al. from Chandigarh (14.3%) [10] and Ramachandran et al. from Gujarat (11.7%) [24]. This may be due to INH prophylactic therapy (IPT) given to patients without ruling out active TB among HIV positives. IPT can increase chances of drug resistant TB [25].

Inefficiency in TB control programmes and irregular antitubercular drug usage leading to accumulation and multiplication of resistant strains is supported by remarkable increase in drug resistance among retreated cases. Because of selection bias in hospital, lack of comorbidity and HIV status and robust retrospective data has limited our study.

One most important limitation of this study is previous treatment histories, demographics, and other data like IPT,

and information about second line drug susceptibility like quinolones were not available for analysis, restricting our ability to derive concrete conclusions. Other limitations are data as they are not representative of the whole community and are limited to one hospital. A community based multicenter study, which includes all parts of the country and uses the full spectrum of drugs, is needed to describe the true prevalence of MDRTB in India.

5. Conclusion

The major problem in the treatment of pulmonary tuberculosis is multidrug resistance. Emergence of MDRTB can be reduced by detecting the drug resistance pattern and by treating with the second line antituberculous drugs in appropriate regimens in failure and relapse cases. MDR rate in our study was significantly higher among treatment failures compared to relapses and treatment after default cases, underlying the need for early identification of treatment failure by early referral for culture and drug susceptibility testing and initiation of appropriate treatment.

Emphasis should be laid on prompt case detection, routine and quality assured DST facilities for high risk patients, prompt administration of anti-TB drugs, and strengthening the coordination of nongovernmental organizations (NGOs) and private practitioners as per the guidelines laid down by RNTCP. Additional studies detecting the drug resistance pattern is the need of the hour to delineate risk factors and to formulate plans for future management of tuberculosis in high MDRTB settings.

Acknowledgments

The authors would like to express their profound gratitude to all the participants for the cooperation and for the immense faith the participants reposed in them.

References

[1] World Health Organization, *Global Tuberculosis Report*, World Health Organization, Geneva, Switzerland, 2012.

[2] T. R. Frieden, T. Sterling, A. Pablos-Mendez, J. O. Kilburn, G. M. Cauthen, and S. W. Dooley, "The emergence of drug-resistant tuberculosis in New York City," *The New England Journal of Medicine*, vol. 328, no. 8, pp. 521–526, 1993.

[3] A. Kochi, "The global tuberculosis situation and the new control strategy of the World Health Organization," *Tubercle*, vol. 72, no. 1, pp. 1–6, 1991.

[4] World Health Organization, *WHO Guidelines for the Programmatic Management of Drug Resistant Tuberculosis*, World Health Organization, Geneva, Switzerland, 2006.

[5] S. D. Lawn and R. Wilkinson, "Extensively drug resistant tuberculosis," *British Medical Journal*, vol. 333, no. 7568, pp. 559–560, 2006.

[6] C. Juan, S. C. Palomino, and R. Viviana, *Tuberculosis 2007—From Basic Science to Patient Care*, 2007.

[7] World Health Organization, "Anti-tuberculosis drug resistance in the world (the WHO/IUATLD global project on anti-tuberculosis drug resistance surveillance 1994–1997)," Tech. Rep. WHO/TB/97-229, World Health Organization.

[8] *Revised National Tuberculosis Control Programme Training Manual for Mycobacterium tuberculosis Culture and Drug Susceptibility Testing*, Central Tuberculosis Division, New Delhi, India, 2009.

[9] V. G. Kumar, T. A. Urs, and R. R. Ranganath, "MPT 64 Antigen detection for rapid confirmation of *M.tuberculosis* isolates," *BMC Research Notes*, vol. 4, article 79, 2011.

[10] S. Sethi, A. Mewara, S. K. Dhatwalia et al., "Prevalence of multidrug resistance in *Mycobacterium tuberculosis* isolates from HIV seropositive and seronegative patients with pulmonary tuberculosis in north India," *BioMed Central Infectious Disease*, vol. 13, article 137, 2013.

[11] C. N. Paramasivan, K. Bhaskaran, P. Venkataraman, V. Chandrasekaran, and P. R. Narayanan, "Surveillance of drug resistance in tuberculosis in the state of Tamil Nadu," *Indian Journal of Tuberculosis*, vol. 47, pp. 27–33, 2000.

[12] D. Lina, M. Priya, and C. Sweta, "Drug resistance in tuberculosis," *Bombay Hospital Journal*, 1999, http://bhj.org/journal/1999_4103_july99/original_253.htm.

[13] S. S. Trivedi and S. G. Desai, "Primary antituberculosis drug resistance and acquired rifampicin resistance in Gujarat, India," *Tubercle*, vol. 69, no. 1, pp. 37–42, 1988.

[14] J. Rawat, G. Sindhwani, and R. Dua, "Five-year trend of acquired antitubercular drug resistance in patients attending a tertiary care hospital at Dehradun (Uttarakhand)," *Lung India*, vol. 26, no. 4, pp. 106–108, 2009.

[15] A. Khanna, V. S. Raj, B. Tarai et al., "Emergence and molecular characterization of extensively drug-resistant *Mycobacterium tuberculosis* clinical isolates from the Delhi region in India," *Antimicrobial Agents and Chemotherapy*, vol. 54, no. 11, pp. 4789–4793, 2010.

[16] P. Narang et al., Personal communication.

[17] N. K. Jain, K. K. Chopra, and G. Prasad, "Initial and acquired Isoniazid and Rifampicin resistance to *M. tuberculosis* and its implications for treatment," *Indian Journal of Tuberculosis*, vol. 39, no. 2, pp. 121–124, 1992.

[18] S. Vijay, V. H. Balasangameshwara, P. S. Jagannatha, V. N. Saroja, B. Shivashankar, and P. Jagota, "Re-treatment outcome of smear positive tuberculosis cases under DOTs in Bangalore city," *Indian Journal of Tuberculosis*, vol. 49, pp. 195–204, 2002.

[19] T. Dam, M. Isa, and M. Bose, "Drug-sensitivity profile of clinical *Mycobacterium tuberculosis* isolates—a retrospective study from a chest-disease institute in India," *Journal of Medical Microbiology*, vol. 54, no. 3, pp. 269–271, 2005.

[20] C. N. Paramasivan, R. Venkataraman, V. Chandrasekaran, S. Bhat, and R. R. Narayanan, "Surveillance of drug resistance in tuberculosis in two districts of South India," *International Journal of Tuberculosis and Lung Disease*, vol. 6, no. 6, pp. 479–484, 2002.

[21] P. G. Gopi, R. S. Vallishayee, B. N. Appegowda et al., "A tuberculosis prevalence survey based on symptoms questioning and sputum examination," *Indian Journal of Tuberculosis*, vol. 44, pp. 171–180, 1997.

[22] A. K. Janmeja and B. Raj, "Acquired drug resistance in tuberculosis in Harayana, India," *Journal of Association of Physicians of India*, vol. 46, no. 2, pp. 194–198, 1998.

[23] S. S. Negi, S. Gupta, and S. Lal, "Drug resistance in tuberculosis in Delhi: a 2 year profile (2001-2002)," *Journal of Communicable Diseases*, vol. 35, no. 2, pp. 74–81, 2003.

[24] R. Ramachandran, S. Nalini, V. Chandrasekar et al., "Surveillance of drug-resistant tuberculosis in the state of Gujarat, India," *International Journal of Tuberculosis and Lung Disease*, vol. 13, no. 9, pp. 1154–1160, 2009.

[25] World Health Organization, "Policy statement on preventive therapy against tuberculosis in people living with HIV," Tech. Rep. WHO/TB/98.255, World Health Organization, Geneva, Switzerland, 1998.

20

Are Shopkeepers Suffering from Pulmonary Tuberculosis in Bahir Dar City, Northwest Ethiopia: *A Cross-Sectional Survey*

Mulusew Andualem Asemahagn

School of Public Health, College of Medicine and Health Sciences, Bahir Dar University, Bahir Dar, Ethiopia

Correspondence should be addressed to Mulusew Andualem Asemahagn; muler.hi@gmail.com

Academic Editor: David C. Perlman

Background. Despite several interventions, tuberculosis (TB) continues to be a major public health concern in developing countries. *Objective.* To determine pulmonary TB prevalence and associated factors among shopkeepers in Bahir Dar City, Ethiopia. *Methods.* A cross-sectional study was conducted in 2016 among 520 shopkeepers who had TB signs and symptoms using questionnaire interview and sputum samples processing. Shopkeepers were considered TB positive if two sputum slides became positive. Data were edited and analyzed using SPSS version 23. Multivariable logistic regression analysis was used to identify factors. *Results.* A total of 520 shopkeepers were interviewed and gave sputum samples. About 256 (49.2%) of them were under the ≤30 years' age category, 22.0% can read and write, 65.0% were Muslims, and 32.0% originated from rural areas. Pulmonary TB prevalence was 7.0% (37/520), and positivity proportion was 57.0% (21/37) in males and 70.0% (26/37) in urban residents. Smaller (44.0%) shopkeepers got health education on TB. Illiteracy, no health education, contact history, cigarette smoking, nonventilated shops, and comorbidities were factors to TB infection (p value < 0.05). *Conclusions.* Significant numbers of shopkeepers were infected by TB. Factors to TB infection were either personal or related to comorbidities or the environment. Therefore, TB officials need to specially emphasize awareness creation, occupational health, and early screening to prevent TB.

1. Introduction

Despite several international and national anti-TB interventions, TB continues to be the ninth leading cause of global morbidity and the leading cause of a single infectious agent, ranking above HIV/AIDS [1]. TB is the first killer contagious disease among people living with HIV/AIDS [1, 2]. Based on the WHO 2017 report, there were 10.4 million new TB cases: 90% adults, 65% men, and 10% people living with HIV/AIDS (74% from Africa). There were also about 1.3 million global TB deaths among HIV negatives and 374 000 deaths among HIV positives in 2016. Similarly, five countries (India, Indonesia, China, the Philippines, and Pakistan) accounted for 56% of the global TB incidence cases [1].

The 2017 WHO report also showed varied distribution of TB incidence cases across the WHO regions in 2016: 45% of TB cases occurred in the WHO Southeast Asia Region and 25% in the WHO African Region followed by the 17% in the WHO Western Pacific Region [1]. Likewise, Nigeria and

South Africa each accounted for 4% of the global total. Poor socioeconomy, high HIV/AIDS burden, malnutrition, poor community awareness, poor healthcare services, and low TB case detection could be potential explanations for high TB incidence in the sub-Saharan Africa [1–6].

Although several anti-TB interventions have been made in Ethiopia, the country continues to be the 7th country in TB incidence among the 22 high TB burden countries globally and 4th from Africa. Ethiopia is also among the top 20 countries with TB-HIV and drug resistance TB (MDR-TB) from the 30 high TB-HIV and MDR-TB burden countries [1, 2]. According to the Ethiopian Federal Ministry of Health hospital statistics evidence, pulmonary TB was the third leading cause of hospital admission (7.8%) and the first leading cause of in-patient deaths (10.1%) [7]. Even though the Ethiopian government has expanded TB diagnosis and treatment services to both the public and private healthcare facilities since 2004, TB is still major public health concern. This may be due to the emergency of drug resistance TB, malnutrition, low community awareness, inaccessibility/ quality of TB services, and high comorbidity rates (HIV AIDS, malaria, and diabetes mellitus) [1–12].

Shopkeepers, people who serve as seller in any shop either for a full or part time, are assumed high risk population groups to TB infection as a result of double infection sources: frequent contact with different customers whose health status is unknown and family or community sources. In addition, overcrowdedness of shops and absence of occupational health safeties such as access to healthcare services including early screening to TB, HIV/AIDS, and others and health insurance may aggravate the risk of acquiring TB infection shopkeepers, mainly in the developing countries. Hence, shopkeepers not only are among the high risk population groups to acquire TB infection but are also high source of TB infection to their families, friends, and the rest of the community.

Although shopkeepers are at high risk of getting TB infection and there are several types of shops where shop-keepers are working in Ethiopia, almost all do not get special attention on TB prevention from the healthcare facilities and TB control program. This may contribute more for the presence of high TB infection burden in Ethiopia. According to my knowledge and search, there is no study conducted on TB infection among shopkeepers in Africa and Ethiopia.

Therefore, this study was aimed at determining the prevalence of pulmonary TB infection and identifying factors associated with TB infection among shopkeepers in Bahir Dar City, Northwest Ethiopia. This will serve as crucial evidence to Ethiopian Federal Ministry of Health, Amhara Regional Health Bureau, Bahir Dar City administration health office, and the nongovernmental organizations working on TB prevention to know the burden of TB infection on shopkeepers and identify associated risk factors so that they will have evidence based intervention plan. It will also be important source to the coming researchers who are interested in TB prevention.

2. Materials and Methods

2.1. Study Design and Area. A cross-sectional study was conducted between October and December 2016 among shop-keepers in Bahir Dar City, Northwest Ethiopia. Bahir Dar City is the capital city of Amhara Regional State and located 565 kilometers to the Northwest of Addis Ababa, the capital city of Ethiopia. The city has nine administrative subcities, two public hospitals, and six public health centers. The Amhara Regional Health Bureau and Regional Public Health Institute are found in the city. More than 2400 legally recognized shops were found in the city. Majority of the shops are located at the center of the city, "Tana Market center" and around it [9].

2.2. Sample Size Determination and Technique. Due to time, feasibility, and resource constraints, only one-third of the total shops (800 out of 2400) were included in the study through simple random sampling technique by taking the sampling frame from the Amhara Region trade office. After assessing the presence of signs and symptoms including presence of cough for 14 days and above, only 520 out of 1600 shopkeepers working in 800 shops were included in the study.

2.3. Data Collection Tools and Procedures

2.3.1. Sociodemographic Data and Risk Factors Assessment. Data on the sociodemographic and associated risk factors were collected using pretested structured questionnaire. Three bachelor nurses collected data through interviewer-administered approach. The questionnaire was comprised of data on sociodemographic data (age, sex, education level, family size, income level, religion, residence, etc.) and risk assessment on TB infection (crowdedness, previous TB contact, awareness/health education access, room size, comorbidity, personal behavior/smoking, khat chewing, alcohol intake, and cough duration). Shopkeepers who either smoke or drink alcohol or chew khat in any amount in a daily manner were considered as poor personal behavior since they have a direct or indirect linkage to TB infection. Awareness of study participants was assessed via access to health education by healthcare workers or media on TB transmission, risk factors, signs and symptoms, and prevention mechanisms. Those who got health education on TB at least one time were considered as having awareness on TB transmission and prevention. The ventilation and crowdedness of the shops were estimated by observation. On the other hand, data on shops' room size were collected through measuring the size by a meter scale.

2.3.2. Sputum Samples Collection, Processing, and Examination. Three laboratory technicians collected sputum data. They informed interviewed shopkeepers how to collect sputum samples and gave them clean, labeled, and dry tightly caped sputum caps to bring samples. Study participants provided three sputum samples (spot-morning-spot) for Acid-Fast staining. Sputum sample collection, smear preparation, AFB staining, and smear examination were done according to the Ethiopian National TB and Leprosy prevention and control standard guideline [3]. Then, stained smears were examined through Olympus microscope and shopkeepers were grouped under TB positives if at least two AFB sputum smear slides were positive.

2.4. Data Quality Assurance and Analysis. Training of data collectors, questionnaire validation, providing information on sample collection, labeling sputum caps/slides, running quality control slides parallel to the sputum samples, reread-ing of all positive sputum slides and 15% of the negative slides by the experienced laboratory technicians, and following the national guideline in all steps were major quality assurance activities. Data were edited and analyzed using the SPSS version 22 software. Different descriptive statistics (percentages, proportions, count, etc.) and binary logistic regression analyses were computed to describe study objectives and identify factors associated with TB infection among shop-keepers, respectively. Odds ratio at 95% confidence level was used to describe statistical association between the study and outcome variables.

2.5. Ethical Consideration. The study was ethically cleared and approved by the ethical review committee of Amhara Regional Health Bureau. A support letter was taken from the

TABLE 1: Sociodemographic variables of shopkeepers in Bahir Dar City, Ethiopia, 2017.

Variable	Responses	Frequency	Percent (%)
Age	≤30	256	49.0
	>30	264	51.0
Sex	Male	224	43.0
	Female	296	57.0
Religion	Christians	183	35.0
	Muslims	337	65.0
Marital status	Single	203	39.0
	Married	317	61.0
Residence	Rural	167	32.0
	Urban	353	68.0
Education level	Cannot read and write	63	12.0
	Can read and write	457	88.0
Work experience	≤5 years	281	54.0
	>5 years	239	46.0
Contact with TB cases	Yes	219	42.0
	No	301	58.0
Got health education on TB	Yes	229	44.0
	No	291	56.0
Shop size in meter square	≥4	354	68.0
	<4	166	32.0
Shops' condition	Ventilated	156	30.0
	Nonventilated	364	70.0

Bahir Dar City administration Health office after discussing the purpose and data collection procedures of the study. Shop owners and study participants were informed on the study objective, data collection procedures, and data confidentiality issues prior to the data collection. Informed consent was taken from each shopkeeper and participation was fully voluntary. Data confidentiality was kept through anonymity. TB positive shopkeepers were counseled and linked to the nearby health facilities and started their anti-TB treatment according to the Ethiopian national TB treatment guideline.

3. Results

3.1. Sociodemographic Characteristics of the Participants. A total of 520 shopkeepers (224 males and 296 females) participated in this study. Nearly half, 256 (49.2%), of the shopkeepers were under the age category of ≤30 years. The mean age and standard deviation of the shopkeepers were 30 ± 5 years. Large number of respondents (61.0%) were married in marital status. About two-thirds (65.0%) of the shopkeepers were Muslims and 32.0% originated from the rural areas. Only 12.0% of the shopkeepers cannot read and write and 42.0% had contact history with known TB cases. Less than half (44.0%) of shopkeepers got health education on TB infection from health extension workers. More than half (54.0%) of them had ≤5 years of work experience as shopkeeper. Nearly three-fourths (70.0%) of the shops were nonventilated/crowded by goods and there was no adequate space/window for air circulation. Over two-thirds (68.0%) of the shops had ≥4 square meter area size (Table 1).

Personal behavior of shopkeepers was described in terms of alcohol intake (any type), smoking, and khat chewing in any amount daily. Over a third, 191 (36.7%), of the shopkeepers had history of alcohol intake of any type daily. Likewise, 222 (42.7%) and 203 (39.0%) of them were cigarette smokers and khat chewers daily, respectively. Regarding comorbidity history, 182 (35%) of the shopkeepers had history of HIV/AIDS and/or DM (Table 2).

3.2. Results of Sputum Microscopy. The prevalence of smear positive pulmonary TB among shopkeepers who had cough for 14 days and above was 7.0% (37/520); 4.0% (21/520) males; and 3.0% (16/520) females. The proportion of TB positivity rate was higher among shopkeepers with age category of ≤30 years: 62.2% (23/37). Similarly, the proportion of TB positivity rate was higher among male, Muslims, urban residents, married, and smokers and from nonventilated shop respondents. Only 10% of the respondents did TB screening before this study. Over a third (35.0%) of the shopkeepers had comorbidity history such as HIV/AIDS and/or diabetes mellitus (DM) (Table 2).

3.3. Risk Factors Associated with TB Infection of Shopkeepers. Education level (illiterate), cigarette smoking, having contact with TB patients, not getting health education on TB, having comorbidity (HIV/AIDS and/or DM), and being in poorly ventilated shops were found to be statistically significant risk factors to acquire TB infection among shopkeepers (p value < 0.05). The odds of acquiring TB infection were double times among illiterate shopkeepers compared to shopkeepers

TABLE 2: TB infection and its determinant factors among shopkeepers in Bahir Dar City, Ethiopia, 2017.

Variables	TB status		COR (95 CI)	AOR (95% CI)	p value
	Positive (%)	Negative (%)			
Age in years					
≤30	23 (4.4)	233 (44.8)	1.76 [0.89–3.51]	0.85 [0.27–2.64]	0.103
>30	14 (2.7)	250 (48.1)	1	1	
Sex					
Male	21 (4.0)	203 (39.0)	1.81 [0.92–3.56]	0.86 [0.17–2.41]	0.081
Female	16 (3.0)	280 (54.0)	1	1	
Marital status					
Single	15 (2.9)	188 (36.2)	1.10 [0.54–2.11]	0.46 [0.15–1.83]	0.846
Married	22 (4.2)	295 (56.7)	1	1	
Residence					
Rural	11 (2.1)	156 (30.0)	0.88 [0.43–1.84]	0.52 [0.21–1.53]	0.747
Urban	26 (5.0)	327 (62.9)	1	1	
Religion					
Christians	9 (1.7)	173 (33.3)	0.58 [0.26–1.25]	0.24 [0.14–1.20]	0.158
Muslims	28 (5.4)	310 (59.6)	1	1	
Education level					
Illiterate	10 (1.9)	53 (10.2)	3.01 [1.38–6.55]	2.14 [1.21–4.75]	0.004
Can read and write	27 (5.2)	430 (82.7)	1	1	
Alcohol intake					
Yes	17 (3.3)	174 (33.5)	1.51 [0.77–2.96]	0.89 [0.32–2.16]	0.228
No	20 (3.8)	309 (59.4)	1	1	
Cigarette smoking					
Yes	23 (4.4)	198 (38.1)	2.40 [1.19–4.71]	2.16 [1.14–3.45]	0.012
No	14 (2.7)	285 (84.8)	1	1	
Khat chewing					
Yes	19	184	1.71 [0.87–3.35]	0.75 [0.42–2.36]	0.111
No	18	299	1	1	
Contact with TB cases					
Yes	23 (4.4)	196 (37.7)	2.41 [1.21–4.79]	1.85 [1.16–3.69]	0.010
No	14 (2.7)	287 (55.2)	1	1	
Got TB Health education					
Yes	10 (1.9)	219 (42.11)	0.45 [0.21–0.94]	0.36 [0.16–0.69]	0.030
No	27 (5.2)	264 (50.80)	1	1	
Work experience					
≤5 years	16 (3.1)	265 (51.0)	0.63 [0.32–1.24]	0.41 [0.26–1.17]	0.172
>5 years	21 (4.0)	218 (41.9)	1	1	
Shops' condition					
Ventilated	5 (1.0)	151 (29.0)	0.35 [0.13–0.89]	0.30 [0.11–0.58]	0.023
Not ventilated	32 (6.1)	332 (63.9)	1	1	
Has comorbidity					
Yes	20 (3.8)	162 (31.2)	2.33 [1.19–4.57]	1.96 [1.14–3.22]	0.012
No	17 (3.3)	321 (61.7)	1	1	

who can read and write (OR = 2.14, 95% CI = [1.21–4.75], p value = 0.004). Similarly, TB infection was found higher among shopkeepers who had contact history with confirmed TB cases compared to their counterparts (OR = 1.85, 95% CI = [1.16–3.69], p value = 0.010). Shopkeepers who had cigarette smoking habits were twice in acquiring TB infection than nonsmoker shopkeepers; OR = 2.16, 95% CI = [1.14–3.45],

p value = 0.012. Likewise, the odds of getting TB infection were 64% times less likely among shopkeepers who got health education on TB than those who did not get health education (AOR = 0.36, 95% CI = [0.16–0.62], p value = 0.030). Also, nonventilated shops were found to be determinant factor in getting TB infection among shopkeepers; those who worked inside the ventilated shops were 70% times less likely to acquire TB infection than the respective groups (OR = 0.30, 95% CI = 0.11–0.58, p value = 0.023). Shopkeepers with HIV/AIDS and/or DM were 1.96 times more likely to be TB positive compared to shopkeepers with no comorbidity history (OR = 1.96, 95% CI = [1.14–3.22], p value = 0.012) (Table 2).

4. Discussion

The current study revealed that pulmonary TB prevalence is important health problem among shopkeepers in Bahir Dar City (7.0%: 7 in 100). This clearly indicates that shopkeepers are at the high risk of getting TB infection, because they have double infection sources: from the customers and families/community. It means that they have high chance of getting conformed and nonconfirmed TB cases without taking care to prevent them from getting the infection. In addition, education level (illiteracy), working inside the nonventilated rooms, low awareness of TB transmission, and comorbidity with other chronic diseases such as HIV/AIDS and DM were statistically significant factors to acquire TB infection among shopkeepers (Table 2). All these were reported challenges to the END TB program in 2015 by the WHO [2] and other studies [5–10].

The situation among shopkeepers is serious in TB transmission due to the nature of their work which will highly expose them to contacting more people per day with minimal or no precautions compared to other institutions. This makes the condition severe because they can easily get TB infection and become potential sources of infection to their families, customers, and the community at large. Hence, TB infection may continue to be the most prevalent among shopkeepers and become big challenge to the END TB program unless appropriate interventions such as continuous information provision, planning TB screening, and treatment services to the high risk areas, improving rooms' conditions, and managing other comorbidities are made. This obviously shows that TB programmers at different levels need to consider additional TB prevention strategies to address communities who are at the high risk of getting TB infection. This was also one of the recommended strategies of the END TB program by the WHO [1, 2] and Ethiopian Federal Ministry of Health [11].

Due to the absence of published evidences on TB prevalence among shopkeepers, the author tried to discuss present prevalence with studies at the community, facility, and prison levels in Ethiopia; since they have some similarities, they are relatively higher, risky/congregated settings/to acquire TB infection [13]. The current prevalence was found to be higher compared to study findings from Dessie and Debre-Birhan (among homeless participants) [5], people attending spiritual holy water services as the alternative medication to their illnesses [10], and North Gondar [12, 14] where TB prevalence was 2.6%, 2.9%, 5.3%, and 4.9%, respectively. The possible explanation for this variation could be differences in area coverage, comorbidity prevalence, information access, contact status with TB patients, and overcrowdedness. In the current study, poor room ventilation (70%), low health education on TB (44%), and high comorbidity with HIV/AIDS and DM

(35%) were assisting factors to TB infection. Hence, these could be potential sources to the variation of TB prevalence compared to the studies stated above.

Consistently, the current prevalence was also higher compared to study findings from abroad: China, 2.7% [15]; India, 4/1000 [16]; and Tanzania, 3.6% [17]. It could be due to variations in personal awareness, TB programs performance, ventilation status, comorbidity, nutritional status, and overcrowdedness.

On the other hand, TB prevalence among shop keepers was found to be lower compared to study findings from Gamo Gofa zone, Ethiopia (19.4%) [18]; Nigeria (21.15%) [19]; and Brazil (25.2%) [20]. This variation could probably be attributed to differences in study period, study area coverage, study population, and methods employed. For example, culture was used to detect TB cases in the case of Gamo Gofa zone which possibly could increase positivity rate. Similarly, in Brazil, Tuberculin skin test was used in addition to sputum microscopy.

In this study, the odds of acquiring TB infection were higher among illiterate shopkeepers (OR = 2.14, 95% CI [1.21–4.75]) compared to those who can read and write. It is known that literacy level is crucial to prevent TB infection because it can determine the understanding level of individuals on TB transmission, prevention, and information searching skills. Evidences by the WHO [2] and other studies [11, 21] also revealed that education level was determinant factor to TB infection.

Correspondingly, TB prevalence was higher among shopkeepers who had cigarette smoking history than the nonsmoker participants (Table 2). This fact was in line with study findings from Ethiopia [3, 8, 11, 12] and abroad [2, 22]. The possible justification could be related to the impact of smoking on lung functionality. Smoking could affect the lung and became a predisposing factor to lung diseases and make individuals more susceptible to pulmonary TB infection.

In this study, the odd of acquiring TB infection was almost double among shopkeepers who had previous contact history with confirmed TB cases (Table 2). This was supported by several study findings [2–7, 11, 12, 22, 23]. It is because one of the primary transmission routes to TB infection is long contact/living with untreated TB cases. Therefore, shopkeepers who have longer contact with several people (customers) have the highest chance of acquiring and transmitting TB from/or to the family, neighbors, customers, and the community.

Similarly, health education was found to be preventive strategy for TB infection; shopkeepers who got health education by the healthcare workers in the past two years about TB transmission and prevention were 64% times less likely to get TB infection compared to the counterparts. The WHO also strongly recommended the importance of awareness creation, and health promotion on TB prevention [2]. It is also one of the basic strategies in Ethiopian health sector transformation plan [8]. This is because health education can facilitate health information dissemination and awareness creation among the community. Thus, they can prevent TB infection through either avoiding the predisposing factors or early diagnosis and treatment of TB infection. Hence, TB programmers in Ethiopia and Bahir Dar City need to think of planning special strategies on accessing health education to shop keepers and people in similar settings since they have lesser chance of getting health education given by the health extension workers at the household levels due to spending their time at shops, and the percentage of health education among shopkeepers was lower (44%).

Another important determinant factor to TB infection was comorbidity history of shopkeepers. The odd of getting TB infection was nearly twofold among shopkeepers who had comorbidity (HIV/AIDS and/or DM) compared to those who had no comorbidity history (Table 2). Almost all studies, reports, and guidelines supported this idea [1–8]. It is because comorbidities such as HIV/AIDS and DM can compromise human immune system and make individuals more susceptible to TB infection. Therefore, regular health education and early screening for TB, HIV, DM, and other chronic diseases are vital among high risk population groups such as shopkeepers.

In addition to the above-mentioned risk factors, shop conditions showed statistically significant association with TB infection in this study: shopkeepers working in ventilated shops were 70% times less likely to acquire TB infection than their counterparts (Table 2). The most important WHO recommendation to prevent TB infection is to have ventilated areas anywhere (working places, homes, hotels, transportation, and public service places). This is because the primary transmission route of TB infection is through air droplets and if the rooms have no two-way parallel air circulations, everyone who enter or stay there can potentially get TB infection. For this case, shops are typical examples since most (32%) were very narrow (less than 4-square meter area), overcrowded/no air circulation (Tables 1 and 2). This clearly shows that special attention is required to make shops occupationally safe to shopkeepers and customers with the emphasis on preventing them from acquiring communicable diseases, particularly TB. In addition, it is better to implement occupational health strategies in such settings to increase individuals' safety.

5. Conclusions and Recommendations

Based on this study, pulmonary TB is found to be an important health problem among shopkeepers (7 in 100). Being unable to read and write, cigarette smoking, not getting health education, previous contact with TB cases, comorbidity (HIV/AIDS and/or DM), and shops' condition were statistical significant factors of TB infection among shopkeepers in Bahir Dar City. Thus, special attention on awareness creation, early screening, treatment (TB, HIV/AIDS, and DM), interventions on poor personal behaviors (cigarette smoking, etc.), implementing occupational health strategies, and improving shops ventilation are crucial for preventing TB infection.

6. Limitations and Implications

In this study, only quantitative data and sputum microscopy were used as data collecting tools which may have limitation on identifying associated risk factors and determining the TB positivity rate among shopkeepers, respectively. Absence of literature on TB infection among shopkeepers was also another limitation to this research work.

Abbreviations

AFB: Acid-Fast Bacilli
AOR: Adjusted odds ratio
CI: Confidence interval
COR: Crude odds ratio
DM: Diabetes mellitus
HIV/AIDS: Human immune virus/acquired immune
           deficiency syndrome
MDR-TB: Multidrug resistance-tuberculosis
OR: Odds ratio
SPSS: Statistical Packages for Social Sciences
TB: Tuberculosis
WHO: World Health Organization.

Ethical Approval

The study was ethically approved by the ethical review committee of Amhara Regional Health Bureau.

Authors' Contributions

Mulusew Andualem Asemahagn took the central role in all parts of the research work through the consultation and assistance of senior researchers and TB control experts.

Acknowledgments

The author would like to acknowledge Amhara Regional Health Bureau, Bahir Dar City Health Office and thank data collectors, sputum processors, and shopkeepers for their candid help to this research work.

References

[1] World Health Organization (WHO), "Global Tuberculosis report," 2017.

[2] WHO, "The Global TB report," 2015.

[3] Federal Democratic Republic of Ethiopia Ministry of Health, *Tuberculosis, Leprosy and TB/HIV prevention and control program manual*, 4th edition, 2008.

[4] S. D. Hamusse, M. Demissie, and B. Lindtjørn, "Trends in TB case notification over fifteen years: the case notification of 25 Districts of Arsi Zone of Oromia Regional State, Central Ethiopia," *BMC Public Health*, vol. 14, no. 1, article no. 304, 2014.

[5] T. Semunigus, B. Tessema, S. Eshetie, and F. Moges, "Smear positive pulmonary tuberculosis and associated factors among homeless individuals in Dessie and Debre Birhan towns, Northeast Ethiopia," *Annals of Clinical Microbiology and Antimicrobials*, vol. 15, no. 1, article no. 50, 2016.

[6] G. Berhe, F. Enqueselassie, E. Hailu et al., "Population-based prevalence survey of tuberculosis in the Tigray region of Ethiopia," *BMC Infectious Diseases*, vol. 13, no. 1, article 448, 2013.

[7] S. Hamusse, M. Demissie, D. Teshome, M. S. Hassen, and B. Lindtjørn, "Prevalence and Incidence of Smear-Positive Pulmonary Tuberculosis in the Hetosa District of Arsi Zone, Oromia Regional State of Central Ethiopia," *BMC Infectious Diseases*, vol. 17, no. 1, article no. 214, 2017.

[8] Ethiopian Federal Ministry of Health. The Ethiopian Health Sector Transformation Plan from, 2015.

[9] Amhara Region Trade Office, "The 2016 annual report of Amhara Region trade office," 2016.

[10] D. Derseh, F. Moges, and B. Tessema, "Smear positive pulmonary tuberculosis and associated risk factors among tuberculosis suspects attending spiritual holy water sites in Northwest Ethiopia," *BMC Infectious Diseases*, vol. 17, no. 1, article 100, 2017.

[11] Ethiopian Federal Ministry of Health, Federal Ministry of Health 16th National Annual Review Meeting Group Discussion: Why TB? Evaluating the National TB Control Program: Challenges and ways forward, 2014.

[12] T. Gebrecherkos, B. Gelaw, and B. Tessema, "Smear positive pulmonary tuberculosis and HIV co-infection in prison settings of North Gondar Zone, Northwest Ethiopia," *BMC Public Health*, vol. 16, no. 1, pp. 1–10, 2016.

[13] M. H. Dangiso, *Tuberculosis control in Sidama Region [Ph.D. dissertation]*, 2016.

[14] T. Tadesse, M. Demissie, Y. Berhane, Y. Kebede, and M. Abebe, "Two-thirds of smear-positive tuberculosis cases in the community were undiagnosed in Northwest Ethiopia: population based cross-sectional study," *PLoS ONE*, vol. 6, no. 12, Article ID e28258, 2011.

[15] Z. Jia, S. Cheng, Y. Ma et al., "Tuberculosis burden in China: a high prevalence of pulmonary tuberculosis in household contacts with and without symptoms," *BMC Infectious Diseases*, vol. 14, article 64, 2014.

[16] A. D. Meundi, M. D. Meundi, B. B. Dhabadi, M. I. Ismail, M. Amruth, and A. G. Kulkarni, "Prevalence of Pulmonary Tuberculosis among Inmates and Staff of Three Indian Prisons," *British Journal of Medicine & Medical Research*, vol. 11, no. 4, 2016.

[17] V. M. Mmbaga, *Prevalence and factors associated with pulmonary Tuberculosis among prisoners in Dar Salaam, Tanzania [Unpublished dissertation]*, 2012.

[18] Z. Zerdo, M. Girmay, W. Adane, and A. Gobena, "Prevalence of Pulmonary Tuberculosis and Associated Risk Factors in Prisons of Gamo Goffa Zone, South Ethiopia: A Cross-Sectional Study," *American Journal of Health Research*, vol. 2, no. 5, pp. 291–297, 2014.

[19] E. O. Ekundayo, O. Onuka, G. Mustapha, and M. Geoffrey, "Active Case Finding of Pulmonary Tuberculosis among Prison Inmates in Aba Federal Prison, Abia State, Nigeria," *Advances in Infectious Diseases*, vol. 5, no. 1, pp. 57–62, 2015.

[20] P. D. De Navarro, I. N. De Almeida, A. L. Kritski et al., "Prevalence of latent mycobacterium tuberculosis infection in prisoners," *Jornal Brasileiro de Pneumologia*, vol. 42, no. 5, pp. 348–355, 2016.

[21] *Federal ministry of health and Ethiopian health and nutrition research institute. First Ethiopian national population based Tuberculosis survey*, Addis Ababa, 2011.

[22] A. Jurcev-Savicevic, R. Mulic, B. Ban et al., "Risk factors for pulmonary tuberculosis in Croatia: A matched case-control study," *BMC Public Health*, vol. 13, no. 1, article no. 991, 2013.

[23] X. Zhang, H. Jia, F. Liu et al., "Prevalence and risk factors for latent tuberculosis infection among health care workers in China: a cross-sectional study," *PLoS ONE*, vol. 8, no. 6, Article ID e66412, 2013.

21

Assessment of Anti-TB Drug Nonadherence and Associated Factors among TB Patients Attending TB Clinics in Arba Minch Governmental Health Institutions, Southern Ethiopia

Addisu Alemayehu Gube (D),[1] **Megbaru Debalkie** (D),[2] **Kalid Seid** (D),[2] **Kiberalem Bisete** (D),[2] **Asfaw Mengesha** (D),[2] **Abubeker Zeynu** (D),[2] **Freselam Shimelis** (D),[2] and **Feleke Gebremeskel**[1]

[1]*Department of Public Health, College of Medicine and Health Sciences, Arba Minch University, P.O. Box 21, Arba Minch, Ethiopia*
[2]*Department of Nursing, College of Medicine and Health Sciences, Arba Minch University, P.O. Box 21, Arba Minch, Ethiopia*

Correspondence should be addressed to Addisu Alemayehu Gube; addis166@gmail.com

Academic Editor: Vincent Jarlier

Background. Tuberculosis (TB) is an infectious disease caused by the bacillus *Mycobacterium tuberculosis.* Nonadherence to anti-TB treatment may result in the emergence of multidrug-resistant TB, prolonged infectiousness, and poor tuberculosis treatment outcomes. Ethiopia is one of the seven countries that reported lower rates of treatment success (84%). This study assessed anti-TB drug nonadherence and associated factors among TB patients in Arba Minch governmental health institutions. *Methods.* An institution based cross-sectional study design was conducted from April 15 to May 30, 2017. A systematic sampling technique was employed to select the study subjects. Data was collected using a semistructured questionnaire with Morisky Medication Adherence Scale-8 (MMAS-8) and was entered, cleaned, and analyzed in SPSS version 20. *Results.* The study included 271 TB patients with a response rate of 96.4%; 58.3% were males and 64.9% were Gamo by ethnicity. The overall nonadherence was 67 (24.7%) (CI = 20.0–30.4). Nonadherence was high if the patients experienced side effects (AOR = 13.332; 95% CI = 2.282–77.905), were far from the health facility (AOR = 21.830; 95% CI = 0.054–77.500), and experienced prolonged waiting time to get medical services (AOR = 14.260; 95% CI = 2.135–95.241). *Conclusions.* The proportion of TB patients that did not adhere to anti-TB drugs was high in Arba Minch governmental health institutions.

1. Introduction

Tuberculosis is an infectious disease caused by the bacillus *Mycobacterium tuberculosis.* It typically affects the lungs (pulmonary TB) but can also affect other sites (extrapulmonary TB). The disease is spread when people sick with pulmonary TB expel bacteria to the air, for example, by coughing. Overall, a relatively small proportion (5–15%) of the estimated 2-3 billion people infected with *Mycobacterium tuberculosis* will develop TB disease during their lifetime [1]. The prevalence of TB among close contacts of infectious patients can be about 2.5 times higher than in the general population [2]. If TB is detected early and fully treated, people with disease quickly become noninfectious and are eventually cured [3].

The WHO, in its global plan to stop TB, reports that poor treatment has resulted in the evolution of Mycobacterium *tuberculosis* strains that do not respond to treatment with the standard first-line combination of anti-TB medicines, resulting in the emergence of multidrug-resistant TB in almost every country of the world [4]. One of the greatest dilemmas and challenges facing most TB programs is a patient that does not complete TB treatment for one reason or another [5].

Poor adherence to treatment of chronic diseases including TB is a worldwide problem of striking magnitude [6]. However, patients with TB are expected to have adherence levels greater than 90% in order to facilitate cure. Failure of cure increases the risk of development of drug-resistant strains and spread of TB in the community, and this in turn increases morbidity and mortality [7, 8]. TB in 2015 was one of the top 10 causes of death worldwide. The best estimates are that there were 1.4 million TB deaths in 2015 and an additional 0.4 million deaths resulting from TB disease among HIV-positive people [1]. According to recent estimates, Ethiopia stands 7th in the list of high TB burden countries. In Ethiopia, TB is the leading cause of morbidity, the third cause of hospital admissions, and the second cause of death. The estimated TB incidence of Ethiopia was 261/100,000 inhabitants in 2011. The lifetime risk of developing TB in Ethiopia is estimated to be 50–60% for HIV-infected people and only 10% for HIV-negative counterparts [9, 10]. In many countries, globally, the adoption of Directly Observed Treatment (DOT) has been associated with reduced rate of treatment failure, relapse, and drug resistance. However, its impact on reducing TB incidence has been limited by noncompliance to DOT, which occurs when patients do not turn up for treatment at the health facility or community DOT point [11].

Despite the implementation of an internationally recommended strategy (DOT) in almost all parts of WHO regions and many national and international efforts exerted against TB prevention and control, still the patients fail to complete their treatment to be declared "cured" or "completed the treatment" [12–14]. Current WHO reports show that a considerable number of TB cases failed after several treatments; many relapsed after completion of the treatment, many had to undergo retreatment after completion of treatment, and many developed MDR-TB among retreatment cases (20%) throughout the world [15]. For this, most probably, treatment nonadherence and loss to followup are the main responsible factors [16]. Nonadherence to anti-TB treatment may result in the emergence of multidrug-resistant TB (MDR-TB), prolonged infectiousness, and poor TB treatment outcomes [17, 18]. In sub-Saharan Africa, there is a high rate of loss to followup of TB patients that ranged from 11.3% to 29.6% [19]. Ethiopia is one of the seven countries that reported lower rates of treatment success (84%) [9].

In Ethiopia, even though TB drugs are given free of charge, TB continues to be a major health problem and cause of death. The Ethiopian national program for TB control recommends DOT as the main strategy for disease control, but its utilization differs due to local health institutions' capacities to guarantee patient supervision. Hence, this study will assess the level of nonadherence to anti-TB therapy and associated factors among TB patients in Arba Minch, Ethiopia.

2. Methods and Materials

2.1. Study Area and Period. The study was conducted in Arba Minch town, Gamo Gofa Zone SNNPR, Ethiopia. The town is located at 505 km from Addis Ababa and 275 km from Hawassa, capital city of Southern Ethiopia. The town is 30° 56′ north and 37° 44′ west, and it is located to the west of Lake Abaya. It covers 514 km^2 and is generally located at the altitude of 1200 through 1400 meters above sea level. Based on the 2007 Ethiopian national population and housing census, the population of the town is projected to be about 86,405. The town has three public facilities: two health centers

and one general hospital. Arba Minch General Hospital was established and started its full function in 1961 EC (Ethiopian Calendar). The hospital and the health centers are now providing several health services including TB treatment program for the community. The study was conducted from April 15 to May 30, 2017.

2.2. Study Population. The study population included all TB patients on anti-TB medication at least for a month at tuberculosis followup clinics in Arba Minch governmental health institutions.

2.3. Inclusion Criteria. All TB patients that were at least 15 years of age, regardless of the site or the smear status of their TB, and have taken anti-TB medication at least for a month were included.

2.4. Sample Size and Sampling Techniques. The sample size was calculated based on a single population proportion formula using the following assumptions: P = 21% [20], with 95% confidence level and 5% level of precision. And by adding 10% for nonresponse rate, the final sample size was 281. In order to draw the sample, average flow of TB patients in each health institution per day was taken as a reference to estimate the client load. Based on the information, proportionate allocation to size was made in each institution. Therefore, 52% (146) of the sample was drawn from Arba Minch General Hospital, 32% (90) from Sikella Health Center, and the rest (16%, 45) from Shecha Health Center. Since TB patients receive the same TB clinic service. Systematic random sampling was used, and by dividing the total 436 patients to 281 patients, every 2nd TB patient was selected. The first study subject was determined randomly.

2.5. Data Collection Instrument and Procedures. Data was collected using a pretested and semistructured questionnaire. It was in English and was translated to Amharic and then back to English to check for consistency and completeness. Then, it was collected through a face-to-face exit interview.

2.6. Operational Definitions. Nonadherence to anti-TB drugs means an individual whose score > 2 points in the Morisky Medication Adherence Scale-8.

MMAS-8 consists of eight items, with a scoring scheme of "yes" = 0 and "no" = 1 for the first seven items, but for the last item, a five-point Likert scale response will be used with options of "never," "once in a while," "sometimes," "usually," and "always." In this Likert scale, values ranging from 0 to 1 were given at a specified interval of 0.25 with "0" given for "never" and "1" given for "always." The degree of adherence was determined according to the score resulting from the sum of all the correct answers to a maximum score of 8. For the purpose of data analysis, the three original categories of adherence were recategorized into two. Accordingly, high and medium adherence were reassigned as adherent with a score of less than or equal to 2 and low adherence will be regarded as nonadherent with a score of greater than 2.

2.7. Data Processing and Analysis. After checking for completeness and consistency, data was entered into SPSS (IBM 20) for descriptive and inferential analysis. Binary logistic regression was used to determine the dependent variable on the basis of continuous and/or categorical independent variables, and factors with *P* value ≤ 0.25 in bivariate analysis were candidates for multivariate analysis and factors with *P* < 0.05 in the final model were statistically significant. The degree of association between dependent and independent variables was assessed using AOR at 95% CI.

2.8. Ethical Consideration. Ethical clearance was obtained from the ethical review committee of the College of Medicine and Health Sciences, Arba Minch University. A formal letter was given to each of the public health institutions in Arba Minch town. In addition, informed consent was obtained from study participants to confirm their willingness for participation after explaining the objective of the study. And the respondents were notified that they have the right to withdraw at any point of the interview.

3. Results

3.1. Sociodemographic Characteristics of the Study Participants. From 281 selected participants, 271 were involved in the study with a response rate of 96.4%. Of these, 142 (52.4%) were aged 25–34, with a mean age of 32.19 (±11.291 SD) years. Of 271, 158 (58.3%) were males and 170 (62.7%) were protestants. 190 (70.1%) of the participants were married and 176 (64.9%) were Gamo by ethnicity. 82 (30.3%) of the study participants attended grades 7–12, 183 (67.5%) were self-employed, and 169 (62.4%) got more than 501 birr as a monthly income (Table 1).

3.2. Behavioral Risk Factors of Study Participants. 249 (91.9%) of the study participants had no smoking habit and 227 (83.8%) never drank alcohol before. 15 (5.5%) of the study participants had no treatment supporter (Table 2).

3.3. Healthcare System Related Characteristics of the Study Participants. 150 (55.3%) stated that their preferable TB clinic opening time was from 2:00 AM to 6:00 PM local time, and for 225 (83.0%), the waiting time at the health facility was <1 hour. 56 (20.7%) of the participants reported that it took them more than 5 kms and 5 birr to reach the nearby TB clinic.

44 (16.2%) of the study participants stated that no one supervised them while taking their TB medication. 208 (76.8%) reported that the health workers were friendly to them.

259 (95.6%) participants had good knowledge about TB but 12 (4.4%) participants did not know the symptoms of TB at all. 46 (17.0%) of the participants reported that they stopped taking their anti-TB medication when they felt better. 249 (91.9%) disclosed their illness to their relatives, and all those who did not disclose had fear of stigma and discrimination (Table 3).

3.4. Disease and Medicine Related Factors. 30 (11.1%) of the TB patients reported some kind of anti-TB medication

TABLE 1: Sociodemographic characteristics of the TB patients that attended TB clinics at governmental health institutions of Arba Minch town, Southern Ethiopia, 2017 (*N* = 271).

Variable	Frequency	Percent
Age		
15–24	65	24
25–34	142	52.4
35–44	30	11
>=45	34	12.6
Sex		
Male	158	58.3
Female	113	41.7
Marital status		
Married	190	70.1
Single	50	18.5
Divorced	21	7.7
Widowed	10	3.7
Religion		
Protestant	170	62.7
Orthodox	90	33.2
Muslim	11	4.1
Ethnicity		
Gamo	176	64.9
Wolaita	80	29.5
Gofa	15	5.5
Educational status		
Cannot read and write	25	9.2
Can read and write	62	22.9
Grades 1–6	75	27.7
Grades 7–12	82	30.3
Diploma and above	27	10.0
Occupational status		
Employee	57	21
Self-employed	183	67.5
No job	31	11.4
Monthly income		
<501 birr	102	37.6
>=501 birr	169	62.4

adverse effects: of these, 10 (33.4%), 9 (30%), 7 (23.3%), and 4 (13.3%) participants complained of minor adverse effects, that is, vomiting and diarrhea, numbness of feet and hands, headache and dizziness, and skin rash, respectively. 257 (94.8%) of the participants reported that they felt better in less than 2 months' time after starting anti-TB medication.

229 (84.5%) of the TB patients were screened for HIV and 6 (2.2%) of them were positive. 14 (5.2%) of the TB patients have taken drugs other than anti-TB medication: of these, 6 (42.8%) for HIV, 2 (14.3%) for pneumonia, 1 (7.1%) for STI, and 5 (35.8%) for fungal diseases (Table 4).

3.5. Prevalence of Nonadherence to Anti-TB Medication. The overall calculated nonadherence in this study was 67 (24.7%) with a confidence interval (CI) of 20.0–30.4 (Figure 1).

TABLE 2: Behavioral characteristics of the TB patients that attended TB clinics at governmental health institutions of Arba Minch town, Southern Ethiopia, 2017 ($N = 271$).

Variable	Frequency	Percent
Smoking		
Yes	22	8.1
No	249	91.9
Alcohol		
Yes	44	16.2
No	227	83.8
Treatment supporter		
Yes	256	94.5
No	15	5.5

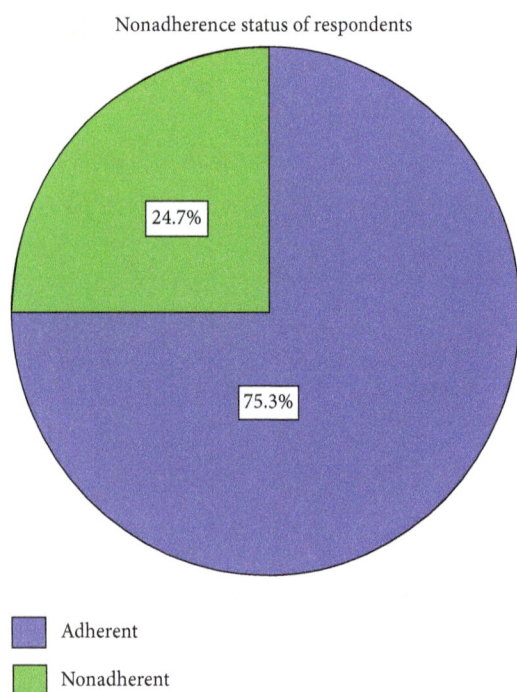

FIGURE 1: Adherence status of the TB patients that attended TB clinics at governmental health institutions of Arba Minch town, Southern Ethiopia, 2017 ($N = 271$).

TABLE 3: Healthcare system related characteristics of the TB patients that attended TB clinics at governmental health institutions of Arba Minch town, Southern Ethiopia, 2017 ($N = 271$).

Variable	Frequency	Percent
Preferable time for TB clinic		
2:00–6:00 AM	150	55.3
8:00–11:00 AM	120	44.3
After 2 PM	1	0.4
Waiting time at health facility		
<1 hr	225	83.0
1-2 hr	46	17.0
Distance to health facility		
0–5 km	215	79.3
>5 km	56	20.7
Transport cost		
0–5 birr	215	79.3
>5 birr	56	20.7
Supervision		
None	44	16.2
Family member	17	6.3
Health worker	210	77.5
Relationship with health worker		
Very friendly	22	8.1
Friendly	208	76.8
Indifferent	32	11.8
Unfriendly	9	3.3
Knowledge on symptoms of TB		
All	144	53.2
Some	115	42.4
Not knowing	12	4.4
Time to stop TB medication		
6–24 months	132	48.7
8–24 months	93	34.3
When feeling better	46	17.0
TB status disclosure		
Yes	249	91.9
No	22	8.1
Reason for not disclosing		
Fear of stigma and discrimination	22	100

3.6. Factors Associated with Nonadherence to Anti-TB Treatment. In bivariate analysis, sex, educational status, waiting time at health facility, distance to health facility, side effects of the drugs, smoking, alcohol use, treatment supporter, and monthly income were significantly associated with nonadherence to anti-TB medication. But in multivariate analysis, patients who experienced drug side effects, those who were far from the health facility, and those that experienced a prolonged waiting time to get medical services remained significantly and independently associated with anti-TB medication nonadherence. Those patients that experienced side effects were thirteen times more likely (AOR = 13.332; 95% CI: 2.282–77.905) to be nonadherent than their counterparts. In addition, patients that came from a far distance to the health facility to get medical services (AOR = 21.830; 95%

CI: 0.0–554–77.500) and those who experienced a prolonged waiting time at the health facility to get medical services (AOR = 14.260; 95% CI: 2.135–95.241) were also at a higher risk of nonadherence than those who were near the health facility and those that waited for a short period of time, respectively (Table 5).

4. Discussion

This study assessed anti-TB drug nonadherence and the associated factors among TB patients in Arba Minch governmental health institutions. Even if it is recommended that every TB patient should adhere to anti-TB medication by following DOT strategy [1], the findings of this study showed

TABLE 4: Disease and medicine related characteristics of the TB patients that attended TB clinics at governmental health institutions of Arba Minch town, Southern Ethiopia, 2017 (N = 271).

Variable	Frequency	Percent
Experience of side effects		
Yes	30	11.1
No	241	88.9
Type of side effects		
Vomiting and diarrhea	10	33.4
Headache and dizziness	7	23.4
Skin rash	4	13.3
Numbness of feet and hands	9	30
Duration to feel better		
<2 months	257	94.8
2–4 months	9	3.3
5-6 months	5	1.8
Missing of anti-TB medication		
Yes	69	25.5
No	202	74.5
Reason for missing anti-TB medication		
Forgetfulness	15	21.7
Vomiting and diarrhea	4	5.9
Cost of transport	5	7.2
Health professional attitude	3	4.3
Stigma and discrimination	7	10.1
Feeling better	35	50.8
HIV status		
Positive	6	2.2
Negative	223	82.3
Not tested	42	15.5
Taking drugs other than anti-Tb medication		
Yes	14	5.2
No	257	94.8
Reason of taking another drug		
HIV/AIDS	6	42.8
Pneumonia	2	14.3
STI	1	7.1
Fungal disease	5	35.8

that 24.7% of TB patients did not adhere to anti-TB drugs. This finding is almost in line with the finding of the study conducted in a tertiary health institution in Southeast Nigeria and in South Ethiopia where nonadherence for anti-TB drugs was 24.2% and 24.5%, respectively [21, 22]. In this study, the proportion of TB patients that do not adhere to anti-TB drugs is higher compared to the findings of the study conducted in Southwest Ethiopia and Northwest Ethiopia where the nonadherence was 20.8% and 10%, respectively [20, 23]. This discrepancy could be, in the first case, because the study was conducted in three big towns in North Ethiopia and, in the second case, could be because the study finding only represents the result from a single hospital and only few patients. In the current study, the number of TB patients that did not adhere to anti-TB drugs is relatively smaller than

that found by a study conducted in Hadiya Zone, Southern Ethiopia, where nonadherence was 30% [24]. This might be attributable to the fact that the finding of the study conducted in Hadiya Zone represents TB patients both in higher health facilities and in rural health facilities, whereas our study was only restricted to patients from health facilities located in an urban setting, which is Arba Minch town.

In this study, one reason for nonadherence of anti-TB drugs is the waiting time at the health facility. While only 10.2% of TB patients waiting for less than 1 hour did not adhere to anti-TB drugs, 95.7% of TB patients waiting for 1-2 hours did not adhere. This is similar to the finding of the study conducted in Hadiya Zone, Southern Ethiopia, where the probability of complying with DOT is 2.5 times higher for TB patients waiting for less than 30 minutes compared to their counterparts [24].

The other important reason for anti-TB nonadherence among TB patients is distance to the health facility. While only 8.4% of TB patients 0–5 kms away from health facility did not adhere to anti-TB drugs, 87.5% of TB patients greater than 5 kms away from the health facility did not adhere. Similarly, the study conducted in South Ethiopia has depicted that the likelihood of not adhering to anti-TB drugs for TB patients faraway from DOT center is 5.7 times higher than TB patients nearer to the center [22].

Side effects of the drugs are also an important reason for anti-TB drug nonadherence among TB patients. While the likelihood of not adhering to anti-TB drugs among TB patients with side effects of the drugs is 90%, only 16.6% of TB patients without the side effects of the drugs did not adhere to anti-TB drugs. This finding is in line with the finding of the study carried out in Tigray, Northern Ethiopia, where the probability of adhering to anti-TB drugs among TB patients without drugs side effects was 3 times higher than in those with drugs side effects [25]. Similarly, in a study carried out in Alamata District, Northeast Ethiopia, one of the main reasons for nonadherence was the presence of drugs side effects among TB patients [26].

In this study, some variables which were significant during bivariate analysis were not found to be statistically significant during multivariate analysis and were not independent determinants of anti-TB drug nonadherence among TB patients. One of such variables was sex, which in this study has no effect on anti-TB drug nonadherence among TB patients. Similarly, studies conducted in Southeast Nigeria and Plateau State, Nigeria, have shown that sex has no significant effect on anti-TB drug nonadherence among TB patients [21, 27]. On the contrary, the study conducted in Argentina has shown that difference in sex has an effect on anti-TB drug nonadherence among TB patients [28]. The other variable with no effect on anti-TB drug nonadherence in this study was educational status. In the same manner, studies carried out in South Ethiopia and Plateau State, Nigeria, have indicated that the educational status of TB patients has no effect on anti-TB drug nonadherence [22, 27]. But studies conducted in Southwest Ethiopia and Southeast Nigeria have shown that educational status has a significant effect on anti-TB drug nonadherence among TB patients [20, 21]. Similarly, having a treatment supporter in this study

TABLE 5: Factors associated with nonadherence of anti-TB drug treatment among TB patients that attended TB clinics at governmental health institutions of Arba Minch town, Southern Ethiopia ($N = 271$).

Variables	Nonadherence		Crude OR	Adjusted OR
	Yes	No		
Sex				
Male	50 (31.6%)	108 (68.4%)	1	1
Female	17 (15.0%)	96 (85.0%)	0.383 (0.207, 0.708)	3.023 (0.071, 11.335)
Educational status				
Cannot read and write	15 (60.0%)	10 (40.0%)	5.250 (1.566, 17.601)	1.923 (0.023, 8.013)
Can read and write	13 (21.0%)	49 (79.0%)	0.929 (0.311, 2.773)	0.745 (0.154, 3.257)
Grades 1–6	19 (25.3%)	56 (74.7%)	1.187 (0.417, 3.380)	0.247 (0.099, 6.227)
Grades 7–12	14 (17.1%)	68 (82.9%)	0.721 (0.246, 2.110)	2.016 (0.085, 11.663)
Diploma and above	6 (22.2%)	21 (77.8%)	1	1
Waiting time at health facility				
<1 hour	23 (10.2%)	202 (89.8%)	1	1
1-2 hours	44 (95.7%)	2 (4.3%)	193.217 (43.929, 849.847)	**14.260 (2.135, 95.241)**[*]
Distance to health facility				
0–5 km	18 (8.4%)	197 (91.6%)	1	1
>5 km	49 (87.5%)	7 (12.5%)	76.611 (30.306, 193.669)	**21.830 (5.278, 90.284)**[*]
Side effects of the drugs				
Yes	27 (90%)	3 (10%)	45.000 (13.020, 155.528)	**13.332 (2.282, 77.905)**[*]
No	40 (16.6%)	201 (83.4%)	1	1
Smoking				
Yes	20 (90.9%)	2 (9.1%)	42.979 (9.708, 190.282)	0.903 (0.080, 10.200)
No	47 (18.9%)	202 (81.1%)	1	1
Alcohol				
Yes	43 (97.7%)	1 (2.3%)	363.708 (47.899, 2761.726)	2.665 (0.897, 9.776)
No	24 (10.6%)	203 (89.4%)	1	1
Treatment supporter				
Yes	53 (20.7%)	203 (79.3%)	1	1
No	14 (93.3%)	1 (6.7%)	53.623 (6.895, 417.018)	2.044 (0.054, 77.500)
Monthly income				
<501 birr	51 (50%)	51 (50%)	9.562 (5.018, 18.223)	2.267 (0.795, 6.468)
>=501 birr	16 (9.5%)	153 (90.5%)	1	1

[*] Significant association.

has no effect on anti-TB drug nonadherence, which is also in line with the finding of the study conducted in South Ethiopia [22]. The other variable that does not affect anti-TB drug nonadherence status in this study was alcohol use. In the same way, studies carried out in South Ethiopia and Plateau State, Nigeria, have revealed that alcohol use has no significant effect on anti-TB drug nonadherence [22, 27]. Cigarette smoking was another variable in this study that does not affect anti-TB drug nonadherence status, but the study conducted in Plateau State, Nigeria, has shown that cigarette smoking is significantly associated with anti-TB drug nonadherence among TB patients [27]. The last variable that is not associated with anti-TB drug adherence status among TB patients in this study was monthly income of TB patients, which is contrary to the finding of the study carried out in Southeast Nigeria where the average monthly income has significantly affected anti-TB drug adherence status of TB patients [21].

5. Conclusions

In general, this study revealed that the level of nonadherence to anti-TB drugs among TB patients in Arba Minch governmental health institutions is high. The waiting time at the health facility, the distance to the health facility, and the side effects of the drugs were significant determinants of nonadherence to anti-TB drugs. The other variables such as sex, educational status, smoking, alcohol use, treatment supporter, and monthly income were only significantly associated with nonadherence to anti-TB medication during bivariate analysis. And they were not found to be statistically significant during multivariate analysis.

Acknowledgments

The authors' sincere thanks go to Arba Minch University for provision of the opportunity to conduct the research. They would also like to give their deepest gratitude to Gamo Gofa Zone Health Department for providing baseline information. Lastly, their thanks go to data collectors and all research participants who took part in the study.

References

[1] WHO, *WHO Global Tuberculosis Report 2016*, WHO Press, Geneva, Switzerland, 2016.

[2] A. C. Lemos, E. D. Matos, D. B. Pedral-Sampaio, and E. M. Netto, "Risk of tuberculosis among household contacts in Salvador, Bahia," *The Brazilian Journal of Infectious Diseases*, vol. 8, no. 6, pp. 424–430, 2004.

[3] J. A. Caminero, "A tuberculosis guide for specialist physicians," *International Union Against Tuberculosis and Lung Diseases*, vol. 24, 2003.

[4] WHO, *The Global Plan to Stop TB 2006–2015*, World Health Organization, Geneva, Switzerland, 2006.

[5] L. H. Rieder, "Interventions for tuberculosis control and elimination," *Journal of International Union against Tuberculosis and Lung Diseases*, vol. 5, 2002.

[6] E. Sabate, *Adherence to Long-Term Therapies: Evidence for Action*, WHO, Geneva, Switzerland, 2003.

[7] A. Harries, D. Maher, and S. Graham, *TB/HIV: A Clinical Manual*, World Health Organization, Geneva, Switzerland, 2004.

[8] N. Awofeso, "Anti tuberculosis medication side-effects constitute major factor for poor adherence to tuberculosis treatment," *Bulletin of the World Health Organization*, vol. 86, no. 3, 2008.

[9] WHO, *WHO report 2011/Global Tuberculosis Control*, WHO, France, Europe, 2011.

[10] Ethiopia FMoH Tuberculosis, Leprosy and TB/HIV Prevention and Control Programme. Addis Ababa, Ethiopia 207 p, 2008.

[11] Ch. Kudakwashe, "Factor affecting compliance to tuberculosis treatment in Andra Kanvango region in Namibia," *Journal of compliance to TB treatment*, pp. 5-6, 2010.

[12] WHO, *Global Tuberculosis Control: Surveillance, Planning, Financing*, WHO Press, Geneva, Switzerland, 2008.

[13] Z. Obermeyer, J. Abbott-Klafter, and C. J. L. Murray, "Has the DOTS strategy improved case finding or treatment success? an empirical assessment," *PLoS ONE*, vol. 3, no. 3, Article ID e1721, 2008.

[14] X. Yin, X. Tu, Y. Tong, R. Yang, Y. Wang, S. Cao et al., "Development and validation of a tuberculosis medication adherence scale," *PLoS ONE*, vol. 7, no. 12, Article ID e50328, 2012.

[15] WHO, *Global Tuberculosis Control Report of 2011*, WHO Press, Geneva, Switzerland, 2012.

[16] H. H. Tola, A. Tol, D. Shojaeizadeh, and G. Garmaroudi, "Tuberculosis treatment non -adherence and lost to Follow up among TB patients with or without HIV in Developing countries: a systematic review," *Iranian Journal of Public Health*, vol. 44, no. 1, pp. 1–11, 2015.

[17] P. Charles, "Felton national tuberculosis center. adherence to treatment for latent tuberculosis infection," *A Manual for Health Care Providers*, 2005.

[18] M. F. Franke, S. C. Appleton, F. Arteaga et al., "Risk factors and mortality associated with default from multidrug-resistant tuberculosis treatment," *Clinical Infectious Diseases*, vol. 48, no. 12, pp. 1844–1851, 2008.

[19] B. Castelnuovo, "A review of compliance to anti tuberculosis treatment and risk factors for defaulting treatment in Sub Saharan Africa," *African Health Sciences*, vol. 10, no. 4, pp. 320–324, 2010.

[20] A. Kebede and N. T. Wabe, "Medication adherence and its determinants among patients on concomitant tuberculosis and antiretroviral therapy in South West Ethiopia," *North American Journal of Medical Sciences*, vol. 4, no. 2, pp. 67–71, 2012.

[21] C. F. Ubajaka, E. C. Azuike, J. O. Ugoji et al., "Adherence to drug medications amongst tuberculosis patients in a tertiary health institution in South East Nigeria," *International Journal of Clinical Medicine*, vol. 06, no. 06, pp. 399–406, 2015.

[22] T. T. Woimo, W. K. Yimer, T. Bati, and H. A. Gesesew, "The prevalence and factors associated for anti-tuberculosis treatment non-adherence among pulmonary tuberculosis patients in public health care facilities in South Ethiopia: a cross-sectional study," *BMC Public Health*, vol. 17, no. 1, article no. 269, 2017.

[23] A. A. Adane, K. A. Alene, D. N. Koye, and B. M. Zeleke, "Non-adherence to anti-tuberculosis treatment and determinant factors among patients with tuberculosis in Northwest Ethiopia," *PLoS ONE*, vol. 8, no. 11, Article ID e78791, 2013.

[24] B. Bayu, A. Lonsako, and L. Tegene, "Directly observed treatment short-course compliance and associated factors among adult tuberculosis cases in public health institutions of Hadiya zone, Southern Ethiopia," *Journal of Infectious Diseases and Immunity*, vol. 8, no. 1, pp. 1–9, 2016.

[25] Y. K. Kiros, T. Teklu, F. Desalegn, M. Tesfay, E. Klinkenberg, and A. Mulugeta, "Adherence to anti-tuberculosis treatment in Tigray, Northern Ethiopia," *Public Health Action*, vol. 4, no. 4, pp. 531–536, 2014.

[26] G. Tesfahuneygn, G. Medhin, and M. Legesse, "Adherence to anti-tuberculosis treatment and treatment outcomes among tuberculosis patients in Alamata District, Northeast Ethiopia," *BMC Research Notes*, vol. 8, no. 503, 2015.

[27] L. M. Ibrahim, I. S. Hadejia, P. Nguku et al., "Factors associated with interruption of treatment among Pulmonary Tuberculosis patients in Plateau State, Nigeria. 2011," *Pan African Medical Journal*, vol. 17, no. 78, 2014.

[28] M. B. Herrero, S. Ramos, and S. Arrossi, "Determinants of non adherence to tuberculosis treatment in argentina: Barriers related to access to treatment," *Revista Brasileira de Epidemiologia*, vol. 18, no. 2, pp. 287–298, 2015.

22

Evaluation of a U.S. Public Health Laboratory Service for the Molecular Detection of Drug Resistant Tuberculosis

Mitchell A. Yakrus, Beverly Metchock, and Angela M. Starks

Centers for Disease Control and Prevention, Atlanta, GA 30329-4027, USA

Correspondence should be addressed to Mitchell A. Yakrus; may2@cdc.gov

Academic Editor: Paul R. Klatser

Crucial to interrupting the spread of tuberculosis (TB) is prompt implementation of effective treatment regimens. We evaluated satisfaction, comfort with interpretation, and use of molecular results from a public health service provided by the Centers for Disease Control and Prevention (CDC) for the molecular detection of drug resistant *Mycobacterium tuberculosis* complex (MTBC). An electronic survey instrument was used to collect information anonymously from U.S. Public Health Laboratories (PHL) that submitted at least one isolate of MTBC to CDC from September 2009 through February 2011. Over 97% of those responding expressed satisfaction with the turnaround time for receiving results. Twenty-six PHL (74%) reported molecular results to healthcare providers in less than two business days. When comparing the molecular results from CDC with their own phenotypic drug susceptibility testing, 50% of PHL observed discordance. No respondents found the molecular results difficult to interpret and 82% were comfortably discussing them with TB program officials and healthcare providers. Survey results indicate PHL were satisfied with CDC's ability to rapidly provide interpretable molecular results for isolates of MTBC submitted for determination of drug resistance. To develop educational materials and strategies for service improvement, reasons for discordant results and areas of confusion need to be identified.

1. Introduction

Prompt identification of new cases and implementation of effective treatment regimens are crucial to interrupt the transmission of tuberculosis (TB) and to prevent the emergence of drug resistant forms of the disease. The first-line antituberculosis regimen combines four first-line drugs: isoniazid (INH), rifampin (RMP), pyrazinamide (PZA), and ethambutol (EMB). Multidrug-resistant (MDR) isolates of *Mycobacterium tuberculosis* complex (MTBC) are defined as resistant to at least RMP and INH. Patients with MDR TB must be placed on regimens containing second-line antituberculosis drugs that are more costly and have more potential for adverse side effects. For 2012, the Centers for Disease Control and Prevention (CDC) reported 9,945 cases of TB in the United States [1]. For 7,188 of these cases, initial drug susceptibility to first-line antituberculosis drugs was reported; 660 (9.2%) were INH resistant and 83 (1.2%) were MDR TB.

CDC offers a nationally available service for the molecular detection of drug resistance (MDDR) by rapidly identifying mutations associated with MDR TB [2, 3]. The service is available by request in coordination with state PHL for isolates and clinical specimens positive by nucleic acid amplification testing for MTBC meeting defined submission criteria [4]. DNA sequencing is used for detection of mutations most frequently associated with RMP, INH, EMB, and PZA drug resistance as well as resistance to the most effective second-line drugs: fluoroquinolones and the second-line injectables amikacin, kanamycin, and capreomycin. All isolates concurrently undergo phenotypic drug susceptibility testing (DST) for a full panel of first and second-line drugs [5]. Submitting laboratories receive an interim report describing molecular test results. Upon completion of phenotypic DST, a final report is issued that includes DST results along with interpretive comments to correlate molecular results with DST results. From a recent study [6], the mean turnaround time (range) for completion of molecular testing through this

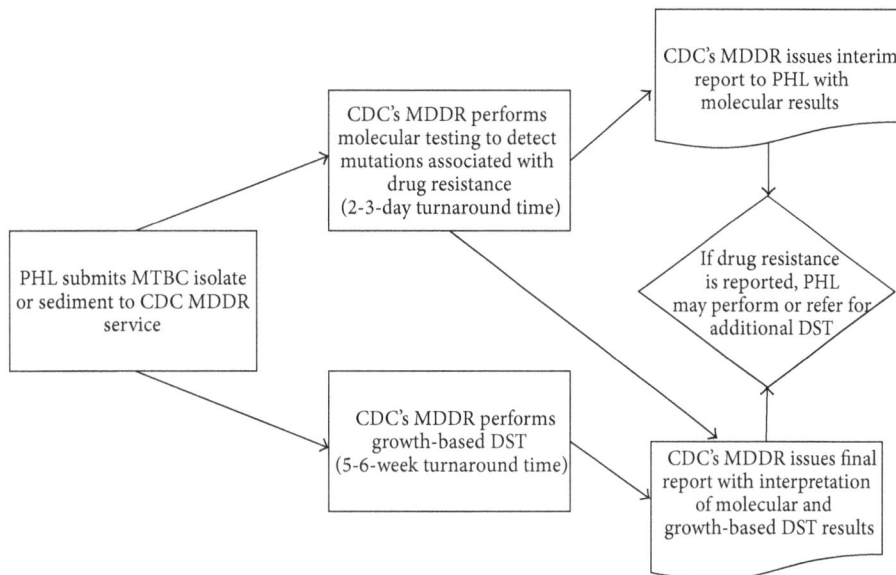

FIGURE 1: Workflow for MTBC isolates and sediments submitted by PHL to the CDC MDDR service for detection or confirmation of drug resistance. MTBC = *Mycobacterium tuberculosis* complex. PHL = Public Health Laboratory. CDC = Centers for Disease Control and Prevention. MDDR = molecular detection of drug resistance. DST = drug susceptibility testing.

service was 2.3 d (1–8 d) and for phenotypic DST was 41 d (14–117 d).

In the United States, PHL usually perform first-line DST in their own laboratory using phenotypic methods. Therefore, PHL may receive molecular results from CDC's MDDR before completion of their own testing. If the interim CDC report detailing molecular results or local phenotypic DST indicates resistance to one or more first-line antituberculosis drugs, the submitting PHL may either initiate additional testing in their own laboratory using a panel of second-line drugs or refer the isolate to another laboratory for additional testing. The general workflow for MTBC isolates and sediments submitted by PHL to CDC's MDDR is shown in Figure 1.

To measure program effectiveness, it is necessary to determine how molecular and phenotypic DST results are interpreted and used by PHL submitting samples to CDC. Evaluation of the service is essential to ascertain if the intended purpose to rapidly identify drug resistance and provide easy to interpret results to stakeholders is being achieved. Elements of difficulty interpreting results from CDC's MDDR need to be identified along with actions taken by PHL to resolve these issues. In addition, PHL awareness and satisfaction with CDC's MDDR need to be measured to determine effectiveness of service delivery and to identify areas for improvement.

2. Materials and Methods

2.1. Survey Design. A survey instrument was designed to elicit information from PHL directors or their designees regarding their interpretation and application of test results from CDC's MDDR. In addition, respondents were asked

questions regarding how they first learned about the service, who in their jurisdiction is responsible for initiating requests for using the service, and customer satisfaction. CDC determined that this activity was public health program evaluation rather than research. Institutional review board approval for human subject research was not required. The survey was piloted by nine randomly selected PHL directors or their designees, who submitted samples to CDC's MDDR between September 2009 and February 2011. Feedback from this group was used to refine questions as needed and establish the estimated time required to complete the survey. The final instrument consisted of 18 multiple-choice questions and respondents were required to answer each question by selecting either one choice or all that applied as indicated in the survey. An open-ended response option was available for some questions. This data collection effort received expedited approval under an Office of Management and Budget (OMB) generic clearance package (Information Collections to Advance State, Tribal, Local and Territorial Governmental Agency System Performance, Capacity, and Program Delivery; OMB number 0920-0879).

2.2. Survey Distribution. The survey instrument was distributed electronically using Snap Surveys version Snap 10 Professional software [7] (http://www.snapsurveys.com) by emailing potential respondents a link to summit responses online. The sampling frame comprised 43 PHL who had submitted at least one isolate of MTBC to CDC's MDDR.

3. Results and Discussion

A total of 35 PHL participated in the survey for an overall response rate of 81%. Responses to the survey questions are presented in Table 1.

TABLE 1: Survey responses from PHL officials who utilized CDC's MDDR.

Variable	Number	Percent
Where information first obtained on CDC's MDDR		
CDC website	1/35	3
"Dear Colleague" letter	6/35	18
Conference call with CDC	3/35	9
Professional meeting	9/35	26
Regional Training and Medical Consultation Center (RTMCC)	0/35	0
TB control program	7/35	20
Another public health laboratory	1/35	3
CDC TB laboratory consultant	8/35	23
Initiates requests for using CDC's MDDR		
Health care provider	12/35	34
TB control program	25/35	71
Laboratory	17/35	49
Laboratory only after consultation with program staff	10/35	29
Other	2/35	6
Satisfaction with turnaround time for receiving results from CDC's MDDR		
Very satisfied	26/35	74
Satisfied	8/35	23
Neither satisfied nor dissatisfied	1/35	3
Dissatisfied	0/35	0
Very dissatisfied	0/35	0
Usual time frame to report molecular results from CDC's MDDR to health care providers		
Reported within one business day	21/35	60
Reported within two business days	5/35	14
Reporting time varies depending on circumstances	1/35	3
Results are reported to health care provider by TB control program	8/35	23
Not applicable. Health care provider receives separate report from CDC's MDDR	0/35	0
Withhold reporting molecular results from CDC's MDDR to health care providers until phenotypic DST is completed by CDC		
Yes	0/35	0
Sometimes	0/35	0
No, results reported as soon as possible	30/35	86
Not applicable. Results are reported to health care provider by TB control program	5/35	14
Not applicable. Health care provider receives separate report from CDC's MDDR	0/35	0
Withhold reporting molecular results from CDC's MDDR to health care providers until phenotypic DST is completed by your laboratory		
Yes	0/35	0
Sometimes	0/35	0
No, molecular results reported as soon as possible	29/35	83
Not applicable. Results are reported to health care provider by TB control program	6/35	17
Not applicable. Health care provider receives separate report from CDC's MDDR	0/35	0
Method (s) for reporting results from CDC's MDDR to health care providers		
Verbally	9/35	26
Copy of CDC report is provided	31/35	89
CDC results transcribed into LIMS for reporting	1/35	3
Not applicable. Results are not reported by our laboratory	3/35	9

Table 1: Continued.

Variable	Number	Percent
Comparison of molecular results from CDC's MDDR with own phenotypic DST for first-line drugs		
Yes, we always compare molecular results from CDC with our phenotypic DST for first-line drugs	30/35	86
Sometimes we compare molecular results from CDC with our own phenotypic DST for first-line drugs	2/35	6
No, we report molecular results from CDC without comparing to our own phenotypic DST first-line drugs	1/35	3
Not applicable. We do not perform phenotypic DST for first-line drugs	2/35	6
Reasons for comparing molecular results from CDC's MDDR with own phenotypic DST for first-line drugs		
Results compared for quality assurance	27/32	84
Results compared to increase understanding of molecular testing	23/32	72
Results are compared to find discordance	29/32	91
Results are compared to prepare for consultation with health care provider or TB control program	20/32	63
Found discordance when molecular results from CDC's MDDR compared to own phenotypic DST for first-line drugs		
Yes, we found potentially discordant results	16/32	50
No, we have not found any potentially discordant results	16/32	50
Actions taken when discordance found between molecular results from CDC's MDDR and own phenotypic DST for first-line drugs		
No action taken	2/16	13
Contacted CDC to discuss results	9/16	56
Retested isolate in our laboratory	10/16	63
Withheld sending CDC results to health care provider or TB control	0/16	0
Notified TB control program of potential discordance	13/16	81
Initiated a corrective plan in our laboratory	1/16	6
Referred isolate from patient to another laboratory other than CDC for molecular testing	0/16	0
Action taken dependent on which drug has discordant test results	2/16	13
Comparison of molecular results from CDC's MDDR with own phenotypic DST for second-line drugs		
Yes, we always compare molecular results from CDC with our phenotypic DST for second-line drugs	13/35	37
Sometimes we compare molecular results from CDC with our own phenotypic DST for second-line drugs	2/35	6
No, we do not perform second-line DST	20/35	57
No, we perform second-line DST but do not compare with molecular results from CDC	0/35	0
Impact on your local phenotypic DST when first available results are molecular results from CDC's MDDR		
Results have no impact on local phenotypic DST	24/35	69
Local results are discarded	0/35	0
If resistance is indicated by molecular results, isolate is referred to another laboratory other than CDC's MDDR for additional testing	3/35	9
Other	8/35	23
Observed discordance between the molecular results and the phenotypic DST on the final report from CDC's MDDR		
Yes, we have observed discordance	12/35	34
No, we have not observed discordance	20/35	57
No, we do not examine CDC's MDDR results for discordance	3/35	9
Actions taken when discordance observed between molecular results and phenotypic results reported by CDC's MDDR		
No additional actions taken	3/12	25
Contacted CDC to discuss results	5/12	42
Retested isolate in our laboratory	6/12	50
Withheld sending CDC results to health care provider or TB control	0/12	0
Contacted TB control program to notify them of potential discordance	10/12	83
Referred an isolate from the patient to another laboratory other than CDC for molecular testing	1/35	8
Referred an isolate from the patient to another laboratory other than CDC for phenotypic DST	1/35	8
Action taken dependent on which drug has discordant results	2/35	17

TABLE 1: Continued.

Variable	Number	Percent
Difficulty interpreting molecular results from CDC's MDDR		
Results were very difficult to interpret	0/35	0
Results somewhat difficult to interpret	9/35	26
Results were not difficult to interpret	17/35	49
Results were very easy to interpret	9/35	26
Comfort discussing interpretation of molecular results from CDC's MDDR with health care providers or TB control		
Very comfortable when discussing the results	23/35	66
Had some difficulty discussing the results	5/35	14
In most instances, not contacted for help interpreting the results	7/35	20
Sought help interpreting results from CDC's MDDR		
Contacted CDC for help interpreting results	16/35	46
Visited CDC website for more information on molecular testing	5/35	14
Consulted with clinician	2/35	6
Did my own research to find information on molecular testing	7/35	20
Contacted local TB program	5/35	14
Contacted Regional Training and Medical Consultation Center (RTMCC)	1/35	3
I did not seek help	14/35	40

PHL = Public Health Laboratory.
CDC = Centers for Disease Control and Prevention.
MDDR = molecular detection of drug resistance.
DST = drug susceptibility testing.
LIMS = Laboratory Information Management System.

3.1. Customer Awareness and Satisfaction. Most respondents indicated they first obtained information on CDC's MDDR at a professional meeting (26%), a CDC-assigned TB laboratory consultant (23%), or their jurisdictional TB program (20%). Only 17% of respondents indicated first becoming aware of the service through a formal communication (i.e., letter via email) from CDC. When asked who initiates test requests, PHL officials collectively indicated that most requests originated from the jurisdictional TB program (71%) followed by the laboratory (49%) and health care providers (34%). Over 97% of PHL officials indicated they were either very satisfied or satisfied with the turnaround time for receiving test results.

3.2. Reporting Results to Health Care Providers. Over 74% of PHL officials indicated that molecular results from CDC's MDDR are provided to health care providers in less than two business days after receipt of the report. However, 23% of PHL officials indicated results are reported to health care providers by their TB program and not the PHL. In these instances, the time frame for health care providers to receive molecular results could not be determined using this survey. Ideally, with expanded access to electronic reporting, molecular results could be provided simultaneously to submitting laboratories and for population of electronic medical records to avoid potential delays in initiation of effective treatment regimens.

PHL providing results from CDC directly to health care providers did not withhold the interim report of molecular results until phenotypic DST was completed by either CDC or their own laboratory. When reporting results to health care providers, PHL most often provided a copy of the CDC report (89%) but frequently verbally communicated results as well (26%).

3.3. Comparison of Molecular Results from CDC's MDDR with Phenotypic DST from PHL. Thirty (86%) of the respondents indicated that they always compare molecular results from CDC's MDDR with phenotypic DST performed in their own laboratory with the primary intent to identify any discordant results for first-line drugs. Of the 32 PHL who compared molecular results from CDC's MDDR with their own phenotypic DST, 16 (50%) reported to have observed discordant results. Most PHL observing potential discordance took multiple actions with the most frequent being to notify their TB program authorities of the discordant results (81%), retesting the isolate in their own laboratory (63%), and contacting CDC directly to discuss the results (56%). Two PHL reported taking no additional action when they observed potential discordance. Of 15 PHL that performed second-line phenotypic DST in-house, 13 (87%) always compared their results with molecular results from CDC's MDDR. The most frequent action selected among those performing second-line testing was to notify their TB program of the potential discordance (83%). Twelve of 35 PHL (34%) responding observed discordance between the molecular results and phenotypic DST performed and reported by CDC's MDDR.

The high frequency of observed discordance contradicts findings from a recently published study where molecular results from CDC's MDDR were compared to local phenotypic DST results collected from submitting PHL [6]. This previous report found 90.1% concordance between CDC molecular and local phenotypic DST results. Discordance between molecular testing and phenotypic DST was due to not detecting mutations in loci associated with resistance in isolates that were later determined to be drug resistant by phenotypic DST. However, this prior study only compared molecular and phenotypic results for RMP and INH. In the present study, respondents needed to consider discordance between CDC's MDDR molecular results and their local phenotypic DST results for detection of drug resistance for all first-line and second line drugs used in testing procedures. This would increase the odds of discovering discordance between testing methods. When potential discordance was noticed by PHL, nearly all contacted their TB program but on occasion some took no further action. This circumstance requires further inquiry because discordant laboratory results should be addressed in the process of clinical decision making.

3.4. Impact of Molecular Results on Phenotypic DST Performed by PHL. PHL officials were asked if there was any impact on their own local phenotypic DST when the first available results were the molecular results from CDC's MDDR. Of these, 24 (69%) indicated that there was no impact on their own phenotypic DST. Three PHL (9%) acknowledged that when resistance was indicated by molecular results, they would refer the isolate to another laboratory other than CDC for additional testing. Among the open responses to this question, three PHL officials (9%) indicated they would initiate additional second-line phenotypic DST if the molecular results from CDC's MDDR indicated drug resistance.

Since CDC's MDDR uses agar proportion for phenotypic DST that can take five weeks or more to complete, PHL may choose to use a more rapid phenotypic method to confirm drug resistance and not wait for a final report from CDC. In addition, PHL may be seeking information about additional drugs not in the panel used by CDC's MDDR at the request of jurisdictional TB programs or healthcare providers.

3.5. Interpretation of Molecular Results. Twenty-six (74%) respondents reported molecular results were either not difficult or very easy to interpret. PHL officials were also comfortable discussing results with either healthcare providers or TB program staff. Among 28 PHL officials contacted to help interpret molecular results, 23 (82%) were comfortable in these discussions. When asked what resources they sought for help with interpreting results, 14 (40%) responded that they did not seek help. For 21 PHL officials who did seek assistance with interpreting molecular results, 16 (76%) contacted CDC. PHL officials sought help less frequently from other sources. Seven (33%) reported doing their own research to find information on molecular testing.

4. Conclusions

Based on survey responses, CDC's MDDR has been successful in providing rapid results for detection of drug resistance

and interpretable molecular results to PHL submitting isolates of MTBC. Whether this translates into prompt initiation of effective TB treatment and subsequent interruption of disease transmission remains to be determined.

Though none of the PHL officials responding to this survey thought the molecular results from CDC's MDDR were very difficult to interpret, 60% did seek some form of assistance using various sources. Areas of confusion need to be identified and addressed by clarifying reporting language and providing either educational materials or training opportunities to increase understanding of molecular testing. CDC is collaborating with partners to develop training modules designed to increase understanding of molecular diagnostics by PHL staff.

To accurately measure the impact of CDC's MDDR on the goal of eliminating TB, it is important to determine how results from the program are influencing clinical decision making. One limitation of this study was that only PHL officials were queried about use of results from CDC's MDDR and not TB program officials and health care providers. Data needs to be collected from patient medical charts and through healthcare provider interview to determine the degree of influence CDC's MDDR had on initiation or changes to treatment regimens and patient outcomes. CDC has completed a separate survey of state TB program officials to assess their use of reported results for implementation of patient treatment. More importantly, CDC has initiated a study to collect data on the outcome of patients from whom PHL submitted samples for MDDR.

Disclosure

The findings and conclusions in this report are those of the authors and do not necessarily represent the views of the Centers for Disease Control and Prevention or the Agency for Toxic Substances and Disease Registry.

Acknowledgments

The authors gratefully acknowledge the contributions of Public Health Laboratories for their time and effort committed to this study and the elimination of tuberculosis.

References

[1] Centers for Disease Control and Prevention (US), "Reported tuberculosis in the United States," 2012, http://www.cdc.gov/tb/statistics/reports/2012/default.htm.

[2] P. J. Campbell, G. P. Morlock, R. D. Sikes et al., "Molecular detection of mutations associated with first- and second-line drug resistance compared with conventional drug susceptibility testing of *Mycobacterium tuberculosis*," *Antimicrobial Agents and Chemotherapy*, vol. 55, no. 5, pp. 2032–2041, 2011.

[3] J. Driscoll, A. Lentz, D. Sikes, D. Hartline, and B. Metchock, "The first month of a new diagnostic service for the molecular detection of MDR and XDR tuberculosis," *American Journal of Respiratory and Critical Care Medicine*, vol. 181, Article ID A2259, 2010.

[4] Centers for Disease Control and Prevention (US), "Molecular detection of drug resistance request form," 2013, http://www.cdc.gov/tb/topic/laboratory/MDDRsubmission-form.pdf.

[5] Clinical and Laboratory Standards Institute, "Susceptibility testing of Mycobacteria, Nocardia, and Other Aerobic Actino-mycetes," Approved Standard. In: CLSI. 2nd ed, M24A2E, vol 31, no 5; 2011.

[6] M. A. Yakrus, J. Driscoll, A. J. Lentz et al., "Concordance between molecular and phenotypic testing of *Mycobacterium tuberculosis* complex isolates for resistance to rifampin and isoniazid in the United States," *Journal of Clinical Microbiology*, vol. 52, no. 6, pp. 1932–1937, 2014.

[7] SnapSurveys, *Version Snap 10 Professional*, SnapSurveys, Portsmouth, NH, USA, 2009.

23

Delay for First Consultation and Its Associated Factors among New Pulmonary Tuberculosis Patients of Central Nepal

**Wongsa Laohasiriwong,[1,2] Roshan Kumar Mahato,[2]
Rajendra Koju,[3] and Kriangsak Vaeteewootacharn[2]**

[1]Board Committee of Research and Training Centre for Enhancing Quality of Life of Working Age People (REQW),
 Khon Kaen University, Khon Kaen, Thailand
[2]Faculty of Public Health, Khon Kaen University, Khon Kaen, Thailand
[3]Departments of Internal Medicine, Dhulikhel Hospital, Kathmandu University Hospital, Dhulikhel, Nepal

Correspondence should be addressed to Wongsa Laohasiriwong; drwongsa@gmail.com

Academic Editor: William N. Rom

Tuberculosis (TB) is still a major public health challenge in Nepal and worldwide. Most transmissions occur between the onset of symptoms and the consultation with formal health care centers. This study aimed to determine the duration of delay for the first consultation and its associated factors with unacceptable delay among the new sputum pulmonary tuberculosis cases in the central development region of Nepal. An analytical cross-sectional study was conducted in the central development region of Nepal between January and May 2015. New pulmonary sputum positive tuberculosis patients were interviewed by using a structured questionnaire and their medical records were reviewed. Among a total of 374 patients, the magnitude of patient delay was 53.21% (95% CI: 48.12–58.28%) with a median delay of 32 days and an interquartile range of 11–70 days. The factors associated with unacceptable patient delay (duration $\geq$ 30 days) were residence in the rural area (adj. OR = 3.10, 95% CI: 1.10–8.72; p value = 0.032) and DOTS center located more than 5 km away from their residences (adj. OR = 5.53, 95% CI: 2.18–13.99; p value < 0.001). Unemployed patients were more likely to have patient delay (adj. OR = 7.79, 95% CI: 1.64–37.00; p value = 0.010) when controlled for other variables.

1. Background

TB ranks as the second leading cause of death from an infectious disease after the Human Immunodeficiency Virus (HIV) worldwide (126 cases per a population of 100000 individuals) [1, 2]. In the South Asia region alone, it accounts for 39% of total global burden of TB [3]. Nepal is a landlocked country between India and China with one-fourth of the total population of 26.6 million under the poverty line and 83% living in the rural areas. TB is one of the major public health challenges in Nepal [4–6]. About 45% of the total population are infected, among which 60% are adults. Every year, 45,000 people are estimated to develop active TB, 50% of which develops into infectious pulmonary disease and is the main cause for spreading the disease [7].

Complete treatment consists of a 6-month drug regimen resulting in a negative sputum smear [8]. If diagnosed between 2 and 3 weeks after the onset of clinical symptoms, it is considered as early diagnosis, while a diagnosis beyond 4 weeks of onset is considered as delayed diagnosis [9]. However, incomplete treatment regimens of tuberculosis patients are as high as 20%–50% in both high and low income countries [10, 11].

Delayed diagnosis or incomplete treatment results in prolonged infectiousness, drug resistance, relapse, and even death [10, 12–14]. Patients with undiagnosed pulmonary TB primarily act as reservoirs for transmission. The contagion parameter suggests that, where TB is endemic, each infectious case will result in 20–28 secondary infections [11]. The related literature has revealed that patients' first presentation to health facilities after more than 30 days is associated with geographical condition, health service, age, poverty, sex, alcoholism, substance abuse, history of immigration, educational status, awareness of TB, social beliefs, self-treatment, and stigma [2, 12, 13, 15–17]. Thus, there are many factors that need to be addressed in order to achieve the goal of reducing the TB burden. These types of studies have not been conducted in the study area. Therefore, this study aimed to investigate the duration of delay for the first consultation and associated factors among the new sputum pulmonary tuberculosis cases in central Nepal.

2. Materials and Methods

2.1. Study Design and Period. An analytical cross-sectional study was conducted on new pulmonary sputum positive pulmonary tuberculosis patients at DOTS centers from January to May 2015.

2.2. Study Setting. The study was conducted in central development region (CDR) of Nepal which is one of the five development regions of Nepal that spans all three ecological regions: mountain, hilly, and terai (plain landscape south of the outer foothills of the Himalaya). Headquartered in Hetauda (Makwanpur district), the CDR comprises three administrative zones (Bagmati, Narayani and Janakpur) and 19 districts. The population density in the CDR is 293 inhabitants per square kilometre, which is the highest among all five development regions and significantly above the national average of 157 inhabitants per square kilometre. The CDR consists of 36.81% of the total population of Nepal. The Human Development Index (HDI) of the CDR (0.531) is higher than the national average of 0.509 [4, 5]. This region constitutes 366 TB treatment centers, 1008 treatment subcenters, 4 drug resistant (DR) treatment centers, 37 DR treatment subcenters, and 198 microscopy centers [18].

This region was selected randomly from the five developmental regions. We then randomly selected 5 districts, one from each ecological region. Finally, the data were collected from treatment centers of each selected district by using systematic random sampling.

2.3. Sample Size and Sampling Procedure. The sample size of 374 was determined by using the formula for multiple logistic regression ($n = [P(1 - P)(Z1 - \alpha + Z1 - \beta)^2/B(1 - B)(P0 - P1)^2 * 1/(1 - P)2])$ [19]. The proportion was obtained from a previous study in Uganda [20] where P (69%) is proportion of delay in diagnosis, $P0$ (97%) is the proportion of delay in patients who had visited the private facilities, $P1$ (60%) is the proportion of delay in patients who had visited the public facilities, B (75%) is proportion of perceiving visiting to the public facilities, $\alpha = 5\%$, and $1 - \beta = 84\%$. New smear positive pulmonary tuberculosis cases above 15 years of age were included in this study, while negative smear, relapse, retreatment, return after defaulter, and patients who had history of prior TB were excluded.

2.4. Data Collection Tools and Quality Assurance. Data were collected using a structured questionnaire which had questions of sociodemographic and economic variables, basic knowledge, attitude and stigmatization on TB, accessibility and availability of TB services, and delay questions. The questionnaire was prepared in English and subsequently translated to the Nepali language. In addition, validity of the questionnaire was checked by three experts. Field activities were conducted to ensure minimum inconvenience to subjects and maximum cooperation was achieved. This involved a trade-off between the need for certain activities and the convenience of the participants. It was important to consider the timing, the place, and the frequency of the activities. The participants were not interrupted unnecessarily in their daily work. The working hours of the enumerators therefore were tailored to the activities of the study subjects and not the other way around. In addition, this study required additional interviewers apart from the researcher to collect the data. The interviewers were paramedics (health assistants) who had basic training on medicine and surgery for three years after finishing ten years of schooling. They received an interview guideline and formal training before the commencement of the survey.

2.5. Definition of Patient Delay. Patient delay is the time interval from the appearance of the first symptoms of tuberculosis until the first visit to any formal health care facility (health centers, hospitals, or DOTS centers) [9, 12, 13, 20–27]. Symptom onset is referred to the time at which the first symptom (i.e., persistent cough, fever, weakness, and weight loss or chest pain) of the illness in which a patient seeks care began [11, 15]. Most of the study has been dichotomized >30 days as a prolonged delay [11, 28–30], but some studies have considered a >3-week delay as an unacceptable patient delay [20]. In this study, a period ≥30 days was considered as an unacceptable patient delay.

2.6. Statistical Analysis. Data were entered in Epi-Data (Version 3.1) and transferred to STATA (Version 13, Stata Corporation, College Station TX) for analysis. The categorical data were reported as number and percentage. Mean, standard deviation, median, and range (minimum : maximum) were described for continuous variables. The proportion of subjects with ≥30-day delay was estimated. Odds ratios (OR) and their 95% confidence intervals (CI) were estimated using unconditional logistic regression with delay as an outcome. Bivariate analysis was performed to measure the effect of each variable of interest on risk factors of prolonging delay. Regarding the scoring technique that we adopted for this study, the first and foremost step that we took was to reverse the scores before adding them to their domain. It was done so to reflect the increment in the variables that we studied. Moving beyond, we calculated the percentage score for knowledge using the following technique: (Sum of scores obtained/maximum possible score that could be obtained) × 100 [31]. Percentiles scores were computed following the previous step and the studied variables were expressed as lying within a range of 0% to 100%, with the highest percentage reflecting the increase in the characteristic/variable. In addition, scores exceeding 80% were considered as good knowledge of TB. Similarly, to assess the attitude level and stigmatization, we administrated eight and seven questions, respectively. Each question had score of 1–5 (strongly disagree–strongly agree), and a score of >60% was considered to be either a good attitude or an experience of stigma.

Multivariate analysis was performed by multiple logistic regression including variables that showed a significant statistical effect in prediction of prolonging delay in bivariate analysis. Variables associated with delay in the bivariate analysis ($p \leq 0.25$) were included in the model. Statistical significance was taken as $p < 0.05$. These estimations incorporated treatment centers as a cluster variable so that the standard error can be correctly estimated. Logistic regression implemented under the generalized linear model (GLM) was used to control the clustering effect at both bivariate and multivariate analysis.

3. Results

A total of 374 new pulmonary TB patients were interviewed. The median age was 35.03 years. 234 (62.57%) patients were males, 292 (78.07%) were Hindus, and 33.42% were residing in rural areas. As many as 32.89% of the respondents did not finish primary formal education (Table 1). One-fourth of patients were farmers and 26.74% of the respondents were unemployed. The median monthly income was USD 170; however, the lowest earned was only USD 10.

Cough was the most common symptom noticed before diagnosis (69.52%). Less than a quarter (21.56%) of the patients lived more than 5 km away from the facility where TB was diagnosed. More than half (52.67%) of the patients first sought care from a public health facility. Nonpublic health facilities were visited by 159 (42.51%), whereas 4.81% of the patients visited a traditional healer for their first consultation. Only 78 (20.86%) of the respondents consulted chest specialists.

3.1. Patient Delay and Determinants. The median patient delay was 32 (IQR 11–70) days. There was unacceptable patient delay in 199 respondents (53.21%). In the bivariate analysis it was found that the factors independently associated with unacceptable delay included the following (Table 2): being Buddhist (OR = 1.46, 95% CI: 1.17–1.83) and residing in the rural areas of Nepal (OR = 2.15, 95% CI: 1.39–3.33). Chest pain was the only first symptom that showed an association with the unacceptable patient delay (OR = 1.5, 95% CI: 1.04–2.17). In addition, living more than 5 km far from the DOTS center (OR = 2.64, 95% CI: 1.58–4.39), being diagnosed and treated by medical officer (OR = 1.72, 95% CI: 1.24–2.37), and consulting chest specialist (OR = 2.98, 95% CI: 1.44–6.13) were also significantly associated with unacceptable patient delay.

The multivariate analysis shows that (Table 3) those who live in rural areas had 3.10 times higher chance to have an unacceptable patient delay than those who were living in urban areas (adj. OR = 3.10, 95% CI: 1.10–8.72). In addition, unemployment was significantly influencing patient delay (adj. OR = 7.79, 95% CI: 1.64–37.00). Distance to reach a DOTS center was strongly associated with patient delay with adj. OR = 5.53, 95% CI: 2.18–13.99. On the other hand, being Muslim was a protective factor for unacceptable delay

TABLE 1: Baseline characteristics of participants.

Characteristics	Number (%)
Gender	
Male	234 (62.57)
Female	140 (37.43)
Age (years)	
15–29	149 (39.84)
30–44	85 (22.73)
≥45	140 (37.43)
Mean (SD)	39.68 (18.6)
Median (min : max)	35.03 (15.07 : 100.56)
Religion	
Hindu	292 (78.07)
Buddha	60 (16.04)
Muslim	22 (5.88)
Residence	
Urban	249 (66.58)
Rural	125 (33.42)
Education	
Illiterate/read & write	123 (32.89)
Primary	69 (18.45)
Secondary	107 (28.61)
University	75 (20.05)
Occupation	
Agriculture	93 (24.87)
Housewife	42 (11.23)
Service	50 (13.37)
Business	58 (15.51)
Unemployed	100 (26.74)
Labour	31 (8.29)
Income (monthly in USD)	
<50	35 (11.08)
50–75	24 (7.59)
≥75	257 (81.33)
Mean (SD)	270.87 (467.32)
Median (min : max)	170 (10 : 3800)
Number of cigarettes per day	
<5	37 (24.34)
≥5	115 (75.66)
Symptoms present before diagnosis	
Cough	260 (69.52)
Fever	56 (14.97)
Loss of weight	17 (4.55)
Hemoptysis	20 (5.35)
Chest pain	21 (5.61)
Family support	
None	126 (33.69)
Husband/wife	76 (20.32)
Parents	101 (27.01)
Child	71 (18.98)
Distance to reach the TB center	
<5 km	291 (78.44)
≥5 km	80 (21.56)
Mean (SD)	4.25 (11.82)
Median (min : max)	2 (1 : 200)
Centre of first contact	
Traditional healer/self-treated	18 (4.81)
Private practitioner/pharmacist/vendor	159 (42.51)
Government health facilities	197 (52.67)

TABLE 1: Continued.

Characteristics	Number (%)
Categories of HCP for TB diagnosis	
Paramedics	87 (23.26)
Medical officer	209 (55.88)
Chest specialist	78 (20.86)
Patient delay (in days)	199 (53.21)
No delay (<30 days)	175 (46.79)
Delay (≥30 days)	199 (53.21)
Mean (SD)	78.64 (233.94)
Median (IQR)	32 (11–70)

(adj. OR = 0.10, 95% CI: 0.03–0.77), and those who have smoked more than 5 cigarettes per day (adj. OR = 0.22, 95% CI: 0.08–0.65) were less likely to have an unacceptable patient delay when controlled for other covariates.

4. Discussion

This is the first study in central Nepal that assessed the prevalence and determinants of patient delay. Nepal is a low income country and a number of studies have revealed that patient delay varies in countries with relatively lower and middle income. In addition, most studies have revealed that patients often do not clearly notice the symptoms at the onset of the disease, which is one of the reasons for delay [11].

Our study found that the unacceptable patient delay of ≥30 days was 53.21% (95% CI: 48.12–58.28%) which was slightly lower than a study of Nepal in 2009, which showed that 73% of the study population faced patient delay [29]. The differences could be due to the variation in the definition of patient delay and selection of study population. Our study defined the patient delay as the time interval from the appearance of the first symptoms of tuberculosis until the first visit to "any formal health care facility," whereas some studies defined it as "any health facility." On the other hand, this study was only focused on sputum positive pulmonary TB patients, whereas the previous study of Nepal included sputum negative and extrapulmonary TB cases. In addition, the DOTS centers have also been expanded, and simultaneously the educational status of the people improved within these years. Therefore, this study has a lower prevalence of patient delay than that of the previous study. However, the result is similar to the study conducted in Uganda [20, 22] and Ethiopia. Higher unacceptable patient delay has been seen in Tanzania, that is, 90% [32].

We found that the patient delay was significantly associated with those who believed in the Buddhist religion and the people living in the rural areas of Nepal (OR = 2.15, 95% CI: 1.39–3.33). This may be because the people with Buddhist religion were more likely to be living in the rural areas where the availability of the health facilities is very poor. Multiple studies have shown that the place of residence leads to the patient delay [21], including a WHO study [31] conducted in seven developing countries and a study conducted in Nigeria. In addition, the result from multivariate analysis showed that being Muslim was protective factor for unacceptable patient delay. This may be because the Muslim populations

are concentrated in the terai region which has flat topography and the accessibility to the treatment center is far better than that of mountain and hilly regions.

Moreover, this study observed that the unemployment status of patients leads to an unacceptable delay. It has been suggested that the increased delay observed among farmers or people who do not have paid employment may be related to their socioeconomic condition, specifically lower education, and high poverty [21]. In Nepal, one-fourth of the population is still under poverty line [4, 6].

Furthermore, gender, age, and marital status were not significantly associated with patient delay even though some studies have shown that females were more likely to be associated with delay. Some found that the age group > 45 years [21, 22] can significantly prolong delay. Symptoms like chest pain were contributing factors for prolonging delay. This is due to the lack of knowledge regarding tuberculosis and its symptoms. People generally thought that cough and having fever in the evening are the only symptoms of TB. Thus, they ignore the chest pain and face delay.

Another factor associated with prolonged patient delay was the distance between a DOTS center and their residence (adj. OR = 5.53, 95% CI: 2.18–13.99). This may be due to the geographical condition of Nepal. Health facilities are also not sophisticated enough to diagnose and are not convenient in all rural areas. These situations are similar to the findings of a study conducted in Ethiopia [22]. The medical officers and chest specialist who diagnosed the respondents had significantly increased delay, because almost all specialized services are centralized in Nepal. However, patients who smoked more than 5 cigarettes per day significantly reduced unacceptable patient delay. This may indicate that patients may think that they are at high risk from smoking and that their cough might develop into tuberculosis. Therefore, they were more likely to seek medical services as soon as possible, resulting in smoking being a protective factor for unacceptable patient delay.

5. Strength and Limitation of the Study

This study is the first of its kind with a high number of representative samples to be conducted in the study area. Despite the severe geographical challenges posed by different ecological regions, this study has overcome obstacles and covered all three ecozones of the central development region of Nepal. In addition, this study has solely focused on new sputum positive pulmonary tuberculosis patients.

As the study collected the historical data regarding the symptoms of the disease and the first consultation with health facilities, the study might be prone to recall bias.

6. Conclusions

Duration of delay for the first consultation was significantly associated with the patient's occupation, income, and persistence of symptoms. The place of residence, distance of the health center from home, and the center of first contact for diagnosis indicate a lack of availability and accessibility of health services in the central development region, even

TABLE 2: Factors associated with patient delay (PD): bivariate analysis.

Factors	Number (% PD)	Crude OR	95% CI	p value
Gender				0.511
Male	234 (53.85)	1		
Female	140 (52.14)	0.93	0.76 to 1.15	
Age (years)				0.759
15–29	149 (51.01)	1		
30–44	85 (51.76)	1.03	0.75 to 1.43	
≥45	140 (56.43)	1.24	0.68 to 2.28	
Religion				<0.001
Hindu	292 (52.40)	1		
Buddha	60 (61.67)	1.46	1.17 to 1.83	
Muslim	22 (40.91)	0.63	0.38 to 1.03	
Residence				<0.001
Urban	249 (46.99)	1		
Rural	125 (65.60)	2.15	1.39 to 3.33	
Education				<0.001
Illiterate/read & write	123 (62.60)	1		
Primary	69 (57.97)	0.82	0.59 to 1.16	
Secondary	107 (42.06)	0.43	0.32 to 0.59	
University	75 (49.33)	0.58	0.29 to 1.16	
Occupation				<0.001
Agriculture	93 (65.59)	1		
Housewife	42 (47.62)	0.47	0.32 to 0.71	
Service	50 (44.00)	0.41	0.15 to 1.13	
Business	58 (48.28)	0.49	0.15 to 1.56	
Unemployed	100 (52.00)	0.56	0.41 to 0.79	
Labour	31 (51.61)	0.56	0.29 to 1.08	
Income (monthly in NRs)				0.009
<5000	35 (68.57)	1		
5000–7500	24 (58.33)	0.64	0.29 to 1.43	
≥7500	257 (50.58)	0.47	0.27 to 0.79	
Number of cigarettes per day				0.063
<5	37 (70.27)	1		
≥5	115 (53.91)	0.49	0.24 to 1.04	
Symptoms present before diagnosis				<0.001
Cough	260 (51.92)	1		
Fever	56 (57.14)	1.23	0.67 to 2.27	
Loss of weight	17 (52.94)	1.04	0.26 to 4.12	
Hemoptysis	20 (50.00)	0.92	0.61 to 1.41	
Chest pain	21 (61.90)	1.50	1.04 to 2.17	
Family support				0.001
None	126 (55.56)	1		
Husband/wife	76 (53.95)	0.94	0.48 to 1.82	
Parents	101 (42.57)	0.53	0.29 to 1.17	
Child	71 (63.38)	1.38	0.56 to 3.41	
Distance to reach the TB center				<0.001
<5 km	291 (48.45)	1		
≥5 km	80 (71.25)	2.64	1.58 to 4.39	
Centre of first contact				<0.001
Traditional healer/self-treated	18 (72.22)	1		
Private practitioner/pharmacist/vendor	159 (49.69)	0.38	0.10 to 1.39	
Government health facilities	197 (54.31)	0.46	0.13 to 1.64	
Categories of HCP for TB diagnosis				0.002
Paramedics	87 (40.23)	1		
Medical officer	209 (53.59)	1.72	1.24 to 2.37	
Chest specialist	78 (66.67)	2.98	1.44 to 6.13	

TABLE 3: Factors associated with patient delay: multivariate analysis.

Factors	Number (% PD)	Crude OR	Adj. OR	95% CI	p value
Religion					<0.001
Hindu	292 (52.40)	1	1		
Buddha	60 (61.67)	1.46	1.86	0.91 to 3.79	
Muslim	22 (40.91)	0.63	0.10	0.03 to 0.77	
Residence					0.032
Urban	249 (46.99)	1	1		
Rural	125 (65.60)	2.15	3.10	1.10 to 8.72	
Education					0.135
Illiterate/read & write	123 (62.60)	1	1		
Primary	69 (57.97)	0.82	0.89	0.21 to 3.76	
Secondary	107 (42.06)	0.43	0.46	0.06 to 3.79	
University	75 (49.33)	0.58	0.96	0.08 to 11.19	
Occupation					<0.001
Agriculture	93 (65.59)	1	1		
Housewife	42 (47.62)	0.47	1.65	0.18 to 14.97	
Service	50 (44.00)	0.41	3.89	0.35 to 43.32	
Business	58 (48.28)	0.49	1.79	0.05 to 70.94	
Unemployed	100 (52.00)	0.56	7.79	1.64 to 37.00	
Labour	31 (51.61)	0.56	0.830	0.17 to 4.02	
Income (monthly in NRs)					0.116
<5000	35 (68.57)	1	1		
5000–7500	24 (58.33)	0.64	13.34	0.35 to 511.0	
≥7500	257 (50.58)	0.47	0.94	0.04 to 21.41	
Number of cigarettes in a day					0.006
<5	37 (70.27)	1	1		
≥5	115 (53.91)	0.49	0.22	0.08 to 0.65	
Symptoms present before diagnosis					0. 573
Cough	260 (51.92)	1	1		
Fever	56 (57.14)	1.23	1.56	0.58 to 4.20	
Loss of weight	17 (52.94)	1.04	1.24	0.36 to 4.22	
Hemoptysis	20 (50.00)	0.92	0.05	0.06 to 4.14	
Chest pain	21 (61.90)	1.50	3.58	0.13 to 95.89	
Family support					<0.001
None	126 (55.56)	1	1		
Husband/wife	76 (53.95)	0.94	1.19	0.22 to 8.65	
Parents	101 (42.57)	0.53	0.66	0.11 to 2.47	
Child	71 (63.38)	1.38	4.12	0.61 to 27.98	
Distance to reach the TB center					<0.001
<5 km	291 (48.45)	1	1		
≥5 km	80 (71.25)	2.64	5.53	2.18 to 13.99	
Centre of first contact					0.443
Traditional healer/self-treated	18 (72.22)	1	1		
Private practitioner/pharmacist/vendor	159 (49.69)	0.38	0.50	0.12 to 2.09	
Government health facilities	197 (54.31)	0.46	0.97	0.12 to 7.86	
Categories of HCP for TB diagnosis					0.929
Paramedics	87 (40.23)	1	1		
Medical officer	209 (53.59)	1.72	1.29	0.34 to 4.98	
Chest specialist	78 (66.67)	2.98	0.99	0.29 to 3.43	

though the studied region is more developed than other regions of Nepal. Therefore, expansion of the DOTS services and increasing the awareness on TB with assured quality will reduce the burden.

Ethical Approval

Ethical clearance and approval was obtained from the office of the Khon Kaen University ethics committee in human research (Reference no. HE582071), Khon Kaen, Thailand, and Institutional Review Committee, Kathmandu University School of Medical Sciences, Dhulikhel, Nepal (Protocol approved no. 08/15). Permission for this study was obtained from the National Tuberculosis Center, Nepal, Regional Health Directories, CDR, Nepal, and District Health Office of the selected districts.

Competing Interests

The authors declare that they have no competing interests.

Acknowledgments

The authors would like to thank Faculty of Public Health, Khon Kaen University, for providing the opportunity to conduct this study. In addition, they would like to thank National Tuberculosis Center, Nepal, for their dearest support and cooperation throughout the study period. This study was supported by Training Center for Enhancing Quality of Life of Working-Age People, Faculty of Nursing, Khon Kaen University, Khon Kaen, Thailand.

References

[1] WHO, *Global Tuberculosis Report 2014*, World Health Organization, Geneva, Switzerland, 2014.

[2] Y. Li, J. Ehiri, S. Tang et al., "Factors associated with patient, and diagnostic delays in Chinese TB patients: a systematic review and meta-analysis," *BMC Medicine*, vol. 11, article 156, 2013.

[3] SEARO and WHO, *Tuberculosis Control in the South-East Asia Region Annual Report Indraprastha Estate*, World Health Organization, Regional Office for South-East Asia, New Delhi, India, 2014.

[4] Government of Nepal National Planning Commission Secretariat Central Bureau Statistics, *National Population and Housing Census 2011*, Central Bureau of Statistic, Kathmandu, Nepal, 2011.

[5] Ministry of Health and Population, New ERA, and ICF International, *Nepal Demographic and Health Survey 2011*, Ministry of Health and Population, New ERA, Kathmandu, Nepal; ICF International, Calverton, Md, USA, 2012.

[6] Central Bureau of Statistics Thapathali, "Nepal living standards survey 2010/11," Tech. Rep., Central Bureau of Statistics Thapathali, Kathmandu, Nepal, 2011.

[7] D. O. H. S. Mohp, "Nepal," Annual Report, Department of Health Services, Nepal, Kathmandu, 2014.

[8] WHO, *Treatment of Tuberculosis Guideline*, World Health Organization, Geneva, Switzerland, 4th edition, 2009.

[9] G. N. Deponti, D. R. Silva, A. C. Coelho, A. M. Muller, and P. D. T. R. Dalcin, "Delayed diagnosis and associated factors among new pulmonary tuberculosis patients diagnosed at the emergency department of a tertiary care hospital in Porto Alegre, South Brazil: a prospective patient recruitment study," *BMC Infectious Diseases*, vol. 13, article 538, 2013.

[10] M. Sagbakken, J. C. Frich, and G. Bjune, "Barriers and enablers in the management of tuberculosis treatment in Addis Ababa, Ethiopia: a qualitative study," *BMC Public Health*, vol. 8, article 11, 2008.

[11] L. Segagni Lusignani, G. Quaglio, A. Atzori et al., "Factors associated with patient and health care system delay in diagnosis for tuberculosis in the province of Luanda, Angola," *BMC Infectious Diseases*, vol. 13, no. 1, article 168, 2013.

[12] S. Konda, C. Melo, P. Giri, and A. Behera, "Determinants of delays in diagnosis and treatment of pulmonary tuberculosis in a new urban township in India: a cross-sectional study," *International Journal of Medical Science and Public Health*, vol. 3, no. 2, pp. 140–145, 2014.

[13] Y. A. Mekonnen, "Delay for first consultation and associated factors among tuberculosis patients in Bahir Dar town administration, north west Ethiopia," *American Journal of Health Research*, vol. 2, no. 4, pp. 140–145, 2014.

[14] M. H. Soomro, E. Qadeer, and O. Mørkve, "Barriers in the management of tuberculosis in Rawalpindi, Pakistan: a qualitative study," *Tanaffos*, vol. 12, no. 4, pp. 28–34, 2013.

[15] D. G. Storla, S. Yimer, and G. A. Bjune, "A systematic review of delay in the diagnosis and treatment of tuberculosis," *BMC Public Health*, vol. 8, article 15, 2008.

[16] A. Asefa and W. Teshome, "Total delay in treatment among smear positive pulmonary tuberculosis patients in five primary health centers, Southern Ethiopia: a cross sectional study," *PLoS ONE*, vol. 9, no. 7, Article ID e102884, 2014.

[17] S. G. Hinderaker, S. Madland, M. Ullenes, D. A. Enarson, I. Rusen, and D. Kamara, "Treatment delay among tuberculosis patients in Tanzania: data from the FIDELIS Initiative," *BMC Public Health*, vol. 11, no. 1, article 306, 2011.

[18] National Tuberculosis Center, "National tuberculosis programme annual report," Tech. Rep., National Tuberculosis Center, Bhaktpur, Nepal, 2014.

[19] F. Y. Hsieh, D. A. Bloch, and M. D. Larsen, "A simple method of sample size calculation for linear and logistic regression," *Statistics in Medicine*, vol. 17, no. 14, pp. 1623–1634, 1998.

[20] E. Buregyeya, B. Criel, F. Nuwaha, and R. Colebunders, "Delays in diagnosis and treatment of pulmonary tuberculosis in wakiso and mukono districts, Uganda," *BMC Public Health*, vol. 14, article 586, 2014.

[21] A. A. Fatiregun and C. C. Ejeckam, "Determinants of patient delay in seeking treatment among pulmonary tuberculosis cases in a government specialist hospital in Ibadan, Nigeria," *Tanzania Journal of Health Research*, vol. 12, no. 2, 2010.

[22] S. Yimer, G. Bjune, and G. Alene, "Diagnostic and treatment delay among pulmonary tuberculosis patients in Ethiopia: a cross sectional study," *BMC Infectious Diseases*, vol. 5, article 112, 2005.

[23] M. Demissie, B. Lindtjorn, and Y. Berhane, "Patient and health service delay in the diagnosis of pulmonary tuberculosis in Ethiopia," *BMC Public Health*, vol. 2, article 23, 2002.

[24] A. Saifodine, P. S. Gudo, M. Sidat, and J. Black, "Patient and health system delay among patients with pulmonary tuberculosis in Beira City, Mozambique," *BMC Public Health*, vol. 1, no. 13, p. 559, 2013.

[25] L. Makwakwa, M.-L. Sheu, C.-Y. Chiang, S.-L. Lin, and P. W. Chang, "Patient and heath system delays in the diagnosis and treatment of new and retreatment pulmonary tuberculosis cases in Malawi," *BMC Infectious Diseases*, vol. 14, no. 1, article 132, 2014.

[26] J. Cai, X. Wang, A. Ma, Q. Wang, X. Han, and Y. Li, "Factors associated with patient and provider delays for tuberculosis diagnosis and treatment in Asia: a systematic review and meta-analysis," *PLoS ONE*, vol. 10, no. 3, Article ID e0120088, 2015.

[27] E. Gebeyehu, M. Azage, and G. Abeje, "Factors associated with patient's delay in tuberculosis treatment in Bahir Dar City Administration, Northwest Ethiopia," *BioMed Research International*, vol. 2014, Article ID 701429, 6 pages, 2014.

[28] E. L. N. Maciel, J. E. Golub, R. L. Peres et al., "Delay in diagnosis of pulmonary tuberculosis at a primary health clinic in Vitoria, Brazil," *International Journal of Tuberculosis and Lung Disease*, vol. 14, no. 11, pp. 1403–1410, 2010.

[29] R. Basnet, S. G. Hinderaker, D. Enarson, P. Malla, and O. Mørkve, "Delay in the diagnosis of tuberculosis in Nepal," *BMC Public Health*, vol. 9, article 236, 2009.

[30] R. Rajeswari, V. Chandrasekaran, M. Suhadev, S. Sivasubramaniam, G. Sudha, and G. Renu, "Factors associated with patient and health system delays in the diagnosis of tuberculosis in South India," *The International Journal of Tuberculosis and Lung Disease*, vol. 6, no. 9, pp. 789–795, 2002.

[31] WHO, *Diagnostic and Treatment Delay in Tuberculosis*, WHO, Cairo, Egypt, 2006.

[32] E. R. Wandwalo and O. Mørkve, "Delay in tuberculosis case-finding and treatment in Mwanza, Tanzania," *The International Journal of Tuberculosis and Lung Disease*, vol. 4, no. 2, pp. 133–138, 2000.

24

Tuberculosis Case Finding in Benin, 2000–2014 and Beyond: A Retrospective Cohort and Time Series Study

Serge Ade,[1,2,3] Wilfried Békou,[1] Mênonli Adjobimey,[1] Omer Adjibode,[1] Gabriel Ade,[1] Anthony D. Harries,[3,4] and Séverin Anagonou[1]

[1]Programme National contre la Tuberculose, 01 BP 321 Cotonou, Benin
[2]Faculté de Médecine, Université de Parakou, Parakou, Benin
[3]International Union against Tuberculosis and Lung Disease, Paris, France
[4]London School of Hygiene & Tropical Medicine, London, UK

Correspondence should be addressed to Serge Ade; adeserg@yahoo.fr

Academic Editor: Sarman Singh

Objective. To determine any changes in tuberculosis epidemiology in the last 15 years in Benin, seasonal variations, and forecasted numbers of tuberculosis cases in the next five years. *Materials and Methods.* Retrospective cohort and time series study of all tuberculosis cases notified between 2000 and 2014. The "R" software version 3.2.1 (Institute for Statistics and Mathematics Vienna Austria) and the Box-Jenkins 1976 modeling approach were used for time series analysis. *Results.* Of 246943 presumptive cases, 54303 (22%) were diagnosed with tuberculosis. Annual notified case numbers increased, with the highest reported in 2011. New pulmonary bacteriologically confirmed tuberculosis (NPBCT) represented 78% ± SD 2%. Retreatment cases decreased from 10% to 6% and new pulmonary clinically diagnosed cases increased from 2% to 8%. NPBCT notification rates decreased in males from 2012, in young people aged 15–34 years and in Borgou-Alibori region. There was a seasonal pattern in tuberculosis cases. Over 90% of NPBCT were HIV-tested with a stable HIV prevalence of 13%. The ARIMA best fit model predicted a decrease in tuberculosis cases finding in the next five years. *Conclusion.* Tuberculosis case notifications are predicted to decrease in the next five years if current passive case finding is used. Additional strategies are needed in the country.

1. Introduction

Despite the discovery of the causative agent more than one century ago, a vaccine, highly effective medications, and recent improvements in biological molecular field and genetic engineering, tuberculosis (TB) remains a major public health concern in the world. In 2014, globally, there were estimated 9.6 million incident cases, of which 1.5 million were estimated to have died. The burden of the disease is particularly immense in Africa from where the case rate was reported to be 281 per 100000 people [1].

The year 2016 is an important turn for the TB world, with the World Health Organization (WHO) launching the "End TB Strategy" with ambitious new targets of reducing by 2035 the incidence and the mortality of the disease by 90% and 95%, respectively, compared with 2015 [2]. Success in this new strategy requires additional and relevant actions/strategies at both international and national levels. In countries, such actions/strategies cannot be properly planned without a clear understanding of the past and current local epidemiology of the disease.

Benin is a small country in West Africa with an area of 114763 km^2 for a population of 10008749 inhabitants in 2013 [3]. With activities just restricted to a mass BCG vaccination before 1966, TB care activities in the country significantly improved from 1972 with the establishment of the National TB Programme (NTP). An epidemiological review of TB patients diagnosed in the country between 1995 and 2007 showed an average of notified new pulmonary bacteriologically confirmed TB (NPBCT) cases of 35 per 100000 inhabitants, with a slight increase of 1% per annum. Large variations were observed in notifications of TB cases between the north and the south of the country, in line with population densities. The male-female sex ratio was 1.8 and no change in the age structure was reported. Human Immunodeficiency Virus (HIV) prevalence of the 97% of TB patients that were tested was 14% [4].

As implementation of the "End TB Strategy" commences, it is important to better understand the new challenges and to determine whether the local TB epidemiology has changed over time. There is also no information available within the national tuberculosis control programme on the relationship between seasons and TB case finding. This information may be useful in forecasting the number of TB cases expected in Benin in the coming years.

The current study was therefore undertaken (i) to assess whether there were any changes in the local TB epidemiology the last fifteen years and (ii) to determine the forecasted number of TB cases in the next five years. Specific objectives were to determine, between 2000 and 2014, in Benin (i) the trend of presumptive and notified TB cases; (ii) the trend of the different types and categories of TB cases; (iii) any changes in baseline characteristics and HIV-status of notified NPBCT; (iv) any seasonality in TB case finding in the country; and (v) the forecasted number of TB cases that might be diagnosed within the programme in the next five years.

2. Materials and Methods

2.1. Study Design. This was a retrospective cohort and time series study of notified TB patients, using routinely collected data.

2.2. General Setting and Study Sites

2.2.1. Country. Benin shares borders with Burkina Faso and Niger in the north, Togo in the west, Nigeria in the east, and the Atlantic Ocean in the south. The country is low-income with a Gross National Income per capita estimated at US$ 810 in 2014. The under-five and maternal mortality rates were 85 per 1000 live births and 340 per 100 000 live births, respectively, in 2013 [5]. HIV prevalence among adults aged between 15 and 49 years was 1.1% in 2012 [6]. For decades, BCG vaccination has been implemented in public and also some appointed health facilities in the country. BCG vaccination is recommended within the first two weeks after birth. In 2014, the coverage rate was 96% [7]. BCG vaccination is free of charge.

Administratively, the country is divided into six functional departments: Atacora-Donga and Borgou-Alibori in the north, Zou-Collines in the centre, and Mono-Couffo, Oueme-Plateau, and Atlantique-Littoral in the south. Cotonou the economic capital is located in Atlantique-Littoral. The density of the population gradually increases from the north to the south, with the highest population density reported from Cotonou. Overall in Benin, the climate is hot and humid. There were two rainy seasons (a principal season from April to July and a shorter season from September to November) and two dry seasons (a principal season from December to April and a shorter season from July to September).

2.2.2. The National Tuberculosis Control Programme (NTP)

Organization and Function. The NTP is under the Ministry of Health and has a pyramidal organizational structure with three (central, intermediate, and peripheral) levels, based on the general health system model. Diagnosis, registration, and treatment are decentralized to 57 BMUs (48 public and 9 confessional health facilities) at peripheral levels. Attempts had been made previously to include private clinics but with no success, because the private sector is benefits-oriented, contrary to the programme's objective of making all TB-related activities free of charge (consultations and/or examination charges for diagnosis, treatment, and follow-up). However, these private clinics are not completely excluded from TB activities. Their workers are regularly trained to identify and refer to the closest BMU patients with presumptive symptoms of TB. This system functions well. There is supervision of all the 57 BMUs organized by the central and intermediate levels of the TB Programme on a quarterly basis.

Diagnosis, Treatment, and Case Notification. Diagnosis and treatment are provided in line with the WHO and The Union recommendations [8, 9]. Overall, a passive screening strategy is routinely performed, although in 2011 there was some experimentation with a semiactive case finding strategy named "TB Reach" funded by the WHO. The laboratory network is made up of 57 laboratories in BMUs with 10 additional centres for microscopic diagnosis. In these laboratories, specimens from all presumptive TB cases (regardless of their public, confessional, or private sector origin) are analysed mainly using Ziehl-Neelsen staining and/or fluorescence auramine microscopy. Fluorescent microscopy was first introduced into the largest BMU of the country twenty years ago. Since then, this technology has been scaled up to six regional laboratories in 2010 and to 10 other laboratories with the highest workloads in 2014. With the new Global Fund against AIDS, Tuberculosis and Malaria (GFATM) grant, the rest of the laboratories in the network will be equipped with fluorescent microscopy by 2017.

In addition to microscopy, phenotypic culture on solid medium (Löwenstein-Jensen) followed by identification and drug susceptibility testing is routinely carried out at the mycobacteria national laboratory. Since 2012, Xpert® MTB/RIF (Cepheid Inc., Sunnyvale, CA, USA) has also been available in this laboratory. This technology is not part of the routine diagnosis strategy of all TB cases but is mainly used for (1) detecting patients earlier with resistance to rifampicin, almost synonymous with multidrug-resistant TB and (2) diagnosing HIV-infected patients with presumptive symptoms of TB. On the first targeted population, in Benin, rifampicin resistant patients are mostly found among retreatment TB cases. Thus, all previously treated patients positive on smear microscopy are tested. In 2016, Xpert MTB/RIF (Cepheid Inc., Sunnyvale, CA, USA) was scaled up in the six regional laboratories. In the short term, decentralization of these machines at peripheral levels is not possible because of various technological and other constraints (e.g., cost, environmental temperatures, shelf-life of cartridges, electricity supplies in a country where electricity is neither stable nor permanent, and the need for annual calibration of the machine) [10].

Once the diagnosis is confirmed, patients are registered in the "TB registers" which are only available in the 57 BMUs. Those, who reside far from the place of diagnosis, are sent to the BMU closest to their domicile and registered in that new BMU.

Treatment is then started and is in line with WHO recommendations. All consultations, bacteriological examinations, treatment, and follow-up are provided free of charge. Anti-TB drugs are not available in private pharmacies but only in BMUs. This presents an advantage for TB notification completeness since patients have to be sent to one of the 57 BMUs and be registered before starting treatment. For all pulmonary TB bacteriologically confirmed cases through microscopy, treatment is directly observed during the intensive phase.

Within the first two weeks after the end of each quarter, a report on TB cases diagnosed during these three months and also outcomes of the cohort of patients put on treatment one year earlier is made by the nurse under the responsibility of the medical doctor. A visit is then made by the supervision team; and the report is checked (and corrected if necessary) before being brought back to the coordinator for national statistics. To date, the notification system is paper based, but the programme is about to move to an electronic notification system (District Health Information System 2 developed by the University of Oslow).

TB/HIV Coinfection Management. Since 2006, all TB cases in the country have been systematically offered HIV testing. Those who are found coinfected with TB and HIV receive cotrimoxazole (CTX) for opportunistic infections prevention. Since 2010, antiretroviral therapy (ART) has been initiated for all coinfected TB/HIV patients, regardless of their CD4 cell counts [11].

Financing. TB activities are funded by the government. However, similar to many other developing countries, an important component of the funding is provided by the International Institutions, especially the Global Fund against AIDS, Tuberculosis and Malaria (GFATM). In 2014, 48% of the national programme needs were internationally funded [12].

2.3. Study Population. All TB patients registered in the NTP between 2000 and 2014 were included in the study.

2.4. Data Variables, Data Sources, Data Validation, and Definitions. Aggregate data were collected for this study and included number of presumptive TB cases, number of notified TB cases (all types), number of NPBCT cases (patients never treated or treated with anti-TB drugs for less than 1 month, whose TB diagnosis was bacteriologically confirmed on sputa by smear microscopy, culture, or WHO-approved rapid diagnostics such as Xpert MTB/RIF), new pulmonary clinically diagnosed TB (patients with pulmonary disease never treated or treated with anti-TB drugs for less than 1 month who did not fulfil the criteria for bacteriological confirmation but were diagnosed with active TB by

a clinician who decided to give the patient a full course of TB treatment), new extrapulmonary TB (patients never treated or treated with anti-TB drugs for less than 1 month with a bacteriological or a clinical diagnosis of TB involving anatomical sites other than the lungs), retreatment TB (or previously treated patients who received 1 month or more of TB treatment in the past. They included relapse, treatment after failure, and treatment after loss to follow-up cases) [13], demographical characteristics of NPBCT cases (sex, age group, and department), and HIV-status of NPBCT (positive, negative, and unknown). These data were collected into paper based quarterly reports and validated during quarterly supervisions. They were then entered into a Microsoft Excel file.

2.5. Analysis and Statistics. Baseline characteristics, types of TB, and HIV-status were described using frequencies and percentages. The notified NPBCT rates in males, females, age groups, and departments were calculated from the general population. For the time series analysis, the number of TB cases notified half-yearly between 2000 and 2014 was derived. The "R" software version 3.2.1 (Institute for Statistics and Mathematics, Vienna, Austria) and the Box-Jenkins (1976) modeling approach were used to analyse the time series and to determine the best suitable model for the time series data. The Ljung-Box-Pierce test was performed to check whether the model was correctly specified. Levels of significance were set at 5%.

2.6. Ethical Considerations. Permission for the study was obtained from the NTP management staff. Approval from the local Ethics Committee "Comité National d'Ethique pour la Recherche en Santé" (http://www.ethique-sante.org/index.htm) was not required because of the retrospective nature of this study according to the country's recommendation. Approval was also not required from the Ethics Advisory Board of the International Union against Tuberculosis and Lung Disease (The Union) because of the use of aggregate not individual data. The study used already collected data. Therefore, written informed consent given by participants was not possible to obtain. Since aggregate data were used for the study, there was no way to recognize participants.

3. Results

3.1. Cases Detection and Types of TB. Between 2000 and 2014, of the 246943 TB presumptive patients, 54303 (22%) were diagnosed with TB. The numbers/trends of presumptive and diagnosed TB patients seen, respectively, over these fifteen years are shown in Figure 1. There was a progressive increase in the number of patients being investigated for TB. In the same manner, the number of diagnosed TB cases also increased. The maximum number of presumptive and diagnosed TB cases was reported in 2011 and this was followed by a decrease the year after. Figure 2 shows the different types of TB diagnosed over the study period. NPBCT through microscopy represented the large majority of TB cases diagnosed (average = 78% [±SD 2%]). Retreatment TB

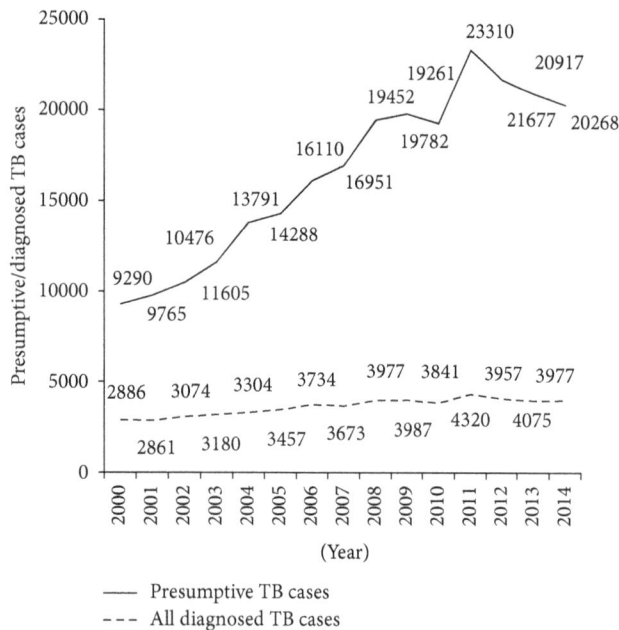

FIGURE 1: Trend of presumptive and notified tuberculosis cases in Benin, 2000–2014.

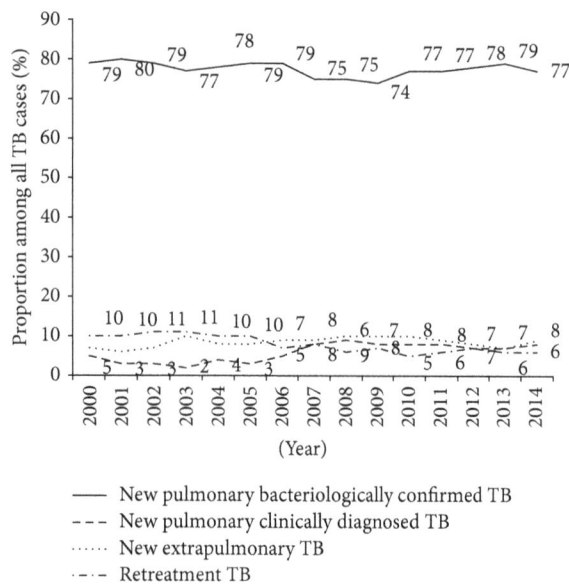

FIGURE 2: Different types of tuberculosis diagnosed in Benin, 2000–2014.

patients declined from at least 10% in the first five years to about 6% in the last few years while new pulmonary clinically diagnosed TB cases slightly increased from 2% to 8%.

3.2. Baseline Characteristics and HIV-Status Variation. Baseline characteristics and HIV-status of patients are shown in Figures 3(a), 3(b), 3(c), and 3(d). Among NPBCT, the notification rate was 1.5 times higher in males compared to females. However, from 2012 onwards there was a decrease in male case numbers (Figure 3(a)). TB case notification rates

TABLE 1: Estimation of the coefficient of the best fit model for the TB case finding time series.

	MA1	AR1	Intercept
	0.6037	0.865	1759.7924
Standard error	0.2232	0.092	163.3689
Best fit model	ARIMA (0, 0, 1) (1, 0, 0) with constant		
Convergence criteria	Log likelihood = −182.67; AIC = 373.33; BIC = 378.94		

Note: MA: moving average; AR: autoregressive.

decreased among young people aged from 15 to 34 years compared with older people (Figure 3(b)). The Atlantique-Littoral region continuously reported the highest rate of TB during the last ten years while a decrease in cases was noticed in Borgou-Alibori (Figure 3(c)). The proportion of TB patients tested for HIV was high (>90%) while the prevalence of HIV positive status among NPBCT cases tested was quite constant each year at 13% (Figure 3(d)).

3.3. Seasonality of TB Case Detection and Forecasted Numbers over the Next Five Years. The time series analysis of TB cases diagnosed between 2000 and 2014 in Benin is shown in Figures 4(a), 4(b), and 4(c). The raw graph of all cases diagnosed each semester showed an overall gradual increase of these cases over the study period, with several peaks suggesting a cyclical seasonal pattern in TB case finding (Figure 4(a)). This assumed that the TB case finding time series was composed of a trend (gradual increase over time), seasonal variations (several peaks at regular intervals), and a residual component. After a profiles method, the additive model was the most appropriate to decompose this time series. The decomposition into trend, seasonality and residual components is shown in Figure 4(b). Trend analysis showed upward-sloping but not linear curve. The seasonality curve described an alternative and regular fluctuation in the interval (52.009; −52.009) over the study period. Overall, in each year, except 2004, 2005, and 2008, the number of TB cases notified for the first semester was higher than that reported for the second semester. The residual component was on average generally constant over the period. The Dickey-Fuller test confirmed that this time series was effectively stationary (Dickey-Fuller = −5.781, Lag order = 3, and P value = 0.01). The Autocorrelation Function (ACF) and the Partial Autocorrelation Function (PACF) suggested an Autoregressive Integrated Moving Average (ARIMA) (2, 0, 3) model (Figure 4(c)). The coefficients of the autoregressive and moving average parts of the best fit model were determined and are presented in Table 1. The best fit model for this time series was therefore ARIMA (0, 0, 1)(1, 0, 0) with a constant. This model was validated using the Ljung-Box-Pierce test (chi-squared = 11.939, df = 1, $P < 0.001$), confirming thereby that the residual components in this time series were white noises (i.e., independent and identically distributed).

Finally, the forecasted number of TB cases per semester between 2015 and 2019 was calculated and is presented in Table 2. The numbers of TB cases are predicted to decrease during these next five years (see Figure 5).

(a)

(b)

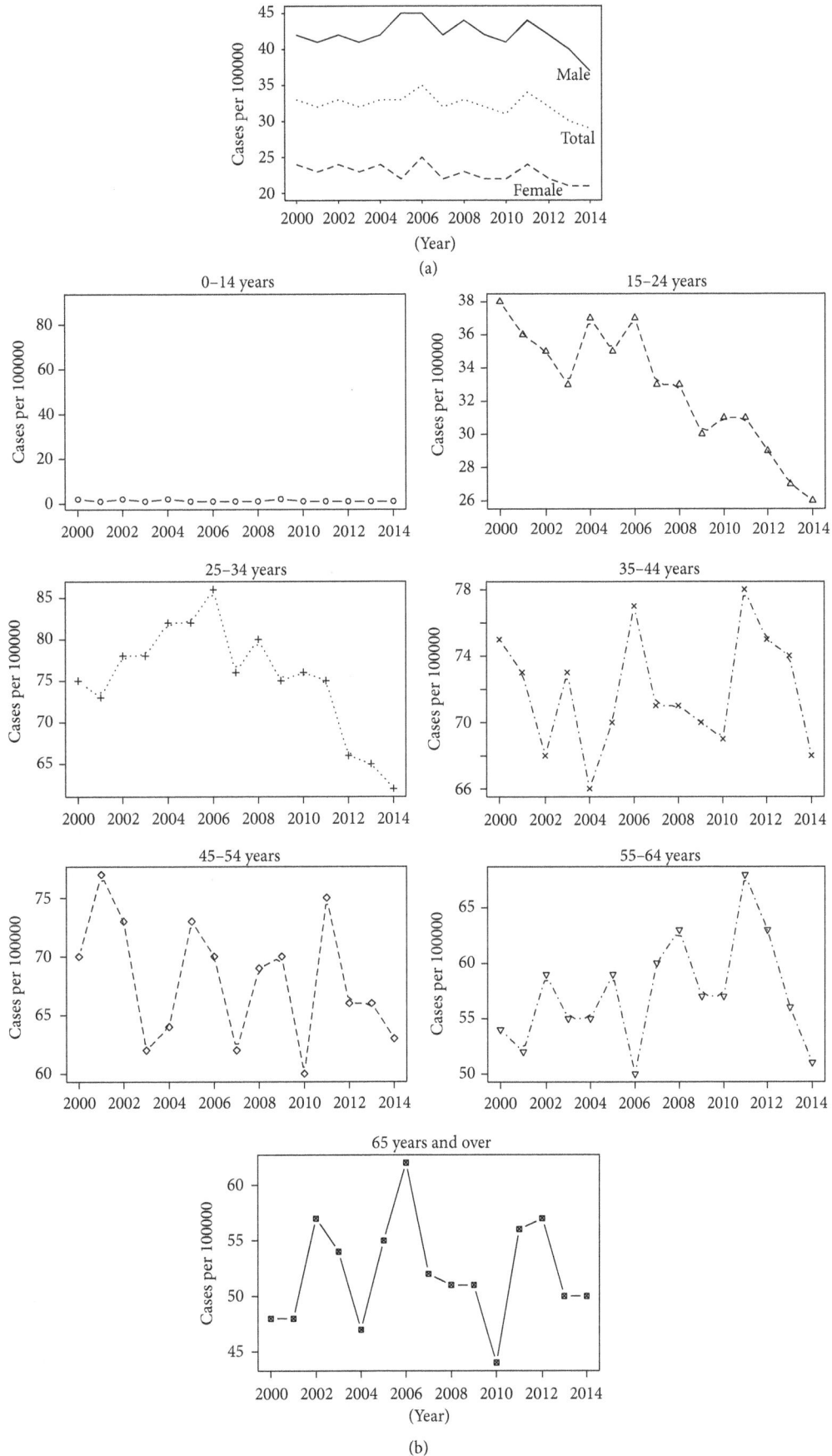

Figure 3: Continued.

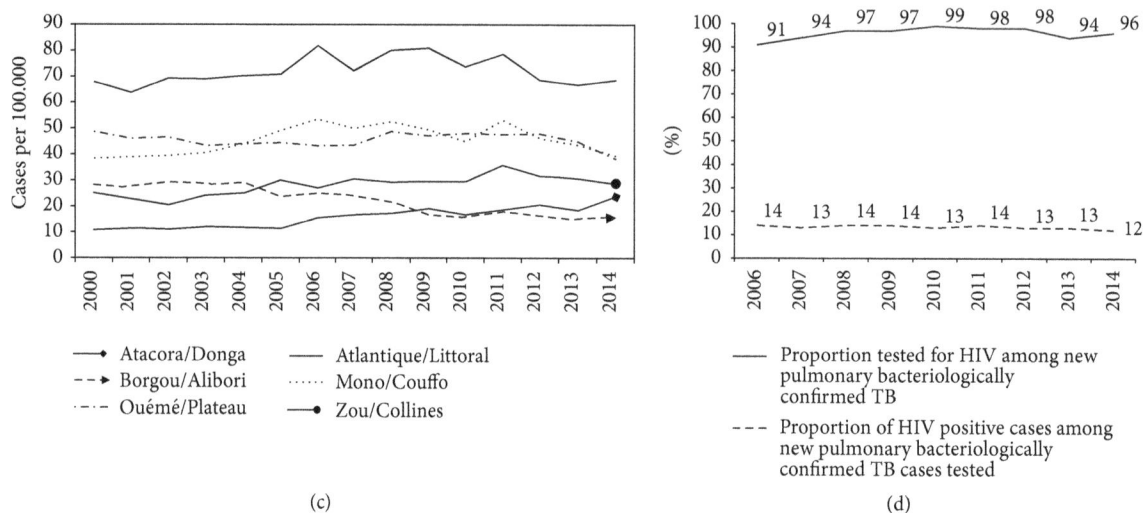

(c)

(d)

FIGURE 3: Trend of baseline characteristics and HIV positive status of tuberculosis patients between 2000 and 2014, Benin. (a) Sex in NPBCT; (b) age group in NPBCT; (c) regions of diagnosis for all TB; (d) HIV prevalence in NPBCT.

TABLE 2: Forecasted number of tuberculosis patients predicted to be diagnosed between 2015 and 2018 in Benin.

	2015		2016		2017		2018		2019	
	S1	S2	S1	S2	S1	S2	S1	S2	S1	S2
Prevision	1989	1917	1958	1896	1931	1877	1908	1861	1888	1848
[IC 95%]	[1788–2189]	[1683–2152]	[1666–2250]	[1586–2206]	[1587–2275]	[1522–2234]	[1529–2287]	[1475–2249]	[1485–2291]	[1439–2257]

Note: S: semester; IC 95%: 95% forecasting interval.

4. Discussion

This study aimed to describe in Benin, at the start of the new Global End TB Strategy, changes that occurred in the epidemiology of TB patients during the previous fifteen years and the predicted trend in TB case finding in the following five years. We found that between 2000 and 2014, the number of presumptive and notified TB cases slightly increased. In contrast to new pulmonary clinically diagnosed TB cases that increased during this time period, the proportion of retreatment TB cases decreased. Patients who were found NPBCT positive on microscopy regularly comprised at least three-quarters of all notified TB cases. With respect to demographic characteristics, the burden of the disease was consistently higher among males compared to females. However, from 2012 onwards, there was a striking decrease in males being notified with TB. The burden of disease also decreased among younger adults aged less than 34 years, who also constituted a large proportion of the TB population. The Atlantique-Littoral region continued to drive the epidemic in the country, while there was a drop in notified cases in Borgou-Alibori.

HIV testing in TB patients was excellent, with each year over 90% of patients tested. Of those who were tested, one in seven was annually found to be coinfected, with no change observed in this proportion over these fifteen years. The findings showed a seasonal variation in TB case finding and

notification, with a higher number of TB cases reported at the end of the first semester of each year. Finally, the forecasted number of TB cases to be diagnosed and notified in the next five years was predicted to decrease if only the current passive screening strategy in the country is applied.

The strengths of this study were that it involved all TB patients in the country who were notified to the NTP and therefore there was no need for any sampling framework. Data used were also previously validated during regular quarterly supervisions which contributed to minimizing errors. The study followed the Strengthening the Reporting of Observational Studies in Epidemiology (STROBE) guidelines [14]. Limitations were related to the retrospective nature of the study.

One of the major concerns that came from our findings was the decrease of TB cases in men and young adults and also the decline in the forecasted numbers that will be notified in the next five years. Taking into account the most important achievement within the programme, that is, a treatment success rate of 90% or more among NPBCT in these last six years [12], it is possible that the programme has significantly cut down transmission of infection from index smear-positive cases leading to a reduction in the burden of TB in the country. However, this belief should be interpreted with caution for several reasons.

First, the programme routinely uses a passive strategy for TB screening. The decrease reported in the study is

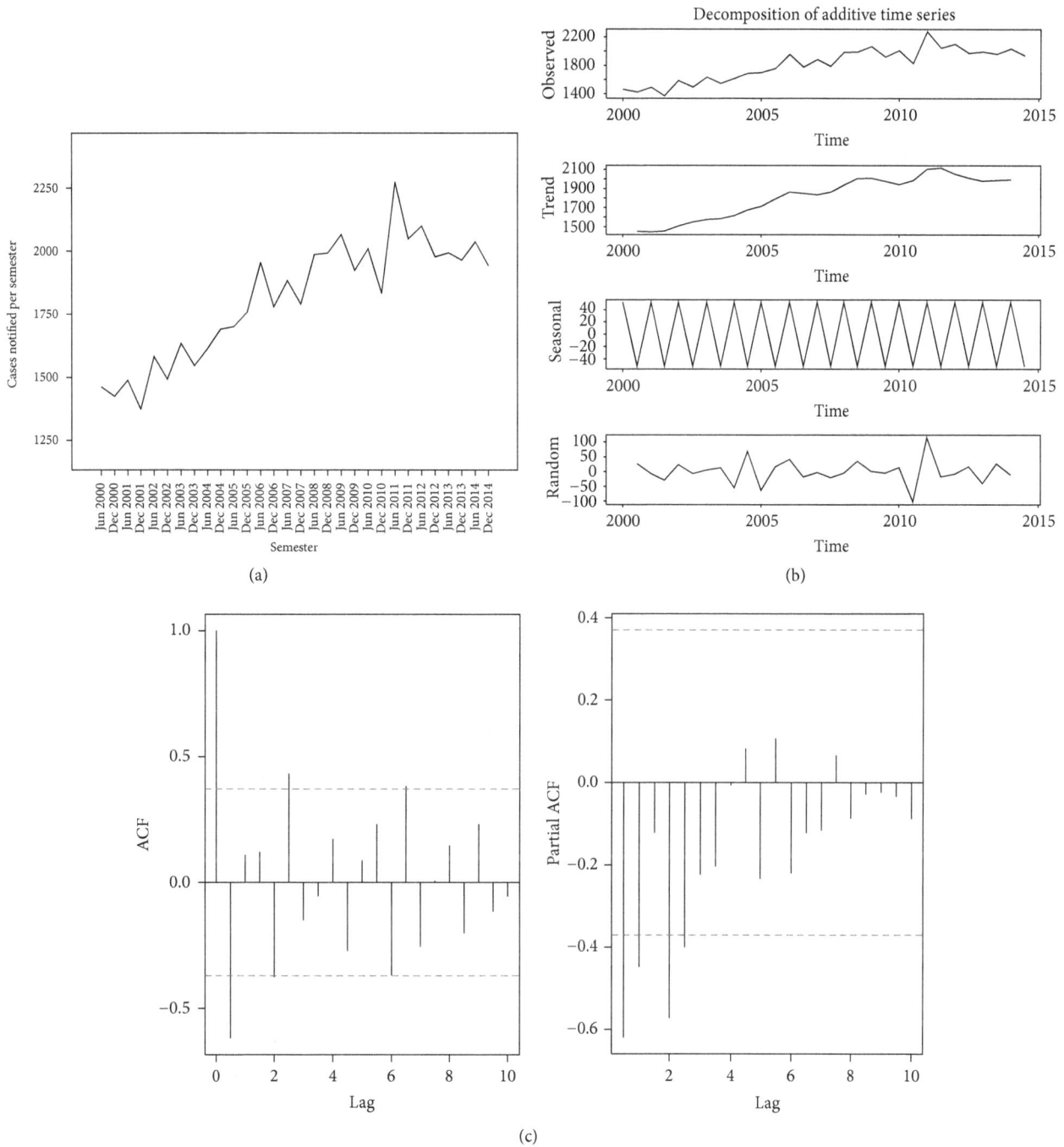

FIGURE 4: Time series analysis of all tuberculosis cases diagnosed, 2000–2014, Benin. (a) Tuberculosis cases diagnosed per semester; (b) decomposition of tuberculosis cases diagnosed with an additive model; (c) Autocorrelation and Partial Autocorrelation Functions of tuberculosis time series.

therefore related to TB cases that reached health facilities. Unfortunately, the utilization of the national health services remains low, estimated at 51.4% in 2013 [15]. In other words, TB cases that occurred in those not accessing TB services will not be diagnosed and notified. The increase in notified TB cases reported in the year of the "TB Reach" experience followed by a decrease after this adds weight to this theory. Advantages of a semiactive case finding strategy have also

been reported elsewhere [16, 17]. The high cost-efficacy of a semiactive case finding strategy does not allow it to be routinely performed in a resource-constrained setting, although this should always be considered. In 2015 and with the positive impact of the "TB Reach" experience on TB case finding, the GFATM authorized the implementation of other active case finding strategies in the country. An additional measure to be taken into account for reaching those who do

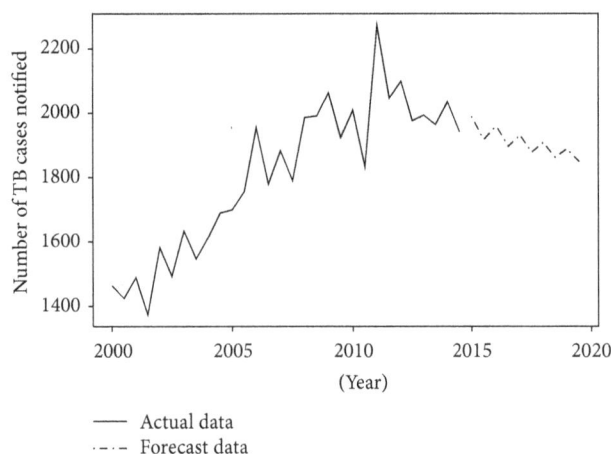

Figure 5: Trend of TB cases in Benin between 2000 and 2014 and forecasted number of TB cases from 2015 to 2019.

not use health facilities could be to strengthen sensitization especially among traditional practitioners who, most of time, are at the front line for providing care.

Second, it is possible that patients of some vulnerable groups such as HIV-infected patients, those with diabetes mellitus, and pregnant women were not diagnosed, since they were not systematically screened by practitioners for TB at each visit, unless they complained themselves of presumptive TB symptoms. Actions to address this shortfall and also implementation of some semiactive case finding sessions have been planned in the next three years' national strategic plan, mainly with the new GFATM grant. All these new activities are expected to increase TB case finding as follows: 5093 cases by 2016, 5449 by 2017, 5613 by 2018, and 5781 by 2019.

Third, because of the strong relationship between TB and poverty, TB reduction/elimination undoubtedly will not be achieved without real improvements in population life conditions. Although the GDP per capital in Benin grew from US$ 339 in 2000 to US$ 810 in 2014, the country remains one of the poorest in the world, with a poverty headcount ratio of 36% in the general population [18, 19]. A significant improvement in population life conditions is probably needed to effectively reverse the TB trend in the country and to achieve the 2035 TB goal of ending TB epidemic.

The high predominance of NPBCT positive cases on microscopy with no apparent decrease over the 15 years confirms the laboratory network efficacy but also raises the question about early diagnosis of TB in the country. A positive result on smear microscopy requires an average concentration of 10000 bacilli per millilitre in sputum specimens [20]. There is a need to advocate for earlier screening and diagnosis through more education, communication, and effective screening of close contacts of smear-positive TB patients [17]. The progressive reduction in the proportion of retreatment TB patients is, however, a favourable observation and is likely to be due to improvements in treatment outcomes of new cases.

We are not surprised that the Atlantique-Littoral region which houses the economic capital and is burdened with rural migrations and promiscuity issues remains the one most affected by the disease; but reasons why the trend of TB notifications is declining in Borgou should be sought and addressed. In the same way, reasons for the apparent seasonality in notified TB cases in the country are not clear. One suggested hypothesis is the variation in health facilities utilization in relation to seasons. Access to health facilities in the rainy season is a problem in many countries, and it might be expected that a decrease in TB case notifications occurs at this time. However, this hypothesis is not supported by our data, since in contrast a higher number of notified TB cases was often reported during the first semester which is when the main rainy season occurs. There may be other determinants contributing to TB case finding and notification seasonality in the country. Seasonality in TB cases finding has also been reported from elsewhere [21–23]. One hypothesis found in the literature which attempted to explain such seasonality has been a variation in Vitamin D, important substance in host defence, which is produced by the body in association with sunshine exposure; it may be a factor [24].

With respect to HIV infection, the proportion of patients with HIV infection has not increased. HIV is an important driver of the TB epidemic in many countries. Benin is a mixed epidemic country. Between 2000 and 2013, there has been a decrease of HIV prevalence in the population aged between 15 and 49 years from 2% to 1.1%. Furthermore, the coverage rate of ART intake that started in 2002 has progressively improved. The proportion of HIV-infected patients on ART increased from 12080 in 2008 to 28850 in 2014 [6, 25]. All of these factors have probably helped in preventing an increase in HIV-associated TB in Benin during the last 15 years.

5. Conclusion

The number of TB cases over the last 15 years in Benin has decreased among males and young adults, and the number of forecasted TB cases predicted to be diagnosed in the next five years will also decrease if only a passive screening strategy is continued. Benin needs to decide whether it needs alternative case finding strategies to meet the End TB Targets by 2035.

Competing Interests

The authors declare that they have no competing interests.

Acknowledgments

The authors thank Professor Martin GNINAFON, the former TB Programme manager, for his great work at the head of the institution during thirty years and all the health workers involved in TB care in the country. The authors also thank the International Union against Tuberculosis and Lung Disease (The Union), Paris, France, for technical support. Serge Ade is a Union Operational Research Fellow. He is part time financially supported by the International Union against Tuberculosis and Lung Disease (The Union),

Paris, France, through an Operational Research Fellowship. Funding was from an anonymous donor and the Department for International Development, UK. The funders had no role in study design, data collection and analysis, decision to publish, or preparation of the paper.

References

[1] World Health Organization, *Global Tuberculosis Report 2015*, WHO/HTM/TB/2015.22, World Health Organization, Geneva, Switzerland, 2015, http://apps.who.int/iris/bitstream/10665/191102/1/9789241565059_eng.pdf?ua=1.

[2] World Health Organization, *The End TB Strategy*, World Health Organization, Geneva, Switzerland, 2015, http://www.who.int/tb/post2015_TBstrategy.pdf.

[3] Institut National de la Statistique et de l'Analyse Economique, Benin en chiffres, http://www.insae-bj.org.

[4] M. Gninafon, A. Trébucq, and H. L. Rieder, "Epidemiology of tuberculosis in Benin," *International Journal of Tuberculosis and Lung Disease*, vol. 15, no. 1, pp. 61–66, 2011.

[5] World Health Organization, *Global Health Observatory. Benin: WHO Statistical Profile*, 2015, http://www.who.int/gho/countries/ben.pdf?ua=1.

[6] UNAIDS, *"Benin,"* http://www.unaids.org/sites/default/files/epidocuments/BEN.pdf.

[7] World Health Organization, *"Baccille Calmette Guérin vaccine, Reported estimates of BCG coverage,"* http://apps.who.int/immunization_monitoring/globalsummary/timeseries/tscoveragebcg.html.

[8] TB CARE I, *International Standards for Tuberculosis Care*, TB CARE I, The Hague, Netherlands, 3rd edition, 2014, http://www.who.int/tb/publications/ISTC_3rdEd.pdf?ua=1.

[9] N. Aït-Khaled, E. Alarcon, R. Armengol et al., *Management of Tuberculosis: A Guide to the Essentials of Good Practice*, International Union Against Tuberculosis and Lung Disease, Paris, France, 2010.

[10] A. Trébucq, D. A. Enarson, C. Y. Chiang et al., "Xpert® MTB/RIF for national tuberculosis programmes in low-income countries: when, where and how?" *International Journal of Tuberculosis and Lung Disease*, vol. 15, no. 12, pp. 1567–1571, 2011.

[11] World Health Organization, *Antiretroviral Therapy for HIV Infection in Adults and Adolescents. Recommendations for a Public Health Approach*, World Health Organization, Geneva, Switzerland, 2010.

[12] World Health Organization, *Tuberculosis Country Profiles: Benin*, World Health Organization, Geneva, Switzerland, 2015, https://extranet.who.int/sree/Reports?op=Replet&name=%2FWHO_HQ_Reports%2FG2%2FPROD%2FEXT%2FTBCountryProfile&ISO2=BJ&LAN=EN&outtype=html.

[13] World Health Organization, "Definitions and reporting framework for tuberculosis—2013 revision," Tech. Rep. WHO/HTM/TB/2013.2, World Health Organization, Geneva, Switzerland, 2013, http://apps.who.int/iris/bitstream/10665/79199/1/9789241505345_eng.pdf.

[14] E. Von Elm, D. G. Altman, M. Egger, S. J. Pocock, P. C. Gøtzsche, and J. P. Vandenbrouckef, "The Strengthening the Reporting of Observational Studies in Epidemiology (STROBE) Statement: guidelines for reporting observational studies," *Bulletin of the World Health Organization*, vol. 85, no. 11, pp. 867–872, 2007.

[15] Ministère de la Santé. Secrétariat Général du Ministère, Direction de la Programmation et de la Prospective, Annuaire des Statistiques Sanitaires 2013, http://www.beninsante.bj/documents/Annuaire_2013.pdf.

[16] D. W. Dowdy, S. Basu, and J. R. Andrews, "Is passive diagnosis enough? The impact of subclinical disease on diagnostic strategies for tuberculosis," *American Journal of Respiratory and Critical Care Medicine*, vol. 187, no. 5, pp. 543–551, 2013.

[17] S. G. Hinderaker, I. D. Rusen, C.-Y. Chiang, L. Yan, E. Heldal, and D. A. Enarson, "The FIDELIS initiative: innovative strategies for increased case finding," *International Journal of Tuberculosis and Lung Disease*, vol. 15, no. 1, pp. 71–76, 2011.

[18] The World Bank, *"Data 2015. GDP per capita,"* http://data.worldbank.org/indicator/NY.GDP.PCAP.CD.

[19] The World Bank, *"Data 2015, Benin,"* http://data.worldbank.org/country/benin.

[20] H. L. Rieder, A. Van Deun, K. M. Kam et al., *Priorities for Tuberculosis Bacteriology Services in Low-Income Countries*, International Union Against Tuberculosis and Lung Disease, Paris, France, 2007.

[21] X. Yang, Q. Duan, J. Wang, Z. Zhang, and G. Jiang, "Seasonal variation of newly notified pulmonary tuberculosis cases from 2004 to 2013 in Wuhan, China," *PLoS ONE*, vol. 9, no. 10, Article ID e108369, 2014.

[22] V. Kumar, A. Singh, M. Adhikary, S. Daral, A. Khokhar, and S. Singh, "Seasonality of tuberculosis in Delhi, India: a time series analysis," *Tuberculosis Research and Treatment*, vol. 2014, Article ID 514093, 5 pages, 2014.

[23] W. Wah, S. Das, A. Earnest et al., "Time series analysis of demographic and temporal trends of tuberculosis in Singapore," *BMC Public Health*, vol. 14, no. 1, article 1121, 2014.

[24] G. C. K. W. Koh, G. Hawthorne, A. M. Turner, H. Kunst, and M. Dedicoat, "Tuberculosis incidence correlates with sunshine: an ecological 28-year time series study," *PLoS ONE*, vol. 8, no. 3, Article ID e57752, 2013.

[25] Comité National de Lutte Contre le Sida, *Rapport de Suivi de la Déclaration de Politique sur le VIH et le Sida au Bénin*, 2015, http://www.unaids.org/sites/default/files/country/documents/BEN_narrative_report_2015.pdf.

25

Comparison of DNA Extraction Protocols and Molecular Targets to Diagnose Tuberculous Meningitis

Flavia Silva Palomo,[1,2] **Martha Gabriela Celle Rivero,**[1]
Milene Gonçalves Quiles,[1] **Fernando Pereira Pinto,**[2]
Antonia Maria de Oliveira Machado,[2] **and Antonio Carlos Campos Pignatari**[1]

[1]*Special Clinical Microbiology Laboratory (LEMC), Federal University of São Paulo (UNIFESP), São Paulo, SP, Brazil*
[2]*Central Laboratory of São Paulo Hospital, Federal University of São Paulo (UNIFESP), São Paulo, SP, Brazil*

Correspondence should be addressed to Flavia Silva Palomo; fla_bio@hotmail.com

Academic Editor: Carlo Garzelli

Tuberculous meningitis (TBM) is a severe form of extrapulmonary tuberculosis. The aims of this study were to evaluate in-house molecular diagnostic protocols of DNA extraction directly from CSF samples and the targets amplified by qPCR as an accurate and fast diagnosis of TBM. One hundred CSF samples from 68 patients suspected of TBM were studied. Four DNA extraction techniques (phenol-chloroform-thiocyanate guanidine, silica thiocyanate guanidine, resin, and resin with ethanol) were compared and CSF samples were used to determine the best target (*IS6110, MPB64,* and *hsp65 KDa*) by qPCR. The extraction protocol using the phenol-chloroform-thiocyanate guanidine showed the best results in terms of quantification and sensitivity of PCR amplification, presenting up to 10 times more DNA than the second best protocol, the silica guanidine thiocyanate. The target that showed the best result for TBM diagnosis was the *IS6110*. This target showed 91% sensitivity and 97% specificity when we analyzed the results by sample and showed 100% sensitivity and 98% specificity when we analyzed the results by patient. The DNA extraction with phenol-chloroform-thiocyanate guanidine followed by *IS6110 target* amplification has been shown to be suitable for diagnosis of TBM in our clinical setting.

1. Background

Tuberculosis is a serious infectious contagious disease that usually affects the lungs but can also affect other organs such as kidney, bone, and central nervous system (CNS) [1]. In 2011, cases of extra pulmonary tuberculosis in Brazil reached almost 16% of all cases of the disease [2] and about 6.3% of these (1.3% of the total) were TBM [3].

The TBM is the most severe form of extra pulmonary tuberculosis that has a high morbidity and mortality [4, 5]. The definitive diagnosis of TBM depends on the *M. tuberculosis* agent detection from cerebrospinal fluid (CSF). Routinely, the survey of *M. tuberculosis* in CSF is carried out by conventional microbiological methods including Ziehl-Neelsen smear, which has low sensitivity (0–20%) and culture, which requires until 65 days to final result [1, 6].

The sensibility for detection of *M. tuberculosis* in CSF samples can be substantially increased from 70% to 100% and the time required to release laboratory results can be significantly decreased with the use molecular methods, including the polymerase chain reaction (PCR). The rapid identification of TBM through molecular analysis of CSF is an important factor for proper and early institution of antimicrobial treatment [7–9].

The aims of this study were to evaluate in-house molecular diagnostic protocols of DNA extraction directly from CSF samples and the targets amplified by qPCR as an accurate and fast diagnosis of TBM.

2. Methods

2.1. Clinical CSF Samples. We utilized the CSF samples sent for mycobacteria culture at the Central Laboratory of São

TABLE 1: Real time PCR targets primers.

Target	Primer	Sequence (5′-3′)	Product	Reference
IS6110	IS-Fw	CGTGAGGGCATCGAGGTGGC	245 bp	[9]
	IS-Rv	CGCTAGGCGTCGGTGACAAA		
Hsp 65 KDa	hsp65-Fw	GAGATCGAGCTGGAGGATCC	383 bp	[7]
	hsp65-Rv	AGCTGCAGCCCAAAGGTGTT		
MPB64	MPB64-Fw	TCCGCTGCCAGTCGTCTTCC	240 bp	[7]
	MPB64-Rv	GTCCTCGCAGTCTAGGCCA		

Note. Fw: forward; Rv: reverse; bp: base pairs of nucleotidis.

Paulo Hospital, Federal University of São Paulo/UNIFESP, Brazil, in the period from January 2011 to June 2014. Aliquots were frozen at −20°C and submitted to molecular tests after being thawed and centrifuged. These samples were also subjected to biochemical and cytological analysis and determination of adenosine deaminase (ADA) levels.

The samples were classified as true positive and negative after a survey in the database "BrazilianTBweb", other laboratory CSF data and evaluation of medical records.

2.2. Microbiological Diagnostic of CSF Samples.

The microbial diagnosis of CSF samples was made in the Central Laboratory of São Paulo Hospital, Federal University of São Paulo/UNIFESP, Brazil. For each CSF a Ziehl-Neelsen smear and mycobacterium culture in Lowenstein Jensen solid medium were done.

2.3. DNA Extraction Protocols.

Four extraction methods were analyzed: phenol-chloroform with guanidine thiocyanate (Brazol®, LabTrade, Brazil), silica-guanidine plus thiocyanate plus guanidine thiocyanate (QIAmp® DNA Mini Kit, Qiagen, USA), resin (Chelex® 100 resin, BioRad, USA), and resin precipitated with ethanol.

Comparison of extraction was determined by a serial 10-fold dilutions prepared in four different diluents (ultrapure water, turbid, xanthochromic, and hemorrhagic CSF pools known negative for TBM) from a 0.5 McFarland (1.5×10^8 CFU/mL) suspension of *M. tuberculosis* ATCC 25177.

The extracted DNA was measured and analyzed by NanoVue ND-100 (*Thermo Fisher Scientific*, Wilmington, USA) and the amplification sensitivity was determined by *IS6110* target. The DNA extraction protocol presenting the best results was chosen for target and clinical samples analysis.

Phenol-Chloroform-Thiocyanate Guanidine (Brazol, Lab-Trade, Brazil) DNA Extraction. An aliquot of 200 μL CSF sample sediment was added to a microtube containing 500 μL of Brazol and mixture. Then ice-cold chloroform (300 μL) was added. The mixture was homogenized and centrifuged at 12,000 rpm for 15 minutes at 8°C. The supernatant was removed and transferred to another microtube containing 500 μL of cold absolute ethanol. The mixture was stirred for 3–5 seconds by vortexing and centrifuged at 12,000 rpm for 15 minutes at 8°C. The supernatant was removed and the "pellet" was washed with 500 μL of ice-cold ethanol and centrifuged

at 12,000 rpm for 15 minutes at 8°C. The supernatant was carefully removed and discarded. The "pellet" was incubated at room temperature to dryness and then dissolved in 30 μL of ultrapure water (Invitrogen Life Technologies, USA) and allowed to dissolve at 65°C for 30 minutes. The samples were frozen at −20°C when not used immediately.

Silica-Guanidine Thiocyanate (QIAamp DNA Mini Kit, Qiagen, USA) DNA Extraction. The protocol recommended by the manufacturer was used with 200 μL of the CSF sediment.

Resin (Resin Chelex100, BioRad, USA) DNA Extraction. A 200 μL aliquot of the CSF sample pellet was placed in 300 μL of a 10% solution Chelex. This mixture was homogenized in vortex for 10 seconds, centrifuged quickly to remove excess fluid from the cover, and incubated at 95°C for 30 minutes in a heat block. The tube was homogenized for 15 sec and centrifuged for 5 minutes at 13000 rpm. The supernatant containing the extracted DNA was transferred to a new tube. When not used immediately, the sample was frozen at −20°C.

Resin Precipitated with Ethanol (Chelex100 Resin, BioRad, USA) DNA Extraction. A 200 μL aliquot of the CSF pellet was placed in 300 μL of 10% solution Chelex. This mixture was homogenized in vortex for 10 seconds and centrifuged quickly to remove excess fluid from the cover. This mixture was incubated at 95°C for 30 minutes in a heat block. The tube was homogenized for 15 sec and centrifuged for 5 minutes at 13000 rpm. The supernatant containing the extracted DNA was transferred to a new tube and 500 μL of cold absolute ethanol was added. The mixture was stirred for 3–5 seconds by vortexing and centrifuged at 12,000 rpm for 15 minutes at 8°C. The "pellet" was washed with 500 μL of ice-cold ethanol and centrifuged at 12,000 rpm for 15 minutes at 8°C. The supernatant was carefully removed and discarded. The "pellet" was incubated at room temperature to dryness and then dissolved in 30 μL of ultrapure water (Invitrogen Life Technologies, USA) and allowed to dissolve at 65°C for 30 minutes. The samples were frozen at −20°C when not utilized immediately.

2.4. Targets and PCR Protocols.

Three different targets were analyzed for *M. tuberculosis* detection by real time PCR: *IS6110* gene, 65 kDa Heat Shock Protein gene *(hsp65 KDa)*, and the MPB64 protein encoding gene *(MPB64)* (Table 1). The reaction was performed on Rotor-Gene 5 plex/HRM

TABLE 2: List of microorganisms used as negative control.

Microorganisms	Origin
Acinetobacter baumannii	ATCC 19606
Candida spp.	Known strain
Cryptococcus neoformans	Known strain
Enterococcus faecalis	ATCC 29212
Enterococcus faecium	Known strain
Escherichia coli	ATCC 35218
Haemophilus influenzae	Known strain
Haemophilus spp.	Known strain
Klebsiella pneumoniae	Known strain
Listeria monocytogenes	Known strain
Mycobacterium chelonae	Known strain
Mycobacterium abscessus	Known strain
Mycobacterium avium	Known strain
Mycobacterium gordonae	Known strain
Mycobacterium intracellulare	Known strain
Mycobacterium kansasii	Known strain
Mycobacterium lentiflavum	Known strain
Neisseria meningitidis	Known strain
Neisseria spp.	Known strain
Nocardia spp.	Known strain
Proteus mirabilis	ATCC 29245
Pseudomonas aeruginosa	ATCC 27853
Salmonella enterica	ATCC 14028
Shigella flexneri	ATCC 12022
Staphylococcus aureus	ATCC 29213
Staphylococcus epidermidis	ATCC 12228
Staphylococcus saprophyticus	ATCC 43867
Streptococcus agalactiae	ATCC 12386
Streptococcus pneumoniae	ATCC 49619
Streptococcus pyogenes	ATCC 19615

ATCC: American Type Collection Culture.

platform (Qiagen, USA) by melting analyses (QuantiFast SYBR Green PCR (Qiagen, USA)) on 20 μL final volume. The limit of detection (LoD) was determined by a serial sevenfold dilutions prepared in ultrapure water (Sigma-Aldrich, Co. Ltd, Saint Louis, US).

The target specificity was carried out by testing the negative control group and CSF samples. The negative control group was made up by ATCC and known strains of bacteria, yeasts, and other mycobacteria (Table 2).

2.5. Real Time PCR Protocol. A reaction containing 10 μL of QuantiFast SYBR Green PCR (Qiagen, USA), 0.5 mM of each primer, and 2 μL of sample was used for *M. tuberculosis* DNA detection directly from the CSF sample. Thermocycling was performed in the PCR system in the real time Rotor-Gene Q 5plex Platform (Qiagen, USA) using the following conditions: an initial cycle of five minutes at 95°C, followed by 45 cycles of 30 seconds at 94°C and 45 seconds at the respective annealing temperature for IS6110 (65°C), hsp65 KDa (62°C), and MPB64 (61°C). At the conclusion of cycling a melting

step ranging from 72°C to 95°C with an increase of 0.5°C per second was added for each gene.

2.6. Statistical Analysis. The results obtained were compared and evaluated clinically and analytically. For each test sensitivity (*S*), specificity (SP), positive predictive value (PPV), negative predictive value (NPV) and accuracy (*A*) were calculated. The *Kappa* index (*k*) was used to analyze the correlation between the tests. For analytical comparison, mycobacteria culture was considered as gold standard. For clinical analysis the patients and their respective samples were classified as true positive and true negative in accordance with the result of mycobacterium culture and clinical and laboratory data. Clinical data of patients were collected from electronic medical records and laboratory reports provided by the Central Laboratory of Hospital São Paulo and records in Brazilian TBweb (http://www.cvetb.saude.sp.gov.br/).

3. Results

Among 100 clinical CSF samples collected from 68 patients, 35 from 16 patients were considered true positive and 65 samples from 52 patients were true negative by clinical parameters.

The DNA extraction protocol using the phenol-chloroform-thiocyanate guanidine presented the highest final DNA concentration among four methods evaluated (Table 3).

From 35 clinical samples considered true positive by clinical parameters for TBM diagnosis, IS6110 PCR was able to detect 32 of them followed by culture and *hsp65 KDa* (16 samples) and *MPB64* (12 samples). (Table 4).

Sixty-five samples were considered as true negative by clinical parameters for TBM diagnosis and culture was negative for all of them while 63 samples were negative by *IS6110, MBP64,* and *hsp65 KDa* PCR. (Table 4).

From 16 patients considered true positive by clinical parameters for TBM diagnosis, *IS6110* was able to correctly detect all of them followed by *hsp65 KDa* (11 patients), culture (10 patients), and *MBP64* (7 samples). (Table 5).

From 52 patients considered true negative by clinical parameters for TBM diagnosis, the culture was able to detect all of them as negative followed by IS6110 (51 patients), hsp65, and MBP64 (50 samples). (Table 5).

LoD, efficiency, Ct (cycle threshold) median and T_m (temperature of melting) median for *IS6110, MPB 64,* and hsp65 KDa are presented in Table 6. The primers were specific for *M. tuberculosis* and did not show cross reactivity against different microorganisms tested.

4. Discussion

Over the years several studies proposed and validated molecular techniques for diagnosis of TBM [8–14]. These studies considered the importance of developing a simple technique that was easily reproduced in laboratories with minimal resources [10, 11, 13, 15, 16]. The choice of the most appropriate extraction method and the target to be amplified are criteria

TABLE 3: Nanovue results form four extraction protocols.

Diluent	Extraction method	Sensitivity amplification	DNA [ng/μL]	A260/280
Ultrapure water	Phenol Chloroform	10^{-10}	24,5	1,53
	Silica	10^{-9}	2,3	1,18
	Resin	10^{-7}	1,2	0,93
	Resin ethanol	10^{-4}	0,3	0,36
Turbid CSF	Phenol Chloroform	10^{-10}	28,5	1,59
	Silica	10^{-10}	22,2	1,45
	Resin	10^{-7}	19	1,08
	Resin ethanol	10^{-3}	0,1	0,01
Xanthochromic CSF	Phenol Chloroform	10^{-10}	53	1,56
	Silica	10^{-9}	21	1,8
	Resin	10^{-7}	24,5	1,09
	Resin ethanol	10^{-6}	0,12	1,4
Hemorrhagic CSF	Phenol Chloroform	10^{-10}	64,5	1,55
	Silica	10^{-10}	60,8	1,76
	Resin	10^{-7}	67	1,22
	Resin ethanol	10^{-6}	0,1	2,19

TABLE 4: Culture and real time PCR results for 100 samples included on the study.

	S	SP	PPV	NPV	A	K
Culture	46%	100%	100%	77%	81%	0,52 (Weak)
INS6110	91%	97%	94%	95%	95%	0,89 (Strong)
MPB64	34%	97%	86%	73%	75%	0,36 (Minimal)
hsp65 KDa	46%	97%	89%	77%	79%	0,48 (Weak)

Note. S: sensitivity; SP: specificity; PPV: positive predictive value; NPV: negative predictive value; A: accuracy; k: Kappa index.

TABLE 5: Culture and real time PCR results for 100 samples included on the study.

	S	SP	PPV	NPV	A	K
Culture	63%	100%	100%	90%	91%	0,72 (moderate)
INS6110	100%	98%	94%	100%	99%	0,96 (almost perfect)
MPB64	44%	96%	78%	85%	84%	0,47 (weak)
hsp65 KDa	69%	96%	85%	91%	90%	0,69 (moderate)

Note. S: sensitivity; SP: specificity; PPV: positive predictive value; NPV: negative predictive value; A: accuracy; k: Kappa index.

TABLE 6: LoD, efficiency, Ct, and Tm results for real time PCR.

Target	LoD (CFU)	Efficiency	Ct Median	T_m Median
IS6110	10^0	1,07	31,09	89,8
Hsp 65 KDa	10^2	1,02	25,78	86,8
MPB64	10^3	1,07	35,07	90,7

LoD: limit of detection; Ct: cycle threshold; T_m: temperature of melting.

that improve the precision, sensitivity and specificity of the PCR test [16–18].

The complexity of rich cell wall lipids of mycobacteria is a limiting factor for the success of some DNA extraction techniques [19–22], besides the fact that the microorganism is an intracellular pathogen, which can hinder the isolation of these microorganisms in clinical samples [19, 22]. Since the CSF samples from patients with TBM are usually paucibacillary it is recommended to recover the greatest amount of DNA as possible.

The extraction protocol using the phenol-chloroform-thiocyanate guanidine showed the best results in terms of quantification and sensitivity of PCR amplification, presenting up to 10 times more DNA than the second best protocol, the silica guanidine thiocyanate.

The techniques using phenol-chloroform, silica, and thiocyanate guanidine are described as excellent choices for DNA extraction in different biological materials, in addition to being inexpensive and simple [8–13].

The methodology of phenol-chloroform extraction and DNA purification utilized the Brazol, which has in its composition in addition to phenol, guanidine thiocyanate, a chaotropic agent that inactivates endonucleases and prevents DNA binding to other molecules and facilitates the separation of cellular debris [23–26]. Furthermore, the phenol which is a potent proteolytic agent, corrosive and caustic, contributes to lysis of the cell envelope of mycobacteria. In phenol extraction, solubilization and denaturation of proteins and lipids occur efficiently [26]. The chloroform used in this method is also a good protein denaturing detergent and a major solvent of fats, which probably contributed to the removal of the lipid layer of the mycobacteria cell wall. Regarding the biohazard risk of phenol-chloroform, all tests were done following the biosafety manuals and chemical waste disposal regulations of our country.

The target that showed the best amplification results was the IS6110 qPCR with a sensitivity of 100% and specificity of 79%, when compared to culture. The sample analysis for IS6110 qPCR amplification showed 91% sensitivity and 97% specificity with the clinical diagnosis. When this analysis was grouped by patient, we showed a very good agreement with the clinical diagnosis with 100% sensitivity and 98% specificity.

These results can be explained since the gene encoding the MPB64 protein and the encoding gene heat shock protein (hsp65 KDa) have single copies in mycobacteria genome while the insertion gene IS6110 has multiple copies which makes the reaction more sensitive [7–9].

The IS6110 target sequence is a repetitive insertion of 1,350 base pairs present in M. tuberculosis complex species with different numbers of copies integrated into various chromosomal sites [9, 27, 28]. This molecular target promotes an increase in the sensitivity of the technique, which is an advantage over other targets. Only three patients had positive CSF samples for target IS6110 undiagnosed for TBM, but when we evaluated other laboratory criteria or clinical characteristics of these patients two of them had TBM and only one remained doubtful.

Commercial molecular tests for pulmonary tuberculosis diagnosis such as XpertMTB/RIF represent a significant advance, since it is automated and provides fast results. However, for TBM diagnosis its sensitivity is around 60% to 80%. [29–31]. Other targets also can be used for M. tuberculosis molecular diagnosis, including the TRC4 primer a conserved repetitive element with specificity for M. tuberculosis complex [32].

There are few reports of M. tuberculosis lacking the IS6110 that eventually could be responsible for false negative results [32, 33]; however, we considered that the benefit of a greater sensitivity of the IS6110 gene that can be found repeatedly in the genome M. tuberculosis justifies its use [11, 32, 33].

Thus, we believe we have demonstrated the feasibility of a molecular test for the diagnosis of TBM by an in-house real time PCR with analytical and clinical correlation to be used in laboratories with adequate cost benefit. Studies comparing other molecular methods of DNA extraction, other molecular targets, in-house protocols, and commercial platforms are warranted.

5. Conclusion

The combination of DNA extraction by phenol-chloroform and guanidine thiocyanate, (Brazol) and qPCR by IS6110 target amplification could be an effective tool for M. tuberculosis diagnosis directly from CSF samples.

Acknowledgments

This study was supported by a grant from Coordenação de Aperfeiçoamento de Pessoal de Nível Superior, Capes, Brazil.

References

[1] G. E. Thwaites, T. T. H. Chau, K. Stepniewska, and etal., "Diagnosis of adult tuberculous meningitis by use of clinical and laboratory features," The Lancet, vol. 360, no. 9342, pp. 1287–1292, 2002.

[2] T. C. de Oliveira, "Implementação de ações de vigilância epidemiológica em nível regional," Revista de Saúde Pública, vol. 23, no. 1, pp. 79–81, 1989.

[3] D. M. Mota, H. B. M. Beltrão, T. M. Lanzieri, L. C. Vieira, and M. Machado, "Avaliação econômica da rubéola e de estratégia de controle em situação de surto em Fortaleza (Ceará)," Saúde e Sociedade, vol. 20, no. 3, 2011.

[4] A. Cherian and S. V. Thomas, "Central nervous system tuberculosis," African Health Sciences, vol. 11, no. 1, 2011.

[5] D. H. Kennedy and R. J. Fallón, "Tuberculous meningitis," Journal of American Medical Association, vol. 241, no. 3, pp. 264–268, 1979.

[6] D. Heemskerk, J. Day, T. T. H. Chau et al., "Intensified treatment with high dose rifampicin and levofloxacin compared to standard treatment for adult patients with tuberculous meningitis (tbm-it): protocol for a randomized controlled trial," Trials, vol. 12, no. 1, 2011.

[7] L. M. Wildner, C. L. Nogueira, da. Silva Souza, B. S. G. Senna, R. M. da Silva, and M. L. Bazzo, "Micobacterias: epidemiologia e diagnóstico," Revista De Patologia Tropical, vol. 40, no. 3, pp. 207–230, 2011.

[8] B. W. Lee, J. A. M. A. Tan, S. C. Wong et al., "DNA amplification by the polymerase chain reaction for the rapid diagnosis of tuberculous meningitis. Comparison of protocols involving three mycobacterial DNA sequences, IS6110, 65 kDa antigen, and MPB64," Journal of the Neurological Sciences, vol. 123, no. 1, pp. 173–179, 1994.

[9] A. W. Mir, A. Kirmani, R. Eachkoti, and M. A. Siddiqi, "Improved diagnosis of central nervous system tuberculosis by MPB64-target PCR," *Brazilian Journal of Microbiology*, vol. 39, no. 2, pp. 209–213, 2008.

[10] P. W. Hermans, D. Van Soolingen, J. W. Dale et al., "Insertion element IS986 from Mycobacterium tuberculosis: a useful tool for diagnosis and epidemiology of tuberculosis," *Journal of Clinical Microbiology*, vol. 28, no. 9, pp. 2051–2058, 1990.

[11] L. Chaidir, A. R. Ganiem, A. vander Zanden et al., "Comparison of real time IS6110-PCR, microscopy, and culture for diagnosis of tuberculous meningitis in a cohort of adult patients in indonesia," *Plos ONE*, vol. 7, no. 12, Article ID e52001, 2012.

[12] S. Haldar, N. Sharma, V. K. Gupta, and J. S. Tyagi, "Efficient diagnosis of tuberculous meningitis by detection of Mycobacterium tuberculosis DNA in cerebrospinal fluid filtrates using PCR," *Journal of Medical Microbiology*, vol. 58, no. 5, pp. 616–624, 2009.

[13] F. C. D. Q. Mello and J. Fonseca-Costa, "A utilidade da biologia molecular no diagnóstico da," *Jornal Brasileiro De Pneumologia*, vol. 31, no. 3, 188 pages, 2005.

[14] T. Takahashi, M. Tamura, Y. Asami et al., "Novel wide-range quantitative nested real-time PCR assay for Mycobactenum tuberculosis DNA: clinical application for diagnosis of tuberculous meningitis," *Journal of Clinical Microbiology*, vol. 46, no. 5, pp. 1698–1707, 2008.

[15] T. Takahashi, M. Tamura, and T. Takasu, "The PCR-based diagnosis of central nervous system tuberculosis: up to date," *Tuberculosis Research and Treatment*, 2012.

[16] V. R. Bollela, D. N. Sato, and B. A. L. Fonseca, "Problems in the standardization of the polymerase chain reaction for the diagnosis of pulmonary tuberculosis," *Revista de Saúde Pública*, vol. 33, no. 3, pp. 281–286, 1999.

[17] C. M. Baratto and F. Megiolaro, "Comparação de diferentes protocolos de extração de dna de bactérias para utilização em RAPD-PCR," *Ciência-ACET*, vol. 3, no. 1, pp. 121–130, 2012.

[18] A. P. Adams, S. R. Bolin, A. E. Fine, C. A. Bolin, and J. B. Kaneene, "Comparison of PCR versus culture for detection of Mycobacterium bovis after experimental inoculation of various matrices held under environmental conditions for extended periods," *Applied and Environmental Microbiology*, vol. 79, no. 20, pp. 6501–6506, 2013.

[19] J. Sambrook and D. W. Russell, *Molecular Cloning. A Laboratory Manual*, Cold Spring Harbor Laboratory Press, New York, NY, USA, 3rd edition, 2001.

[20] M. J. Zumárraga, V. Meikle, A. Bernardelli et al., "Use of touch-down polymerase chain reaction to enhance the sensitivity of mycobacterium bovis detection," *Journal of Veterinary Diagnostic Investigation*, vol. 17, no. 3, pp. 232–238, 2005.

[21] Z.-Q. Zhang and M. Ishaque, "Evaluation of methods for isolation of DNA from slowly and rapidly growing mycobacteria," *International Journal of Leprosy and Other Mycobacterial Diseases*, vol. 65, no. 4, pp. 469–476, 1997.

[22] M. Jaber, A. Rattan, A. Verma, J. Tyagi, and R. Kumar, "A simple method of DNA extraction from mycobacterium tuberculosis," *Tubercle and Lung Disease*, vol. 76, no. 6, pp. 578–581, 1995.

[23] B. J. Wards, D. M. Collins, and G. W. de Lisle, "Detection of mycobacterium bovis in tissues by polymerase chain reaction," *Veterinary Microbiology*, vol. 43, no. 2, pp. 227–240, 1995.

[24] R. Boom, C. Sol, M. Beld, J. Weel, J. Goudsmit, and P. Wertheim-Van Dillen, "Improved silica-guanidiniumthiocyanate DNA isolation procedure based on selective binding of bovine alpha-casein to silica particles," *Journal of Clinical Microbiology*, vol. 37, no. 3, pp. 615–619, 1999.

[25] I. N. De Almeida, W. Da Silva Carvalho, M. L. Rossetti, E. R. D. Costa, and S. S. De Miranda, "Evaluation of six different DNA extraction methods for detection of Mycobacterium tuberculosis by means of PCR-IS6110: preliminary study," *BMC Research Notes*, vol. 6, no. 1, Article 561, 2013.

[26] P. Chomczynski and N. Sacchi, "Single-step method of RNA isolation by acid guanidinium thiocyanate-phenol-chloroform extraction," *Analytical Biochemistry*, vol. 162, no. 1, pp. 156–159, 1987.

[27] A. S. Goldsborough and M. R. Bates, *U.S. Patent Application No. 14/193*, p. 680, 2014.

[28] D. Van Soolingen, P. W. Hermans, P. E. W. De Haas, D. R. Soll, and J. D. A. Van Embden, "Occurrence and stability of insertion sequences in Mycobacterium tuberculosis complex strains: evaluation of an insertion sequence-dependent dna polymorphism as a tool in the epidemiology of tuberculosis," *Journal of Clinical Microbiology*, vol. 29, no. 11, pp. 2578–2586, 1991.

[29] N. C. S. De Assis, M. L. Lopes, N. C. Cardoso, M. M. Da Costa, C. D. O. Sousa, and K. V. B. Lima, "Molecular diagnosis of pulmonary tuberculosis," *Jornal Brasileiro De Patologia E Medicina Laboratorial*, vol. 43, no. 1, pp. 1–7, 2007.

[30] N. T. Q. Nhu, D. Heemskerk, T. T. H. Chau et al., "Evaluation of GeneXpert MTB/RIF for diagnosis of tuberculous meningitis," *Journal of Clinical Microbiology*, vol. 52, no. 1, pp. 226–233, 2014.

[31] V. B. Patel, G. Theron, L. Lenders et al., "Diagnostic accuracy of quantitative PCR (Xpert MTB/RIF) for tuberculous meningitis in a high burden setting: a prospective study," *PLoS Med*, vol. 10, no. 10, Article ID e1001536, 2013.

[32] A. N. I. Sattar, S. K. Setu, A. A. Saleh, and S. Ahmed, "TRC4 gene based PCR assay in diagnosis of tuberculous meningitis," *Journal of Medical Microbiology*, vol. 8, no. 2, pp. 19–22, 2017.

[33] A. Berwal, K. Chawla, S. Vishwanath, and V. P. Shenoy, "Role of multiplex polymerase chain reaction in diagnosing tubercular meningitis," *Journal of Laboratory Physicians*, vol. 9, no. 2, pp. 145–147, 2017.

26

The Role of *Foxp3*-Expressing Regulatory T Cells and T Helpers in Immunopathogenesis of Multidrug Resistant Pulmonary Tuberculosis

E. G. Churina, O. I. Urazova, and V. V. Novitskiy

SBEI-HPE "Siberian State Medical University of the Ministry of Health Care and Social Development of the Russian Federation", Tomsk, Russia

Correspondence should be addressed to E. G. Churina, lena1236@yandex.ru

Academic Editor: Giovanni Battista Migliori

Subpopulation structure of regulatory T cells and T helpers of peripheral blood in patients with newly diagnosed pulmonary tuberculosis depending on the clinical form of disease and sensitivity of *Mycobacterium tuberculosis* to antituberculosis drugs has been analyzed in this work. It has been shown that the leading part in immune suppression at infiltrative, dissemination, and fibrosis-cavity pulmonary tuberculosis is played by natural regulatory CD4$^+$CD25$^+$Foxp3$^+$-T lymphocytes. Thus we estimate increase of their number in blood by drug-resistance and drug-susceptible patients. It has been demonstrated that in patients with fibrocavernous and infiltrative form of the disease and drug-resistant pulmonary tuberculosis the number of CD4$^+$CD25$^-$Foxp3$^+$-regulatory T cells was increasing. In patients with infiltrative pulmonary tuberculosis, including multidrug-resistant *M. tuberculosis*, an increased number of CD3$^+$CD4$^+$CD25$^-$ T helpers is determined by the pathogenic features of the development of the tuberculosis infection and is connected with the activation of Th1-dependent immune response. Reduction in the number of T-helpers in the blood of patients with dissemination and fibrosis-cavity pulmonary tuberculosis mediates inefficient implementation of cell-mediated protective immunity.

1. Introduction

Drug-resistant pulmonary tuberculosis (DR-TB) is a case of tuberculosis caused by *M. tuberculosis* strains (MBTs) which are drug resistant to the effect of antituberculosis drugs (ATDs). It is supposed that drug-resistance (DR) is, above all, connected with accumulation of mutations in *M. tuberculosis* genes [1]. Multidrug-resistant tuberculosis (MDR-TB) is a special form of drug-resistant TB. It develops in case of resistance of *M. tuberculosis* at least to isoniazid and rifampicin—the two most powerful ATDs [2]. The problem of multidrug resistance of a tuberculosis causative agent to ATD in newly detected patients has lately gained global importance [3, 4]. According to the data of World Health Organization (2010), based on the information received from 114 countries around the world, primary MDR of MBT comprises about 4% from all newly detected TB cases, whereas on the territory of the CIS countries (Russia,

Belarus, Ukraine, Kazakhstan, Armenia, and Azerbaijan) this indicator is 3–6 times higher [2].

Increase in morbidity of cases with primary DR-TB in patients who earlier did not receive ATD is especially alarming [5, 6]. Primary DR-TB develops as a result of primary infection by drug-resistant *M. tuberculosis* strains. In some regions of Russia secondary (acquired) DR-TB to ATD among earlier treated patients reaches 88% [5, 7]. Besides, an unfavorable tendency towards the increase in specific gravity of polyresistance and the decrease in specific gravity of monoresistance to ATD is marked; that is, at present MDR-TB is encountered more frequently among TB patients than DR-TB [5, 6]. A serious problem is a rise in the number of cases of primary DR to the most active chemical drugs—isoniazid and rifampicin—which, in combination with resistance to other first-line ATD or without it, is classified as MDR-TB, whereas in combination with resistance to second-line drugs, including fluoroquinolones and one of the injectable drugs (such as kanamycin or capreomycin), it is classified as XDR-TB [3, 5].

Clinical treatment of patients with MDR-TB is 3 times less than of those with TB whose causative agent is sensitive to ATD, in other words, effectiveness of treatment of such patients, which is determined by the cease in bacterioexcretion, is 3 times lower in MDR-TB than in drug-resistant variants of the disease. Besides, the frequency of termination of selection of ATD-sensitive MBT in patients reaches 92,5%, whereas in cases of TB caused by resistant strains of the causative agent only 58,1% [5, 8]. Therefore, ATD-multiresistant MBT becomes the major component of TB morbidity and mortality, which poses a serious threat to the whole mankind [2–5].

It is obvious that the above-stated problem requires many-sided and integrated approaches to its solution, the main of which is studying of immunopathogenic processes accompanying the course of pulmonary tuberculosis. Nowadays it is commonly believed that the development and the progressive course of the tubercular infection are impossible without functional defects in the protective cell immunity system [9]. Enhanced proliferation and excessive activity of regulatory T cells, which tend to weaken the anti-infectious organism immunity, are at present viewed as one of the mechanisms of Th-1-dependent immune response suppression, aimed at elimination of pathogens of various nature [10–12]. From all the identified regulatory T cells (Treg) subpopulations, Treg, expressing intracellular transcription factor *Foxp3*, which is the most precise marker of regulatory T-lymphocyte identification, has today the most functional activity in the aspect of implementation of immunosuppressive mechanisms. It is worth mentioning that *Foxp3*-positive regulatory T cells can be both natural (formed in the course of antigen-dependent differentiation in the thymus) and induced in the periphery in the process of adaptive immune system [13, 14]. One of the major indicators of Treg functional activity is their suppression of proliferation of T-helper effector clones, which mediates T-cell anergy formation.

The Objective of the Work. To define the role of *Foxp3*-expressing regulatory T cells and T helpers in immunopathogenesis of multidrug-resistant pulmonary tuberculosis.

2. Materials and Methods

The diagnosis of pulmonary tuberculosis was put on the basis of the clinical picture of the disease as well as X-ray lungs examination and data of microscopic and bacteriological sputum tests. The causative agent of tuberculosis was detected by means of direct light microscopy of the sputum smear, with the use of Ziehl-Neelsen stain, by the method of fluorescence microscopy with the use of fluorochromes (auramine). For species identification of *M. tuberculosis* and definition of sensitivity to anti-TB chemodrugs (a method of absolute concentration), we conducted sputum culture on dense Lowenstein-Jensen and Finn-2 media.

2.1. Microbiological Research Methods. To determine drug resistance of *M. tuberculosis* to basic ATD (rifampicin (RIF), isoniazid (INH), streptomycin, and ethambutol), we used the traditional bacteriological method of absolute concentrations. To carry out microbiological tests, we collected sputum in sterile 50 mL plastic test tubes with hermetically sealed screw caps. After sputum decontamination and MTB concentrating, the washed MTB sediment was used for culture on dense Lowenstein-Jensen medium with further detection of MTB sensitivity to RIF, INH, streptomycin, and ethambutol using the bacteriological absolute concentration method.

Mononuclear cells of peripheral blood, which was taken in the quantity of 10 mL from the cubital vein on an empty stomach in the morning, before the course of specific antitubercular therapy, served as the material of the research. Mononuclear cells of peripheral blood were isolated by gradient centrifugation [15].

2.2. Isolation of Mononuclear Leucocytes from Whole Blood. Heparinized venous blood (25 units/mL) was kept at the temperature of 37°C for 30 min to separate plasma from erythrocytes. The obtained plasma was layered on Ficoll-urografin (ρ = 1077 g/cm^3) density gradient ("MP Biomedical, LLC", USA) in a 1 : 2 ratio and centrifuged at 1500 rev/min for 20 min. The resulting interphase ring consisting of a mixture of mononuclear cells was collected with a pipette and then thrice washed with RPMI-1640 medium ("Vektor," Russia), which was supplemented with 100 mkg/mL of gentamicin and 5% inactivated fetal calf serum ("BioloT LLC", Russia), being consistently resuspended and centrifuged once every 10 min at 1500 rev/min. When using the gradient with the above-stated density, 90–95% of all the isolated mononuclear cells were lymphocytes.

2.3. Determination of the Quantity of $CD4^+CD25^+Foxp3^+$, $CD4^+CD25^+FoxP3^-$, and $CD4^+CD25^-FoxP3$ Regulatory T Cells in Peripheral Blood. To define CD4, CD25 superficial receptors and *Foxp3* intracellular marker of immunosuppression activity in peripheral blood lymphocytes, we used the method of laser three-color cytometry with the use of fluorescently labeled multichannel antibodies (MCAB). Staining of superficial (CD4, CD25) and intracellular (*Foxp3*) markers was conducted according to the protocol of the manufacturing company ("Becton Dickinson (BD)," USA).

Course of Work. After isolation, the mononuclear leucocytes were twice washed with phosphate-saline buffer (pH = 7,4) the amount of cells in the suspension was standardized to 10×10^6 cells/mL. To stain superficial markers (CD4, CD25) of the peripheral blood leucocytes, 20 mcl of the corresponding fluorescently labeled MCAB was added to the suspension of mononuclear leucocytes: to CD4—FITC-labeled, to CD25—PE-Cy5-labeled ("Becton Dickinson (BD)", USA) and then incubated at room temperature for 20 min, while providing protection from light. To stain the intracellular marker *Foxp3* the process of cell permeabilization was conducted. For this we alternately added working solutions of standard buffers to every test tube: Human *FoxP3* Buffer A and Human *FoxP3* Buffer C from the set BD Pharmingen Human *FoxP3* Buffer Set Cat. No. 560098. The buffers were diluted according to the instruction (cat. No. 560098). Leucocytes have been incubated for 30 min in a dark place at room temperature. Then the cells were twice washed with 2 mL of phosphate-saline buffer (PH = 7,4). PE-labeled antibodies in the amount of 20 mcl were added in the resuspended sediment to the intracellular marker *Foxp3*. This solution has been incubated for 30 min in a dark place at room temperature. Then the cells were twice washed with 2 mL of phosphate saline buffer (PH = 7,4).

Measurements were carried out on a cytofluorimeter FACSCalibur (Becton Dickinson, USA), which has a laser with 488 nm wavelength as well as standard filters. The analysis of the obtained data was performed by means of a software application BD Cell CellQuest for Mac OS X.

2.4. Determination of the Amount of CD3$^+$CD4$^+$CD25$^-$ T Helpers in Peripheral Blood. To determine the level of expression of superficial receptors CD3, CD4, and CD25 in peripheral blood lymphocytes, we used the method of laser three-color flow cytometry with fluorescently labeled MCAB.

Staining of the markers CD3, CD4, and CD25 was conducted according to the protocol of the manufacturing company ("Becton Dickinson (BD)," USA).

The Course of Work. After isolation, mononuclear leucocytes were twice washed with phosphate saline buffer (pH = 7,4), every time having been resuspended and centrifuged for 10 min at 1500 rev/min. Then the supernatant was drained off, the remaining sediment was resuspended in phosphate-saline buffer, and the amount of cells was standardized in the suspension to 10×10^6 cells/mL. To stain lymphocytes, we added 50 mcl of the mononuclear leucocyte suspension and 20 mcl of conjugated MCAB-CD3 (PerCP-Cy5,5)/CD4 (FITC)/CD25 (PE) ("Becton Dickinson (BD)", USA, cat. No. 333170) to every cytometric test tube, mixed on vortex and incubated for 15 min in a dark place at room temperature.

Measurements were carried out on a cytometer FACSCalibur (Becton Dickinson, USA), which has an argon laser with 488 nm wavelength as well as standard filters. The analysis of the obtained data was conducted by means of a software application BD CellQuest for Mac OS X.

2.5. Statistical Processing of the Research Results. Analysis of the primary data was conducted using the methods of statistical description and verification of statistical hypotheses. All quantitative indicators were tested for normal distribution using Shapiro-Wilks test. For normally distributed samples, we calculated average sample characteristics: arithmetic average (X), mean square deviation (σ), and error of mean (m). For the samples which distribution differed from normal one we calculated median (M) as well as the first and the third quartiles (Q_1, Q_3).

When the feature in the researched samples corresponded with the normal law of distribution, verification of hypotheses about equality of average sample values was

conducted using unifactor variance analysis. To evaluate certainty of differences of the sample numerical characteristics which are not subject to normal distribution, we used the Kruskal-Wallis test. For pairwise comparison of indicators in the researched groups, we used the Mann-Whitney test for independent groups. The difference in indicators in the compared groups was considered statistically significant at the significant level $P \leq 0,05$. Calculations were performed using the program Statistica 6.0.

3. Results and Discussion

115 patients with advanced destructive forms of newly detected pulmonary tuberculosis (85 men and 30 women at the age of 18–55, average age 44 ± 12 years) have been examined. All patients were divided into 3 groups according to the clinical form of the disease: a group with infiltrative pulmonary tuberculosis (ITB) contained 65 people, with disseminated pulmonary tuberculosis (DTB) 31 people, with fibrous-cavernous pulmonary tuberculosis (FCTB) 19 people. When dividing the patients into groups, we took into account drug sensitivity of the causative agent to the basic ATD: the group of patients having MBT sensitive to basic ATD contained 68 people and the second group included 47 patients with MBT resistant to the first-line ATD (such as isoniazid, rifampicin, streptomycin, and ethambutol).

The control group included 26 healthy donors with similar sex and age characteristics (16 men and 10 women at the age of 18–55, average age 44 ± 12 years).

The carried-out research allowed us to conclude that the amount of T helpers in blood of TB patients is changing multidirectionally depending on the clinical form of the disease and sensitivity of *M. tuberculosis* to ATD. It has been revealed that the increase in the number of lymphocytes with immunophenotype CD3$^+$CD4$^+$CD25$^-$ (T-helpers) is registered in the group of ITB patients (in comparison with the group of healthy donors), whereas in the groups of disseminated and fibrous-cavernous TB patients the number of CD3$^+$CD4$^+$CD25$^-$ cells is decreasing (Table 1). Under TB with MDR-TB, the amount of T helpers is bigger in the group of ITB and DTB than in that of DS TB patients, whereas under FCTB the presence or absence of drug resistance of *M. tuberculosis* does not affect the amount of T helpers (Table 1).

It should be noticed that the above-stated subpopulation of T lymphocytes is heterogeneous and forms the general idea of the amount of T helpers in blood of TB patients. Initially it was thought that T helpers are differentiated into two stable subpopulations: T helpers (Th) Th1 and Th2, the characteristic feature of which is production of immunoregulatory cytokines, multidirectional in their spectrum of action [16]. However, the research carried out in recent years allowed us to determine that among CD-4-positive T lymphocytes there are other cells which have "helper" functions. In particular, it was demonstrated that among CD4$^+$ T lymphocytes there are Th17, Treg, and adaptive regulatory T cells: Th3, Tr1, and Foxp3$^+$ Treg, which are formed in the course of immune response, as well as Th-activated cells and recently identified follicular T-helpers

TABLE 1: Relative amount of T helpers ($CD3^+CD4^+CD25^-$) in peripheral blood of patients suffering from pulmonary tuberculosis, depending on the form of the disease and sensitivity of the causative agent to antitubercular drugs (%), Me (Q_1–Q_3).

Type of a researched patients	Relative amount of T helpers in the group	Relative amount of T helpers in the group depending on sensitivity of the causative agent to antitubercular drugs	
		DS TB	MDR TB
Healthy donors	35,38 (32,74–38,74)		
Patients with ITB	45,47 (43,07–47,82) $p_1 = 0,038$	38,20 (33,04–47,88)	54,41 (54,38–54,89) $p_1 = 0,042$ $p_4 = 0,036$
Patients with DTB	31,61 (29,33–34,41) $p_1 = 0,042$ $p_2 = 0,042$	23,90 (16,84–26,66) $p_1 = 0,043$ $p_2 = 0,041$	39,38 (24,57–48,75) $p_1 = 0,049$ $p_2 = 0,041$ $p_4 = 0,048$
Patients with FCTB	25,46 (21,38–32,86) $p_1 = 0,029$ $p_2 = 0,048$ $p_3 = 0,035$	24,4 (22,38–25,35) $p_1 = 0,037$ $p_2 = 0,045$	26,0 (21,20–28,70) $p_1 = 0,041$ $p_2 = 0,028$ $p_3 = 0,039$

Note: p_1: the level of statistical significance of differences in comparison with the group of healthy donors; p_2: in ITB patients; p_3: in DTB patients; p_4: in DS TB patients.

(T_{FH}), whose function presumably lies in protection from extracellular pathogens [13, 17]. A peculiar feature of specific immune response under ITB is relatively adequate realization of Th1-dependent inflammatory response, the effector cells of which are $CD4^+$ T lymphocytes. In connection with this, the increase in the number of $CD4^+$ T-cells under ITB is viewed as a logical fact. At the same time the above-shown decrease in the total amount of T-helpers in blood of DTB and FCTB patients is the evidence of inhibition of clonal proliferation of $CD4^+$ T cells (Table 1).

As for the patients with infiltrative and disseminated MDR TB, where the biggest amount of T helpers was detected in comparison with DS TB and healthy donors, is it likely that drug-resistant strains of MBT do not have a pathological effect on the process of T lymphocyte differentiation and proliferation under acute and subacute MDR TB, which include ITB and DTB? Nevertheless, to answer this question, further more profound studying of the subpopulation composition of T-helpers in TB patients is necessary.

As is known, natural Treg cells with the phenotype $CD4^+CD25^+Foxp3^+$ and adaptive regulatory $CD4^+CD25^-Foxp3^+$ T-lymphocytes are key suppressor cells of the immune response [13, 14]. The analysis of the amount of Foxp3-expressing regulatory T cells has shown that in all TB patients, irrespective of the clinical form of the disease, the increase in the number of $CD4^+CD25^+Foxp3^+$ Treg is defined in comparison with the group of healthy donors, whereas the number of CD25-negative regulatory T cells, containing the Foxp3 molecule, is rising only in

FCTB patients (Table 2). In Figures 1, 2, 3, and 4 Treg cells with the phenotype $CD4^+CD25^+Foxp3^+$ are localized in the right upper quadrants and $CD4^+CD25^-Foxp3^+$ cells in the left-upper quadrants.

This fact allows us to suggest that in the case of chronic destructive process in Treg-mediated specific immunosuppression, regulatory T cells, both natural as well as formed, are involved in the course of the adaptive immune response.

Tuberculosis, with the exception of acutely progressive forms, is considered to be "slow" infection, whose feature is long-flowing, but unfortunately, poor immune response against the background of abundance of a constantly persistent antigen. The previous studies we conducted have shown that dysregulation of cytokine production is met in patients with TB, and, in particular, the hypersecretion of immunoregulatory cytokines with suppressor activity (IFNγ, IL-4, IL-10, TGF-β) against the background of reduction of the secretion of IL-2 has been found out [18]. In this regard, as demonstrated in this study, the reduction in the number of T lymphocytes with the phenotype $CD4^+CD25^+Foxp3^-$ in all clinical forms of TB (Table 2) is more likely connected with imbalance of cytokine production with a predominance of secretion of immunosuppressive cytokines and, consequently, the inhibition of not only proliferation, but also differentiation of Th0 into activated antigenspecific Th1-lymphocytes. In Figures 1, 2, 3, and 4 the $CD4^+CD25^+Foxp3^-$ cells are localized in the right-lower quadrants. Interestingly, the fate of selection occurring in the thymus of Foxr3-negative $CD4^+CD25^+$ regulatory T cells by activation of endogenous (mitochondrial) apoptosis after

TABLE 2: Subpopulation composition of regulatory T cells of peripheral blood in patients suffering from pulmonary tuberculosis, depending on a clinical form of the disease (%), Me (Q_1–Q_3).

Groups of the researched patients	Relative content of regulatory T-cell subpopulations		
	$CD4^+CD25^+Foxp3^+$	$CD4^+CD25^-Foxp3^+$	$CD4^+CD25^+Foxp3^-$
Healthy donors	2,63	5,12	25,45
	(2,00–3,29)	(4,76–9,75)	(22,30–27,60)
ITB patients	4,48	6,95	17,52
	(3,10–6,00)	(5,50–11,20)	(9,400–22,60)
	$p_1 = 0,047$		$p_1 = 0,036$
DTB patients	5,35	6,30	13,50
	(3,75–7,14)	(5,50–8,00)	(8,400–17,20)
	$p_1 = 0,014$		$p_1 = 0,005$
			$p_2 = 0,026$
FCTB patients	4,80	8,50	19,50
	(3,20–6,00)	(4,20–11,50)	(13,400–24,30)
	$p_1 = 0,045$	$p_1 = 0,049$	$p_1 = 0,038$
			$p_2 = 0,047$
			$p_3 = 0,049$

Note: p_1: the level of statistical significance of differences in comparison with the group of healthy donors; p_2: in ITB patients; p_3: in DTB patients.

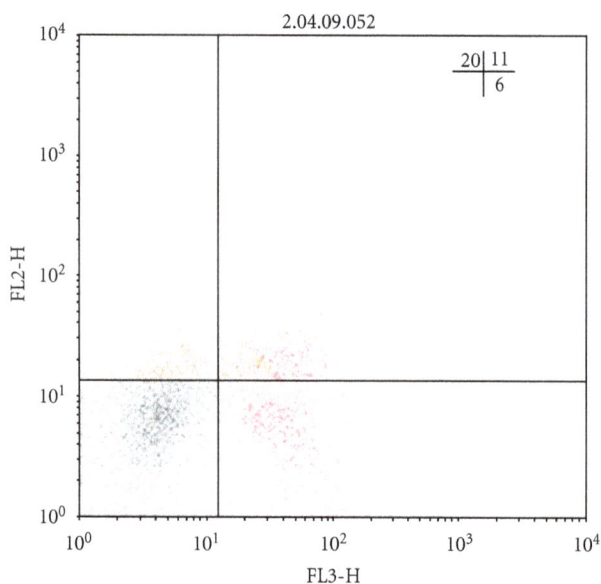

FIGURE 1: Individual bar chart of distribution of regulatory T cells in a population of CD4-positive blood lymphocytes, expressing CD25 and Foxp3, in a healthy person. Relative content of $CD4^+CD25^+Foxp3^+$ cells (upper-right quadrant) 3,02%, $CD4^+CD25^-Foxp3^+$ cells (upper-left quadrant)—6%, $CD4^+CD25^+Foxp3^-$ cells (lower-right quadrant)—26%.

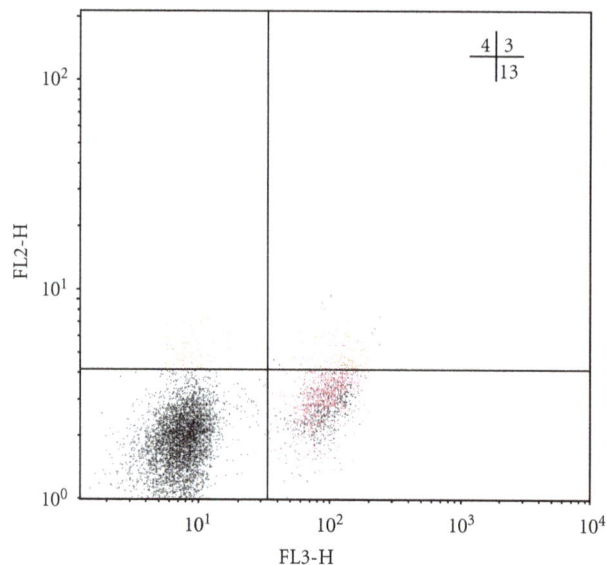

FIGURE 2: Individual bar chart of distribution of regulatory T cells in a population of CD4-positive lymphocytes of blood, expressing CD25 and Foxp3, in a patient with infiltrative pulmonary tuberculosis (patient N., 39 years old, diagnosed with infiltrative tuberculosis S_{1-2} of the right lung in a phase of decay and semination, MTB (+)). The relative abundance of $CD4^+CD25^{+hi}Foxp3^+$ cells (upper-right quadrant) is 5%, $CD4^+CD25^-Foxp3^+$ cells (upper-left quadrant) is 7%, $CD4^+CD25^+Foxp3^-$ cells (lower-right quadrant) is 13.5%.

their migration into the circulating blood and secondary lymphoid organs is further determined by different mechanisms of immune regulation, many of which are still not established [19, 20].

As our studies have shown, the number of $CD4^+CD25^+Foxp3^+$ Treg lymphocytes in the blood of patients with ITB and DTB, regardless of the drug sensitivity of the causative agent to anti-tuberculosis drugs before specific therapy, that is, in the acute phase of tuberculous infection, has been rising with respect to the number of $CD4^+CD25^+Foxp3^+$ Treg lymphocytes in healthy donors, as well as in general in the groups (Tables 2 and 3).

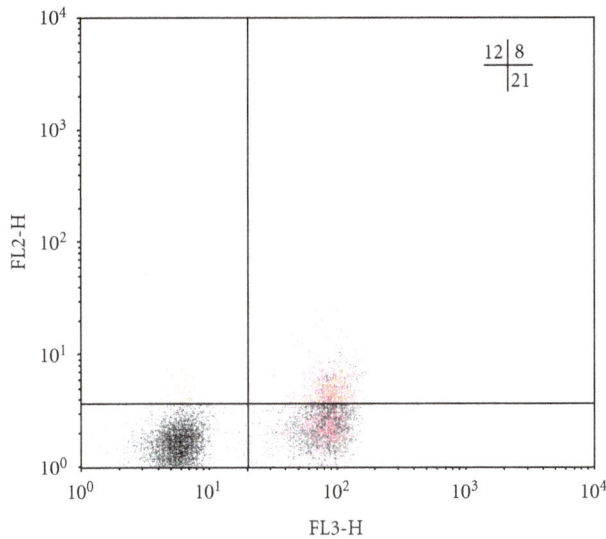

FIGURE 3: Individual bar chart of distribution of regulatory T cells in a population of CD4-positive lymphocytes of blood, expressing CD25 and Foxp3, in a patient with disseminated pulmonary tuberculosis (patient S., 28 years old, diagnosed with subacute disseminated pulmonary tuberculosis in the phase of infiltration and decay, MTB (+)). The relative content of CD4$^+$CD25^{+hi}Foxp3$^+$ cells (upper-right quadrant) is 8%, CD4$^+$CD25$^-$Foxp3$^+$ cells (upper-left quadrant) is 11,5%, CD4$^+$CD25$^+$Foxp3$^-$ cells (lower-right quadrant) is 23.3%.

FIGURE 4: Individual bar chart of distribution of regulatory T cells in a population of CD4-positive lymphocytes of blood, expressing CD25 and Foxp3, in a patient with fibrous-cavernous pulmonary tuberculosis (patient S., 53 years old, diagnosed with fibrous-cavernous tuberculosis of the upper lobe of the left lung in a phase of infiltration and semination, MTB (+)). The relative content of CD4$^+$CD25^{+hi}Foxp3$^+$ cells (upper-right quadrant) is 11%, CD4$^+$CD25$^-$Foxp3$^+$ cells (upper-left quadrant) is 13,5%, CD4$^+$CD25$^+$ Foxp3$^-$ cells (lower-right quadrant) is 25.3%.

A similar pattern was also observed in FCTB with MDR of the causative agent (Table 3).

In our opinion, such changes primarily contribute to the formation of suppression of Th1-response to prevent the development of hyperergic immune responses and damage of lung tissue. For example, in the studies of Raghvan and Holgren [21] and Lee et al., [10] the deterrent role of Treg in the development of intensive immune inflammation and immune pathology accompanying various infectious processes has been shown [21, 22].

However, in the long run, this, to some extent, compensatory reaction associated with increased proliferation and differentiation of Treg, leads to negative consequences in the form of weakening of the effectiveness of protective immunity, promoting generalization and chronicity of infection [23].

It is clear that increasing numbers of CD4$^+$CD25$^+$Foxp3$^+$ Treg in blood of patients with TB are an unfavorable factor. The main way of realization of the effect of Treg is through the implementation of triple-contact interaction, in which, together with Treg and target cells, the tolerogenic dendritic cells (TDCs) are involved [13, 24]. TDC and Treg have mutually activating properties, presumably by contacting "cell-to-cell." Perhaps, Treg prevents the formation of the immune synapse between TDC and effector T cell. It is assumed that the basis of this mechanism is competitive interaction of the negative activator CTLA-4 (cytotoxic T-lymphocyte antigen-1) with costimulatory molecules B7 (CD80/86) on the surface of target cells, promoting the formation of T-cell anergy [13].

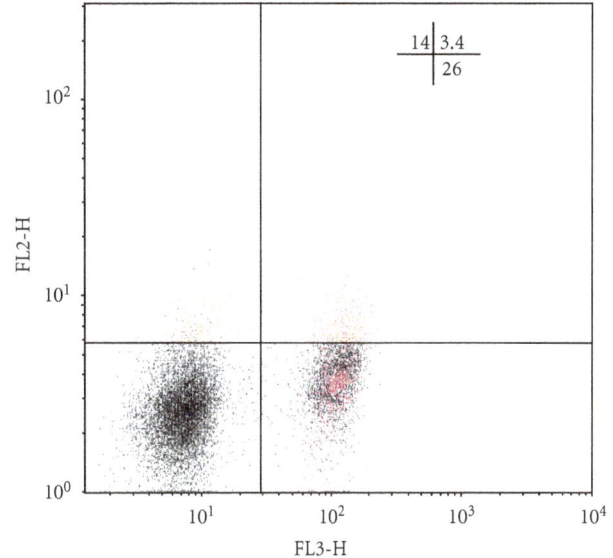

Thus, an increasing number of Treg in almost all clinical forms and variants of the TB course lets us suggest that they carry out major immunosuppressive function in tuberculosis infection.

It is known that Treg cells with the phenotype CD4$^+$ CD25$^+$Foxp3$^+$ "are trained" in the thymus at the stage of negative selection and leave the thymus as the population of natural Treg, which has maximum suppressor activity. At the same time it is shown that a subpopulation CD4$^+$CD25$^+$Foxp3$^+$ Treg is replenished in the peripheral section of immune system at the expense of their development from CD4$^+$CD25$^-$ T cells (the conversion of T-helpers into the regulatory T-cells) as a result of intercellular interactions with participation of costimulatory molecules with action of TGF-β and in the presence of TDC [13]. Conversion is a manifestation of the expression of the *Foxp3* molecule within a cell, as well as molecules CD25 and CTLA-4 on its surface [19]. In connection with the above-mentioned information, it is logical to assume that rather high number of adaptive regulatory T cells in the blood of patients with TB is caused not only by activation of intercellular interactions, but also by the enhanced production of cytokine-inductor Treg-TGF-β in pulmonary tuberculosis [18]. In addition, the source of CD4$^+$CD25$^+$Foxp3$^+$ T cells could also be CD4$^+$CD25$^-$Foxp3$^-$ T-helpers, which are differentiated in the thymus and which form a reserve pool for the formation of CD25$^+$ Treg lymphocytes [11, 24].

Table 3: Subpopulation composition of regulatory T cells of peripheral blood in patients suffering from pulmonary tuberculosis, depending on a clinical form of the disease and sensitivity of the causative to antituberculosis drugs (%), Me (Q_1–Q_3).

Groups of patients		Relative content of regulatory T-cell subpopulations		
		$CD4^+CD25^+Foxp3^+$	$CD4^+CD25^-Foxp3^+$	$CD4^+CD25^+Foxp3^-$
Healthy donors		2,63 (2,00–3,29)	5,12 (4,76–9,75)	25,45 (22,30–27,60)
ITB patients	DS TB	4,32 (4,12–8,25) $p_1 = 0,007$	5,81 (4,12–9,63)	9,72 (7,14–21,69) $p_1 = 0,003$
	MDR TB	5,08 (3,12–7,42) $p_1 = 0,039$	8,41 (5,62–11,58) $p_1 = 0,005$ $p_4 = 0,037$	16,27 (9,13–25,92) $p_1 = 0,048$ $p_4 = 0,017$
DTB patients	DS TB	5,31 (2,84–9,48) $p_1 = 0,015$	5,63 (3,79–8,47)	13,71 (9,64–17,08) $p_1 = 0,006$
	MDR TB	4,42 (3,17–7,53) $p_1 = 0,038$	6,75 (4,82–8,16)	13,98 (7,52–17,80) $p_1 = 0,006$
FCTB patients	DS TB	2,72 (2,09–3,66) $p_3 = 0,013$	3,25 (2,17–5,82) $p_2 = 0,014$	19,62 (11,31–31,75) $p_3 = 0,018$
	MDR TB	6,82 (3,17–10,42) $p_1 = 0,003$ $p_4 = 0,039$	12,27 (8,45–13,09) $p_1 = 0,017$ $p_4 = 0,015$	17,68 (12,42–23,19)

Note: p_1: the level of statistical significance of differences in comparison with features of healthy donors; p_2: in ITB patients; p_3: in DTB patients; p_4: in DS TB patients.

Regulatory T cells with the phenotype $CD4^+CD25^-Foxp3^+$ in the absence of expression on the surface of CD25 marker are considered to be induced, that is, generated on the periphery under the influence of TGF-β, as the expressions of the Foxr3 marker largely contribute to TGF-β among all the cytokines suppressors [9, 25]. We found the increase in the number of $CD4^+CD25^-Foxp3^+$ regulatory T cells in patients with MDR TB compared to drug-sensitive variant of the disease in ITB and FCTB patients (Table 3).

Perhaps this could be induced by the mycobacteria themselves. Thus, Sahno et al. [26] suggested that the strains of mycobacteria, resistant to standard chemotherapy, have special properties with respect to induction of $CD4^+CD25^{+hi}$ regulatory T cells with suppressor activity [26]. Thus, we cannot exclude the fact that in MDR TB, on the one hand, the activation of mechanisms of immunosuppression takes place due to both natural and adaptive regulatory T cells, and on the other hand, the drug-resistant strains of the MBT may contribute to suppression of immune response by means of induction of Treg.

As for the role of Treg in immunopathogenesis of drug-resistant TB, in this case it is difficult to underestimate it from the point of formation of the suppressor regime of immunoregulation in pulmonary TB in general. From this point of view the increase in the number of Treg at the periphery among patients with drug-resistant TB is also considered as a prognostically unfavourable factor leading to prolonged course of the disease as well as immunological discredit of the patient.

It is known that the main target cells of the influence of Treg are the activated $CD4^+$ and $CD8^+$ T cells, the key effector cells of antituberculosis immunity. Naive T cells are more sensitive to Treg than Th1 and Th2 lymphocytes [27, 28]. The identified reduced content of T lymphocytes with immunophenotype $CD4^+CD25^+$, which do not express the transcription factor Foxr3, in patients with TB, regardless of clinical forms of the disease and with no association with drug sensitivity of the MBT to anti-tuberculosis drugs, in comparison with the group of healthy donors (Tables 2 and 3), can probably be determined by the inhibition of proliferation and differentiation of T helpers, as well as by the influence of regulatory Foxp3$^+$ T-cells with suppressor activity and which could affect the $CD4^+$ and $CD8^+$ T-lymphocytes by direct contact "cell-to-cell."

At the same time, the reduction of $CD4^+CD25^+Foxp3^-$ T lymphocytes in peripheral blood under TB can be considered as manifestation of T cell immunodeficiency associated with either the initial disintegration of the immune system in patients with TB, or with the formation of immune deficiency against the background of the spreading TB infection.

As mentioned above, *Foxp3*-negative T cells may be of thymic origin, as well as generated at the periphery. In addition, this subpopulation of lymphocytes is heterogeneous and, along with regulatory T cells, involves activated T helpers. Thus, we can assume that the decrease in the number of T lymphocytes with the phenotype CD4$^+$CD25$^+$Foxp3$^-$ in blood in FCTB is determined by the deficiency of activated T helpers.

It is known, that in case Treg come into action by contact-dependent way towards the CD4$^+$-cells, the target cells themselves gain suppressor functions: they gain the ability to secrete cytokines inhibitors, thus, inhibiting the proliferative and secretory activity of the secondary targets [29, 30]. In light of the shown changes and given the data from literature, it is obvious that the maintenance of the effective immune response in such a situation becomes impossible, which will inevitably lead to an unfavorable clinical course of TB.

4. Summary

(1) The mechanism of immunologic deficiency, accompanying the course of pulmonary tuberculosis, is associated with the increase of *Foxp3*-expressing regulatory T cells with suppressor activity in blood, and is associated with the reduction in the number of CD4$^+$CD25$^+$Foxp3$^-$ T lymphocytes (*Foxp3*-negative regulatory T cells and activated T helpers).

(2) Imbalance of subpopulation composition of *Foxp3*-expressing regulatory T cells in patients with different clinical forms of multiple drug-resistant pulmonary tuberculosis is determined by higher content of CD4$^+$CD25$^+$Foxp3$^+$ Treg in blood in the case of DTB and is combined with the increase in the number of CD4$^+$CD25$^-$Foxp3$^+$ adaptive regulatory T cells in the case of ITB and FCTB.

(3) In patients with ITB, including multidrug-resistant *M. tuberculosis*, an increased number of CD3$^+$ CD4$^+$CD25$^-$ T helpers is determined by the pathogenic features of the development of the tuberculosis infection and is connected with the activation of Th1-dependent immune response. Reduction in the number of T helpers in the blood of patients with DTB and FCTB mediates inefficient implementation of cell-mediated protective immunity.

References

[1] O. A. Manicheva, E. B. Lasunskya, V. Y. Zhuravlev et al., "Drug sensitivity of *Mycobacteria tuberculosis* in contrast to their viability, citotoxicity, genotype and flow of the disease in respiratory tuberculosis patients," *Problems of Tuberculosis and Lung Diseases*, vol. 12, pp. 18–21, 2008.

[2] "Multidrug and extensively drug-resistant TB (M/XDR-TB): 2010 global report on surveillance and response," WHO Global Report, 2010, 71 c.

[3] J. A. Caminero, "Multidrug-resistant tuberculosis: epidemiology, risk factors and case finding," *International Journal of*

Tuberculosis and Lung Disease, vol. 14, no. 4, pp. 382–390, 2010.

[4] A. Wright, M. Zignol, A. Van Deun et al., "Epidemiology of antituberculosis drug resistance 2002–07: an updated analysis of the global project on anti-tuberculosis drug resistance surveillance," *The Lancet*, vol. 373, no. 9678, pp. 1861–1873, 2009.

[5] O. V. Filinyuk, *Risl factors associated with multidrug-resistant tuberculosis*, Ph.D.dissertation, Novosibirsk, Russia, 2011.

[6] I. P. Zinovyev, N. A. Esaulova, V. G. Novikova et al., "Primary drug resistance of *M. Tuberculosis* in patients with newly detected destructive pulmonary tuberculosis," *Problems of Tuberculosis and Lung Diseases*, vol. 4, pp. 37–39, 2009.

[7] Y. Balabanova, M. Radi, K. Gram et al., "Analysis of risk factors of emergence of drug resistance in tuberculosis patients living in civil and penitentiary sectors in Samara region in Russia," *Problems of Tuberculosis and Lung Diseases*, vol. 5, pp. 25–31, 2005.

[8] V. Y. Mishin, V. I. Chukanov, Y. Grigoryev et al., *Pulmonary Tuberculosis with Drug Resistance of the Causative Agent.M*, Geotar-Media, 2009.

[9] A. S. Simbirtsev, *Interleukin-1. Physiology. Pathology. Clinic*, Foliant, 2011.

[10] D. C. Lee, J. A. Harker, J. S. Tregoning et al., "CD25$^+$ natural regulatory T cells are critical in limiting innate and adaptive immunity and resolving disease following respiratory syncytial virus infection," *Journal of Virology*, vol. 84, no. 17, pp. 8790–8798, 2010.

[11] G. Darrasse-Jèze, S. Deroubaix, H. Mouquet et al., "Feedback control of regulatory T cell homeostasis by dendritic cells in vivo," *The Journal of Experimental Medicine*, vol. 206, no. 4, pp. 741–750, 2009.

[12] K. S. Lee, N. Bosco, B. Malissen, R. Ceredig, and A. Rolink, "Expansion of peripheral naturally occurring T regulatory cells by Fms-like tyrosine kinase 3 ligand treatment," *Blood*, vol. 113, no. 25, pp. 6277–6287, 2009.

[13] R. M. Haitov, A. A. Yarilin, and B. V. Pinegin, *Immunology*, Geotar-Media, 2011.

[14] S. V. Haidukov and A. V. Zurochka, "Cytometric analysis of subpopulations of T-helpers (Th1, Th2, Treg, Th17, T-helpers activated," *Medical Immunology*, vol. 13, no. 1, pp. 7–16, 2011.

[15] A. Böyum, "Separation of leukocytes from blood and bone marrow," *Scandinavian Journal of Clinical and Laboratory Investigation, Supplement*, vol. 21, pp. 1–9, 1968.

[16] K. Nagata, K. Tanaka, K. Ogawa et al., "Selective expression of a novel surface molecule by human Th2 cells in vivo," *Journal of Immunology*, vol. 162, no. 3, pp. 1278–1286, 1999.

[17] S.A. Ketlinskiy, "Th17 as a new line of differentiation of T-helpers: data review," *Cytokines and Inflammation*, vol. 8, no. 2, pp. 3–15, 2009.

[18] E. G. Churina, O. I. Urazova, V. V. Novitskiy et al., "Peculiarities of secretion of pro- and anti-inflammatory cytokines in vitro in tuberculin-negative patients with various clinical forms of pulmonary tuberculosis," *Pulmonology*, vol. 5, pp. 46–50, 2010.

[19] D. Male, G. Brostoff, D. B. Rott et al., *Immunology*, Logosfera, 2007.

[20] C. Mottet and D. Golshayan, "CD4$^+$CD25$^+$Foxp3$^+$ regulatory T cells: from basic research to potential therapeutic use," *Swiss Medical Weekly*, vol. 137, no. 45-46, pp. 625–634, 2007.

[21] S. Raghvan and J. Holgren, "CD4$^+$CD25$^+$ suppressor T cells regulate pathogen induced inflammation and disease," *FEMS Immunology and Medical Microbiology*, vol. 44, pp. 121–127, 2005.

[22] K. E. Webster, S. Walters, R. E. Kohler et al., "In vivo expansion of t reg cells with il-2-mab complexes: induction of resistance to eae and long-term acceptance of islet allografts without immunosuppression," *Journal of Experimental Medicine*, vol. 206, no. 4, pp. 751–760, 2009.

[23] D. A. Vignali, L. W. Collison, and C. J. Workman, "How regulatory T cells work," *Nature Reviews Immunology*, vol. 8, no. 7, pp. 523–532, 2008.

[24] S. Klein, C. C. Kretz, V. Ruland et al., "Reduction of regulatory T cells in skin lesions but not in peripheral blood of patients with systemic scleroderma," *Annals of the Rheumatic Diseases*, vol. 70, no. 8, pp. 1475–1481, 2011.

[25] S. M. Pop, C. P. Wong, D. A. Culton, S. H. Clarke, and R. Tisch, "Single cell analysis shows decreasing FoxP3 and TGFβ1 coexpressing CD4$^+$CD25$^+$ regulatory T cells during autoimmune diabetes," *Journal of Experimental Medicine*, vol. 201, no. 8, pp. 1333–1346, 2005.

[26] L.V. Sahno, M. A. Tikhonova, E. V. Kurganova et al., "T-cell anergy in pathogenesis of immune insufficiency under pulmonary tuberculosis," *Problems of Tuberculosis and Lung Diseases*, vol. 11, pp. 23–28, 2004.

[27] S. Sakaguchi, T. Yamaguchi, T. Nomura, and M. Ono, "Regulatory T cells and immune tolerance," *Cell*, vol. 133, no. 5, pp. 775–787, 2008.

[28] D. Dieckmann, H. Plöttner, S. Dotterweich, and G. Schuler, "Activated CD4$^+$ CD25$^+$ T cells suppress antigen-specific CD4$^+$ and CD8$^+$ T cells but induce a suppressive phenotype only in CD4$^+$ T cells," *Immunology*, vol. 115, no. 3, pp. 305–314, 2005.

[29] L. Pace, C. Pioli, and G. Doria, "IL-4 modulation of CD4$^+$CD25$^+$ T regulatory cell-mediated suppression," *Journal of Immunology*, vol. 174, no. 12, pp. 7645–7653, 2005.

[30] S. Fichtner-Feigl, W. Strober, K. Kawakami, R. K. Puri, and A. Kitani, "IL-13 signaling through the IL-13α2 receptor is involved in induction of TGF-β1 production and fibrosis," *Nature Medicine*, vol. 12, no. 1, pp. 99–106, 2006.

27

Prognostic Factors in Tuberculosis Related Mortalities in Hospitalized Patients

Ghazal Haque, Ashok Kumar, Fatima Saifuddin, Shafaq Ismail, Nadeem Rizvi, Shaista Ghazal, and Sadhna Notani

Department of Chest Medicine, Jinnah Postgraduate Medical Centre, Rafiqui H J Shaheed Road, Karachi 75510, Pakistan

Correspondence should be addressed to Ashok Kumar; ashoka_pj@yahoo.com

Academic Editor: José R. Lapa e Silva

Setting. The study was undertaken at the Department of Pulmonology at a public, tertiary care centre in Karachi, Pakistan. *Objectives.* To evaluate factors concerned with in-hospital deaths in patients admitted with pulmonary tuberculosis (TB). *Design.* A retrospective case-control audit was performed for 120 patients hospitalised with pulmonary TB. Sixty of those discharged after treatment were compared to sixty who did not survive. Radiological findings, clinical indicators, and laboratory values were compared between the two groups to identify factors related to poor prognosis. *Results.* Factors concerned with in-hospital mortality listed late presentation of disease ($P < 0.01$), noncompliance to antituberculosis therapy ($P < 0.01$), smoking ($P < 0.01$), longer duration of illness prior to treatment ($P < 0.01$), and low body weight ($P < 0.01$). Most deaths occurred during the first week of admission ($P < 0.01$) indicating late referrals as significant. Immunocompromised status and multi-drug resistance were not implicated in higher mortality. *Conclusions.* Poor prognosis was associated with noncompliance to therapy resulting in longer duration of illness, late patient referrals to care centres, and development of complications. Early diagnosis, timely referrals, and monitored compliance may help reduce mortality. Adherence to a more radically effective treatment regimen is required to eliminate TB early during disease onset.

1. Introduction

Tuberculosis (TB) has been a declared worldwide health emergency since the last two decades. With an estimated 9 million new cases and 1.4 million deaths occurring annually, TB still stands to be a major global health risk despite rigorous efforts to contain its spread and implementation of effective treatment strategies [1].

Worldwide, Pakistan stands among the 22 countries that are most affected by TB. As of 2011, with an estimated population of 177 million, there were approximately 400,000 incident TB cases annually with about 59,000 deaths [2]. Every year, 15,000 new multi-drug resistant (MDR; resistant to isoniazid and rifampicin; first-line drugs) TB cases are reported in the country and an unprecedented number of cases remain unreported. Despite the availability of effective treatment regimens and clear regulations for their placement, active TB and its complications are a common cause of hospital admissions and TB related fatalities continue to persist. The reasons for these are widely distributed. While immunocompromised conditions [3, 4], disseminated disease [5], and environmental factors such as poor living and work conditions [6] are considered significant parameters, undernourishment [7] and anaemic [8] status, constant exposure to infected individuals, and disruption in treatment [9, 10] are also implicated.

To assess the factors associated with mortality, a holistic study is required to the weighing in all aspects of patient demographic, disease progression, treatment practices, and clinical and laboratory indicators. A retrospective case control study was carried out with patient data from February 2009 to March 2010 to analyse the implications of these elements on inpatient mortality.

2. Methods

The study was conducted at the department of Chest Medicine of the Jinnah Postgraduate Medical Centre (JPMC)

in Karachi, Pakistan; a 1800-bed, public, tertiary care centre hosting 16 specialist facilities and 5 Intensive Care Units, admitting patients through outpatient clinics, and referrals. Patients included those with active TB in various treatment categories; requiring extensive treatment for complications of TB, multi-drug resistance, and TB with associated diseases.

A retrospective case control study was carried out on patients admitted to the hospital between February 2009 and March 2010 who were diagnosed with TB or its complications (Table 1). Patients' data were compared between two groups of 60 patients each: case patients who expired during hospitalization and controls who were discharged from the centre following treatment. Data were anonymously collected on a uniform, standardized questionnaire from filed records of patients who fulfilled the inclusion criteria. The hospital receives patients referred by primary and secondary care facilities from throughout the country, usually in advanced disease stages or with severe comorbid conditions; hence it was difficult to obtain follow up data on 68.3% controls who were unreachable after treatment. Compared cases and controls included those admitted to the centre in the same month of the year, with a positive diagnosis for TB, thus attempting to minimise bias since demographic, clinical, radiological, and other parameters were compared for their role in mortality. Inpatient records were examined for age and sex variations, clinical history and examination, chest radiographs obtained at the time of admission, and the subsequent treatment provided while hospitalised. The diagnosis for TB was made based on an initial evaluation by the admitting doctor and supported with clinical indicators for active TB in the history and examination: chronic (over months), persistent lowgrade fever with night sweats, productive cough resistant to antibiotic treatment, and weight loss and anorexia. Posteroanterior chest radiographs were studied to ascertain region of lung involvement and areas showing evidence of infiltration; cavitations or fibrosis was accounted as zones of involvement. Sputum smears tested for acid-fast bacilli (AFB) on Ziehl-Neelsen (ZN) stain and sputum cultures were used for confirmation wherever performed. Documentary proof of smears and cultures from a majority of the case patients was unavailable due to absent records and inadequate time between admission and death to perform fresh tests. However, evidence of previous ATT administration (complete or incomplete) was considered confirmatory for TB in such patients. Sputum cultures were received with all established cases of MDR-TB. TB was confirmed after a final assessment for the presence of one or more satisfactory diagnostic parameters by the resident postgraduate doctor.

Since the study was conducted at a dedicated pulmonology ward, cases of uniquely extrapulmonary TB were not available for inclusion. However, pulmonary TB cases that also exhibited extrapulmonary manifestations were discerned for significance. Further data recovered from patient files included duration of symptoms, comorbidities, history of TB contact and infection, smoking, disease and treatment status, weight at the time of admission, electrolyte and renal function panel, complete blood count, and blood gases.

TABLE 1: Diagnostic, inclusion, and exclusion criteria for cases and controls*.

Parameters for TB diagnosis
Positive sputum smear and/or culture for AFB
CXR with evidence of cavitations, infiltration, and/or fibrosis
Clinical indicators of TB, chronic persistent: low-grade fever with night sweats, productive cough, weight loss, and anorexia
Inclusion criteria
Fulfilling two or more diagnostic parameters for pulmonary TB
Patients admitted within the same month of the year
Exclusion criteria
No clear evidence of active pulmonary TB
Exclusively extrapulmonary TB
Cause of death other than TB (for cases)

*TB: tuberculosis; AFB: acid-fast bacilli; CXR: chest X-ray.

It was difficult to obtain accurate histories of past TB infection and/or treatment due to unreliable patient accounts, improper documentation, and patient illiteracy. However, patients having received ATT with positive smears any time in the past were considered positive for a history of TB.

Those requiring category I ATT (new patients) were placed on a standard daily treatment [11] of isoniazid, rifampicin, pyrazinamide, and ethambutol for a two-month initial phase followed by a four-month continuation phase with isoniazid and rifampicin, while category II ATT (relapse or treatment default) added streptomycin to the initial phase and a five-month continuation phase with the addition of ethambutol. Patients with known drug resistances (category I failure or MDR-TB) were treated according to the reported drug sensitivity. Wherever possible, laboratory testing was performed via standardized procedures at the local lab conforming to ISO 9001:2008 certification.

Data collected were analyzed using PASW Statistics version 16. Categorical values were compared between cases and controls for risk estimation and odds ratios were reported with 95% confidence interval. Continuous values from laboratory data were analyzed through independent t-tests. A P value of <0.05 was considered significant.

3. Results

A total of 120 admitted patients who were diagnosed with TB were compared with each other: 60 case patients who did not survive hospitalization and 60 controls who were discharged after treatment (Table 2). Overall, there were 52 women (43.3%) and 68 men (56.6%). The male to female ratio was 1.14 : 1 and 1.5 : 1 among cases and controls, respectively, ($P = 0.46$). The mean age for controls was 32.9 years and 47 years for cases ($P < 0.01$). Most deaths occurred in the >40 age group with 35 fatalities of the 51 (68.6%, $P < 0.01$). On- admission body weights presented a mean of 48.8 kg for controls and 36.8 kg for cases ($P < 0.01$).

A past history of TB was found in 19 (31.6%) controls and 32 (53.3%) cases; 38 (63.3%) controls and 21 (35%) cases were primary diagnoses, while 3 controls and 7 cases could not

TABLE 2: Patient particulars on admission with odds ratio[*].

Factor	Cases	Controls	P	OR (95% CI)
Female sex, N (%)	28 (46.6)	24 (40)	0.46	0.76 (0.36–1.57)
Age, mean years (range)	47 (14–95)	32.97 (15–75)	0.04	n/a
Weight, mean kg (range)	36.82 (28–65)	48.83 (25–81)	<0.01	n/a
Smokers, N (%)	32 (53.3)	11 (18.3)	<0.01	0.19 (0.08–0.44)
Past TB history, N(%)	32 (53.3)	19 (31.6)	0.04	0.32 (0.15–0.71)
Pulmonary TB, N (%)	39 (65)	16 (26.6)	<0.01	0.19 (0.09–0.42)
Bilateral lung involvement, N (%)	31 (51.6)	7 (11.6)	<0.01	8.09 (3.17–20.6)
Not taking ATT, N (%)	48 (80)	04 (6.6)	<0.01	56 (16.9–185.0)
Smear positive, N	15/25	39/56	<0.01	n/a
HIV positive, N (%)	1/54	00	0.02	n/a
TLC $\times 10^9$/L, mean	12.91	8.27	<0.01	n/a
Neutrophils, mean %	82.60	77.07	0.02	n/a
Lymphocytes, mean %	12.49	18.27	<0.01	n/a
Serum protein U/L, mean	5.01	6.48	<0.01	n/a

[*] OR: odds ratio; CI: confidence interval; TB: tuberculosis; ATT: anti-tuberculosis treatment; HIV: human immunodeficiency virus; TLC: total leukocyte count; n/a: not applicable.

provide the information ($P < 0.01$). History of close contact with a TB patient was reported in 18 (30%) patients from each group, while 42 (60%) controls and 28 (46.6%) case patients had no such contact. Data were unavailable for 14 of the case patients ($P < 0.01$).

Bilateral lung disease emerged as a significant factor, 31 cases (51.6%) showed bilateral disease and unilateral lung involvement was seen in 53 controls (88.3%, $P < 0.01$).

Sputum smears were positive for AFB in 39 (65%) controls, 17 (25%) tested negative, and smears were unavailable for 4 controls. Smears were reported on only 25 case patients out of which 15 were AFB-positive. MDR-TB was reported in 4 controls and 8 cases ($P < 0.01$). On admission, 56 (82.4%) controls and only 12 (17.6%) cases were taking ATT ($P < 0.01$). These included 46 controls and 6 cases on category I, 6 controls and 1 case on category II, and 4 controls and 5 cases were on MDR treatment ($P < 0.01$) [11].

Pulmonary TB limited to lung parenchyma was present in 39 (65%) case patients and only 16 (26.6%) controls. Both pulmonary and extrapulmonary TB were found in 44 (73.3%) controls and 21 (35%) cases ($P < 0.01$). Complications of TB were seen on admission in some patients including high risk factors such as type II respiratory failure, pulmonary fibrosis, and dissemination (Table 3). Other recorded conditions included systemic arterial hypertension (12 cases and 5 controls) and diabetes (8 cases and 3 controls). Two patients had asthma, 3 had COPD, 2 had hepatitis C, and 1 had carcinoma of the lung; all of these were case patients. Save for 6 case patients, test for human immunodeficiency virus (HIV) was performed on all participants and only 1 case patient tested positive ($P = 0.02$).

A positive history of tobacco use was found in 11 (18.3%) controls and 32 (53.3%) cases ($P < 0.01$). Mean pack years for controls were 4.5 and 13.9 for cases ($P < 0.01$). A large number of smokers (60.5%) contracted pulmonary TB alone while 62.3% (48 of 77) of nonsmokers had both pulmonary and extrapulmonary TB ($P = 0.01$). Passive smoking was

TABLE 3: Complications and variations of TB, N (%).

	Cases	Controls	P^*
Complication of TB			
Type II respiratory failure	18 (30)	1 (1.6)	<0.01
Pulmonary fibrosis	19 (31.6)	8 (13.3)	0.01
Disseminated TB	11 (18.3)	3 (5)	0.02
Post-TB bronchiectasis	12 (20)	7 (11.6)	0.21
Variation of TB			
Pleural effusion	9 (15)	27 (45)	<0.01
Hydropneumothorax	2 (3.3)	12 (20)	<0.01
Miliary TB	1 (1.6)	3 (5)	<0.01
Empyema	1 (1.6)	2 (3.3)	<0.01
Lymph node TB	1 (1.6)	0 (0)	<0.01
Multiple sites	7 (11.6)	0 (0)	<0.01

[*] P value for variations of TB is within observed instances of extrapulmonary TB.

reported in 18 (30%) controls and 44 (73.3%) cases and was associated with high mortality ($P < 0.01$). A comparative profile of smokers and nonsmokers is given (Table 4).

The mean duration of symptoms among controls was 19 months and for cases was 5 years ($P < 0.01$). Shorter duration of symptoms before admission was associated with better chances of survival. In the group of patients with less than 6 months duration of symptoms, 37 of 53 (69.8%) survived treatment ($P < 0.01$).

A majority of deaths (78.3% of cases) occurred in the first week ($P < 0.01$), indicating that most patients reached the centre at terminal stages of disease (Figure 1). Mean hospital stay for controls was 17.73 days (range 3–74 days) while that for case patients was 5.83 days (range 0–29 days, $P < 0.01$).

At the time of admission raised leukocytes, neutrophilia, lymphocytopaenia, and low serum protein were found significantly related to mortality (Table 1).

TABLE 4: Patient profile: smokers versus nonsmokers*.

Feature	Smoker	Nonsmoker	P	OR (95% CI)
Patients, N (%)	43/120 (35.8)	77/120 (64.1)	<0.01	n/a
Cases, N (%)	32/43 (74.4)	28/77 (36.4)	<0.01	2.04 (1.45–2.88)
Controls, N (%)	11/43 (25.6)	49/77 (63.6)	<0.01	0.40 (0.23–0.68)
Age, mean years	48.49	35.23	<0.01	n/a
Weight, mean kg	41.74	43.43	0.46	n/a
Male sex, N (%)	34/43 (79.1)	34/77 (50)	<0.01	0.20 (0.08–0.49)
Bilateral lung involvement, N (%)	18/43 (41.9)	20/77 (26)	0.07	0.48 (0.22–1.07)
Pulmonary fibrosis, N (%)	12/43 (27.9)	15/77 (19.5)	0.28	1.60 (0.66–3.83)
Type II respiratory failure, N (%)	10/43 (23.3)	9/77 (11.7)	0.09	2.29 (0.84–6.17)
Duration of hospital stay, mean days	8.8	13.4	0.02	n/a
TLC $\times 10^9$/L, mean	11.7	9.9	0.12	n/a
Neutrophils, mean %	84.0	78.1	0.02	n/a
Serum protein U/L, mean	5.09	6.11	<0.01	n/a

*OR: odds ratio; CI: confidence interval; TLC: total leukocyte count; n/a: not applicable.

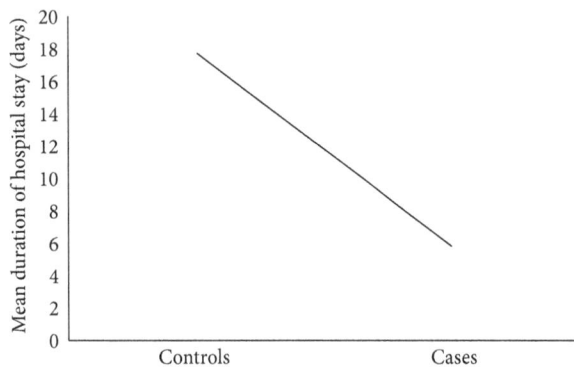

FIGURE 1: Relationship between mean number of hospitalization days and patient outcome.

4. Discussion

Tuberculosis stands as the second leading cause of death worldwide despite the enforcement of comprehensive prevention, detection, and treatment measures. Although the mortality rate of TB has reduced by 41% in the last two decades, many countries with a high burden of TB still have a long way to go in disease eradication [1]. Incidences of HIV coinfection [12], MDR-TB, and extensively drug-resistant TB (XDR-TB; resistance to at least isoniazid and rifampicin, any fluoroquinolone, and to injectable amikacin, capreomycin, or kanamycin) have raised concerns in many regional treatment strategies [13]. Pakistan ranks among countries with both a high burden of TB and MDR-TB and encounters a high mortality rate from TB [2]. Efforts have been made in the past to analyze the causes of high mortality in TB patients and for their poor prognosis [14–18], especially in hospitalized patients [12, 19, 20]. HIV and other immunocompromised status [21], MDR-TB [22], late referrals [23], and increased age of patients [24] have been implicated, but these factors

can vary regionally. Our research aimed to analyze these factors from a local perspective to examine the causes of poor prognosis in hospitalized TB patients in Karachi.

While studies [4–6, 12, 15–19, 21] from most countries have reported concomitant HIV to be an important factor in TB mortality, Pakistan fortunately escapes the list of countries with a high HIV burden and thus, it is not considered a major risk factor for high mortality with pulmonary TB [25, 26]. In the course of this study, HIV was detected in only one case patient and hence no significant association could be established.

Patients belonging to the >40-age group were more at risk compared to younger subjects. The combination of advanced age, deferred treatment, and frequent complications was a marker of poor prognosis. The male to female ratio was very slightly higher for cases. Low body weight was an important factor compounded by association with undernourishment and anaemia. Although no statistical significance resulted between mortality and low haemoglobin levels, clinical anaemia was observed in over half of the cases and under half of the controls. Moreover, a majority of the patients had lymphocytopenia and hypoproteinaemia, suggesting a generally malnourished, disease-susceptible patient outlook [7].

With a high burden environment for TB and scarce resources, sputum smears were observed when a clinical and radiological diagnosis was uncertain. Although nearly 3/4 of patients receiving ATT had positive smears, there was also a small number of retreated patients who had to be placed on category II treatment [27]. However, over 90% of those who were not taking ATT died. This can be accounted to illiteracy, low awareness regarding ATT, nonadherence to directly observed treatment (DOT) programmes, and low level of social support. Most patients hailed from low-income, rural settings and cited lack of infrastructural support as a reason for noncompliance [28]. MDR-TB has presented treatment challenges for countries with a high burden of MDR-TB [29]. We received 12 patients with established drug-resistant isolates on culture and only 4 of them survived. Notably, failure of getting followup exams and sputum smears likely results in a good number of relapse and MDR cases going undetected in our setting.

Poor record keeping and widespread reliance on nondigital filing systems presented difficulties in obtaining accurate treatment and disease histories and patient accounts were largely unreliable. However, nearly half of the patients in the study were new TB cases while a majority of the other half was cases of interrupted treatment or default. A surprisingly long duration of symptoms was seen in all the patients. This was attributed to the patients' neglect to report and seek medical assistance early on during the disease due to lack of awareness, resources, and social stigma. Long-established cultural practices among patients of visiting unqualified persons and quacks resulted in delayed detection and treatment [10].

Indigenous pulmonary TB and bilateral lung involvement were poor prognostic factors for hospitalized patients, usually associated with the development of complications. Conversely, patients with TB-involving sites other than the lung parenchyma fared better. Long-term complications of TB significantly raised the risk of mortality for inpatients [30, 31] at times requiring intensive care or ventilation support [32, 33]. Long-term sequelae of TB such as pulmonary fibrosis, type II respiratory failure, and disseminated disease were indicators of poor prognosis. Most deaths occurred within the first week of admission implicating late referrals and subsequent complications since these patients could not benefit from further treatment.

Various studies [34–36] have reported a strong association between tobacco use and increased risk of TB incidence and mortality. Passive smoking too is considered a health risk [37], yet Pakistan remains in the top five countries in the world with both a high burden of TB and tobacco usage. Our study revealed 75% mortality from TB among smokers. Moreover, these patients exhibited lower body weight, bilateral lung involvement, increased risk of infections, and developing life-threatening complications when compared to their nonsmoking counterparts.

5. Conclusions

The conclusions drawn from this study indicate delayed and interrupted treatment, failure to refer complications, nonadherence to treatment programmes, and tobacco usage as risk factors for increased TB mortality in hospitalized patients. We recommend stringent implementation of standardized treatment regimens [11] in tandem with local restrictions in their practice. Concrete statistical data on the incidence of these factors needs to be meticulously obtained to outline remedial lines of action. Awareness programmes and stricter regulations for TB and antitobacco use are pertinent to reduction in TB incidence. Simple corrective measures such as better record keeping, educating patients and caregivers regarding treatment, and creating awareness regarding TB and tobacco use can go a long way in preventing high mortality and curtailing this epidemic.

Authors' Contribution

The project was funded and supervised by Nadeem Rizvi, MB BS, MRCP, MCPS, and FRCP. Data collection was performed by Fatima Saifuddin, MB BS and MD; Ghazal Haque, MB BS; Shafaq Ismail, MB BS; and Sadhna Notani, MB BS. The final paper was prepared by Ghazal Haque and Ashok Kumar, MB BS.

Acknowledgments

Gratitude is due to Salman Bashir for his assistance with the data analysis and Ammara Abdul Majeed for her help.

References

[1] World Health Organization, *Global Tuberculosis Report 2012*, WHO/HTM/TB/2012.6, World Health Organization, Geneva, Switzerland, 2012.

[2] World Health Organization, *Global Tuberculosis Report 2012 Annex 2: Country Profiles*, WHO/HTM/TB/2012.6, World Health Organization, Geneva, Switzerland, 2012.

[3] World Health Organization, "TB/HIV facts 2012-13," http://www.who.int/hiv/topics/tb/tbhiv_facts_2013/en/index.html.

[4] L. E. Kivihya-Ndugga, J. J. Ochola, G. Otieno, L. N. Muthami, and S. Gathua, "Clinical and immunological markers in Kenyan pulmonary tuberculosis patients with and without HIV-1," *East African Medical Journal*, vol. 71, no. 6, pp. 373–375, 1994.

[5] N. T. Burton, A. Forson, M. N. Lurie, S. Kudzawu, E. Kwarteng, and A. Kwara, "Factors associated with mortality and default among patients with tuberculosis attending a teaching hospital clinic in Accra, Ghana," *Transactions of the Royal Society of Tropical Medicine and Hygiene*, vol. 105, no. 12, pp. 675–682, 2011.

[6] K. Lönnroth, E. Jaramillo, B. G. Williams, C. Dye, and M. Raviglione, "Drivers of tuberculosis epidemics: the role of risk factors and social determinants," *Social Science and Medicine*, vol. 68, no. 12, pp. 2240–2246, 2009.

[7] H.-J. Kim, C.-H. Lee, S. Shin et al., "The impact of nutritional deficit on mortality of in-patients with pulmonary tuberculosis," *International Journal of Tuberculosis and Lung Disease*, vol. 14, no. 1, pp. 79–85, 2010.

[8] S. Isanaka, S. Aboud, F. Mugusi et al., "Iron status predicts treatment failure and mortality in tuberculosis patients: a prospective cohort study from Dar es Salaam, Tanzania," *PLoS ONE*, vol. 7, no. 5, Article ID e37350, 2012.

[9] K. Kliiman and A. Altraja, "Predictors and mortality associated with treatment default in pulmonary tuberculosis," *International Journal of Tuberculosis and Lung Disease*, vol. 14, no. 4, pp. 454–463, 2010.

[10] A. Finlay, J. Lancaster, T. H. Holtz, K. Weyer, A. Miranda, and M. Van Der Walt, "Patient- and provider-level risk factors associated with default from tuberculosis treatment, South Africa, 2002: a case-control study," *BMC Public Health*, vol. 12, no. 1, article 56, 2012.

[11] World Health Organization, *Treatment of Tuberculosis: Guidelines—4th Edition. WHO Report 2010*, (WHO/HTM/TB/

2009.420), World Health Organization, Geneva, Switzerland, 2010.

[12] L. V. Sacks and S. Pendle, "Factors related to in-hospital deaths in patients with tuberculosis," *Archives of Internal Medicine*, vol. 158, no. 17, pp. 1916–1922, 1998.

[13] P. Glaziou, K. Floyd, E. L. Korenromp et al., "Lives saved by tuberculosis control and prospects for achieving the 2015 global target for reducing tuberculosis mortality," *Bulletin of the World Health Organization*, vol. 89, no. 8, pp. 573–582, 2011.

[14] E. W. Tiemersma, M. J. van der Werf, M. W. Borgdorff, B. G. Williams, and N. J. D. Nagelkerke, "Natural history of tuberculosis: duration and fatality of untreated pulmonary tuberculosis in HIV negative patients: a systematic review," *PLoS ONE*, vol. 6, no. 4, Article ID e17601, 2011.

[15] A. H. van't Hoog, J. Williamson, M. Sewe et al., "Risk factors for excess mortality and death in adults with tuberculosis in Western Kenya," *The International Journal of Tuberculosis and Lung Disease*, vol. 16, no. 12, pp. 1649–1656, 2012.

[16] C. J. Waitt and S. B. Squire, "A systematic review of risk factors for death in adults during and after tuberculosis treatment," *International Journal of Tuberculosis and Lung Disease*, vol. 15, no. 7, pp. 871–885, 2011.

[17] L. Selig, M. T. C. T. Belo, E. G. Teixeira et al., "The study of tuberculosis-attributed deaths as a tool for disease control planning in Rio de Janeiro, Brazil," *International Journal of Tuberculosis and Lung Disease*, vol. 7, no. 9, pp. 855–859, 2003.

[18] L. Selig, R. Guedes, A. Kritski et al., "Uses of tuberculosis mortality surveillance to identify programme errors and improve database reporting," *International Journal of Tuberculosis and Lung Disease*, vol. 13, no. 8, pp. 982–988, 2009.

[19] R. Alavi-Naini, A. Moghtaderi, M. Metanat, M. Mohammadi, and M. Zabetian, "Factors associated with mortality in tuberculosis patients.," *Journal of Research in Medical Sciences*, vol. 18, pp. 52–55, 2013.

[20] N. Horita, N. Miyazawa, T. Yoshiyama et al., "Development and validation of a tuberculosis prognostic score for smear-positive in-patients in Japan," *The International Journal of Tuberculosis and Lung Disease*, vol. 17, no. 1, pp. 54–60, 2013.

[21] P. Nahid, L. G. Jarlsberg, I. Rudoy et al., "Factors associated with mortality in patients with drug-susceptible pulmonary tuberculosis," *BMC Infectious Diseases*, vol. 11, article 1, 2011.

[22] P. R. Donald and P. D. Van Helden, "The global burden of tuberculosis—combating drug resistance in difficult times," *New England Journal of Medicine*, vol. 360, no. 23, pp. 2393–2395, 2009.

[23] Y.-C. Liu, H.-H. Lin, Y.-S. Chen et al., "Reduced health provider delay and tuberculosis mortality due to an improved hospital programme," *International Journal of Tuberculosis and Lung Disease*, vol. 14, no. 1, pp. 72–78, 2010.

[24] J.-Y. Feng, W.-J. Su, Y.-C. Chiu et al., "Initial presentations predict mortality in pulmonary tuberculosis patients—a prospective observational study," *PLoS ONE*, vol. 6, no. 9, Article ID e23715, 2011.

[25] Z. A. Syed, M. I. Khan, M. Aslam, and I. H. Taseer, "Frequency of HIV infection in patients of pulmonary tuberculosis and various cancers at Nishtar Hospital Multan," *Pakistan Journal of Medical Research*, vol. 42, no. 4, pp. 45–48, 2003.

[26] M. K. Chaudhry, Z. A. Syed, and M. Younus, "Prevalence of Human Immunodeficiency Virus infection in patients with pulmonary tuberculosis," *Pakistan Journal of Chest Medicine*, vol. 15, no. 3, p. 4, 2009.

[27] F. M. Marx, R. Dunbar, D. A. Enarson, and N. Beyers, "The rate of sputum smear-positive tuberculosis after treatment default in a high-burden setting: a retrospective cohort study," *PLoS ONE*, vol. 7, no. 9, Article ID e45724, 2013.

[28] C. N. Deivanayagam, "The challenges of tuberculosis," *The Indian Journal of Chest Diseases & Allied Sciences*, vol. 48, no. 4, pp. 245–247, 2006.

[29] E. Nathanson, P. Nunn, M. Uplekar et al., "MDR tuberculosis—critical steps for prevention and control," *New England Journal of Medicine*, vol. 363, no. 11, pp. 1050–1058, 2010.

[30] Y. J. Ryu, J. H. Lee, E.-M. Chun, J. H. Chang, and S. S. Shim, "Clinical outcomes and prognostic factors in patients with tuberculous destroyed lung," *International Journal of Tuberculosis and Lung Disease*, vol. 15, no. 2, pp. 246–250, 2011.

[31] H. Y. Kim, K.-S. Song, J. M. Goo, J. S. Lee, K. S. Lee, and T.-H. Lim, "Thoracic sequelae and complications of tuberculosis," *Radiographics*, vol. 21, no. 4, pp. 839–860, 2001.

[32] J.-R. Zahar, E. Azoulay, E. Klement et al., "Delayed treatment contributes to mortality in ICU patients with severe active pulmonary tuberculosis and acute respiratory failure," *Intensive Care Medicine*, vol. 27, no. 3, pp. 513–520, 2001.

[33] D. R. Silva, D. M. Menegotto, L. F. Schulz, M. B. Gazzana, and P. T. R. Dalcin, "Mortality among patients with tuberculosis requiring intensive care: a retrospective cohort study," *BMC Infectious Diseases*, vol. 10, article 54, 2010.

[34] World Health Organization and International Union Against Tuberculosis and Lung Disease, *A WHO/The Union Monograph on TB and Tobacco Control: Joining Efforts to Control Two Related Global Epidemics*, WHO Report 2007, (WHO/HTM/TB/2007.390), World Health Organization, Geneva, Switzerland, 2007.

[35] M. Underner and J. Perriot, "Smoking and tuberculosis," *Presse Medicale*, vol. 41, no. 12, Part 1, pp. 1171–1180, 2012.

[36] H.-H. Lin, M. Ezzati, H.-Y. Chang, and M. Murray, "Association between tobacco smoking and active tuberculosis in Taiwan: Prospective cohort study," *The American Journal of Respiratory and Critical Care Medicine*, vol. 180, no. 5, pp. 475–480, 2009.

[37] C. C. Leung, T. H. Lam, K. S. Ho et al., "Passive smoking and tuberculosis," *Archives of Internal Medicine*, vol. 170, no. 3, pp. 287–292, 2010.

28

Factors Associated with Mortality among Patients on TB Treatment in the Southern Region of Zimbabwe, 2013

Kudakwashe C. Takarinda,[1,2] **Charles Sandy,**[1] **Nyasha Masuka,**[3]
Patrick Hazangwe,[4] **Regis C. Choto,**[1] **Tsitsi Mutasa-Apollo,**[1] **Brilliant Nkomo,**[1]
Edwin Sibanda,[5] **Owen Mugurungi,**[1] **Anthony D. Harries,**[2,6] **and Nicholas Siziba**[1]

[1]*AIDS & TB Department, Ministry of Health & Child Care, Harare, Zimbabwe*
[2]*International Union against Tuberculosis and Lung Disease, Paris, France*
[3]*Ministry of Health and Child Care, Harare, Zimbabwe*
[4]*World Health Organisation Country Office, Harare, Zimbabwe*
[5]*Health Services Department, Bulawayo, Zimbabwe*
[6]*Department of Clinical Research, London School of Hygiene and Tropical Medicine, London, UK*

Correspondence should be addressed to Kudakwashe C. Takarinda; ktakarinda@theunion.org

Academic Editor: Brian Eley

Background. In 2013, the tuberculosis (TB) mortality rate was highest in southern Zimbabwe at 16%. We therefore sought to determine factors associated with mortality among registered TB patients in this region. *Methodology.* This was a retrospective record review of registered patients receiving anti-TB treatment in 2013. *Results.* Of 1,971 registered TB patients, 1,653 (84%) were new cases compared with 314 (16%) retreatment cases. There were 1,538 (78%) TB/human immunodeficiency virus (HIV) coinfected patients, of whom 1,399 (91%) were on antiretroviral therapy (ART) with median pre ART CD4 count of 133 cells/uL (IQR, 46–282). Overall, 428 (22%) TB patients died. Factors associated with increased mortality included being ≥65 years old [adjusted relative risk (ARR) = 2.48 (95% CI 1.35–4.55)], a retreatment TB case [ARR = 1.34 (95% CI, 1.10–1.63)], and being HIV-positive [ARR = 1.87 (95% CI, 1.44–2.42)] whilst ART initiation was protective [ARR = 0.25 (95% CI, 0.22–0.29)]. Cumulative mortality rates were 10%, 14%, and 21% at one, two, and six months, respectively, after starting TB treatment. *Conclusion.* There was high mortality especially in the first two months of anti-TB treatment, with risk factors being recurrent TB and being HIV-infected, despite a high uptake of ART.

1. Introduction

Tuberculosis remains one of the world's biggest public health threats and now ranks alongside HIV as the world's leading infectious cause of death. In 2014, there were an estimated 9.6 million people diagnosed with TB globally, of whom 1.5 million died from the disease in the same year (0.4 million were HIV-positive). Despite this, TB incidence has slowly declined by 18% since 2000 and it is estimated that 43 million lives were saved between 2000 and 2014 through effective diagnosis and treatment [1]. However, given that most deaths from TB are preventable, the death toll from the disease is still unacceptably high and efforts to combat this must be continuously accelerated beyond the Millennium Development Goal (MDG) targets, in line with the recently set Sustainable Development Goal (SDG) and the End TB strategy targets [2]. By 2030, the ambition is to reduce TB mortality by 90% compared with 2015. Of the 6 million new cases of TB notified to World Health Organisation (WHO) in 2014, 21% were from the African region which had the highest burden of TB at 281 cases per 100,000 population compared to the global average of 133 cases per 100,000 population [1].

Zimbabwe, which is in the Southern African region, is among the 30 high-burden TB, HIV, and MDR-TB countries in the world and it also has a high HIV prevalence of 15% [3]. In 2014, Zimbabwe had an estimated TB incidence of 278 (193–379) cases per 100,000 population inclusive of HIV-positive TB cases, whilst TB prevalence in the same year was 292 (158–465) cases per 100,000 population [1]. Furthermore, the estimated TB mortality in 2014 stood at 50 (34–68) cases per 100,000 population, although Zimbabwe was notably one of the only 11 high-burden countries to meet the target of halving the TB mortality rate by 2015 compared to 1990. The high burden of TB in Zimbabwe is mostly associated with HIV, with 69% of TB patients having HIV coinfection in 2014 [1]. Thus, national ART guidelines state that all TB/HIV coinfected patients are eligible for ART and cotrimoxazole preventive therapy (CPT) in order to improve TB treatment success rates [4].

The TB treatment success rate for newly registered cases in 2012 was 81% [5], which is below the 85% target recommended by WHO. According to national data, one of the contributors to this low treatment success rate was a high mortality rate of 8% among patients on TB treatment regardless of type and category of TB. Further analysis of this data showed that death rates were highest in the three southern region provinces of Zimbabwe which are Matabeleland North, Matabeleland South, and Bulawayo, each recording case fatalities of 16%, 18%, and 14%, respectively (source: National TB Programme). Death rates in these three provinces have been consistently high in previous years. Given these high mortality rates, we set out to determine among TB patients registered in the three provinces in 2013: (i) their demographic and clinical characteristics, (ii) factors associated with mortality, and (iii) among those who died their time from start of anti-TB treatment to death.

2. Methods

2.1. Study Design. This was a retrospective cohort study using routinely collected data on patients receiving TB treatment.

2.2. Setting: General and Study Site. Selected for this study were three districts from each of the three provinces with the highest TB mortality rates in Zimbabwe in 2013 (nine districts alltogether). Matabeleland South, Matabeleland North, and Bulawayo provinces jointly constitute 16% of Zimbabwe's population according to the Zimbabwe 2012 national census results [6] and have populations of 685,046, 743,871, and 655,675, respectively. Matabeleland South and North provinces are divided into 7 rural districts. Each of these districts has a district hospital and in some instances, there are also mission hospitals at the second level of the health delivery tiered system where there are medical doctors and laboratory facilities enabling the diagnosis of TB through direct smear microscopy and of late GeneXpert MTB/RIF.

The two provinces each have a provincial hospital where referrals from district level are sent. Bulawayo city is Zimbabwe's second largest city where three of the country's central hospitals are located. In addition, there are a number of polyclinics which fall under the Bulawayo City Health Directorate and which are responsible for TB treatment in Bulawayo city. All health facilities in the three provinces offer general health services including TB treatment services as part of an integrated care package.

2.3. Management of TB Cases and HIV Coinfection in Zimbabwe. In Zimbabwe, all public health facilities offer TB treatment services integrated with general health services. First, all presumptive pulmonary TB cases at each health centre have their sputum collected, and sputum specimens are sent to the nearest TB diagnosis laboratory for direct smear microscopy or GeneXpert MTB/RIF with results expected to return to their respective health centres within 2 days. Patients diagnosed with TB are then entered in the health facility DOT register and started on TB treatment. Those with smears positive for acid-fast bacilli are diagnosed as smear-positive PTB, whilst those with negative smears or smears not done are referred for a chest radiograph. If the latter is suggestive of TB, the patients may be diagnosed as smear-negative PTB or PTB with smears not done. Extrapulmonary TB (EPTB) is mainly diagnosed on clinical grounds and circumstantial evidence along with supporting specific diagnostic tests [7].

Patients are also classified and recorded by category of TB as follows: (i) new case defined as a patient who has never had treatment for TB or who has taken anti-TB drugs for less than 1 month, or (ii) previously treated case defined as a patient who has received 1 month or more of anti-TB drugs in the past. Patients who are previously treated for TB (named as "retreatment cases") are further classified by the outcome of their most recent course of treatment either as relapse, treatment after default, treatment after failure, transfer-in, or retreatment others [8].

Upon starting TB treatment, patients take directly observed treatment (DOT) using standardized anti-TB regimens [8], regardless of HIV status. Monitoring is done bacteriologically for all forms of TB since all patients on anti-TB treatment are supposed to have their sputum tested at 2, 4, and 5 months. Smear-negative patients who complete treatment and smear-positive patients who complete treatment with negative smears are regarded as "successfully completing treatment."

All presumptive TB patients are offered HIV counselling and testing (opt-out provider-initiated) [9] and, if found to have TB/HIV coinfection, CPT is started together with anti-TB treatment, provided there is no contraindication. After starting TB treatment, all HIV coinfected patients should be referred for ART initiation and provision of HIV/AIDS care and support within that health facility or alternatively to the nearest ART initiating clinic within their district if ART services are not available on site.

According to national guidelines, ART should be started at least two weeks after the start of TB therapy that is during the intensive phase when the patient has stabilized on anti-TB treatment regardless of the CD4 cell count status. However, for severely immunosuppressed patients (those with CD4 < 50 cells/uL), ART is initiated within the first two weeks of initiating TB treatment. In 2013, ART initiation services were found at all district, mission, and rural hospitals and selected primary care facilities in the three provinces although as of 2015 all health facilities are now offering ART services.

2.4. Study Population. All TB patients who were registered in the district TB registers from the nine selected districts in the three provinces and started on TB treatment between 1 January and 31 December 2013 were included in the study.

2.5. Data Variables, Sources of Data, and Data Collection Procedures. Sources of data included TB and ART registers and, in cases of missing data for ART initiation, the ART patient files. Data were abstracted from routinely existing health facility records into structured forms by three teams of trained and experienced data collectors, each consisting of 5 people. First, data were abstracted from district TB registers for each selected district and variables collected from these registers included TB treatment start date, patient age and sex, TB category and type, TB treatment outcome, other comorbidities, HIV status, pre-ART CD4 cell count, WHO stage, and whether the patient was on ART or not. Patient names were also collected and used to follow up and search for missing information about pre-ART CD4 cell count, WHO clinical staging, and ART status. These names were used to search ART registers and individual ART care booklets from the respective health facilities in each district where these patients were registered and receiving anti-TB treatment.

2.6. Statistical Analysis. Patient data collected in the structured report form was coded and single-entered by six data entry clerks into EpiData version 3.1 (EpiData, Odense, Denmark) and later cleaned for errors and analysed using STATA, version 13.1 (Stata Corporation, College Station, Texas). Proportions and their 95% confidence intervals (CIs) were reported for categorical variables whilst medians and interquartile ranges were reported for continuous skewed variables. Associations between categorical variables were determined using the chi-square test or alternatively Fisher's Exact test.

Univariate and multivariate-adjusted risk ratios together with their 95% CIs and aimed at determining factors associated with mortality were calculated using generalized linear models with a log link and binomial distribution. If there was a convergence problem with the regression models, STATA's *"binreg"* command was implemented. Variables included in the multivariate generalized linear models were those with a *p* value < 0.25. The multivariate generalized linear model for HIV status, classification, and category of TB included all study participants and were adjusted for age and level of healthcare facility. However, separate multivariate generalized linear models for the variables *ART use recorded, ART initiation in relation to start of TB treatment, WHO staging, and CD4 cell count at ART initiation* whilst adjusting for age, level of healthcare, and TB category were run separately to avoid collinearity and were also restricted to those HIV-positive since they did not apply to those HIV-negative.

For survival analysis, we used date of starting TB treatment as time of entry and follow-up was censored at either

date of death or date last seen or date of completing TB treatment. Time-to-event data were complete for 98% of all individuals who successfully completed TB treatment or who died after excluding those who were lost to follow-up, were not evaluated, and were still on MDR-TB treatment. Whilst those excluded should have been included in the survival analysis as censored, this was not possible because their dates of last DOT visit were not recorded in the TB registers. Stratified Kaplan-Meier curves were used to graphically assess survival proportions and calculate the median survival time on TB treatment. A *p* value < 0.05 was considered to indicate statistical significance.

2.7. Ethical Considerations. Ethics approval was granted locally by the Medical Research Council of Zimbabwe and the International Union against Tuberculosis and Lung Disease (The Union) Ethics Advisory Group, Paris, France. Privacy and confidentiality of information drawn from the hospital registers were ensured by excluding patient names from the electronic data entry. All data abstracted were kept in a safe and secure place accessible only to the investigator.

3. Results

There were 1,971 patients who were registered and started on TB treatment between 1 January and 31 December 2013 in the selected districts of the three southern provinces. Demographic and clinical characteristics of TB patients in the southern region provinces are shown in Tables 1 and 2, respectively. Males constituted 1,075 (55%) of all patients whilst the overall median age of patients was 34 years (IQR, 28–44). Close to half of all patients were receiving anti-TB treatment at rural health clinics, whilst 436 (22%) and 341 (17%) were registered at district/provincial hospitals and mission/rural hospitals, respectively. Only 63 (3%) of all patients had a recorded history of travel outside Zimbabwe, and of these 57 (90%) had been to South Africa.

Clinical characteristics of TB patients are shown in Table 2. Of all TB patients, 1,653 (84%) were newly registered TB patients, and of these the majority (44%) were smear-negative pulmonary TB cases whilst 37% were smear-positive PTB cases. Of the retreatment TB cases, 191 (62%) were "retreatment others" whilst 78 (25%) were relapse TB cases. Close to all patients had an HIV test result, of whom 1,538 (78%) were HIV-positive. Of these, 1,399 (91%) were recorded as receiving ART. More than half of all HIV-positive patients had missing WHO clinical staging and baseline CD4 cell counts at ART initiation. Of those with recorded WHO clinical staging, 84% had advanced HIV disease whilst the median CD4 cell count was 133 cells/uL (IQR, 46–282). Of those patients with documented ART status, 584 (42%) were on ART prior to starting TB treatment whilst 543 (39%) initiated ART within 2 weeks of commencing TB treatment.

As shown in Figure 1, 1,419 (72%) of all TB patients had a treatment success whilst death (22%) was the most common adverse TB treatment outcome. Table 3 shows relative risks and their 95% CIs for factors associated with mortality. Patients aged 65 years and older compared to those

TABLE 1: Demographic characteristics of TB patients in southern Zimbabwe, 2013.

Characteristics	n	N	% (95% CI)
Sex			
Female	891	1,966	45.3 (43.1–47.5)
Male	1,075	1,966	54.7 (52.5–56.9)
Missing	5	1,971	0.3
Age (in years)			
0–4	67	1,967	3.4 (2.7–4.3)
5–14	70	1,967	3.6 (2.8–4.5)
15–44	1,353	1,967	68.8 (66.7–70.8)
45–64	366	1,967	18.6 (16.9–20.4)
65+	111	1,967	5.6 (4.7–6.8)
Missing	4	1,971	0.2
Median (IQR)		*34 (28–44)*	
Type of health facility			
Rural health clinic	922	1,965	46.9 (44.7–49.1)
Mission/rural hospital	341	1,965	17.4 (15.7–19.1)
Polyclinic	266	1,965	13.5 (12.1–15.1)
District/provincial hospital	436	1,965	22.2 (20.4–24.1)
Missing	6	1,971	0.3
Recorded history of travel outside Zimbabwe prior to TB treatment			
Yes	63	1,971	3.2 (2.5–4.1)
No	1,908	1,971	96.8 (95.9–97.5)

IQR = interquartile range; TB = tuberculosis.

<5 years old and having retreatment TB compared to newly treated TB were associated with higher risk of mortality in all multivariate regression models. However accessing treatment from a polyclinic or higher level health centre and having CD4 count >50 cells/mL versus ≤50 cells/mL were associated with lower risk of mortality. Being HIV-positive was associated with higher mortality compared to being HIV-negative [adjusted relative risk (ARR) = 1.87 (95% CI, 1.44–2.42)], but among those who were HIV-positive, those on ART had lower mortality [ARR = 0.25 (95% CI, 0.22–0.29)] compared with those not on ART. Compared to those who initiated ART > 3 months prior to starting TB treatment, those who initiated ART within 2 weeks [ARR = 0.73 (95% CI, 0.54–0.98)] were less likely to die whilst those initiated on ART 0–3 months prior to TB treatment were more likely to die [ARR = 1.80 (95% CI, 1.34–2.43)].

The overall mortality incidence rate was 49.1 (44.5–54.2) per 100 person-years. Figure 2 shows the overall Kaplan-Meier survival estimates for all patients enrolled on TB treatment. The mortality rate increased rapidly in the first two months of TB treatment from 10% at one month to 14% at two months and eventually increased slowly over time to 21% at the 6-month end-point. Kaplan-Meier survival estimates for the HIV-negative compared to those HIV-positive on ART and those HIV-positive but not documented on ART are shown in Figure 3: 10% of the respective cohorts had died by 13 weeks, by 7 weeks, and by less than one week, respectively ($p < 0.001$). In relation to median survival time, this could not be estimated for those HIV-negative and those HIV-positive on ART. However, median survival time among

those HIV-positive and not on ART was 3.3 weeks (95% CI, 2.3–5.4).

4. Discussion

We conducted a retrospective review of data collected on patients receiving anti-TB treatment in a routine programme setting in the southern region of Zimbabwe where the TB mortality rate is the highest in the country. This region, where the average TB mortality rate is more than double that of the national average of 10% [1], is a cause for concern and attention is needed to address this huge problem. We observed that TB coinfection with HIV among patients on anti-TB treatment was eleven percent higher than the national average in Zimbabwe [5]. This correlates with HIV prevalence figures in this region which are the highest in the country at 21%, 18%, and 19% for Matabeleland South, Matabeleland North, and Bulawayo, respectively, compared to the national HIV prevalence of 15.2% according to the 2010-11 Zimbabwe Demographic and Health Survey [3].

Whilst only a quarter of TB/HIV coinfected patients had a documented CD4 cell count, we observed that these patients presented late with low CD4 cell counts and this is similar to previous local findings [10]. These late presentations occur despite national guidelines recommending over the years an increased CD4 cell count eligibility for starting ART: from a CD4 cell count threshold of <200 cells/mL before 2010 to <350 cells/mL from 2011 to 2013 and eventually to <500 cells/mL from 2014 onwards in accordance with WHO guidelines [11–13]. We also observed that the elderly, those

TABLE 2: Clinical characteristics of TB patients in southern Zimbabwe, 2013.

Characteristics	n	N	Percentage (95% CI)
TB category			
New	1,653	1,969	84.0 (82.3–85.5)
Retreatment	314	1,969	15.9 (14.4–17.6)
MDR-TB	2	1,969	0.1 (0.0–0.4)
Missing data	2	1,971	0.1
Type of new TB			
Smear-positive PTB	603	1,651	36.5 (34.2–38.9)
Smear-negative PTB	720	1,651	43.6 (41.2–46.0)
EPTB	227	1,651	13.7 (12.2–15.5)
Smear-not-performed PTB	101	1,651	6.1 (5.1–7.4)
Missing	2	1,653	0.12
Type of retreatment TB			
Treatment after default	29	308	9.4 (6.6–13.2)
Retreatment others	191	308	62.0 (56.4–67.3)
Relapse	78	308	25.3 (20.8–30.5)
Treatment after failure	10	308	3.2 (1.7–5.9)
Missing data	6	314	1.9
HIV status			
HIV-negative	419	1,971	21.3 (19.5–23.1)
HIV-positive	1,538	1,971	78.0 (76.1–79.8)
Unknown	14	1,971	0.7 (0.4–1.2)
WHO clinical staging at ART initiation[*]			
I	30	638	4.7 (3.3–6.7)
II	75	638	11.8 (9.5–14.5)
III	494	638	77.4 (74.0–80.5)
IV	39	638	6.1 (4.5–8.3)
Missing data	900	1,538	58.5
CD4 count (cells/mL) at ART initiation[*]			
≤50	96	364	26.4 (22.1–31.2)
51–200	137	364	37.6 (32.8–42.8)
201–350	74	364	20.3 (16.5–24.8)
351–500	28	364	7.7 (5.4–10.9)
>500	29	364	8.0 (5.6–11.2)
Missing data	1,174	1,538	76.3
Median (IQR)		*132.5 (46; 282)*	
ART use recorded[*]			
No	139	1,538	9.0 (7.7–10.6)
Yes	1,399	1,538	91.0 (89.4–92.3)
ART initiation in relation to start of TB treatment[*]			
>3 months before TB treatment	412	1,399	29.4 (27.1–31.9)
0–3 months before TB treatment	172	1,399	12.3 (10.7–14.1)
<2 weeks after TB treatment	543	1,399	38.8 (36.3–41.4)
2–8 weeks after TB treatment	15	1,399	1.1 (0.6–1.8)
Not recorded	257	1,399	18.4 (16.4–20.5)

CI = confidence interval; TB = tuberculosis; MDR-TB = multidrug resistant TB; PTB = pulmonary TB; EPTB = extrapulmonary PTB; HIV = human immunodeficiency virus; WHO = World Health Organisation; IQR = interquartile range; ART = antiretroviral therapy.
[*]These variables refer only to those who were diagnosed as HIV-positive.

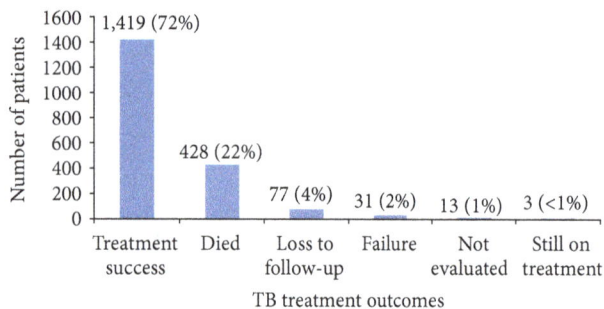

FIGURE 1: Overall TB treatment outcomes among enrolled patient on TB treatment in southern Zimbabwe, 2013. TB = tuberculosis.

with recurrent TB, those diagnosed HIV-positive, those HIV-positive with no documentation of ART, and those HIV-positive presenting with lower CD4 cell counts were more likely to die during anti-TB treatment. Of particular note was the fact that mortality was most common in the intensive phase of anti-TB treatment particularly for those who were HIV-positive without documented ART initiation.

A major strength of this study is that data were an exhaustive sample of all registered cases on anti-TB treatment in the high mortality burden districts of the three highest TB death rate provinces, and hence this study was well powered. Data were obtained from routinely existing programme data which make the study representative of TB patients receiving treatment in public health facilities in southern Zimbabwe. Study limitations include access to few variables that may not exhaustively provide information on mortality-associated factors and also possibilities of incomplete recording of important patient information such as whether an HIV-positive patient was on ART and when they initiated ART, dates of death, and the presence or absence of other comorbidities (such as diabetes mellitus) which may account for mortality among patients who received anti-TB treatment. Another study limitation was that there were no postmortem facilities or access to sophisticated laboratory diagnostic facilities and therefore the exact cause(s) of death could not be determined.

Being HIV-positive was the most common risk factor for mortality whilst on anti-TB treatment and this has been reported in studies from different parts of the world such as in Cameroon [14], the United States [15], South Africa [16], and Ghana [17]. HIV-positive individuals with latent TB are known to be approximately 20–30 times more likely to develop TB disease than those who are HIV negative, at a rate of 8–10% per year [1], because of their suppressed immune system which can result in an increase odds of mortality with further progression of the HIV disease killing 1 in 3 patients [18]. Starting TB treatment with a low CD4 cell count, particularly those with CD4 cell counts <50 cells/mL, was associated with higher mortality and this is a well-established risk factor for early mortality [19]. The declining CD4 cell count influences both the frequency and severity of active TB disease [20], and active TB disease may be associated with a higher HIV viral load and more rapid progression of HIV disease [21]. Such cases presenting for TB treatment with

advanced HIV infection are also likely to present with other AIDS-defining diseases which further add to the risk of dying [22].

In this study we observed a reduction in mortality among HIV-positive TB patients who had documented ART use and this clearly highlights the protective effects of ART from mortality. Similar findings by Agbor et al. [14] showed that those who were HIV coinfected and not receiving antiretroviral therapy were more than twofold likely to die. Among those HIV-infected, starting ART in the intensive phase of TB treatment was also associated with lower mortality compared to those who were previously on ART. These findings concur with SAPiT [23], CAMELIA [24], and STRIDE [25] clinical trials which informed WHO guidance and collectively demonstrated that early initiation of ART can reduce mortality and AIDS progression, notwithstanding the risk of increased immune reconstitution inflammatory syndrome (IRIS) in patients with active TB and with very low CD4 cell counts (i.e., <50 cells/mL). Those who had started TB treatment within 3 months of ART initiation had an almost twofold higher risk of mortality during anti-TB treatment and this may be attributed to late presentation for ART initiation with advanced HIV disease which is associated with "unmasking" TB-IRIS [26] and early mortality within the first three months of ART initiation [19]. It is also possible that there are delays in laboratory diagnosis and start of TB treatment among presumptive TB patients identified through intensified TB-case finding using the WHO recommended four-symptom TB checklist within ART clinics and this requires further investigation in future studies.

Late presentation with advanced HIV disease and low CD4 cell counts at the time of starting anti-TB treatment are often anecdotally reported by health workers in these southern regions of Zimbabwe as the major reason for the high mortality rates. Many of these patients are said to reside as migrant workers in neighbouring South Africa where they do not seek HIV testing and HIV treatment and care services and commonly return to their homes to seek treatment when they are very sick and bed-ridden. Whilst this records review study also sought to determine the proportion of patients who had a history of travel to South Africa as a proxy indicator of these HIV late presentation cases, less than five percent had this information documented and we also did not find it to be a significant risk factor for mortality. It is likely that this information may have been underreported since TB and HIV data collection tools are not standardized to collect this data.

Whilst male gender has commonly been reported as a risk factor for mortality among TB patients in other studies [15, 16, 27], this was not the case in our study. As with other studies, in Sub-Saharan Africa, there was higher mortality among those with pulmonary TB for which sputum smear status was unknown [17] and smear-negative pulmonary PTB [16]. In addition to most smear-negative PTB cases being HIV-positive, there are potential time delays in diagnosis, after receipt of negative sputum smears, which include undergoing a chest radiograph (CXR) that is performed, read, and interpreted by a clinician and a clinical assessment. These diagnosis delays [28] can be associated with progression of disease and worse treatment outcomes. Smear-not-performed PTB

TABLE 3: Factors associated with mortality among TB patients in southern Zimbabwe, 2013.

Characteristics	N	Died, n (%)	Univariate RR (95% CI)	Multivariate-adjusted RR (95% CI)[‡]			
				Model 1	Model 2	Model 3	Model 4
Total	1,847	428 (23.2)	—	—	—	—	—
Age (in years)							
<5	63	11 (17.5)	Reference	Reference	Reference	Reference	Reference
5–14	69	11 (15.9)	0.91 (0.43–1.96)	0.91 (0.42–1.99)	0.89 (0.43–2.00)	1.76 (0.66–4.66)	1.07 (0.39–2.94)
15–44	1,257	290 (23.1)	1.32 (0.77–2.28)	1.17 (0.65–2.10)	1.16 (0.64–2.09)	2.17 (0.97–4.84)	1.12 (0.47–2.65)
45–64	347	74 (21.3)	1.22 (0.69–2.17)	1.10 (0.60–2.01)	1.12 (0.61–2.4)	2.02 (0.91–4.51)	0.95 (0.39–2.32)
65+	107	41 (38.3)	**2.19 (1.22–3.95)**	**2.48 (1.35–4.55)**	**2.47 (1.35–4.57)**	**3.13 (1.4–6.98)**	1.37 (0.5–3.8)
Missing data	4	1 (25)	—	—	—	—	—
Type of health facility	1847						
Rural health clinic	870	214 (24.6)	Reference	Reference	Reference	Reference	Reference
Mission/rural hospital	319	79 (24.8)	1.01 (0.80–1.26)	0.96 (0.77–1.20)	1.04 (0.62–1.76)	**0.94 (0.94–0.94)**	0.91 (0.68–1.21)
Polyclinic	254	35 (13.8)	**0.56 (0.40–0.78)**	**0.56 (0.40–0.78)**	**0.22 (0.07–0.7)**	**0.55 (0.39–0.77)**	0.57 (0.39–0.85)
District/provincial hospital	398	98 (24.6)	1.00 (0.81–1.23)	0.99 (0.81–1.21)	**0.33 (0.12–0.9)**	**0.9 (0.9–0.9)**	0.78 (0.59–1.02)
Missing data	6	2 (33.3)	—	—	—	—	—
TB category							
New TB	1557	337 (21.6)	Reference	Reference	Reference	Reference	Reference
Retreatment TB	288	90 (31.3)	**1.44 (1.19–1.76)**	**1.34 (1.10–1.63)**	1.2 (0.65–2.22)	**1.53 (1.39–1.68)**	**1.59 (1.24–2.04)**
Missing data	2	1 (50)	—	—	—	—	—
HIV status							
HIV-negative	396	59 (14.9)	Reference	Reference	Reference	Reference	Reference
HIV-positive	1439	364 (25.3)	**1.70 (1.32–2.18)**	**1.87 (1.44–2.42)**	—	—	—
HIV unknown	1	1 (100)	—	—	—	—	—
Missing data	11	4 (36.4)	—	—	—	—	—
*WHO clinical staging at ART initiation**							
I	27	3 (11.1)	Reference	Reference	Reference	Reference	Reference
II	70	9 (12.9)	1.16 (0.34–3.95)	—	0.65 (0.17–2.43)	—	—
III	470	69 (14.7)	1.32 (0.44–3.93)	—	1.22 (0.45–3.31)	—	—
IV	39	5 (12.8)	1.15 (0.30–4.43)	—	1.29 (0.36–4.58)	—	—
Missing data	831	278 (33.4)	—	—	—	—	—
*CD4 count at ART initiation(cells/mL)**							
≤50	94	28 (29.8)	Reference	—	Reference	Reference	Reference
51–200	132	15 (11.4)	**0.38 (0.22–0.67)**	—	**0.40 (0.23–0.7)**	—	—
201–350	68	9 (13.2)	**0.44 (0.22–0.88)**	—	**0.47 (0.24–0.91)**	—	—
351–500	27	1 (3.7)	**0.12 (0.02–0.87)**	—	**0.13 (0.02–0.88)**	—	—
>500	29	5 (17.2)	0.58 (0.25–1.36)	—	0.61 (0.26–1.46)	—	—
Missing data	1,089	306 (28.1)	—	—	—	—	—
*ART use recorded**							
No	117	90 (76.9)	Reference	—	Reference	Reference	Reference
Yes	1,322	274 (20.7)	**0.27 (0.23–0.31)**	—	—	**0.25 (0.22–0.29)**	—

TABLE 3: Continued.

Characteristics	N	Died, n (%)	Univariate RR (95% CI)	Multivariate-adjusted RR (95% CI)[‡]			
				Model 1	Model 2	Model 3	Model 4
ART initiation in relation to start of TB treatment[*]							
>3 months before TB treatment	392	83 (21.2)	Reference	Reference	Reference	Reference	Reference
0–3 months before TB treatment	165	56 (33.9)	**0.84 (0.63–1.12)**	—	—	—	**1.8 (1.34–2.43)**
<2 weeks after TB treatment	515	73 (14.2)	**1.34 (0.99–1.82)**	—	—	—	**0.73 (0.54–0.98)**
2–8 weeks after TB treatment	13	2 (15.4)	**0.56 (0.41–0.76)**	—	—	—	0.88 (0.24–3.19)
Not recorded	237	60 (25.3)	—	—	—	—	—

RR = relative risk; CI = confidence interval; TB = tuberculosis; PTB = pulmonary TB; EPTB = extrapulmonary PTB; HIV = human immunodeficiency virus; WHO = World Health Organisation; ART = antiretroviral therapy.

[*]These variables refer only to those who were diagnosed as HIV-positive.

[‡]Multivariate generalized linear regression models 2, 3, and 4 exclude HIV-negative and HIV unknown patients.

Model 1 assesses HIV status whilst adjusting for the potential confounding effects of age, type of health facility, and TB category.

Model 2 assesses WHO clinical staging and CD4 count at ART initiation whilst adjusting for the potential confounding effect of age, type of health facility, and TB category.

Model 3 assesses ART use (yes/no) whilst adjusting for the potential confounding effect of age, type of health facility, and TB category.

Model 4 assesses "ART timing in relation to start of TB treatment" whilst adjusting for potential confounding effect of age, type of health facility, and TB category.

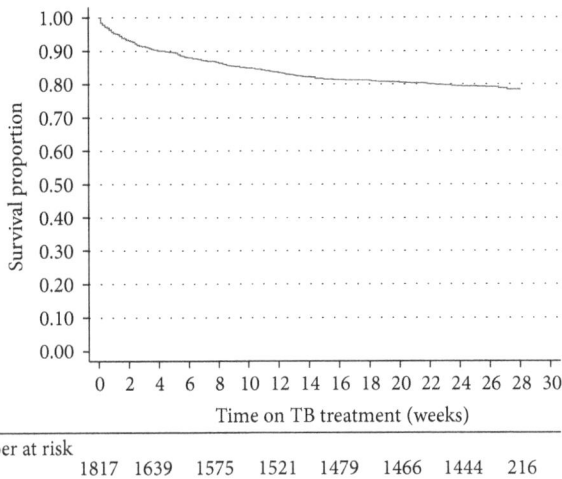

Number at risk

1817	1639	1575	1521	1479	1466	1444	216

FIGURE 2: Overall Kaplan-Meier survival estimates among patients on TB treatment. TB = tuberculosis.

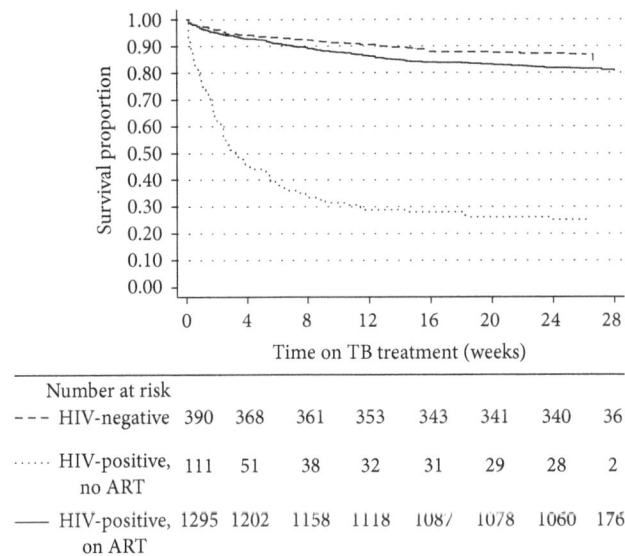

Number at risk

- - - HIV-negative	390	368	361	353	343	341	340	36
······ HIV-positive, no ART	111	51	38	32	31	29	28	2
—— HIV-positive, on ART	1295	1202	1158	1118	1087	1078	1060	176

FIGURE 3: Kaplan-Meier survival estimates stratified by HIV status and ART initiation. TB = tuberculosis; HIV = human immunodeficiency virus; ART = antiretroviral therapy. Note: the numbers of HIV-negative patients and those HIV-positive on ART and not on ART differ from those presented in Table 1 because some patients were excluded from survival analysis because of missing outcome status dates.

cases did not follow national guidelines which recommend TB diagnosis with two sputum smear examinations, and this may result in overdiagnosis of TB disease and underdiagnosis of other respiratory diseases thus increasing mortality risk.

Mortality was also notably higher among patients with recurrent TB [16, 27, 29] who have a strong association with HIV infection, whether on ART or with unknown ART status [30]. Such patients are also more likely to be noncompliant to TB treatment and hence linked with drug-resistant TB [31]. Multidrug-resistant (MDR-TB) poses a threat to TB control worldwide, and globally an estimated 3.5% (95% CI: 2.2–4.7%) of new cases and 20.5% (95% CI: 13.6–27.5%) of

previously treated cases have MDR-TB. In 2013, neighbouring South Africa was one of the countries with the highest number of notified MDR-TB or Rifampicin-resistant TB (RR-TB) cases who were eligible for MDR-TB treatment. Only 41% of those diagnosed were enrolled to treatment [5], and this is of great concern given that Zimbabwe had the largest number of registered immigrants in South Africa from the Africa region in 2013 [32]. The incidence of MDR-TB is also increasing in high human immunodeficiency virus (HIV) prevalence settings, with high associated mortality. A recent meta-analysis of treatment outcomes for HIV and MDR-TB coinfected adults and children showed that treatment success rates were low, mortality was 38% in adults (95% CI 28–48.1) and 11.4% (95% CI 5.8–17.1) in children, and loss to follow-up was also higher among adults (16.1%, 95% CI 9–23.2) than among children (3.9%, 95% CI 0.9–6.9) [33]. In our setting, it is possible that mortality among TB patients may be partly driven by undiagnosed drug-resistant TB and hence it is important to scale up the use of Xpert MTB/RIF assays for TB diagnosis especially in HIV settings.

Mortality was also notably higher in those aged >65 years and this could possibly be attributed to diabetes mellitus which is common among the elderly and causes immuno-suppression thus increasing the risk of TB disease [34]. The prevalence of diabetes mellitus (DM) in adults for Zimbabwe is unexplored and therefore requires investigation. The association between diabetes mellitus and TB has been well documented, and some studies report that smear-negative PTB is more common in people with diabetes, although this association may require rigorous studies to prove an association [35]. This may pave the way for interventions such as active case finding and treatment of latent TB and efforts to diagnose, detect, and treat DM may have a beneficial impact on TB control. It is also possible that rifampicin-, isoniazid-, and pyrazinamide-containing regimens led to anti-TB drug-induced liver disease in these elderly patients [36], and this in turn can lead to drug induced acute liver failure which is associated with high mortality [37]. This also will require further exploration in future studies.

There are a number of programmatic implications from this study. First it is important to continue doing HIV testing for all presumptive TB patients given the high HIV coinfection in these settings and subsequently ensuring that all TB patients who are HIV-infected are started on ART as soon as possible after anti-TB treatment. Second, with most clinical management and initiation on ART and TB treatment being done by nurses, it is important to ensure that there is continued clinical mentorship and training of these cadres to manage any arising drug interactions in the treatment of HIV-associated TB or TB-related IRIS given the complexities of patients presenting for TB treatment with advanced HIV disease. Third, it is necessary to scale up the use of the Xpert MTB/RIF assay technology to diagnose TB among HIV-infected patients in order to identify drug-resistant TB so that these patients receive appropriate treatment. This will reduce reliance on the use of sputum smear microscopy which is also less sensitive among HIV-infected TB patients with low CD4 cell counts. Finally, it may be worthwhile exploring the burden of DM among TB patients, particularly among the elderly who are at higher risk of noncommunicable diseases, in order to enable appropriate management.

Competing Interests

The authors declare that there is no conflict of interests regarding the publication of this paper.

Authors' Contributions

Kudakwashe C. Takarinda, Charles Sandy, Patrick Hazangwe, Tsitsi Mutasa-Apollo, and Anthony D. Harries were involved in the design of the study and data collection. Kudakwashe C. Takarinda analysed the data, wrote the first draft, and subsequently coordinated the writing of the subsequent drafts and the final paper. Charles Sandy, Nyasha Masuka, Patrick Hazangwe, Regis C. Choto, Tsitsi Mutasa-Apollo, Brilliant Nkomo, Edwin Sibanda, Owen Mugurungi, Anthony D. Harries, and Nicholas Siziba contributed to the review of all subsequent drafts of the paper. All authors read and approved the final paper.

Acknowledgments

Funding for the study was obtained from the Global Fund HIV and AIDS Grant in Zimbabwe. Technical support in writing this paper was provided through the International Union against Tuberculosis and Lung Disease. Kudakwashe C. Takarinda is supported as an operational research fellow from the Centre for Operational Research at The Union, Paris, France.

References

[1] World Health Organisation (WHO), *WHO Glocal Tuberculosis Report 2015*, WHO, Geneva, Switzerland, 2015.

[2] World Health Organisation, "Regional Office for Africa. The End TB Strategy," http://www.who.int/tb/post2015_TBstrategy .pdf?ua=1.

[3] Zimbabwe National Statistics Agency (ZIMSTAT) and ICF International, *Zimbabwe Demographic and Health Survey 2010-11*, ZIMSTAT and ICF International, Calverton, Md, USA, 2012.

[4] National Medicine and Therapeutics Policy Advisory Committee (NMTPAC) and The AIDS and TB Directorate M of H and CC (MoHCC), *Guidelines for Antiretroviral Therapy for the Prevention and Treatment of HIV in Guidelines for Prevention and Treatment of HIV*, NMTPAC and The AIDS and TB Directorate, MoHCC, Harare, Zimbabwe, 2013.

[5] WHO, Global tuberculosis report 2014 (WHO/HTM/TB/2014.08), 2014.

[6] Zimbabwe National Statistics Agency (ZIMStat), *Census 2012: Preliminary Report*, Zimbabwe National Statistics Agency (ZIMStat), Harare, Zimbabwe, 2013.

[7] Ministry of Health and Child Care NTP, *Ministry of Health and Child Welfare: Zimbabwe National Tuberculosis Control Programme Manual*, Ministry of Health and Child Care, National Tuberculosis Programme, Harare, Zimbabwe, 3rd edition, 2007.

[8] World Health Organization, *Treatment of Tuberculosis: Guidelines*, World Health Organization (WHO), Geneva, Switzerland,

4th edition, 2010, http://apps.who.int/iris/bitstream/10665/44165/1/9789241547833_eng.pdf.

[9] Ministry of Health and Child Care, *National HIV Testing and Counselling Training Manual*, Ministry of Health and Child Care, Harare, Zimbabwe, 2007.

[10] T. Mutasa-Apollo, R. W. Shiraishi, K. C. Takarinda et al., "Patient retention, clinical outcomes and attrition-associated factors of HIV-infected patients enrolled in Zimbabwe's National Antiretroviral Therapy Programme, 2007–2010," *PLoS ONE*, vol. 9, no. 1, Article ID e86305, 2014.

[11] World Health Organisation, *Antiretroviral Therapy for HIV Infection in Adults and Adolescents: Recommendations for a Public Health Approach-2006 Revision*, WHO, Geneva, Switzerland, 2006, http://www.who.int/hiv/pub/guidelines/artadult-guidelines.pdf.

[12] World Health Organization (WHO), *Antiretroviral Therapy for HIV Infection in Adults and Adolescents: Recommendations for a Public Health Approach—2010 Revision*, vol. 4911, WHO, Geneva, Switzerland, 2010, http://www.who.int/hiv/pub/arv/adult2010/en/index.html.

[13] World Health Organisation (WHO), *Consolidated Guidelines on the Use of Antiretroviral Drugs for Treating and Preventing HIV Infection: Recommendations for a Public Health Approach*, WHO, Geneva, Switzerland, 2013, http://apps.who.int/iris/bitstream/10665/85321/1/9789241505727_eng.pdf.

[14] A. A. Agbor, J. J. R. Bigna, S. C. Billong et al., "Factors associated with death during tuberculosis treatment of patients co-infected with HIV at the Yaoundé Central Hospital, Cameroon: an 8-year hospital-based retrospective cohort study (2006–2013)," *PLoS ONE*, vol. 9, no. 12, Article ID e115211, 2014.

[15] D. J. Horne, R. Hubbard, M. Narita, A. Exarchos, D. R. Park, and C. H. Goss, "Factors associated with mortality in patients with tuberculosis," *BMC Infectious Diseases*, vol. 10, article 258, 2010.

[16] T. E. Mabunda, N. J. Ramalivhana, and Y. M. Dambisya, "Mortality associated with tuberculosis/HIV co-infection among patients on TB treatment in the Limpopo province, South Africa," *African Health Sciences*, vol. 14, no. 4, pp. 849–854, 2014.

[17] N. T. Burton, A. Forson, M. N. Lurie, S. Kudzawu, E. Kwarteng, and A. Kwara, "Factors associated with mortality and default among patients with tuberculosis attending a teaching hospital clinic in Accra, Ghana," *Transactions of the Royal Society of Tropical Medicine and Hygiene*, vol. 105, no. 12, pp. 675–682, 2011.

[18] J. Zwang, M. Garenne, K. Kahn, M. Collinson, and S. M. Tollman, "Trends in mortality from pulmonary tuberculosis and HIV/AIDS co-infection in rural South Africa (Agincourt)," *Transactions of the Royal Society of Tropical Medicine and Hygiene*, vol. 101, no. 9, pp. 893–898, 2007.

[19] R. Zachariah, M. Fitzgerald, M. Massaquoi et al., "Risk factors for high early mortality in patients on antiretroviral treatment in a rural district of Malawi," *AIDS*, vol. 20, no. 18, pp. 2355–2360, 2006.

[20] B. E. Jones, S. M. M. Young, D. Antoniskis, P. T. Davidson, F. Kramer, and P. F. Barnes, "Relationship of the manifestations of tuberculosis to CD4 cell counts in patients with human immunodeficiency virus infection," *American Review of Respiratory Disease*, vol. 148, no. 5, pp. 1292–1297, 1993.

[21] C. Whalen, C. R. Horsburgh, D. Hom, C. Lahart, M. Simberkoff, and J. Ellner, "Accelerated course of human immunodeficiency virus infection after tuberculosis," *American Journal of Respiratory and Critical Care Medicine*, vol. 151, no. 1, pp. 129–135, 1995.

[22] The Opportunistic Infections Project Team of the Collaboration of Observational HIV Epidemiological Research in Europe (COHERE) in EuroCoord, "CD4 cell count and the risk of AIDS or death in HIV-Infected adults on combination antiretroviral therapy with a suppressed viral load: a longitudinal cohort study from COHERE," *PLOS Medicine*, vol. 9, no. 3, Article ID e1001194, 2012.

[23] S. S. Abdool Karim, K. Naidoo, A. Grobler et al., "Timing of initiation of antiretroviral drugs during tuberculosis therapy," *New England Journal of Medicine*, vol. 362, no. 8, pp. 697–706, 2010.

[24] F.-X. Blanc, T. Sok, D. Laureillard et al., "Earlier versus later start of antiretroviral therapy in HIV-infected adults with tuberculosis," *New England Journal of Medicine*, vol. 365, no. 16, pp. 1471–1481, 2011.

[25] D. V. Havlir, M. A. Kendall, P. Ive et al., "Timing of antiretroviral therapy for HIV-1 infection and tuberculosis," *The New England Journal of Medicine*, vol. 365, no. 16, pp. 1482–1491, 2011.

[26] K. Viskovic and J. Begovac, "Tuberculosis-associated immune reconstruction inflammatory syndrome (TB-IRIS) in HIV-infected patients: report of two cases and the literature overview," *Case Reports in Infectious Diseases*, vol. 2013, Article ID 323208, 7 pages, 2013.

[27] T. Santha, R. Garg, T. R. Frieden et al., "Risk factors associated with default, failure and death among tuberculosis patients treated in a DOTS programme in Tiruvallur District, South India, 2000," *International Journal of Tuberculosis and Lung Disease*, vol. 6, no. 9, pp. 780–788, 2002.

[28] F. M. L. Salaniponi, F. Gausi, J. H. Kwanjana, and A. D. Harries, "Time between sputum examination and treatment in patients with smear- negative pulmonary tuberculosis," *International Journal of Tuberculosis and Lung Disease*, vol. 4, no. 6, pp. 581–583, 2000.

[29] R. Alavi-Naini, A. Moghtaderi, M. Metanat, M. Mohammadi, and M. Zabetian, "Factors associated with mortality in tuberculosis patients," *Journal of Research in Medical Sciences*, vol. 18, no. 1, pp. 52–55, 2013.

[30] G. M. C. Louwagie and O. A. Ayo-Yusuf, "Factors associated with retreatment tuberculosis in Tshwane, South Africa: the role of tobacco smoking," *Southern African Journal of Infectious Diseases*, vol. 29, no. 2, pp. 87–90, 2014.

[31] K. Abdella, K. Abdissa, W. Kebede, and G. Abebe, "Drug resistance patterns of Mycobacterium tuberculosis complex and associated factors among retreatment cases around Jimma, Southwest Ethiopia," *BMC Public Health*, vol. 15, no. 1, article 599, 2015.

[32] Statistics South Africa, *Statistical Release: Documented Immigrants in South Africa, 2014*, Statistics South Africa, Pretoria, South Africa, 2013, http://www.statssa.gov.za/publications/P03514/P035142012.pdf.

[33] P. Isaakidis, E. C. Casas, M. Das, X. Tseretopoulou, E. E. Ntzani, and N. Ford, "Treatment outcomes for HIV and MDR-TB co-infected adults and children: systematic review and meta-analysis," *International Journal of Tuberculosis and Lung Disease*, vol. 19, no. 8, pp. 969–978, 2015.

[34] A. D. Harries, A. M. V. Kumar, S. Satyanarayana et al., "Addressing diabetes mellitus as part of the strategy for ending TB," *Transactions of the Royal Society of Tropical Medicine and Hygiene*, vol. 110, no. 3, pp. 173–179, 2015.

[35] C. Y. Jeon and M. B. Murray, "Diabetes mellitus increases the risk of active tuberculosis: a systematic review of 13 observational studies," *PLoS Medicine*, vol. 5, no. 7, article e152, 2008.

[36] L. Huang-Shen, C.-W. Cheng, M.-S. Lin et al., "The clinical outcomes of oldest old patients with tuberculosis treated by regimens containing rifampicin, isoniazid, and pyrazinamide," *Clinical Interventions in Aging*, vol. 11, pp. 299–306, 2016.

[37] H. Devarbhavi, R. Singh, M. Patil, K. Sheth, C. K. Adarsh, and G. Balaraju, "Outcome and determinants of mortality in 269 patients with combination anti-tuberculosis drug-induced liver injury," *Journal of Gastroenterology and Hepatology (Australia)*, vol. 28, no. 1, pp. 161–167, 2013.

29

Nurses' Roles and Experiences with Enhancing Adherence to Tuberculosis Treatment among Patients in Burundi: A Qualitative Study

Marie Carlsson,[1] **Stina Johansson,**[1] **Remy-Paul Bosela Eale,**[2] **and Berthollet Bwira Kaboru**[1]

[1] *School of Health and Medical Sciences, Örebro University, 701 82 Örebro, Sweden*
[2] *International Leadership University in Burundi, P.O. Box 2330, Bujumbura, Burundi*

Correspondence should be addressed to Berthollet Bwira Kaboru; berthollet.kaboru@oru.se

Academic Editor: Vincent Jarlier

Background. In TB control, poor treatment adherence is a major cause of relapse and drug resistance. Nurses have a critical role in supporting patients in TB treatment process. Yet, very little research has been done to inform policymakers and practitioners on nurses' experiences of treatment adherence among patients with TB. *Aim*. To describe nurses' experiences of supporting treatment adherence among patients with tuberculosis in Burundi. *Method*. The study adopted qualitative approach with a descriptive design. A purposive sampling was performed. Eight nurses were selected from two TB treatment centers in Burundi. Content analysis was used to analyze the data. *Result*. According to the nurses, most patients complete their treatment. Educating patients, providing the medication, observing and following up treatment, and communicating with the patients were the key tasks by nurses to support adherence. Causes for interruption were medication-related difficulties, poverty, and patients' indiscipline. Treatment adherence could also be affected by patients' and nurses' feelings. Providing transportation and meals could enhance treatment compliance. *Conclusion*. Nurses are critical resources to TB treatment success. In a poverty stricken setting, nurses' work could be facilitated and adherence further could be enhanced if socioeconomic problems (transportation and nutritional support) were alleviated.

1. Introduction

1.1. Global Tuberculosis, TB Treatment, and TB/HIV. TB is one of the most spread diseases in the world. TB is an infectious disease, and second to HIV/AIDS it is the greatest killer worldwide due to a single infectious agent. In 2012, 8,9 million people had symptoms from TB and 1,3 million died from the disease. Over 95% of the people that succumb to the disease are from low- and middle-income countries in Asia and Africa. The reasons are the standard of living and the large spread of HIV/AIDS in these areas. However, thanks to the global efforts within the framework of the Millennium Development Goals (MDGs), TB death rate has dropped by 45% from 1990 to 2012. This is partly because of the implementation of the comprehensive "Stop TB Strategy" promoted by the World Health Organization (WHO). Directly Observed Treatment Short-course (DOTS)

is the essential element that has presumably saved over 22 million lives. Because of this strategy, the world is on track to achieve the objective of reversing the spread of TB by 2015 [1, 2].

First-line anti-TB drugs have been used for a long time and resistance to the medicines is growing. Multidrug resistant TB (MDR-TB) is caused by bacteria that do not respond to first-line anti-TB drugs. There are medicines to treat MDR-TB but this second-line treatment is more complicated and has harder side-effects on the patient. The drugs have lower effect and are more expensive than the first-line treatment. The options of second-line treatment are limited and recommended medicines are not always available. The second-line treatment includes extensive chemotherapy up to two years which is more costly and can produce severe side-effect reactions in patients. In 2012 about 450,000 people in the world developed MDR-TB [1].

People with reduced immune systems like HIV/AIDS patients are more sensitive to the bacteria and suffer a 30% greater risk of developing an active TB, compared to people without HIV/AIDS. At least one-third of the people with HIV/AIDS also have the TB bacteria active or latent. In combination, the two diseases make the immune system weaken faster. Almost 25% of all deaths among HIV/AIDS-patients are due to TB. Sub-Saharan Africa accounts for largest population with HIV in the world; 1 in 20 adults is living with the disease. Thus, prevalence of HIV/AIDS is one of the largest contributing factors of the spread of TB in that region [1].

1.2. TB Treatment Approach: DOTS. Until 50 years ago, there were no medicines to cure TB. But today TB is a curable disease. The treatment of drug-sensitive TB consists of four antimicrobial drugs, information, supervision, and support to the patient by health workers or trained volunteers. Treatment adherence can be difficult without such supervision and support. The majority of TB cases can be cured when medicines are provided and taken properly [1]. The drugs are taken once a day and it is a strict treatment that is ongoing for at least 6 months, but if the patient's sputum is still positive for active TB after 2 months the treatment is extended to 9 months. Inappropriate or incorrect use of antimicrobial drugs or premature treatment interruption can cause drug resistance and the chances of relapse are increased. Also the use of poor quality medicines can be a contributing factor to drug resistance. MDR-TB can be transmitted in the same ways as drug-sensitive TB [3]. DOT involves observing patients during their intake of medication. This is supposed to enhance treatment adherence among patients, to help them take their medicines regularly, and to successfully complete their treatment. This also prevents the development of MDR-TB. Depending on the local conditions, the supervision can vary from case to case. It may be undertaken at a health facility, in the workplace, in the community, or at home. The supervisors have to be approved by the patients and have to be trained and taught by health staff to be able to supervise [4].

Treatment adherence is essential not only from the perspective of the patient as an individual but also from the community level and preventive perspective. It is known that interrupted treatment is a major cause of relapse and multidrug resistant tuberculosis. It is important that the patients treatment adherence is as high as possible so that as many as possible can be cured and that the incidence of TB can be decreased [1]. For many reasons, adherence is not easy to achieve and National Tuberculosis Control Programs (NTPs) have a responsibility to ensure that the health systems are supportive of patients from diagnosis throughout the treatment. Due to their proximity with the patients in environments characterized by shortages of human health for health, nurses are critical health professionals playing an important role in supporting the patients in their treatment process. However, their experiences with respect to this task are rarely investigated. This study is therefore seeking answers to the following questions. What

are the nurses' experiences of treatment adherence among patients with TB? What is the main reason for interrupted TB treatment according to nurses? What do nurses do in supporting patients under TB treatment? What can and could nurses do to increase the adherence among patients with tuberculosis?

2. Aim

The aim of the study was to identify nurses' roles and experiences in relation to their work with supporting patients under tuberculosis treatment in Burundi.

3. Methods

3.1. Setting. Burundi is one of the smallest countries in Africa with a surface of about 27800, km^2 [5]. The population was, in 2012, around 9.8 million people. During 2012 the TB prevalence in the country was 199 per 100 000, which means that about 19 500 people in Burundi suffered from TB (this includes patients with TB and TB/HIV). There were 6711 new cases of tuberculosis and 305 retreatment cases reported. The retreatment cases include relapses, treatment after failure, and treatment after default. New smear-positive and/or culture-positive cases had a success rate of 92% in 2012 and new smear-negative/extra pulmonary 84%, and among the retreatment cases the success rate was 85%. According to WHO, the treatment success rate among TB patients has been increasing since 2005. As to TB/HIV coinfection, 82% of all the patients with tuberculosis in 2012 also reported a known HIV status, which is a relatively high proportion [2].

In Burundi NTP is called The National Leprosy Tuberculosis Program (PNLT). PNLT is structured according to three levels of a health pyramid: peripheral level, intermediate level, and central level. There are a total of 606 health centres in Burundi; 165 of these are Centres for Screening and Treatment (CDTs), of which 138 are functional treatment centres. In addition to peripheral CDTs, there is one centre in Kibumbu which is the National Reference Centre for Multiresistant TB. All multiresistant TB cases confirmed or suspected at the peripheral levels are referred to this national reference centre.

With regard to human resources, health workers of the CDTs are overseen by multidisciplinary supervision teams at District Health Offices (DHO), which coordinate the peripheral level. These teams are supervised by the intermediate level supported by the central level [6]. In 2009 there were a total of 7576 health workers in Burundi, 4241 nurses and midwives, 255 physicians, and 159 laboratory technicians [7]. The peripheral CDTs are staffed by nurses only, whereas the staff at the MDR centre in Kibumbu is made of a majority of nurses, including nutritionists and a few physicians.

3.2. Study Design. This is a qualitative study with a descriptive design. Descriptive qualitative studies are common in nursing and the goal of this type of research is to develop a rich understanding of a phenomenon [8]. Qualitative semistructured interviews have been used in this study and the purpose of these types of interviews is to get complex answers with a lot of information [9].

3.3. Sampling.

A purposive sampling of nurses from two different centers of tuberculosis in Burundi was performed. One center was located in the city of Bujumbura and the other center was located in the country-side in Kibumbu. The center in Bujumbura treated patients with different types of tuberculosis except for patients with multidrug resistant tuberculosis; they were sent to the center in Kibumbu. The latter treated only patients with drug resistant tuberculosis. Contact was taken with the two centers to see if there were any nurses who were interested in participating in the study. In order to be selected, one needed to be qualified nurse (university graduate) and must have been working with TB treatment issues for at least one year, including the year prior to the interview.

A total of eight nurses were included, four nurses from each center. The participating nurses were between 33 and 52 years old; they had been working as nurses between six and 25 years and with tuberculosis between six and 22 years. Two participants were men and six were women.

3.4. Data Collection Process.

Data has been collected with qualitative semistructured interviews during a two-week period in January 2014. The purposes of qualitative interviews are to understand how the participants are thinking and feeling, what experiences they have, and how their world looks like [9]. The interviews were held in each of the two different TB treatment centers. A guide with questions was used, and the interviews were recorded. A guide of questions can be used to make sure that the authors do not forget any of the topics [9]. Each nurse was interviewed once for 15 to 40 minutes. No back translation of the interview guide was done as the questions were deemed easy to understand, generic, and rather straightforward. Instead, focus was put on the interpreter to ensure she perfectly understood the questions. The interpreter had previous experience of interpretation in qualitative research interviewing. The interviews were conducted in English, with interpretation from English to French. The first two authors were present during the interviews as well as an interpreter. The interpreter was a student from the partner university in Bujumbura. One author held the interview while the other took notes. To start the interview the nurses were asked to describe a typical treatment of TB. This was meant to make them feel comfortable and to feel that the authors were there to learn from them. In the end of the interviews, the author who had been taking notes was able to ask some complementing questions.

The authors who conducted the interviews felt that saturation was reached during the seventh interview, which was conducted at the MDR centre in Kibumbu. It was realized that all the data was redundant and no new information was coming out. The 8th interview was conducted to see if any new insights could emerge, but this was not the case. It was then concluded that saturation had been reached.

3.5. Processing and Analysis of Data.

The interviews were transcribed before they were analyzed using content analysis approach inspired by Burnard [10]. The purpose of performing a qualitative content analysis is to convert large masses of data into smaller segments and then to put those segments together into meaningful conceptual patterns [8].

Content analysis is suitable for semistructured or open-ended interviews but it is also suggested that the method can be used for more clearly structured interviews. To use this method the interviews have to be recorded and transcribed. The analysis consisted of 14 steps which were the base for the analysis in this study. Through these steps, themes and issues were identified and linked together under appropriate categories and subcategories [11]. To analyze the transcribed interviews the authors followed some of these steps and the interview transcript was broken down into relevant data. The authors read the transcribed data several times during this step and changed the coding to what was most appropriate. This is called open coding. The open coding still contained a lot of information. In the following step, the open coding that contained the same information was organized into broader subcategories which were then summarized together into categories. The authors performed these steps together and discussed what could be relevant names for the subcategories and categories; which codes should be put together into the same categories was also discussed. The interviews were read through repeatedly to make sure that the categories reflected the data [10]. The authors also discussed the collected data during the time of the analysis to get a relation between the small parts and the whole context. After this, another coauthor who did not participate in the interviews read through the material to ensure the validity. To put everything together, the subcategories and categories were marked with different colors, which made it easier to put the information with the same content into the corresponding unit. The categories were constantly checked against the aim of the study to make sure that they answered the purpose.

3.6. Ethical Considerations.

Ethical approval was given by the National Tuberculosis Control Program in Burundi which is under the Ministry of Health. The participation was voluntary and the nurses were able to choose the time and place for the interviews. The nurses were given verbal information about the study in their local language. The nurses also received information in writing regarding the purpose of the study, their ethical rights, and their participation. All information was handled with confidentiality and the participating nurses have been unidentified in the result. Each nurse has been given a number instead of their names and the numbers do not depend on the order of which the interviews were held. The nurses were told that they could stop their participation at any time without any consequences. The interviews were recorded but after they had been transcribed they were deleted. The nurses were given information about where the result was going to be published and how they would be able to reach it.

TABLE 1: Presentation of categories and subcategories.

Subcategory	Category
(i) Treatment adherence overall situation	Understanding of treatment adherence
(ii) Understanding of the impact of gender issues on treatment	
(iii) Understanding of HIV/AIDS effects on TB incidence and treatment	
(iv) Understanding of prerequisites for increased adherence	
(i) Enhancing knowledge through education and information to patients	Practical work to support treatment
(ii) Provision of medication, DOT, and treatment followup	
(iii) Maintaining a positive attitude and relationship with patients	
(i) Food insecurity	Perceived reasons for interrupted treatment
(ii) Relief from symptoms	
(iii) Poverty	
(iv) Indiscipline	
(i) Nurses' personal feelings combined with increased risks of infection	Mixed emotional feelings
(ii) Nurses perception of patients feelings	

4. Results

The analysis resulted in four categories and some subcategories (Table 1).

4.1. Understanding of Treatment Adherence

4.1.1. Treatment Adherence's Overall Situation. The opinion from all of the interviewed nurses was that the majority of patients with TB do complete their treatment. Some of the nurses explained that it is difficult for the patients to follow the treatment throughout but that most of the patients try their very best to complete.

> "*Most of the patients that we have complete the treatment but besides this obviously there are others who do not complete their treatment. Because of different reasons*" (Nurse 1).

4.1.2. Understanding of the Impact of Gender Issues on Treatment. Six of the respondents stated that it is more usual that women follow the treatment better than men. A few reasons were given to explain this difference, including the fact that women are more emotional than men; they care about their families and are afraid of affecting others in their surroundings. Women also show more courage to keep up with the treatment than men.

> "*Women are more touched than men. More emotional, because when you tell them they have TB, that they have to take care of this and take the medication, because if you do not you are going to affect other people. So when you tell them they get scared and fear. And that is why they have to take their medication, because at least they care about their families around them. For the men that is not the same, it is different*" (Nurse 1).

4.1.3. Understanding of HIV/AIDS Effects on TB Incidence and Treatment. The prevalence of HIV/AIDS among patients

with tuberculosis is increasing according to four of the interviewed nurses. There was a difference in how the nurses explained the treatment adherence among patients suffering from both TB and HIV/AIDS. Some nurses thought that it is easier for those patients to follow the treatment than for the patients suffering only from TB, whereas some nurses believed that it is the other way around. There were a few different explanations to why it is easy for the patients suffering from both diseases to follow the treatment. The explanations included that the treatment makes the patients feel better and therefore they want to continue, that patients have a schedule for when the medicines are supposed to be taken, that the patients only come to collect their medication for HIV/AIDS once a month, and that these patients get help from a certain group of people. The nurses who described that they do not think it is easy for these patients also mentioned different reasons. Five nurses described that these patients have to take a lot of medication. Some also described that the medicines are taken at different times during the day and that the medications might give the patients side effects and make them weaker.

> "*It is hard for them because of the medicines. You find that it is too much for one person to take. At times these medicines cause them to have pain, and at some point may become weaker*" (Nurse 8).

4.1.4. Understanding of Prerequisites for Increased Adherence. The participants described what they thought could help patients get better adherence to the treatment. One nurse talked about the importance of visiting patients in their home and that they would need more transportation to be able to do more visits. Some of the nurses also explained that it would be helpful if they could offer some food for the patients in combination with the medicine because the medication increases appetite. It was also described that daily communication between nurses and patients is helpful to increase compliance. One nurse believed that it could be helpful if patients who live far away from the centres could be offered accommodation in case of difficulties to reach the centres every day.

4.2. Practical Work to Support Treatment

4.2.1. Enhancing Knowledge through Education and Information to Patients. Four of eight nurses described education and information to patients as something important in their job to support the patients. The patients are informed and educated about the disease, how to behave and how to prevent transmission of the disease to other people. They are also taught about the advantage of good adherence and the risks associated with interrupted treatment. The nurses also educate patients about side effects and that they should not mix medication with substances like alcohol or other drugs. One nurse mentioned that counseling is important and available for patients whenever they want to talk to somebody.

> "I teach these patients, and tell them how they are supposed to behave and how to take their medications and how to prevent themselves from infected others" (Nurse 1).

4.2.2. Provision of Medication, DOT, and Treatment Followup. To support the patients with their treatment, nurses describe a number of helpful actions. Almost all, seven out of eight nurses, explained that they follow up the treatment to see how it is going, if the patients improve or if the situation is becoming worse, how the patients feel, if they feel any side effects, and also to see if the patients are taking their medication every day. Four nurses said that they give out the medication to the patients and three of them explained that the patients should take the medication in their presence.

> "I follow up and then I make sure that I communicate daily with the patient that I am dealing with to find out if they took the medication and if it had any side effects on the patient. And then I follow up to find out if the medication that I give the patients is being held, if they are improving or if the situation is becoming worse" (Nurse 2).

One nurse explained that they have an organization of different members outside the centers to help the nurses follow up patients. One nurse also explained that it is important to call the patients if they do not show up to see why and that it is important to visit patients in their homes. Two nurses said that encouraging patients is supporting and one nurse spoke of morale, that you as a nurse should help patients with their morale. One respondent in the center of Kibumbu explained that the patients sign a contract when they arrive; the contract says that they should stay at the center for 9 months and that they should finish the treatment. This nurse believed this to be a supporting factor. In the center of Kibumbu the patients stay for their whole treatment and they get accommodation, food, and medicines. One nurse stated that asking the patients what they want to eat is also a way to encourage them. The nurses believed that this is supporting the patients to follow through their treatments.

4.2.3. Maintaining a Positive Attitude and Relationship with Patients. Four nurses talked about how to receive the patients, that you, as a nurse, should treat all people the same no matter what, rich or poor. You should try to be close to the patients, be calm, and speak normally in every situation even if the patients are not serene. One nurse specifically spoke about loving your patients, that you as a nurse should treat them as any human beings.

> "You try to be closer to the patients... then you have to be cool, because if you react they are also going to react, so you have to be normal when you are talking to them" (Nurse 1).

4.3. Perceived Reasons for Interrupted Treatment. Even though the nurses said that most patients follow through their treatment some also explained that there are those who do not, because of several different reasons.

4.3.1. Food Insecurity. The findings underscored that treatment is demanding in that the patients have to come to the centre every day to pick up the medicines. Two nurses said that the medication causes the patients to have increased appetite and for different reasons this might be a factor that makes them interrupt the treatment. The respondents stated that either the patients could not afford to eat, or they would rather go and look for food instead of going to the centres and take the medicines. It was also common that, due to lack of food, patients would rather stop taking the medication instead of taking the medicine and be even hungrier.

> "Whereby we find that people are making that effort to take their medication but, because it requires them to eat, because when you are taking such kind of medication it causes them to have appetite and then they have the appetite, they are taking the medication but they cannot afford to eat" (Nurse 3).

4.3.2. Interruption due to Relief from Symptoms. One nurse also pointed out that treatment interruption could be once the medicines relieved the symptoms. When the patients feel better they stop taking the medication.

4.3.3. Poverty. Five of the eight interviewed nurses described that one big reason for interrupted treatment is poverty. The fact that patients are poor leads to consequences for the treatment. Five nurses also spoke of the distance as a cause of interruption. That it is difficult for the patients to reach the centre, they cannot get transportation. Two nurses said that it is more important to provide for the family than to go and get the medication. So they would like to do that before they go to get the medication. One nurse described that it is usual that men are supposed to provide for the family and that this might cause them to interrupt the treatment.

> "In almost every home, the men are the heads of the family. However much you are sick, still people will be looking up to you. So they do not want to

waste that energy, first they want to go here and there to maybe get a little bit of money so that they can provide for their family. So they always talk like they first want to get the money and then they will come back and finish..." (Nurse 2).

4.3.4. Indiscipline.

Five nurses described indiscipline as a reason for interrupted treatment and four said that it is men who are often undisciplined. Two nurses explained that there are those types of patients who do not listen to what nurses tell them and that instead they do the opposite of what they are told. One nurse said that even if they explain that the patients should not mix medications with alcohol or other drugs there are people who do not follow the recommendations. According to four nurses, alcohol and other drugs are a big reason for the patients' undisciplined behaviour. Two nurses described that men are more often addicted to alcohol.

"*It is maybe out of ignorance for the men because, for the nurses, we always educate these people and remind them, so the men, they do it out of ignorance. Because maybe you find that most of them are alcohol addicts, you find that when they feel better they think that it is time to stop taking the medicine [and I should] go back and find [my] boos*" (Nurse 8).

Another nurse explained that men are associated with bars. Another reason for interrupted treatment was explained as forced interruption, for example, when patients happen to be imprisoned.

4.4. Mixed Emotional Feelings

4.4.1. Nurses' Personal Feelings Combined with Increased Risks of Infection.

Three respondents described that nurses' and patients' feelings could be a contributing factor for nurses' difficulties in supporting patients. One nurse said that nurses sometimes get scared when patients are furious. Another nurse said that she felt bad when patients harass or insult her.

"*...when they do not give me a positive attitude or they harass me or they insult me, I would feel bad and at times I would even cry*" (Nurse 4).

There was also one nurse who explained that it is a risk for those who treat the patients. The nurse explained that it is a bigger risk for them when the patients are so sick that they cannot go and get the medication themselves. Then the nurses have to go to the patients rooms and the risk of getting infected is increased. When patients suffer from both HIV/AIDS and TB, this causes an even greater risk and the nurses have to be careful when they treat them.

4.4.2. Nurses' Perception of Patients Feelings.

Four nurses explained that they think patients feel discouraged to follow the treatment because of different reasons. Two of these nurses said that poverty is a reason for their lack of motivation. When patients are poor, having no food security and having to come to the centre every day, they are easily discouraged. One nurse described that if patients are seeking help from a hospital, which also treats other diseases, the patients might have to wait for a long time to get help and then they feel discouraged. Two nurses also explained that the patients feel alone and one said that patients might feel that nobody cares about them. Once frustrated, the patients put all their anger on the nurses and no matter how much nurses try to help them they feel that something is missing.

"*...we are dealing with patients who feel alone, it is like they are discouraged, nobody cares about them. So what I do is like, I give them courage, I give them courage, I give them moral*" (Nurse 2).

5. Discussion

The result in this study shows that all of the interviewed nurses had the experience that the majority of the patients follow through the treatment for TB. Nurses are indeed at forefront of TB care and they are critical to informing about opportunities and obstacles to patients' adherence to TB treatment [12]. According to Ugochukwu and colleagues [13], one of the critical roles of nurses in Sub-Saharan Africa is to provide health education to communities, care providers, clients, and patients.

This study shows that nurses in Burundi have an expert knowledge of issues surrounding treatment adherence in Burundi. They have both broad understanding of the magnitude of adherence, issues of adherence among TB and HIV coinfected patients, and reasons for treatment default and possible interventions to improve adherence. Nurses in Burundi report that they are involved in practical work of educating patients on TB and its treatment, providing medication (DOT) and related followup, and ensuring the patients are of good morale to complete their treatment. The latest report from WHO showed that 84–92% of the patients in Burundi had a successful treatment in 2012 [1]. Burundian nurses' support to patients is likely to be a contributing factor to this high adherence.

For nurses to sustain patients' knowledge, they need to be well trained themselves. A study conducted in Ethiopia found that 43% of the patients interrupted their treatment. Patients' knowledge of TB and its treatment was poor but treatment interruption was associated with inadequate supervision of health care providers. One suggested solution was to improve training for service providers [14]. Sagbakken et al. [15] are also describing the lack of knowledge among health workers as a reason for low compliance [15]. Knowledge among patients may not only encourage the patients to higher adherence but also better equip patients for better self-care. According to Orem [16], most activities to maintain health have to come from the individuals themselves. It could be easier for the patients to come up with these activities if they had knowledge about their needs. If the knowledge is lacking, self-care will be deficient, implying increased demand for other people to take over parts of the patients' self-care to compensate for patients' limitations.

The purpose of DOT is to lower the risk of self-care deficit, but the concept does not underscore what the patients can do themselves. DOT is contributing to maintaining self-care requisites but this could be perceived as humiliating for the patients. An article on ethical aspects of DOT conducted in Ethiopia and in Norway showed that in both countries patients with TB were deprived of their autonomy and lacked the opportunity to influence the delivery of their own health care. The patients experienced that they had no power to influence how their treatment was organized, even if they had tried. Patients reported issues with their income during TB treatment which was not flexible and did not take the patients daily routines into consideration. Many patients reported that they had difficulties to keep their job due to DOT requirements [15]. In Burundi there were few reports of interrupted treatment and adherence was reported to be increasing. According to the nurses in Burundi, DOT as an approach is in progress and it is helpful in order to help patients complete the treatment. However, some nurses also explained the inflexibility of DOT and that this could make the treatment harder for patients to follow.

Some patients were reported to feel that the distance they have to go every day for the medication is one of the biggest causes for treatment interruption. Communication between patients and nurses is a key to make DOT work. One way of communication is through community organizations or groups. Engaging a community organisation to help the nurses conduct DOT for those who cannot come to the centres every day may be one way of making the treatment under DOT more flexible. In addition, one reason for increased adherence that was mentioned was improved knowledge about TB in the communities. They also believe that the patients' self-care, the nurses' health work, and the community have to work together to make the treatment successful and to lower the spread of TB.

According to Frieden and Sbarbaro [17] interrupted treatment is not affected by socioeconomic status, educational level, sex, race, severity of illness and dosage, or adverse effects; the only factor affecting the treatment success is the band between patients and the health workers [17]. This study's findings show that poverty, drug regimens' requirements with regard to nutrition, poverty, relief from symptoms, patients' indiscipline, and gender related issues are factors which may affect adherence. Even though treatment and medicines are for free, there are still other aspects of the importance of money during the treatment. The nurses reported that lack of food because of patients' poverty may be one reason for interruption. The nurses explained that they tell the patients that they should eat when they take the medicines and also that the medication may cause increased appetite. Nutritional support provided with the treatment could therefore improve compliance. This support was only available at the MDR-TB center of Kibumbu, as per MDR-TB treatment policy. Another critical problem was a logistical one. Nurses expressed the need for transportation means to help them reach defaulting or irregular patients and to liaise with the communities. Such are recurrent programmatic problems in TB control [18].

Indiscipline among patients was also described as a reason for default or incorrect treatment. The patients do not listen to the nurses when they try to teach them about the disease and the treatment and they do not do as they are told. The respondents did not explain what they thought could help these patients apart from listening and trying to make the patients understand the importance of completing treatment. Individually tailored solutions should be identified. Some nurses also described addiction to alcohol as a type of indiscipline, as patients refuse abiding to recommendations of not mixing alcohol and other drugs with the medicine. Burundi is a postconflict country and people have been traumatized in several ways. Alcohol, drugs, and mental health disorders are likely to affect substantial proportions of the population [19].

The result of this study shows that the nurses believe that there is a difference among men and women regarding adherence to the treatment. All nurses reported observing better adherence among women than men. The authors do not know why this could be and it would be interesting to know if it really is like this.

In Burundi there are 4242 nurses and midwives and 19500 people suffering from TB. According to Cailhol and colleagues, Burundi is in need of more human resources [20]. There is also indication that many nurses are working in Non-Governmental Organizations (NGO) where salaries are higher than in the public sector. DOT requires a high number of human resources to make the system work. At the two centers in Burundi where the research was conducted, adherence was described as good, indicating perhaps that nurses were coping with the amount of patients they are dealing with. Surprisingly, none of the nurses described human resources as a factor that affects the adherence.

The nurses in this study explained that the prevalence of HIV is increasing among patients with TB. This is also strengthened by the latest WHO report of TB/HIV [21]. The result in this study shows that the nurses had different thoughts of whether it was easier or harder for patients suffering from both TB and HIV to follow the treatment compared to patients who suffered only from TB. Both groups of nurses had good arguments as to why it was easier or harder for these patients. The authors' opinion is that it may depend on the patients' personality more than on which types of diseases they are suffering from. WHO explains the importance of integration between the tuberculosis program and the HIV program [22]. The nurses explained that they also provided HIV treatment for patients who were suffering from both diseases. Other nurses also described that patients suffering from both diseases got extra help to manage the respective treatments. The authors of this study got the impression that because of this extra help it is equally difficult/easy for both types of patients to manage the treatment.

Nurses try their best in supporting patients with their treatment but the effort simply costs in terms of feelings and risks. Feelings such as fear were described when the patients express anger and when they harass or insult the nurses. Also, caring for patients with transmissible infectious disease raises fear for contamination. The authors believe that this fear could affect the nurses' support to these patients in a negative way and that their receiving attitude is affected by these feelings. Nurses also explained the patients' feelings and that discourage, demotivation, and loneliness among patients could affect their treatment negatively.

This study might have some limitations. Convenience sampling is not a preferred approach even in qualitative studies but in this study this design was used for several reasons [8]. The time for the study was limited and nurses at the two centers were of limited number. In this particular context, the authors believe that this type of sampling provided valuable information that was sought. As to the sample size, eight nurses were deemed sufficient given the rich amount of information provided, especially since the respondents had long experience of working with TB patients.

The question guide was piloted prior to the interviews. It was adjusted to eliminate ambiguous formulations. Reconstructing the questions might have made the data more reliable. The pilot interview was also useful for the interviewers who did not have any prior experiences of conducting qualitative interviews. This enhanced reliability of the data collection. When presenting the results, quotations were used to demonstrate credibility of the data [8]. In order to ensure confirmability of the interpretation of the data, a third person read through the material to make sure that the study reflects what the participants said.

6. Conclusion

Nurses constitute a key resource in ensuring patients with TB complete their treatment. They provide a range of services and demonstrate a multifaceted understanding of problems surrounding adherence to treatment. Nurses' work could be made easier if they were equipped with transportation means and if they could provide nutritional support to more patients in need.

6.1. Policy Implications and Further Research

(i) Although adherence in Burundi seems to be increasing and according to the nurses the majority of the patients complete the treatment, there are still many people suffering from the disease and there are people who do not complete their treatment as they should. This study shows some reasons for interrupted treatment and what nurses can and could do to support the patients in Burundi. TB being one of the most spread diseases in several countries in Sub-Saharan Africa, it is suggested that the results from this study are, to a greater extent, transferable to other similar settings.

(ii) Policy makers may consider the aspects mentioned in this study (e.g., transportation facilities, nutritional support, etc.) in the formulation of national and local strategies to enhance adherence to TB treatment. There is a need for robust cost-effectiveness studies to see if investments in transport for nurses, for instance, and in provision of food to patients could lead to reduced incidence of drug-sensitive TB and of MDR-TB and associated costs.

(iii) Further studies are needed in Burundi to explain the factors behind the reported increases in treatment success and increases in adherence rates so that policy makers could strengthen them further. Many nurses complained about workload. They work every day and many report being continuously exhausted. It could be interesting to do further research on the nurses' working conditions, including the number of nurses in relation to the number of patients, to see if this could have impact on patients' treatment adherence. The factors explaining gender differences in adherence to TB treatment are another possible area of further research.

Acknowledgments

The authors are grateful to the Swedish International Development Agency (Sida) for funding this study through a grant within the framework of the Minor Field Studies (MFS). Thanks are to Mrs. Annick Bujeje, Secretary of the Vice-Chancellor at ILU Burundi, for assisting with all the necessary contacts to secure ethical and legal permissions to conduct this study in Burundi.

References

[1] WHO, "Global Tuberculosis Report," 2013, http://www.who.int/tb/publications/global_report/en/.

[2] WHO, "Burundi: Tuberculosis profile," 2014, https://extranet.who.int/sree/Reports?op=Replet&name=%2FWHO_HQ_Reports%2FG2%2FPROD%2FEXT%2FTBCountryProfile&ISO2=BI&LAN=EN&outtype=html16.

[3] L.-O. Larsson, R. Bennet, and B. Normann, "Tuberculosis," in Lungs Medicine, I. T. Sandström and A. Eklund, Eds., pp. 85–100, Studentlitteratur, Lund , Sweden, 2009.

[4] WHO, "The five elements of DOTS: element 3," 2013, http://www.who.int/tb/dots/whatisdots/en/index2.html.

[5] Landguiden, "Burundi," http://www.landguiden.se.db.ub.oru.se/Lander/Afrika/Burundi?p=1.

[6] Programme National de Lutte contre la Lèpre et la Tuberculose (PNLT), Plan Stratégique de Lutte Contre la Tuberculose 2011—2015, PNLT, Ministère de la Santé, Bujumbura, Burundi, 2010.

[7] Africa Health Workforce Observatory, "Burundi: HRH fact sheet-Burundi. Health Workforce Observatory," Africa Health Workforce Observatory, http://www.hrh-observatory.afro.who.int/en/country-monitoring/50-burundi.html.

[8] D. F. Polit and C. T. Beck, Essentials of Nursing Research: Appraising Evidence for Nursing Practice, Wolters Kluwers, Philadelphia, Pa, USA, 2013.

[9] J. Trost, Kvalitativa Intervjuer [Qualitative Interviews], Studentlitteratur, Lund, Sweden, 2010.

[10] P. Burnard, "A method of analysing interview transcripts in qualitative research," Nurse Education Today, vol. 11, no. 6, pp. 461–466, 1991.

[11] S. Elo and H. Kyngäs, "The qualitative content analysis process," *Journal of Advanced Nursing*, vol. 62, no. 1, pp. 107–115, 2008.

[12] T. Ghebrehiwet, "Nurses in the forefront of tuberculosis prevention, care and treatment," *International Nursing Review*, vol. 53, no. 4, pp. 239–240, 2006.

[13] C. G. Ugochukwu, L. R. Uys, A. K. Karani et al., "Roles of nurses in Sub-Saharan African region," *International Journal of Nursing and Midwifery*, vol. 5, pp. 117–131, 2013.

[14] M. M. Mesfin, J. N. Newell, J. D. Walley et al., "Quality of tuberculosis care and its association with patient adherence to treatment in eight Ethiopian districts," *Health Policy and Planning*, vol. 24, no. 6, pp. 457–466, 2009.

[15] M. Sagbakken, J. C. Frich, G. A. Bjune, and J. D. H. Porter, "Ethical aspects of directly observed treatment for tuberculosis: a cross-cultural comparison," *BMC Medical Ethics*, vol. 14, article 25, 2013.

[16] M. Kirkevold, *Nursing Theories: Analysis and Evaluation*, Lund Studentlitteratur, 2000.

[17] T. R. Frieden and J. A. Sbarbaro, "Promoting adherence to treatment for tuberculosis: the importance of direct observation," *World Hospitals and Health Services*, vol. 43, pp. 30–33, 2007.

[18] L. J. George, "Self-determination and compliance in directly observed therapy of tuberculosis treatment in the Kingdom of Lesotho," *Social Work in Health Care*, vol. 46, no. 4, pp. 81–99, 2008.

[19] M. Sommers, *Adolescents and Violence: Lessons from Burundi*, University of Antwerp, Antwerp, Belgium, 2013.

[20] J. Cailhol, I. Craveiro, T. Madede et al., "Analysis of human resources for health strategies and policies in 5 countries in Sub-Saharan Africa, in response to GFATM and PEPFAR-funded HIV-activities," *Globalization and Health*, vol. 9, article 52, 2013.

[21] WHO, *WHO Policy on Collaborative TB/HIV Activities: Guidelines for National Programmes and Other Stakeholders*, WHO, Geneva, Switzerland, 2012, http://www.who.int/tb/challenges/hiv/en/index.html.

[22] WHO, *The Stop TB Strategy: Building on and Enhancing DOTS to Meet the TB-Related Millennium Development Goals*, 2006, http://whqlibdoc.who.int/hq/2006/WHO_HTM_STB_2006.368_eng.pdf.

30

Pouched Rats' Detection of Tuberculosis in Human Sputum: Comparison to Culturing and Polymerase Chain Reaction

Amanda Mahoney,[1,2] **Bart J. Weetjens,**[2] **Christophe Cox,**[2] **Negussie Beyene,**[2]
Klaus Reither,[3,4] **George Makingi,**[5] **Maureen Jubitana,**[2] **Rudovick Kazwala,**[5]
Godfrey S. Mfinanga,[6] **Amos Kahwa,**[6] **Amy Durgin,**[1,2] **and Alan Poling**[1,2]

[1] *Department of Psychology, Western Michigan University, Kalamazoo, MI 49008-5200, USA*
[2] *Tuberculosis Research, Anti-Persoonsmijnen Ontmijnende Product Ontwikkeling (APOPO), Morogoro, Tanzania*
[3] *Tuberculosis Research, Swiss Tropical and Public Health Institute, 4051 Basel, Switzerland*
[4] *TB Research and Training Center, Ifakara Health Institute, Bagamoyo, Tanzania*
[5] *Department of Veterinary Medicine, Sokoine University of Agriculture, Morogoro, Tanzania*
[6] *Clinical Research Laboratory, National Institute for Medical Research, Dar es Salaam, Tanzania*

Correspondence should be addressed to Amanda Mahoney, amanda.mahoney@apopo.org

Academic Editor: Soumitesh Chakravorty

Setting. Tanzania. *Objective.* To compare microscopy as conducted in direct observation of treatment, short course centers to pouched rats as detectors of *Mycobacterium tuberculosis. Design.* Ten pouched rats were trained to detect tuberculosis in sputum using operant conditioning techniques. The rats evaluated 910 samples previously evaluated by smear microscopy. All samples were also evaluated through culturing and multiplex polymerase chain reaction was performed on culture growths to classify the bacteria. *Results.* The patientwise sensitivity of microscopy was 58.0%, and the patient-wise specificity was 97.3%. Used as a group of 10 with a cutoff (defined as the number of rat indications to classify a sample as positive for *Mycobacterium tuberculosis*) of 1, the rats increased new case detection by 46.8% relative to microscopy alone. The average samplewise sensitivity of the individual rats was 68.4% (range 61.1–73.8%), and the mean specificity was 87.3% (range 84.7–90.3%). *Conclusion.* These results suggest that pouched rats are a valuable adjunct to, and may be a viable substitute for, sputum smear microscopy as a tuberculosis diagnostic in resource-poor countries.

1. Introduction

A major hurdle in combating tuberculosis (TB) is diagnosing the disease in resource-poor countries. Sputum smear microscopy, the technique typically used, is relatively slow and characteristically has high specificity but low sensitivity [1, 2]; therefore, the international medical community has prioritized developing a quick, accurate, and affordable alternative diagnostic. In an attempt to develop one, researchers recently have investigated the use of scent-detecting pouched rats (*Cricetomys gambianus*) as a TB diagnostic. An initial proof of principle investigation [3] revealed that pouched rats trained through operant conditioning procedures could detect TB in human sputum, and three subsequent studies, involving a total of over 20,000 patients, showed that

using the rats in second-line screening of sputum samples initially screened by smear microscopy at direct observation of treatment—short course (DOTS) centers in Tanzania increased new case detections by 31.4% [4], 44% [5], and 42.8% [6].

These results are promising, but the accuracy of *Cricetomys* in detecting TB has not been extensively evaluated relative to an established reference standard. Culturing is considered the "gold standard" for TB detection [2], and Weetjens et al. [3] reported the results of a study in which two rats, Mandela and Kingston, evaluated 817 sputum samples also evaluated by culturing, which revealed 67 TB-positive samples. Sensitivity relative to culturing for both rats was 73.1%, while specificity was 97% and 97.8% for Mandela and Kingston, respectively. In an attempt to provide more comprehensive information regarding pouched rats' TB-detection accuracy relative to the best available and affordable method, this experiment evaluated 10 rats' performance compared to culture in combination with Multiplex PCR.

2. Method

2.1. Subjects and Materials. Ten adult *Cricetomys* obtained from our breeding colony, 5 males and 5 females, evaluated all sputum samples. The animals were housed and maintained as detailed elsewhere [3, 7]. Ethical clearance to conduct the research was obtained from the Tanzanian National Institute for Medical Research. Some of the rats had been used in previous studies and all of the rats had been evaluating sputum samples for TB for at least one year.

Testing was conducted in a chamber 205 cm long, 55 cm wide, and 55 cm high with clear plastic walls and ceiling and a stainless steel floor. Ten holes with sliding lids 2.5 cm in diameter were spaced equidistance apart along the centerline of the chamber floor's long axis. Pots containing sputum were placed beneath the holes for the rats to evaluate. Edible reinforcers (rewards), consisting of a mixture of mashed banana with ground rodent diet pellets, were delivered through a plastic syringe through feeding holes.

2.2. Collection of Sputum Samples. Sputum samples were collected weekly from eight DOTS centers in Dar es Salaam and Morogoro, Tanzania, using World Health Organization (WHO) recommended sputum containers. Direct smear microscopy after Ziehl-Neelsen staining was conducted at the DOTS centers prior to collection of the samples. Samples of less than 2 mL were excluded to ensure that there was sufficient volume for culturing and rat evaluation. In all, 910 samples from 456 patients (two from each of 454, one from each of two) were evaluated. Before evaluation by rats, an aliquot was taken from each sample for culture purposes, and then sterile phosphate buffered saline solution (5 mL) was added to each sputum sample and microorganisms were inactivated by heating the sample at 90°C in a water bath for 30 min [8]. The samples were then frozen at −20°C until the day of evaluation (up to seven days). Though there is some controversy surrounding the cellular impact of freezing and thawing sputum, past research suggests that samples may be kept frozen without significant alteration of cell quality or cell counts [9]. Furthermore, data collected internally suggest that the rats' performance is unaffected by the freezing procedures employed. Samples were thawed four times for the purpose of this study: once on the day of collection, once to take aliquots for culture, once to evaluate the sputum quantity and add buffer, and once on the day of evaluation by the rats.

2.3. Rats' Evaluation of Samples. Prior to this study, the rats were trained to detect TB as detailed elsewhere [3, 7]. In the present study, each rat evaluated each sample twice, in a different order, across 13 sessions. In each session, 63 samples found negative by microscopy at DOTS centers and seven samples found positive were presented to the rats. The seven

positive samples served as reinforcement opportunities to maintain the rats' indications while the remaining samples were categorized as "unknown". During the sessions, the experimenter opened each hole in the cage as the rat passed over and sniffed. When the rat paused for 5 s (i.e., emitted an indicator response), the experimenter informed a data collector who then stated whether the sample was smear positive according to DOTS-center microscopy. If the rat made an indicator response above a smear-positive sample, the experimenter sounded a click and delivered food, after which the rat then moved to the next hole to continue evaluations. If the rat emitted an indicator response at a smear-negative sample, which is considered an unknown sample, the experimenter closed the hole but did not sound a click or present food.

2.4. Data Analysis of Rat Results. Following evaluations, the rats' performance was assessed relative to the results of culture with *M. tuberculosis* Multiplex PCR. Sensitivity and specificity were calculated for the group of 10 rats, and thus the criterion for counting a rat-positive indication could be an indication on either or both sample presentations by one rat, ten rats, or any number of rats in between, which are referred to hereafter as cutoffs 1–10. At a cutoff of 3, for example, a sample was deemed rat positive if three or more rats indicated it; samples indicated by only 2, 1, or 0 rats were deemed negative.

2.5. Culturing and PCR. Culturing was conducted in accordance with an established and recommended procedure for culturing sputum samples on Lowenstein-Jensen (LJ) solid media (WHO Guidelines on Standard Operating Procedures for Microbiology, Tuberculosis, WHO Regional Office for Southeast Asia, 2006). Decontaminated samples were inoculated onto different tubes of Lowenstein-Jensen solid media, one with pyruvate and the other with glycerol. The tubes were incubated at 37°C and inspected weekly for eight weeks. Media on which microbial growth was observed were scraped, stained by the ZN method, and analyzed by light microscopy. Each specimen which exhibited either AFB-positive culture material or characteristic bacterial growth was further analyzed by Multiplex PCR.

In the first step of PCR [10], Multiplex PCR genus typing was conducted to identify species belonging to the *Mycobacterium* genus. This genotyping distinguished species belonging to the *Mycobacterium tuberculosis* complex (MTC), specifically *M. bovis*, *M. africanum*, *M. tuberculosis*, and *M. microti*, from nontuberculous mycobacteria (*M. avium*, *M. intracellulare*, and others). All bacterial suspensions or DNA extracts containing MTC were subjected to another PCR, deletion typing. This procedure differentiated bacteria that were *M. tuberculosis*, *M. bovis*, or *M. africanum*.

3. Results

All sputum samples were classified as positive or negative for *M. tuberculosis* by microscopy at the DOTS centers, culturing (with PCR as appropriate), and rats' evaluation.

TABLE 1: Samples classified as *M. tuberculosis* and non-*M. tuberculosis* by Multiplex PCR.

	M. tuberculosis	Non *M. tuberculosis*
Total PCR+	129	13
ZN+ glycerol/pyruvate	(102/87)	(2/13)
[a]Rat+	109	10
Smear+ (DOTS)	86	7

[a]A sample was considered rat positive if at least one rat indicated.

TABLE 2: Sample-wise and patient-wise sensitivity and specificity at rat agreements cutoffs 1–10.

Cutoff	Samplewise		Patientwise	
	Sensitivity	Specificity	Sensitivity	Specificity
1	84.50	64.00	85.54	49.06
2	81.40	75.70	81.93	64.61
3	76.00	81.80	75.90	73.99
4	74.40	86.60	73.49	80.70
5	68.20	89.40	66.27	84.18
6	66.70	91.90	65.06	88.47
7	65.10	93.30	63.86	90.88
8	62.80	95.50	62.65	94.64
9	58.90	96.90	60.24	96.51
10	53.50	98.10	54.22	98.12

[a]Relative to Multiplex PCR.

Culture-positive samples were those in which characteristic growth was stained with a Ziehl-Neelsen stain and the presence of acid-fast bacilli confirmed. A sample was further considered PCR-positive if, following amplification, the amplified nucleotide sequence for *M. tuberculosis* was detected (see Table 1 for these results). DOTS centers' microscopy identified 96 positive samples and 49 positive patients, and culture identified 162 positive samples and 104 positive patients. PCR identified 129 positive samples and 81 positive patients. DOTS-centers' microscopy found 86 of the PCR positive samples and 771 of the PCR negative samples. Thus, relative to PCR, sputum smear microscopy conducted at the DOTS centers yielded a sample-wise sensitivity of 66.7% and a specificity of 98.7%.

Table 2 displays rat results relative to PCR at rat cutoffs 1–10. At a cutoff of 1, sample-wise sensitivity was 84.5% and specificity was 64%. As the cutoff increased, specificity characteristically improved while sensitivity worsened. At the largest cutoff, 10 (meaning all rats must indicate upon the sample to score it as rat-positive), sensitivity was 53.5% and specificity was 98.1%. At a cutoff of 7 sample-wise sensitivity was 65.1% and specificity was 93.3%.

Although it is tenable to use 10 rats, using fewer animals would render the evaluation process faster and less expensive. To ascertain the effects of using fewer animals, 36 combinations of randomly selected rats were created from the present data set, 12 combinations of 4 rats, 12 combinations of 3 rats, and 12 combinations of 2 rats. Sample-wise sensitivity and specificity relative to culture/PCR were calculated for each rat combination (Table 3). Using four rats at a cutoff

of one rat, average sensitivity was 79.9% (range 76.2–82.5%) and average specificity was 73.8% (range 71.2–75.4%). When only two rats were used, average sensitivity decreased to 74.9% (range 69–88.1%) while average specificity increased to 81.6% (range 78.1–85.6%). As the cutoff selected is increased, meaning more rat indications are required to count a sample as rat-positive, sensitivity decreases and specificity increases. For example, using four rats at a cutoff of four, sensitivity dropped to 57.8% (from 79.9% at a cutoff of 1) while specificity improved to 96.2% (from 73.8% at a cutoff of 1).

Table 4 shows patient-wise data comparing the sensitivity and specificity of DOTS centers' microscopy to the average for the 10 individual rats. Relative to combined Multiplex PCR and MTB/RIF results, DOTS centers' microscopy identified 47 of 81 positive patients and 407 of 409 negative patients. Therefore, at the patient-wise level, the sensitivity of microscopy at DOTS centers was 58% and the specificity was 99.5%. The rats correctly classified, on average, 57.1 positive and 329.1 negative patients and 104.2 positive and 675 negative samples. For the rats, the mean patient-wise sensitivity was 70.5% (99% confidence interval [CI] .68–.73) and mean specificity was 80.5% (95% CI .78–.83). Predictive values were calculated for patient-wise results of DOTS microscopy and the rats (Table 4). The positive predictive value (i.e., the probability that a patient with a positive test result really does have the condition of interest) was .96 (95% confidence interval [CI] .84–.99) for microscopy and .42 (95% CI .33–.50) for the rats. The negative predictive value (i.e., the probability that a patient with a negative test result really is free of the disease) was .92 (95% CI .89–.95) for microscopy and .93 (95% CI .89–.96) for the rats.

4. Discussion

In this study, 10 adult *Cricetomys* evaluated 910 sputum samples collected from patients suspected for tuberculosis. Weetjens et al. [3] previously reported that each of two pouched rats yielded a sensitivity of 73.1% relative to culturing, and their specificities were 97% and 97.8%. In the present study, which included Multiplex PCR, somewhat lower values were obtained where the mean individual sample-wise sensitivity of 10 rats relative to culture/PCR was 68.4%, and the mean specificity was 87.3%. Nonetheless, each rat's sensitivity exceeded that of ZN smear microscopy performed as part of routine TB screening at DOTS centers, although their specificity was lower. Because the rats can evaluate samples quickly, it is tenable to have several of them evaluate each sputum sample, and this has been done in studies examining their use in second-line screening of samples initially evaluated by ZN microscopy [4–6]. For example, Poling et al. [5] used a cutoff of 2 of 10 rats for identifying a sample as TB-positive. The present data suggest that this is a reasonable criterion in terms of balancing sensitivity and specificity, which were 81.4% and 75.7% when it was used in the present study. Similar values were obtained with cutoffs of 3 of 10 and 4 of 10. With a cutoff of 2, the rats as a group detected 66 of 81 patients found

TABLE 3: Average sensitivity and specificity for 12 groups of 4, 3, and 2 rats.

Cutoff	4 Rats		3 Rats		2 Rats	
	Sensitivity	Specificity	Sensitivity	Specificity	Sensitivity	Specificity
1	79.9	73.8	77.2	77.4	74.9	81.6
2	71.5	86.4	68.8	89.7	63.4	93.4
3	64.8	92.0	60.6	95.6		
4	57.8	96.2				

[a] Relative to culture/PCR.

TABLE 4: Patient-wise smear microscopy and average rat reference results.

	Sensitivity Culture/PCR	Specificity No TB	Pos predictive value Culture/PCR	Neg predictive value No TB
[a] Smear				
Correct/total samples (%)	47/81 (58.0)	407/409 (99.5)	.96	.92
95% confidence interval (CI)	46.6–68.7	98–99.9	.84–.99	.89–.95
Rat (average of 10)				
Correct/total samples (%)	57.1/81 (70.5)	329.1/409 (80.5)	.42	.93
95% CI	68.2–72.8	78.4–82.6	.33–.50	.89–.96

[a] Smear microscopy conducted at DOTS centers.

to be TB-positive by culturing/PCR, whereas DOTS centers' microscopy detected 47 of these patients. Therefore, had the rats been used in second-line screening as in prior studies [5, 6] and their results verified, they would have increased new-case detections by 40.4%.

Results revealed 57 culture-negative and three culture-positive, but PCR-negative samples indicated by six or more rats. To clarify the status of these samples, an internal test was done on all of these plus 100 randomly-selected rat-negative samples using the GeneXpert MTB/RIF (Cephid, Sunnyvale, CA, USA) [11]. Analysis by the GeneXpert revealed 25 positive samples and 23 positive patients that had previously been classified as negative by culture or Multiplex PCR, bringing the combined Multiplex PCR and MTB/RIF positive samples to 154 and positive patients to 98. The test reclassified 18 of the 60 rat-positive samples and 7 of the 100 rat-negative samples. An analysis was conducted including these reclassified participants and revealed a patient-wise sensitivity of microscopy at DOTS centers of 48% and specificity of 98.3%. For the rats, patient-wise sensitivity was 67% (range 62.2–72.5%) while their mean specificity was 93.5% (range 91.1–95.3%). Due to the costs of the cartridges required for the GeneXpert, it was not possible to evaluate all samples and, to avoid a possible bias, these data were not incorporated into the main results. These additional data suggest that the specificity of the rats may be higher than that suggested by the comparison to culture and, to test this possibility these findings, a study is underway that will thoroughly evaluate the rats relative to MTB/RIF.

In prior studies, a second microscopy was used to verify the status of DOTS-negative, rat-positive samples, but such confirmation is weak. The rats identify as positive a relatively high number of TB-negative samples; however, relying on microscopy alone allows a substantial number of patients with TB to go undetected. A better procedure would be to use the GeneXpert to confirm the status of rat-positive, smear-negative samples. Confirmation of samples in this way is likely to reveal a substantial number of TB-positive patients missed with the present procedure and thus slow the spread of transmission. This benefit would seemingly justify the financial cost of using the GeneXpert.

In addition to finding TB-positive patients overlooked by microscopy, the rats may potentially yield savings in time and cost. The rats are faster in evaluation than a lab technician, but require that the samples be transported and processed. These steps are completed with large batches of samples and it is important that future studies clearly demonstrate the cost-efficiency of these procedures relative to microscopy and investigate potential savings in costs and time. Prospectively, should the rats be called upon as a first-line screening tool, research on the MTB/RIF assay indicates that its high cost may limit its global utility [12], and the rats seem particularly well suited to work in conjunction with this technology to reduce costs. The rats screen samples quickly and, if used in areas with prevalence similar to that in which they have been tested, will reduce the number of patients in need of followup. The outcome of such a setup depends largely upon the number of rats used. Extrapolating from the current results, one could expect to recheck about 10% of samples if one rat is used and recheck about 45% of samples if 10 rats are used. The ideal number, as illustrated in Table 4, is probably between 2 and 4 rats as sensitivity remains relatively high while the false alarm rate improves with fewer rats.

A significant limitation of the present study is that no clinical data were available for comparison. TB-positive patients evaluated by TB specialists are more likely to be identified than those diagnosed by smear results alone [13], and so a study is underway at APOPO that will incorporate clinical data. A second limitation is that the HIV status of patients was not available to us; therefore, the sensitivity and specificity of DOTS microscopy and the rats could not be compared in HIV-positive and HIV-negative patients. Further research in this area is planned to make the comparison and to evaluate the value of the rats in detecting TB in children.

5. Conclusions

In this study, DOTS microscopy found 58% of the culture/Multiplex PCR positive patients, which is similar to results found in past studies [2, 11], compared to an average of 70.5% of positive patients found by individual rats. The results presented herein, combined with previously published operational data, demonstrate that the rats are faster than smear microscopy as commonly practiced and can identify more TB-positive patients. There is now substantial evidence that when used for second-line screening, *Cricetomys* can have a large positive impact on TB detection and public health in high-incidence areas, such as sub-Saharan Africa, although future research is necessary to refine training techniques to identify the applications for which the rats are best suited and to ascertain their per-case-detected cost relative to alternative diagnostics.

Authors' Contribution

This work was carried out in collaboration among all authors listed. C. Cox, B. J. Weetjens, A. Poling, G. Makingi, and A. Mahoney conceptualized this research and provided critical intellectual content. R. Kazwala, G. S. Mfinanga, and K. Reither provided expertise on the laboratory operations necessary for carrying out this experiment, contributed to the conceptualization of this research, and participated in the discussion on presentation of the results. A. M. Mahoney, N. Beyene, M. Jubitana, D. Kuipers, and A. Durgin oversaw the laboratory experiments, analyzed the data, and interpreted the results. A. Poling, A. Mahoney, and N. Beyene wrote the paper. All authors have contributed to, seen, and approved this paper.

Acknowledgments

The authors wish to acknowledge the trainers, secretaries, and laboratory technicians in the TB laboratory at APOPO for their hard work throughout this experiment. This work would not have been possible without their support. Financial support for this work was provided by the UBS Optimus Foundation. The authors declare that they have no competing interests, and specifically have no competing interests with respect to the use of the Cepheid GeneXpert.

References

[1] C. Dye, C. J. Watt, D. M. Bleed, S. M. Hosseini, and M. C. Raviglione, "Evolution of tuberculosis control and prospects for reducing tuberculosis incidence, prevalence, and deaths globally," *Journal of the American Medical Association*, vol. 293, no. 22, pp. 2767–2775, 2005.

[2] K. R. Steingart, M. Henry, V. Ng et al., "Fluorescence versus conventional sputum smear microscopy for tuberculosis: a systematic review," *Lancet Infectious Diseases*, vol. 6, no. 9, pp. 570–581, 2006.

[3] B. J. Weetjens, G. F. Mgode, R. S. Machang'u et al., "African pouched rats for the detection of pulmonary tuberculosis in sputum samples," *International Journal of Tuberculosis and Lung Disease*, vol. 13, no. 6, pp. 737–743, 2009.

[4] B. J. Weetjens, G. F. Mgode, W. B. Davis, C. Cox, and N. W. Beyene, "African giant rats for tuberculosis detection: a novel diagnostic technology," in *Global Forum Update on Research for Health*, C. A. Gardner, S. Jupp, S. A. Matlin, and C. Mauroux, Eds., vol. 6 of *Innovating for the Health of All*, Pro-Book, Woolbridge, UK, 2009.

[5] A. Poling, B. Weetjens, C. Cox et al., "Using giant African rats to detect tuberculosis: 2009 findings," *American Journal of Tropical Medicine and Hygiene*, vol. 83, no. 6, pp. 1308–1310, 2010.

[6] A. Mahoney, B. Weetjens, C. Cox et al., "Using giant African pouched rats to detect tuberculosis in human sputum samples: 2010 findings," *The Pan African Medical Journal*, vol. 9, no. 28, 2011.

[7] A. Poling, B. Weetjens, C. Cox, N. Beyene, A. Durgin, and A. Mahoney, "Tuberculosis detection by giant African pouched rats (*Cricetomys gambianus*)," *Behavior Analyst*, vol. 34, no. 1, pp. 47–54, 2011.

[8] C. Doig, A. L. Seagar, B. Watt, and K. J. Forbes, "The efficacy of the heat killing of Mycobacterium tuberculosis," *Journal of Clinical Pathology*, vol. 55, no. 10, pp. 778–779, 2002.

[9] O. Holz, M. Mücke, P. Zarza, D. Loppow, R. A. Jörres, and H. Magnussen, "Freezing of homogenized sputum samples for intermittent storage," *Clinical and Experimental Allergy*, vol. 31, no. 8, pp. 1328–1331, 2001.

[10] S. Berg, *Standard Operating Procedure for Mycobacterium Genus Typing*, VLA Press, London, UK, 2008.

[11] M. D. Perkins, G. Roscigno, and A. Zumla, "Progress towards improved tuberculosis diagnostics for developing countries," *The Lancet*, vol. 367, no. 9514, pp. 942–943, 2006.

[12] P. M. Small and M. Pai, "Tuberculosis diagnosis-time for a game change," *The New England Journal of Medicine*, vol. 363, no. 11, pp. 1070–1071, 2010.

[13] P. K. Lam, P. A. Lobue, and A. Catanzaro, "Clinical diagnosis of tuberculosis by specialists and non-specialists," *International Journal of Tuberculosis and Lung Disease*, vol. 13, no. 5, pp. 659–661, 2009.

Permissions

The contributors of this book come from diverse backgrounds, making this book a truly international effort. This book will bring forth new frontiers with its revolutionizing research information and detailed analysis of the nascent developments around the world.

We would like to thank all the contributing authors for lending their expertise to make the book truly unique. They have played a crucial role in the development of this book. Without their invaluable contributions this book wouldn't have been possible. They have made vital efforts to compile up to date information on the varied aspects of this subject to make this book a valuable addition to the collection of many professionals and students.

This book was conceptualized with the vision of imparting up-to-date information and advanced data in this field. To ensure the same, a matchless editorial board was set up. Every individual on the board went through rigorous rounds of assessment to prove their worth. After which they invested a large part of their time researching and compiling the most relevant data for our readers.

The editorial board has been involved in producing this book since its inception. They have spent rigorous hours researching and exploring the diverse topics which have resulted in the successful publishing of this book. They have passed on their knowledge of decades through this book. To expedite this challenging task, the publisher supported the team at every step. A small team of assistant editors was also appointed to further simplify the editing procedure and attain best results for the readers.

Apart from the editorial board, the designing team has also invested a significant amount of their time in understanding the subject and creating the most relevant covers. They scrutinized every image to scout for the most suitable representation of the subject and create an appropriate cover for the book.

The publishing team has been an ardent support to the editorial, designing and production team. Their endless efforts to recruit the best for this project, has resulted in the accomplishment of this book. They are a veteran in the field of academics and their pool of knowledge is as vast as their experience in printing. Their expertise and guidance has proved useful at every step. Their uncompromising quality standards have made this book an exceptional effort. Their encouragement from time to time has been an inspiration for everyone.

The publisher and the editorial board hope that this book will prove to be a valuable piece of knowledge for researchers, students, practitioners and scholars across the globe.

List of Contributors

Scott K. Heysell and Eric R. Houpt
Division of Infectious Diseases and International Health, University of Virginia, Charlottesville, VA 22908-1340, USA

Jane L. Moore, Debbie Staley and Denise Dodge
Tuberculosis Control and Prevention, Virginia Department of Health, Richmond, VA, USA

Wei-Teng Yang, Tokunbo Akande, Aditya Chandrasekhar and Alan de Lima Pereira
Johns Hopkins Bloomberg School of Public Health, Baltimore, MD 21205, USA

Celine R. Gounder and Katherine N. McIntire
Department of Medicine, Johns Hopkins University School of Medicine, Baltimore, MD 21287, USA

Jan-Walter De Neve
Harvard School of Public Health, Boston, MA 02115, USA

Naveen Gummadi
Narayana Hrudayalaya Hospital, Hyderabad 500055, India

Santanu Samanta
All India Institute of Medical Sciences, New Delhi 110029, India

Amita Gupta
Johns Hopkins Bloomberg School of Public Health, Baltimore, MD 21205, USA
Department of Medicine, Johns Hopkins University School of Medicine, Baltimore, MD 21287, USA
Center for Clinical Global Health Education, 600 NorthWolfe Street, Phipps 540B, Baltimore, MD 21287, USA

Daniel S. Smyk
Institute of Liver Studies, King's College Hospital and Division of Transplantation Immunology and Mucosal Biology, School of Medicine, King's College London, London SE5 9RS, UK

Christos Liaskos
Cellular Immunotherapy and Molecular Immunodiagnostics, Center for Research and Technology Thessaly, 41222 Larissa, Greece

Eirini I. Rigopoulou
Department of Medicine, University Hospital of Larissa, University of Thessaly School of Medicine, 41110 Larissa, Greece

Dimitrios P. Bogdanos
Institute of Liver Studies, King's College Hospital and Division of Transplantation Immunology and Mucosal Biology, School of Medicine, King's College London, London SE5 9RS, UK
Cellular Immunotherapy and Molecular Immunodiagnostics, Center for Research and Technology Thessaly, 41222 Larissa, Greece
Department of Medicine, University Hospital of Larissa, University of Thessaly School of Medicine, 41110 Larissa, Greece

Albert Pares
Liver Unit, Hospital Clínic de Barcelona, IDIBAPS, CIBERehd, University of Barcelona, 08036 Barcelona, Spain

Charalambos Billinis
Faculty of Veterinary Science, University of Thessaly, 43100 Karditsa, Greece

Andrew K. Burroughs
The Royal Free Sheila Sherlock Liver Centre, Royal Free Hospital and Department of Surgery, University Collegue London, London NW32QG, UK

Benjamin Thumamo Pokam
Department of Medical Laboratory Science, University of Buea, Buea, Cameroon

Anne E. Asuquo
Department of Medical Laboratory Science, University of Calabar, Calabar, Nigeria

Lucy Mupfumi, Rumbidzai Manzou, Beauty Makamure and Reggie Mutetwa
Biomedical Research and Training Institute, Harare, Zimbabwe

Tichaona Sagonda, Lovemore Gwanzura and Peter Mason
Biomedical Research and Training Institute, Harare, Zimbabwe
Department of Medical Laboratory Sciences, University of Zimbabwe, Harare, Zimbabwe

Mqondisi Tshabalala
Immunology Department, College of Health Sciences, University of Zimbabwe, Avondale, Harare, Zimbabwe

Rouhollah Keshavarz, Kioomars Soleymani, Fereshteh Sadat Seddighinia, Nader Mosavari and Daryoush Hamedi Asl
PPD Tuberculin Department, Razi Vaccine and Serum Research Institute, Karaj 3197619751, Iran

Saman Soleimanpour
PPD Tuberculin Department, Razi Vaccine and Serum Research Institute, Karaj 3197619751, Iran
Antimicrobial Resistance Research Center, Mashhad University of Medical Sciences, Mashhad, Iran

Keyvan Tadayon
PPD Tuberculin Department, Razi Vaccine and Serum Research Institute, Karaj 3197619751, Iran
Aerobic Bacterial Research and Vaccine Production Department, Razi Vaccine and Serum Research Institute, Karaj, Iran

Ali Asghar Farazi
Arak University of Medical Sciences, Arak, Iran

Samuel Melaku
Department of Public Health Nursing, Jijiga Health Science College, Jijiga, Ethiopia

Hardeep Rai Sharma
Institute of Environmental Studies, Kurukshetra University, Kurukshetra, Haryana 136119, India

Getahun Asres Alemie
Institute of Public Health, University of Gondar, Gondar, Ethiopia

Lisa V. Adams and C. Fordham von Reyn
Dartmouth Medical School, Hanover, NH 03755, USA

Elizabeth A. Talbot
Dartmouth Medical School, Hanover, NH 03755, USA
Infectious Diseases and International Health Section, 1 Medical Center Drive, Lebanon, NH 03756, USA

Isaac Maro, Lillian Mtei and Mecky Matee
Muhimbili University of Health and Allied Sciences, Dar es Salaam, Tanzania

Katherine Ferguson
Dartmouth College, Hanover, NH 03755, USA

Varun Kumar, Abhay Singh, Mrinmoy Adhikary, Shailaja Daral, Anita Khokhar and Saudan Singh
Department of Community Medicine, Vardhman Mahavir Medical College and Safdarjung Hospital, New Delhi 110029, India

Eliana Peresi
Tropical Disease Department, Botucatu School of Medicine, UNESP, São Paulo State University, Botucatu, SP, Brazil
Departamento de Doenças Tropicais e Diagnóstico por Imagem, Faculdade de Medicina de Botucatu, UNESP, Rubião Júnior S/N, Botucatu 18618-970, SP, Brazil

Larissa Ragozo Cardoso Oliveira, Sueli Aparecida Calvi and Érika Alessandra Pellison Nunes da Costa
Tropical Disease Department, Botucatu School of Medicine, UNESP, São Paulo State University, Botucatu, SP, Brazil

Weber Laurentino da Silva and Ana Carla Pereira
Lauro de Souza Lima Institute, Bauru, SP, Brazil

João Pessoa Araujo Jr.
Microbiology and Immunology Department, Bioscience Institute, UNESP, São Paulo State University, Botucatu, SP, Brazil

Jairo Aparecido Ayres
Nursing Department, Botucatu School of Medicine, UNESP, São Paulo State University, Botucatu, SP, Brazil

Maria Rita Parise Fortes
Dermatology and Radiotherapy Department, Botucatu School of Medicine, UNESP, São Paulo State University, Botucatu, SP, Brazil

Edward A. Graviss
The Methodist Hospital Research Institute, Houston, TX, USA

Sarah J. Iribarren
School of Nursing, Columbia University, 630 West 168 Street, New York, NY 10032, USA
Institute for Clinical Effectiveness and Healthcare Policy, Dr. Emilio Ravignani 2024, C1414CPT Buenos Aires, Argentina

Fernando Rubinstein
Institute for Clinical Effectiveness and Healthcare Policy, Dr. Emilio Ravignani 2024, C1414CPT Buenos Aires, Argentina

Vilda Discacciati
Division of Family and Community Medicine, Hospital Italiano de Buenos Aires, Juan D. Perón 4190, C1181ACH Buenos Aires, Argentina

Patricia F. Pearce
School of Nursing, Loyola University, 6363 Saint Charles Avenue, Stallings Hall, New Orleans, LA 70118, USA

Christopher Affusim and Kester Anyanwu
Department of Family Medicine, Ambrose Alli University, PMB 8, Ekpoma, Edo state, Nigeria

Vivien Abah
Department of Family Medicine, University of Benin Teaching Hospital, Benin, Edo State, Nigeria

Emeka B. Kesieme
Department of Surgery, Ambrose Alli University, PMB 8, Ekpoma, Edo state, Nigeria

Taofik A. T. Salami
Department of Internal Medicine, Ambrose Alli University, PMB 8, Ekpoma, Edo state, Nigeria

Reuben Eifediyi
Department of Obstetrics and Gynaecology, Ambrose Alli University, PMB 8, Ekpoma, Edo state, Nigeria

Dawn M. Hunter and Daniel V. Lim
Department of Cell Biology, Microbiology and Molecular Biology, University of South Florida, 4202 E. Fowler Avenue, ISA 2015, Tampa, FL 33620-7115, USA

Minwuyelet Maru, Tekle Airgecho, Endalamaw Gadissa and Abraham Aseffa
Armauer Hansen Research Institute, P.O. Box 1005, Jimma Road, Addis Ababa, Ethiopia

Solomon H. Mariam
Armauer Hansen Research Institute, P.O. Box 1005, Jimma Road, Addis Ababa, Ethiopia
Aklilu Lemma Institute of Pathobiology, Addis Ababa University, P.O. Box 1176, Addis Ababa, Ethiopia

Duc T. M. Nguyen
Department of Pediatrics, University of British Columbia and BC Children's Hospital, 4480 Oak Street, A4-198 AD, Vancouver, BC, Canada V6H 3V4

Hung Q. Nguyen
Department E (HIV Infection), Hospital for Tropical Diseases (HTD), Ho Chi Minh City, Vietnam

R. Palmer Beasley and Lu-Yu Hwang
Division of Epidemiology, Human Genetics and Environmental Sciences, University of Texas School of Public Health (UTSPH), Houston, TX 77030, USA

Charles E. Ford
Division of Biostatistics, University of Texas School of Public Health (UTSPH), Houston, TX 77030, USA

Edward A. Graviss
Division of Epidemiology, Human Genetics and Environmental Sciences, University of Texas School of Public Health (UTSPH), Houston, TX 77030, USA

Department of Pathology and Genomic Medicine, The Methodist Hospital Research Institute (THMRI), Houston, TX 77030, USA

Stella O. Chuke
Northrop Grumman Information Systems Sector, 2800 Century Parkway NE, Atlanta, GA 30345, USA
Division of Tuberculosis Elimination, Centers for Disease Control and Prevention (CDC), Mail Stop E-10, 1600 Clifton Road NE, Atlanta, GA 30333, USA

Nguyen Thi Ngoc Yen, Nguyen Huu Phuoc, Nguyen An Trinh, Duong Thi Cam Nhung, Vo Thi Chi Mai, An Dang Qui, Hoang Hoa Hai and Le Thien Huong Loan
Cho Ray Hospital, 201B Nguyen ChiThanh Street, District 5, Ho Chi Minh City, Vietnam

William C. Whitworth and Gerald H.Mazurek
Division of Tuberculosis Elimination, Centers for Disease Control and Prevention (CDC), Mail Stop E-10, 1600 Clifton Road NE, Atlanta, GA 30333, USA

Kayla F. Laserson
Division of Tuberculosis Elimination, Centers for Disease Control and Prevention (CDC), Mail Stop E-10, 1600 Clifton Road NE, Atlanta, GA 30333, USA
Center for Global Health, CDC, Mail Stop D-68, 1600 Clifton Road NE, Atlanta, GA 30333, USA

Warren G. Jones
International Organization for Migration (IOM), 1B Pham Ngoc Thach District 1, Ho Chi Minh City, Vietnam
International Organization for Migration (IOM), P.O. Box 55040, Westlands, Nairobi 00200, Kenya

John A. Painter
Division of Global Migration and Quarantine, CDC, Mail Stop E-03, 1600 Clifton Road NE, Atlanta, GA 30333, USA

Susan A. Maloney
Center for Global Health, CDC, Mail Stop D-68, 1600 Clifton Road NE, Atlanta, GA 30333, USA
Division of Global Migration and Quarantine, CDC, Mail Stop E-03, 1600 Clifton Road NE, Atlanta, GA 30333, USA

J. Jina Shah
Division of Global Migration and Quarantine, CDC, Mail Stop E-03, 1600 Clifton Road NE, Atlanta, GA 30333, USA
Department of Family and Community Medicine, University of California, San Francisco, 500 Parnassus Avenue, MU 3E, San Francisco, CA 94143, USA
Genentech, Inc., 1 DNA Way, South San Francisco, CA 94080, USA

Tehmina Mustafa
Centre for International Health, Department of Global Public Health and Primary Care, University of Bergen, 5021 Bergen, Norway
Department of Thoracic Medicine, Haukeland University Hospital, 5021 Bergen, Norway

Karl Albert Brokstad
Broegelmann Research Laboratory, Department of Clinical Science, University of Bergen, 5021 Bergen, Norway

Sayoki G. Mfinanga
National Institute for Medical Research, Muhimbili, Tanzania

Harald G.Wiker
The Gade Research Group for Infection and Immunity, Department of Clinical Science, University of Bergen, 5021 Bergen, Norway

Limakatso Lebina, Katlego Motlhaoleng, Modiehi Rakgokong and Pattamukkil Abraham
Perinatal HIV Research Unit, University of Witwatersrand, Johannesburg 2000, South Africa

Nigel Fuller and Tolu Osoba
Public Health, School of Medicine, University of Liverpool, Liverpool L69 7ZX, UK

Lesley Scott
Department of Molecular Medicine and Hematology, University of theWitwatersrand, Johannesburg 2000, South Africa

Ebrahim Variava
Department of Internal Medicine, Klerksdorp/Tshepong Hospital Complex, NorthWest Department of Health and University of the Witwatersrand, Johannesburg 2000, South Africa

Neil Alexander Martinson
Perinatal HIV Research Unit, University of Witwatersrand, Johannesburg 2000, South Africa
DST/NRF Centre of Excellence for Biomedical TB Research, University of the Witwatersrand, Johannesburg 2000, South Africa

Rajani Ranganath
Department of Microbiology, Navodaya Medical College and Research Centre, Raichur, Karnataka, India

Vijay G. S. Kumar
Department of Microbiology, JSS Medical College and Research Centre, Mysore, Karnataka 570 015, India

Ravi Ranganath
Usha Kidney Care, Bellary, Karnataka 583103, India

Gangadhar Goud
Department of Community Medicine, VIMS, Bellary, Karnataka 583104, India

Veerabhadra Javali
Department of Orthopaedics, Navodaya Medical College and Research Centre, Raichur, Tamil Nadu 641043, India

Mulusew Andualem Asemahagn
School of Public Health, College of Medicine and Health Sciences, Bahir Dar University, Bahir Dar, Ethiopia

Addisu Alemayehu Gube and Feleke Gebremeskel
Department of Public Health, College of Medicine and Health Sciences, Arba Minch University, P.O. Box 21, Arba Minch, Ethiopia

Megbaru Debalkie, Kalid Seid, Kiberalem Bisete, Asfaw Mengesha, Abubeker Zeynu and Freselam Shimelis
Department of Nursing, College of Medicine and Health Sciences, Arba Minch University, P.O. Box 21, Arba Minch, Ethiopia

Mitchell A. Yakrus, Beverly Metchock and Angela M. Starks
Centers for Disease Control and Prevention, Atlanta, GA 30329-4027, USA

Wongsa Laohasiriwong
Board Committee of Research and Training Centre for Enhancing Quality of Life of Working Age People (REQW), Khon Kaen University, Khon Kaen, Thailand
Faculty of Public Health, Khon Kaen University, Khon Kaen, Thailand

Roshan Kumar Mahato and Kriangsak Vaeteewootacharn
Faculty of Public Health, Khon Kaen University, Khon Kaen, Thailand

Rajendra Koju
Departments of Internal Medicine, Dhulikhel Hospital, Kathmandu University Hospital, Dhulikhel, Nepal

Wilfried Békou, Mênonli Adjobimey, Omer Adjibode, Gabriel Ade and Séverin Anagonou
Programme National contre la Tuberculose, 01 BP 321 Cotonou, Benin

Serge Ade
Programme National contre la Tuberculose, 01 BP 321 Cotonou, Benin

Faculté de Médecine, Université de Parakou, Parakou, Benin
International Union against Tuberculosis and Lung Disease, Paris, France

Martha Gabriela Celle Rivero, Milene Gonçalves Quiles and Antonio Carlos Campos Pignatari
Special Clinical Microbiology Laboratory (LEMC), Federal University of São Paulo (UNIFESP), São Paulo, SP, Brazil

Fernando Pereira Pinto and Antonia Maria de Oliveira Machado
Central Laboratory of São Paulo Hospital, Federal University of São Paulo (UNIFESP), São Paulo, SP, Brazil

Flavia Silva Palomo
Special Clinical Microbiology Laboratory (LEMC), Federal University of São Paulo (UNIFESP), São Paulo, SP, Brazil
Central Laboratory of São Paulo Hospital, Federal University of São Paulo (UNIFESP), São Paulo, SP, Brazil

E. G. Churina, O. I. Urazova and V. V. Novitskiy
SBEI-HPE "Siberian State Medical University of the Ministry of Health Care and Social Development of the Russian Federation", Tomsk, Russia

Ghazal Haque, Ashok Kumar, Fatima Saifuddin, Shafaq Ismail, Nadeem Rizvi, Shaista Ghazal and Sadhna Notani
Department of Chest Medicine, Jinnah Postgraduate Medical Centre, Rafiqui H J Shaheed Road, Karachi 75510, Pakistan

Charles Sandy, Regis C. Choto, Tsitsi Mutasa-Apollo, Brilliant Nkomo, Owen Mugurungi and Nicholas Siziba
AIDS and TB Department, Ministry of Health and Child Care, Harare, Zimbabwe

Kudakwashe C. Takarinda
AIDS and TB Department, Ministry of Health and Child Care, Harare, Zimbabwe
International Union against Tuberculosis and Lung Disease, Paris, France

Nyasha Masuka
Ministry of Health and Child Care, Harare, Zimbabwe

Patrick Hazangwe
World Health Organisation Country Office, Harare, Zimbabwe

Edwin Sibanda
Health Services Department, Bulawayo, Zimbabwe

Anthony D. Harries
International Union against Tuberculosis and Lung Disease, Paris, France
Department of Clinical Research, London School of Hygiene and Tropical Medicine, London, UK

Marie Carlsson, Stina Johansson and Berthollet Bwira Kaboru
School of Health and Medical Sciences, Örebro University, 701 82 Örebro, Sweden

Remy-Paul Bosela Eale
International Leadership University in Burundi, P.O. Box 2330, Bujumbura, Burundi

Amanda Mahoney, Amy Durgin and Alan Poling
Department of Psychology, Western Michigan University, Kalamazoo, MI 49008-5200, USA
Tuberculosis Research, Anti-Persoonsmijnen Ontmijnende Product Ontwikkeling (APOPO), Morogoro, Tanzania

Bart J. Weetjens, Christophe Cox, Negussie Beyene and Maureen Jubitana
Tuberculosis Research, Anti-Persoonsmijnen Ontmijnende Product Ontwikkeling (APOPO), Morogoro, Tanzania

Klaus Reither
Tuberculosis Research, Swiss Tropical and Public Health Institute, 4051 Basel, Switzerland
TB Research and Training Center, Ifakara Health Institute, Bagamoyo, Tanzania

George Makingi and Rudovick Kazwala
Department of Veterinary Medicine, Sokoine University of Agriculture, Morogoro, Tanzania

Godfrey S. Mfinanga and Amos Kahwa
Clinical Research Laboratory, National Institute for Medical Research, Dar es Salaam, Tanzania

Index

www.ingramcontent.com/pod-product-compliance
Lightning Source LLC
Chambersburg PA
CBHW080514200326
41458CB00012B/4208